HANDBOOK OF

Primary Care
Medicine

HANDBOOK OF

Primary Care Medicine

Editor-in-Chief
Dale Berg, M.D.
Assistant Professor of Medicine
Medical College of Wisconsin
Milwaukee, Wisconsin

Advising Editor
Laura Cantwell, M.D.
Resident in Medicine
Medical College of Wisconsin
Milwaukee, Wisconsin

Contributing Editors
Gustavo Heudebert, M.D.
Assistant Professor of Medicine
Southwestern Medical School
Dallas, Texas

James L. Sebastian, M.D.
Associate Professor of Medicine
Medical College of Wisconsin
Milwaukee, Wisconsin

 J.B. Lippincott Company
Philadelphia

Acquisitions Editor: Richard Winters
Assistant Editor: Jody M. Schott
Indexer: Roger Wall
Interior Designer: Susan Blaker
Cover Designer: Tom Jackson
Production Managers: Lori J. Bainbridge/Mary Kinsella
Production Service: P. M. Gordon Associates, Inc.
Compositor: Achorn Graphic Services, Inc.
Printer/Binder: R.R. Donnelley & Sons
Cover Printer: New England Book Components

6 5 4 3 2

Library of Congress Cataloging-in-Publication Data

Handbook of primary care medicine / editor-in-chief, Dale Berg ; advising
    editor, Laura Cantwell ; contributing editors, Gustavo Heudebert, James
    L. Sebastian.
        p. cm.
    Includes bibliographical references and index.
    ISBN 0–397–51213–9
    1. Primary care (Medicine)—Handbooks, manuals, etc. I. Berg.
    Dale.
        [DNLM: 1. Primary Health Care—handbooks. W 30 H2355 1993]
    RC55.H28 1993
    616—dc20
    DNLM/DLC
    for Library of Congress   93–5547
                                                                            CIP

The authors and publisher have exerted every effort to ensure that drug
selection and dosage set forth in this text are in accord with current
recommendations and practice at the time of publication. However, in
view of ongoing research, changes in government regulations, and the
constant flow of information relating to drug therapy and drug reactions,
the reader is urged to check the package insert for each drug for
any change in indications and dosage and for added warnings and
precautions. This is particularly important when the recommended agent
is a new or infrequently employed drug.

Preface

Primary care medicine is perhaps the quintessential discipline of medicine. The prototypic general practice physician was the turn-of-the-century country doctor who had an unflappable personality, enormous quantities of empathy, a great deal of common sense both in medicine and in life, and the zeal and overriding concern for and of his (her) patients. Although a powerful force for good, the general practice physician was able to intervene only minimally against many of the common disease entities of that time. As medicine has evolved scientifically, new treatment modalities have been developed, many of which have prolonged the length and improved the quality of life. These modalities, including coronary angioplasty and bypass grafting, organ transplantation, and antineoplastic chemotherapy, have impacted significantly on health care. This component in medical evolution and development, however, involved a sub- or even subsubspecialization in medicine in which physicians became experts in one endeavor or specific field of medicine, but allowed other medical and personal skills to atrophy.

Although this subspecialization has overall been positive for health care, it has come at some expense. These expenses include, but are not limited to, a loss of the art of medicine, a decrease in the empathic nature of the physician, a fragmentation of care with a built-in inefficiency both in time and financially, a decrease in emphasis on prevention, and, finally, some would submit, a loss of the common sense inherent to being a physician and not a technician. Medicine, however, has continued to evolve so that therapeutic advances can now be administered by nonspecialists, i.e., primary care providers. The role of a primary care physician will continue to evolve but clearly will continue to be the central component in health care delivery in this and the next millennium.

Based on the above discussion, primary care physicians must have a model to approach a diverse set of medical problems; know how to recognize, evaluate, and manage common problems; have a sense of when to consult other physicians and whom to consult; recognize when patients should be admitted to an inpatient service; and have references in the literature to support these models. This text is designed to fill these needs for the youngest members in medicine—medical students and house staff members. This book is designed with the following features to assist in easy utility:

1. The format is reproducible from section to section.
2. A box outlining the overall approach to common problems appears in each section. These boxes are designed to provide a readily accessible source of focused, on-your-feet type of information, clearly to complement not supplant the text and discussion.
3. References on each major topic are provided at the end of each chapter.
4. Each section ends with an outline of when and with whom to consult. In this section "elective" means as necessary, "required" means within the next month, "urgent" means within the next 24 hours, and "emergent" means within the next hour.
5. At the end of each section is an outline of indications for admission to an inpatient setting.
6. We involved a medical student and now junior house staff member, the advising editor, Laura Cantwell, M.D., to assist us in the design, components, contents, and delivery of the text.

—D.D.B.

Contents

CHAPTER 4

Pulmonary Diseases   199

CHAPTER 5

Hematology/Oncology   258

CHAPTER 6

Infectious Diseases   313

CHAPTER 7

Musculoskeletal Disorders   361

C H A P T E R 8

Dermatology   **457**

C H A P T E R 9

Endocrine Disorders   **515**

C H A P T E R 1 0

Male Genitourinary Tract   **558**

C H A P T E R 1 1

Gynecology/Breast   **568**

HANDBOOK OF

Primary Care
Medicine

Dale Berg, Ed. *Handbook
of Primary Care Medicine.*
Copyright © 1993 J. B.
Lippincott Company.

CHAPTER 1

Cardiology

James L. Sebastian and Dale Berg

Atherosclerotic Heart Disease: Risk Factor Modification

I. **Risk factors**
The **risk factors** for the development of atherosclerotic disease, especially coronary arterial atherosclerotic disease, include the following:
   A. **Cigarette smoking**
   B. **Hypertension,** if uncontrolled
   C. **Diabetes mellitus,** both insulin-resistant and insulin-dependent
   D. **Obesity** (exacerbates other risk factors)
   E. **Family history** of premature atherosclerotic disease in a first-degree relative
   F. **Hyperlipidemia**
   Of these risk factors, the only one that cannot be modified is a family history of premature heart disease. All of the other factors **can and should be modified.** Modification of risk factors slows the development and progression of atherosclerotic disease.
   Strategies for modifying several of these risk factors are discussed in other chapters (cigarette-smoking cessation—Chapter 16, hypertension—Chapter 3, diabetes mellitus—Chapter 9). The strategy to intervene with hyperlipoproteinemias is discussed in Box 1-1.

II. **Consultation**

Problem	Service	Time
Hypothyroidism	Endocrinology	Elective
Refractory hyperlipidemia	Endocrinology	Required

III. **Indications for admission:** None

B O X 1 - 1

Overall Evaluation and Management of the Hyperlipidemias

1. Assess the **risk factor** profile of the patient.
2. Hyperlipidemia is often asymptomatic, and its detection requires screening.
   a. National Institutes of Health (NIH) recommendations for screening for hyperlipidemia: In every individual over age 20 years, a random, nonfasting, total cholesterol level should be determined every 5 years.
      i. If the value is above 240 mg/dL, a full cholesterol evaluation is warranted (see below).
      ii. If the value is 200–239 mg/dL *and* two or more risk factors are present, a full cholesterol evaluation is warranted.
      iii. If the value is less than 199 mg/dL, the test is repeated in 5 years.
   b. The **full cholesterol evaluation** includes:
      i. Looking for **secondary causes** of hyperlipidemias
         (a) Diabetes mellitus (fasting blood glucose)
         (b) Nephrotic syndrome (urinalysis to check for proteinuria)
         (c) Hypothyroidism (TSH, T_3RU, T_4)
         (d) Cholestatic jaundice (total bilirubin, alkaline phosphatase)
      ii. Measuring **fasting plasma triglyceride** (TG), **high density lipoprotein** (HDL), and **total cholesterol** (TC) levels in order to calculate the **low density lipoprotein** (LDL). The equation used to calculate this value is:

      $$LDL = TC - (HDL + TG/5).$$

      iii. A **physical examination** to look for goiter, peripheral signs of hypothyroidism, **xanthomas** (nodules in the skin), or **xanthelasma** (yellow streaking in the infraorbital skin). Xanthomas or xanthelasma may be indicative of cholesterol deposition.
   c. The goals of the **full** cholesterol evaluation include looking for any secondary causes, assessing the degree of lipoprotein elevation, and cate-

   (continued)

B O X 1 - 1 *(continued)*

> gorizing the type of hyperlipidemia (see Tables 1-1 and 1-2).
> 3. **Therapeutic intervention: Goals**
>   a. If hyperlipidemia is the only cardiac risk factor, keep LDL below 160 mg/dL.
>   b. If one of many cardiac risk factors, keep LDL above 130 mg/dL.
>   c. Decrease levels of TC, TG, and LDL overall.
>   d. **Increase** levels of **HDL** overall.
> 4. **Therapeutic intervention: Methods**
>   a. **Dietary changes** (see Table 1-3)
>   b. **Exercise:** Increase aerobic exercise, especially walking, swimming, or jogging.
>   c. **Drug therapy** (see Table 1-4)

Chest Pain

Chest pain is a common problem with many possible causes. Assessment and diagnosis can be difficult. Because several of the underlying causes are disorders that can result in **imminent death,** any chest pain requires an intense evaluation to determine its cause. Diagnosis begins with deciding whether the chest pain is of **cardiac** or **noncardiac origin.**

I. Types of chest pain by origin
   A. **Cardiac origin**
      Chest pain of cardiac origin is assessed clinically to be the result of cardiac ischemia. This type of chest pain is also referred to as **angina pectoris** (see Box 1-2).
      1. **Typical or true angina pectoris** is characterized by a squeezing sensation that is retrosternal, is reproduc-

T A B L E 1 - 1
National Cholesterol Education Project Guidelines

Parameter Measured	Desirable (mg/dL)	Borderline Elevated (mg/dL)	High (mg/dL)
Total cholesterol	<200	200–239	>240
LDL cholesterol	<130	130–159	>160
Triglycerides	250	250–500	>500

T A B L E 1-2
Classification of Hyperlipoproteinemia

Type	Lipoprotein	Elevated Lipid	Incidence (%)	Manifestations	Secondary Causes
I	Chylomicrons	TG	<1	Pancreatitis Xanthomas Lipemia retinalis	Diabetes mellitus
IIa	LDL	Chol.	10	Premature ASHD Xanthomas	Hypothyroidism Nephrotic syndrome Biliary obstruction
IIb	LDL + VLDL	TG + chol.	40	Premature ASHD	Same as for IIa
III	IDL	TG + chol.	<1	Premature ASHD	Hypothyroidism Ethanolism Diabetes mellitus
IV	VLDL	TG + chol.	45	Premature ASHD	Diabetes mellitus Ethanolism Estrogens/steroids
V	VLDL + chylomicrons	TG + chol.	5	Pancreatitis Xanthomas Lipemia retinalis	Diabetes mellitus Ethanol

T A B L E   1 - 3
**American Heart Association's Dietary Therapy
for Hyperlipidemia**

Dietary Component	AHA Step 1 Diet	AHA Step 2 Diet
Total fat	<30% of total calories	Same
Saturated fatty acids	<10% of total calories	<7% of total calories
Polyunsaturated fatty acids	≤10% of total calories	Same
Mono-unsaturated fatty acids	10%–15% of total calories	Same
Carbohydrates	50%–60% of total calories	Same
Protein	10%–20% of total calories	Same
Cholesterol	<300 mg/day	<200 mg/day
Total calories	To achieve and maintain a desirable weight	Same
Ethanol	Maximum 1–2 beverages/day	Same

ibly precipitated or exacerbated by exercise, and is
relieved with rest or sublingual nitroglycerin. Typical
angina pectoris is easily diagnosed from a thorough
history and is virtually diagnostic of atherosclerotic
heart disease (i.e., Heberden's angina pectoris).

2. **Atypical chest pain** has some features of angina but
other features that are quite different from the classic
description. In patients with atypical cardiac chest
pain, no other noncardiac cause of the pain can be
demonstrated, although one might in fact exist. Atypical cardiac chest pain can result from **coronary arterial spasm** (Prinzmetal's angina), from a **diabetic neuropathy,** which can mask the symptoms of cardiac
chest pain, or from **nonischemic cardiac causes** (e.g.,
pericarditis).

B. **Noncardiac origin chest pain** is assessed to be from a
discrete noncardiac source. Some of the more common
causes of noncardiac chest pain are listed in Table 1.5.

II. Diagnosis

Typical and **atypical cardiac chest pain** are clinical diagnoses (see Box 1-2, page 7). Once the chest pain has been categorized (see I, above), further evaluation and management are
necessary.

The **specific evaluation and management** of angina pectoris include determining if the angina is **stable** or **unstable** or
if it is the manifestation of an acute **myocardial infarction.**

T A B L E 1-4
Drug Therapy for Hyperlipidemias

Bile Acid–Binding Agents (Cholestyramine, Colestipol)

Effect:	Reduces LDL levels.
Dose:	5 g PO b.i.d., increasing to 15 g PO b.i.d., as tolerated.
Side effects:	Constipation, bloating, excess flatulence. May interfere with absorption of other drugs. Can cause hypertriglyceridemia.

Gemfibrizol

Effect:	Reduces serum triglycerides (also tends to reduce LDL cholesterol and increase HDL).
Dose:	600 mg PO b.i.d.
Side effects:	Transient increase in transaminase levels. Less frequent side effects include nausea, diarrhea, gallstones, alopecia, and muscle weakness with an elevated CPK.
Note:	Use with caution when combined with HMG CoA reductase inhibitors (see below) because of reports of an increased incidence of myositis.

HMG CoA Reductase Inhibitors (Lovastatin)

Effect:	Reduces LDL cholesterol and plasma triglycerides, mildly elevates HDL.
Dose:	20–40 mg PO once or twice daily.
Side effects:	Transaminase elevations and increased CPK levels in a few patients.

Nicotinic Acid

Effect:	Reduces cholesterol and triglyceride levels, increases HDL cholesterol levels.
Dose:	500–1,500 mg t.i.d.
Side effects:	Flushing, which can be minimized by pretreatment with aspirin. Can also increase uric acid levels, cause mild hepatitis, and increase plasma glucose levels in diabetic patients. Rarely, may produce a dermatologic manifestation, acanthosis nigricans.

T A B L E 1-5
Some Causes of Noncardiac Chest Pain

Skin lesions
  Trauma to the skin
  Herpes zoster
Chest wall trauma
Pulmonary embolism/infarction
Pneumothorax
Pneumonitis
Dissecting thoracic aortic aneurysm
Peptic ulcer disease
Costochondritis (Tietze's syndrome)

B O X 1 - 2

Overall Evaluation and Management of Angina Pectoris

Evaluation

1. Take a **thorough history** to document the nature of the chest pain. **Typical ischemic chest pain** has an **onset** with exertion, is **relieved** with rest, is squeezing and oppressive in **nature**, is substernal in **location**, often **radiates** to the left chest, jaw, and/or upper extremity, and often is accompanied by dyspnea, diaphoresis, and lightheadedness. Further historical data include the patient's profile of risk factors for the development of ASHD.
2. Perform a **physical examination** with emphasis on vital signs. An S_4 gallop can be indicative of cardiac ischemia.
3. Obtain a **12-lead** ECG, looking for any **ischemic** changes (e.g., flipped T-waves) or evidence of **acute injury** (i.e., localized ST-segment elevation) or of old myocardial infarction (i.e., Q-waves).
4. Determine electrolytes, BUN, creatinine, glucose, and CBC for baseline purposes.
5. Monitor **O_2 saturation.** If <90%, obtain arterial blood gas values and place patient on oxygen, 2 L/min, delivered by nasal cannula.
6. Obtain **chest radiographs,** PA and lateral, to look for any cardiomegaly, any pulmonary vascular redistribution, or any potential noncardiac causes of the chest pain.

Management

1. Based on results of the evaluation, **categorize** the chest pain as being cardiac, atypical, or noncardiac in origin.
   a. If **cardiac in origin,** intervention with aspirin, antianginal agents (see Table 1-8, page 13), and cardiac catheterization is indicated. If there is any evidence that the chest pain is unstable or potentially a myocardial infarction, admission for aggressive intervention is mandatory. See text and Table 1-9 (page 14) for details.
   b. If **atypical in nature,** place the patient on aspirin, 325 mg PO q.d., and nitroglycerin, 1/150 gr sl prn
   (continued)

B O X 1 - 2 *(continued)*

and perform a noninvasive test for cardiac ischemia (i.e., a symptom-limited stress test, thallium
stress test, or persantine thallium stress test). Refer to Table 1-6 for specific test characteristics. If
one of these noninvasive tests is positive for coronary arterial disease, referral to a cardiologist for
cardiac angiography is indicated.

   c. If **noncardiac in nature,** treat the underlying
cause. **Musculoskeletal chest pain** responds well
to a nonsteroidal anti-inflammatory agent (e.g.,
ibuprofen, 400–600 mg PO t.i.d.).

2. Assess the **functional capacity** of the patient. One
method is to use the Canadian Cardiovascular Grading System (Table 1-7). This provides a powerful
baseline for future reference and assessment of
therapy.

3. **Chronic therapy** for stable angina is discussed in the
text (see III. Management).

4. The **acute management** of unstable angina and
other acute coronary syndromes is described in the
text (see III. Management).

Referral

Referral to a **cardiologist** is indicated for all patients
with cardiac-origin or atypical chest pain.

III. Management
A. Stable angina pectoris

Stable angina pectoris is present in a patient who has a
history of ASHD and chest pain that is not increasing in
frequency, duration, or intensity. The **specific management** includes the initiation of aspirin, 325 mg PO every
morning, and **antianginal** agents from one or more of the
following categories: nitrates, β-blockers, and/or calcium
channel blockers (see Table 1-8).

   Coronary angiography is clearly indicated if the coronary anatomy is not known. **Surgical intervention** with
bypass grafts is indicated in patients with stable angina
who have **left main** coronary arterial disease or **three-
vessel ASHD,** especially if there is evidence of ventricular
dysfunction as evidenced by a decreased ejection frac-
tion. The goals of treatment are to minimize the episodes

of angina and to prolong life; the combination of medical and surgical interventions will help achieve those goals.

B. **Unstable angina pectoris**

If the angina is of new onset (i.e., began within 6 weeks of presentation) or has been increasing in frequency, duration, or intensity, it is, by definition, **unstable angina pectoris.** Unstable angina requires therapy with antiplatelet agents (i.e., aspirin, 325 mg PO q.d.) and nitrates (e.g., 1 inch of nitroglycerin ointment q.6h.). Other modalities include β-blockers, calcium channel blockers (see Table 1-8), and oxygen.

Admission to a cardiology service is indicated.

If the patient has severe angina that is refractory to first-line therapy, the initiation of intravenous nitroglycerin and/or anticoagulation with heparin is indicated.

In all cases of unstable angina, **coronary angiography** is indicated and will provide a basis for a decision on intervention with angioplasty or surgery.

C. **Myocardial infarction**

Angina that is **not relieved** with nitroglycerin, is present for more than 15 minutes, **and** is accompanied by ST-segment elevation is a **myocardial infarction.** If there is no contraindication, emergency **thrombolysis** with streptokinase or tissue plasminogen activator (tPA) and admission to an intensive care unit is indicated (see Table 1-9). Further acute management schemas are beyond the scope of this text.

IV. **Consultation**

Problem	Service	Time
Stable angina	Cardiology	Required
Unstable angina	Cardiology	Urgent/emergent
Myocardial infarction	Cardiology	Emergent

V. **Indications for admission:** Any degree of instability or any evidence of myocardial infarction. The patient is admitted to the intensive care unit.

Congestive Heart Failure

The heart is a **pump** that provides the flow of blood and therefore oxygen and nutrients to the vital tissues and organs of the body. If the heart fails in its mission, the flow of blood, nutrients, and oxygen to the tissues is markedly decreased. Therefore, failure of the heart will result in failure, to various degrees, of all of the organs, including the brain.

The **overall manifestations** of heart failure are quite diverse and are best categorized by grouping them into those that are the result

TABLE 1-6
Noninvasive Tests for Atherosclerotic Heart Disease

Reference standard is coronary angiography.
Significant disease is defined as a greater than 50% defect in the lumen of a coronary artery.
Sensitivity/specificity: determined when a heart rate above 85% of the target heart rate is reached.

Test	Description and Procedure	Indications	Results/Sensitivity/Specificity
Symptom-limited stress test (SLST)	The patient is placed on a treadmill or bicycle to exercise. Parameters monitored include rhythm, ECG, blood pressure, and development of symptoms attributable to coronary arterial disease (i.e., angina pectoris). The exercise is conducted using a standardized protocol, the most commonly used protocol being that described by Bruce. These protocols allow reproducible tests and the measurement of aerobic respiration (O_2 consumption) in units of METS (metabolic equivalents). One MET = 3.5 mL O_2 consumed/kg/min.	Diagnosis of atypical chest pain Diagnosis of Q-wave MI 6 wk after episode. Cannot be performed if any of the following contraindications exist: Aortic stenosis Asymmetric septal hypertrophy MI in past 6 wk Unstable angina pectoris Decompensated CHF	Diagnosis of ASHD: >2 mm ST-segment depression: Sensitivity: 95% Specificity: 95% 1–2 mm ST-segment depression: Sensitivity: 25%–40% Specificity: 85% Indications to stop SLST: Hypotension ST-segment depression Severe dysrhythmias Angina pectoris

Test	Description	Abnormal resting ECG variant	Interpretation / Results

Stress thallium or sestamibi test	Same as the SLST, plus the administration of a radioisotope, either thallium or Tc-sesta MIBI, in a fixed dose at the peak of exercise. Normally perfused and functioning cardiac myocytes take up the radioisotope; however, nonviable or underperfused areas will not take up the radioisotope. Scintigraphy is performed at the time of initial administration and 3 hr later.	Same as for SLST except that the patient has an abnormal resting ECG.	A *fixed defect*—i.e., one that remains constant at rest—is consistent with nonviable myocardium.
			
			A *reversible defect*—i.e., one that resolves at rest—is consistent with hypoperfusion (i.e., ASHD) in the vessel supplying that area.
			
			    Sensitivity: 84%
			    Specificity: 87%

Dipyridamole thallium or sestamibi stress test	Instead of exercise, the agent dipyridamole is used. This agent causes coronary vasodilation and when used with the radioisotope thallium or Tc-sesta MIBI can scintigraphically assess for uptake. A scintigraphic picture is taken at the time of administration of the radioisotope and 3 hr later.	Same as for SLST except that the patient cannot exercise.	Fixed and reversible defects are as defined above.
			
			    Sensitivity: 85%
			    Specificity: 82%

T A B L E   1 - 7
Canadian Cardiovascular Society Grading Scale
for Angina Pectoris

Class I	Ordinary physical activity does not cause angina: no angina occurs when walking or climbing stairs; angina does occur with strenuous or rapid or prolonged exertion at work or recreation.
Class II	Slight limitation of ordinary activity: angina occurs when walking or climbing stairs rapidly, walking uphill, walking or stair climbing after meals, in the cold, in the wind, under emotional stress, or only during the first few hours after awakening; walking more than two blocks on the level and climbing more than one flight of ordinary stairs at a normal pace and in normal conditions.
Class III	Marked limitation of ordinary physical activity: angina occurs when walking one or two blocks on the level and climbing one flight of stairs in normal conditions and at a normal pace.
Class IV	Inability to carry on any physical activity without discomfort. Anginal symptoms may be present at rest.

of **backward failure** (i.e., pulmonary congestion) versus those that are the result of **forward failure** (i.e., low output). Heart failure of any cause can manifest with any of these manifestations, but quite often the manifestations of backward or forward failure will predominate. The overall manifestations are given in Table 1-10.

I. Categorization of CHF by overall manifestations
A. Backward failure
The **manifestations** of backward failure—i.e., resulting from pulmonary congestion—include dyspnea, tachypnea, orthopnea, paroxysmal nocturnal dyspnea, an S_3 gallop, bilateral crackles, and right-sided failure findings: ascites, bipedal pitting edema, and distended neck veins.
B. Forward failure
The **manifestations** of forward failure—i.e., resulting from pump failure—include hypotension, confusion, lethargy, renal dysfunction, tachycardia, and cool, clammy skin and extremities.

Another method of categorizing heart failure that is central to the **pathophysiology** and management of this syndrome is by **systolic** versus **diastolic dysfunction.** Distinguishing systolic from diastolic dysfunction is difficult when only clinical methods such as the history, physical examination, electrocardiography, and chest x-ray are used.

T A B L E 1-8
Antianginal Agents

Class	Agent/Dose	Mechanism of Action	Side Effects
Antiplatelet	Aspirin, 325 mg PO q. A.M.	Inhibits platelet aggregation	Gastric erosions
Nitrates	Isordil, 10 mg PO t.i.d. to 40 mg PO q.i.d. *or* Nitropaste, 1–2 inches q.6h.	Decreases preload, dilates capacitance vessels	Hypotension, headaches
β-blockers	Atenolol (Tenormin), 50–100 mg PO q.d. *or* Metoprolol (Lopressor), 50–150 mg PO b.i.d. *or* Propranolol (Inderal), 10–40 mg PO t.i.d. to q.i.d.	Decreases heart rate and contractility, therefore decreasing myocardial oxygen demand	AV nodal block, exacerbation of bronchospasm, hypotension, exacerbation of heart failure
Calcium channel blockers	Diltiazem (Cardiazem), 30–120 mg PO q.i.d. *or* Nifedipine (Procardia), 10–40 mg PO t.i.d.	Decreases preload, mildly decreases heart rate, moderate vasodilator Decreases preload, moderate vasodilator	Hypotension; diltiazem can exacerbate AV nodel blocks and heart failure

13

T A B L E 1 - 9
Thrombolytic Therapy for Acute Myocardial Infarction

Agent	Contraindications	Initial Dose	Maintenance Dose
Streptokinase	Active bleeding Hypersensitivity Major surgery in previous 6 wk Cerebrovascular accident in previous 6 wk Use within previous 6 mo.	250,000 units IV bolus	17,000 units/hr IV Concurrent use of heparin in dose below Concurrent use of ASA 325 mg q.d.
Tissue plasminogen activator	Active bleeding Major surgery in previous 6 wk Cerebrovascular accident in previous 6 wk	6 mg bolus IV, then 54 mg IV over 1st hr	20 mg IV over 2nd hr, 20 mg IV over 3rd hr Concurrent use of heparin in dose below Concurrent use of ASA 325 mg PO q.d.
Heparin	Active bleeding History of heparin-related thrombocytopenia Major surgery in previous 6 wk Cerebrovascular accident in previous 6 wk	5,000–10,000 units IV bolus	1,000 units IV/hr Target aPTT: 45–60 sec

T A B L E 1 - 1 0
**Physical Examination Criteria for the Diagnosis
of Congestive Heart Failure**

Major Criteria

Paroxysmal nocturnal dyspnea or orthopnea
Neck vein distention
Rales
Cardiomegaly
Acute pulmonary edema
S_3 gallop
Increased venous pressure (>6 cm H_2O)
Hepatojugular reflux

Minor Criteria

Bilateral ankle edema
Nocturnal cough
Dyspnea on exertion
Hepatomegaly
Pleural effusions, right side greater than left side
Tachycardia, rate >120 beats/min

II. **Categorization of CHF by pathophysiology**
   A. **Systolic dysfunction**
      Systolic dysfunction is characterized by a reduced extent
      of contraction, a decreased ejection fraction, and left ven-
      tricular dilation. It is the most common pathogenesis of
      heart failure. The **most common causes** of systolic heart
      failure include **cardiomyopathy** and **ischemic heart
      disease.**
   B. **Diastolic dysfunction**
      Diastolic dysfunction is a common clinical problem, oc-
      curring in 30%–40% of patients referred for evaluation
      for CHF. The **underlying pathogenesis** of primary dia-
      stolic dysfunction is usually associated with left ventricu-
      lar hypertrophy (LVH) and a normal or supernormal ex-
      tent of contraction and ejection fraction. This results in
      an increased **resistance to diastolic filling** resulting from
      increased left ventricular mass itself and subendocardial
      ischemia, which is often present in patients with LVH.
      The increased resistance to filling results in an **elevated
      diastolic (filling) pressure** which is transmitted to the
      pulmonary capillaries and causes pulmonary congestive
      manifestations.
      One of the **most common causes** of diastolic heart fail-
      ure is a hypertrophied left ventricle, usually as the result
      of long-standing, severe **hypertension.**

C. **Mixed systolic/diastolic dysfunction**

Occasionally diastolic dysfunction develops as an outcome of systolic dysfunction. Secondary diastolic dysfunction may be present when the heart of a patient with severe systolic dysfunction reaches the limit of dilation and distensibility, resulting in an increased resistance to filling.

III. **Management of CHF by clinical category**

The **various clinical categories** of CHF are referenced to the site of the predominant pathology: the endocardium, the pericardium, and the myocardium. Myocardial causes are subgrouped into systolic versus diastolic dysfunction.

A. **Endocardial (valvular) failure**

Evaluation of the **endocardium** is quite useful in documenting the significance of a clinically appreciated murmur. **Manifestations** are specific to the valve involved.

1. **Aortic stenosis**

a. **Manifestations**

Aortic stenosis manifests with a systolic murmur at the base with radiation into the carotids, a decrease in the pulse pressure, and a carotid pulsation that is slow and low (pulsus parvus et tardus). Secondary manifestations include LVH, an S_4 gallop, and syncope.

b. **Evaluation and management**

The **specific evaluation and management** of aortic stenosis include the steps described in Box 1-3. Echocardiography should be performed with Doppler studies. The normal valve size is greater than 2.0 cm². A valve less than 2.0 cm² is considered stenotic, a valve less than 1.0 cm² is severely stenotic, a valve less than 0.5 cm² is critically stenotic. Referral to a cardiologist for cardiac angiography and ventriculography should be performed in preparation for aortic valve replacement. Antibiotic prophylaxis is required for any procedure (see Table 6-4, page 322).

2. **Aortic insufficiency**

a. **Manifestations**

Aortic insufficiency manifests with a diastolic murmur at the base with an increase in pulse pressure and the development of bounding "Corrigan's" or "water hammer" pulses. Secondary manifestations include LVH, an S_4 gallop, and syncope.

b. **Evaluation and management**

The **specific evaluation and management** of aortic insufficiency include the steps listed in Box 1-3. Echocardiography should be performed with

B O X 1 - 3

Overall Evaluation and Management of Congestive Heart Failure

Evaluation

Two questions are integral to the approach, evaluation, and management of heart failure: Why is the patient in heart failure, i.e., what is the etiology? Why is the patient worse now? The evaluation is designed to answer these questions.

1. **History,** including onset of symptoms and the presence of backward or forward manifestations of failure (see text).
2. **Physical examination** for vital signs, crackles, the presence of an S_3 gallop, and to help in assessing the severity of the failure.
3. A 12-lead ECG to look for any acute changes consistent with acute ischemia; any Q-waves, indicative of old infarctions and therefore more systolic dysfunction; and LVH, consistent with diastolic dysfunction.
4. **Chest radiography,** PA and lateral, to look for an enlarged heart. A ratio of heart size to chest size greater than 0.5 is a marker of CHF. In addition, there is often pulmonary vascular redistribution and a right pleural effusion.
5. Attempt to categorize the heart failure as being predominantly **backward or forward, systolic versus diastolic** in nature, and if the site of failure is **endocardial, pericardial, or myocardial.** The most powerful tools to assist in such a grouping are the physical examination and echocardiography.

Management

1. **Acute intervention** in a patient with florid pulmonary edema includes administration of the following agents:
   a. **Oxygen,** to keep PaO_2 > 60 mm Hg.
   b. **Morphine sulfate,** 2 mg IV, to decrease preload, to decrease any chest pain, and to decrease anxiety. This is an agent that is underutilized in the acute management of heart failure.

(continued)

B O X 1 - 3 *(continued)*

> c. If no pericardial process is suspected and if the
>   systolic blood pressure is greater than 100 mm
>   Hg, the clinician can administer **nitroglycerin
>   paste,** 1 inch, to decrease preload, and a **loop di-
>   uretic** (e.g., furosemide [Lasix], 20 mg IV).
> 2. **Admit** patient to inpatient service.
> 3. See text (III. Management of CHF by clinical cate-
>   gory) for chronic management schemas.
>
> *Referral*
>
> Consultation with a cardiologist is necessary.

Doppler studies. The echocardiogram will reveal
the insufficiency. Referral to a cardiologist for cardiac angiography and ventriculography should be
performed in preparation for potential aortic valve
replacement. **Antibiotic prophylaxis** is required
for any procedure (see Table 6-4, page 322).
3. **Mitral regurgitation**
   a. **Manifestations**
      Mitral regurgitation manifests with a systolic mur-
      mur at the apex. Although many patients have be-
      nign mitral insufficiency, mitral insufficiency that
      has been acquired from an MI as the result of dys-
      function or rupture of the papillary muscles may
      manifest with pulmonary edema, hypotension, and
      a loud murmur, i.e., one with an associated palpa-
      ble thrill.
   b. **Evaluation and management**
      The **specific evaluation and management** of mi-
      tral regurgitation include the steps listed in Box
      1-3. Echocardiography should be performed with
      Doppler studies. The echocardiogram will reveal
      the mitral insufficiency and, quite often, an area of
      inferior wall hypokinesis. Referral to a cardiologist
      for cardiac angiography and ventriculography
      should be performed in preparation for potential
      mitral valve replacement. Antibiotic prophylaxis is
      required for any procedure (see Table 6-4, page 322).
B. **Pericardial dysfunction**
   1. **Manifestations**
      The **specific manifestations** of a pericardial effusion
      include those of low-output failure (crackles), an ele-

vated jugular venous pressure, and peripheral edema. The heart tones are usually quite distant, and on the ECG there often is the unique phenomenon of **electrical alternans,** i.e., there is a 2−3 milliamp difference in the amplitude of QRS complexes. **Chest radiography** will show a large cardiac shadow.

2. **Evaluation and management**

   The **specific evaluation and management** of pericardial disease include the steps listed in Box 1-3 and admission to an ICU if the patient is unstable. The echocardiogram will reveal a large pericardial effusion with end-diastolic collapse of the right ventricle. Therapy includes draining the pericardium and determining the underlying etiology. Referral to a cardiologist for pericardiocentesis is indicated on an emergency basis.

C. **Myocardial dysfunction**

   1. **Manifestations**

      The **specific manifestations and pathogenesis** are those described in Box 1-3 and the above discussion. The history, physical examination, and echocardiogram will assist in categorizing the failure into predominantly systolic versus predominantly diastolic. The echocardiogram is pivotal in this differentiation. Although the measurement of ejection fraction is less accurate and precise with echocardiography than with **nuclear cardiography** (MUGA), echocardiography provides an excellent opportunity to visualize the myocardium in action. One can easily differentiate a **predominantly systolic** (low contractility) process from a **predominantly diastolic** (poor filling, good to excellent contractility) process.

   2. **Evaluation and management**

      The **specific evaluation and management** of myocardial etiologies of heart failure include the steps described in Box 1-3 and admission to the inpatient service if the failure is of new onset, is worsening, or is associated with any dysrhythmias, chest pain, syncope, or ECG changes.

   3. **Objectives in management**

      a. **Systolic dysfunction**

         i. **Decrease pulmonary edema** by decreasing preload and improving oxygenation

         ii. **Increase myocardial contractility** to increase cardiac output

         iii. **Decrease afterload** (i.e., systemic resistance) to assist the ventricle in pumping effectiveness and to prolong life

         iv. **Determine the underlying etiology**

METHODS

i. **Decrease pulmonary edema**

Beneficial agents include loop diuretics, e.g., furosemide (Lasix), 20 mg IV; preload reduction with nitropaste, 1 inch q.6h.; and oxygen given by nasal cannula.

ii. **Increase cardiac output**

In severe cases, parenteral dobutamine is effective, but in less serious and in chronic cases, **digoxin,** 0.125–0.250 mg PO q.d., is indicated.

iii. **Decrease afterload**

The use of **angiotensin-converting enzyme (ACE) inhibitors** is of benefit. When the patient is near or at a euvolemic state, an ACE inhibitor should be initiated. One of the best agents is captopril. The starting dose of captopril is 6.25 mg PO q.6–8h., increasing slowly and titrating to systolic blood pressure to a maximum of 50 mg PO q.8h. The use of an ACE inhibitor is the only medical intervention proven to prolong life in patients with significant systolic heart failure. The use of captopril has been especially important in the postacute myocardial infarction period.

iv. **Determine the underlying etiology**

Referral to a cardiologist for assessment of the underlying etiology of the systolic failure, usually by coronary angiography, is indicated.

b. **Diastolic dysfunction**

The management objectives for diastolic dysfunction are similar to those for systolic dysfunction, with the following caveats:

i. **Diuretics** and **nitrates** should be used judiciously. Overuse may exacerbate this type of failure by decreasing preload and embarrassing the filling of the ventricles.

ii. **Digoxin** and other inotropic agents are relatively **contraindicated.** Digoxin should be used only if needed for control of atrial fibrillation.

iii. Optimal **control of hypertension** is necessary. The best agents to use are beta-blockers or calcium channel blockers. **Beta-blockers** control hypertension and decrease the heart rate, affording an increase in ventricular filling. **Calcium channel blockers,** in addition to the af-

fects described for beta-blockers, may assist in
ventricular relaxation. Refer to Table 3-4 (page
155) for dosing details.

   iv. As with systolic dysfunction, referral to a
cardiologist for assessment of the underlying
etiology, usually with coronary angiography,
is indicated.

IV. Consultation

Problem	Service	Time
Any new heart failure	Cardiology	Required
Valvular disease	Cardiology and cardiovascular surgery	Required
Pericardial effusion	Cardiology	Emergent

  V. **Indications for admission:** Any new-onset heart failure, any
acute decompensation of chronic heart failure, any concurrent unstable angina pectoris, any syncope or hemodynamically unstable tachydysrhythmias or bradydysrhythmias.

Syncope

Syncope is defined as transient, sudden loss of consciousness that
resolves spontaneously. Because there are many potential causes
for syncope in adults, it is important to approach this problem
systematically with an appreciation for the various **pathophysiologic mechanisms** that might be involved in producing an individual patient's manifestations.

The critical question to address in patients with syncope is
whether or not the syncope appears to be associated with a **cardiac cause.** Such patients tend to have a **worse prognosis** than
patients with syncope not associated with cardiac causes or those
with syncope of undetermined etiology. The latter group may
comprise up to 50% of all syncope patients evaluated in some
large series.

   I. **Differential diagnosis** (Table 1-14)

The most common causes of syncope, although multiple and
varied, can be categorized into vasovagal causes, cardiac
causes, orthostatic hypotension, neurologic causes, and electrolyte disturbances.

     A. **Vasovagal causes**

Vasovagal reactions, also known as a simple faint, are a
specific, quite common cause of syncope. The **underlying
pathogenesis** of this entity is a massive surge in the parasympathetic system resulting in transient hypotension
and syncope.

Specific manifestations include a preceding emotionally traumatic event with the patient spontaneously and very transiently having a complete loss of consciousness. There are no associated symptoms or any signs on physical examination.

B. Cardiac causes

The **cardiac causes** of syncope are quite diverse. The underlying pathogenesis is a decrease in the ability of the heart to perfuse the brain, resulting in syncope. Categories of etiologies include those associated with **rhythm** disturbances and those associated with **structural** cardiac abnormalities. The rhythm disturbances include **bradycardias** (e.g., third-degree AV nodal block) and **tachycardias** (e.g., atrial fibrillation or ventricular tachycardia). The structural abnormalities include **aortic stenosis, ASH,** and ventricular dysfunction as a result of ischemic heart disease.

C. Orthostatic hypotension

Orthostatic hypotension is one of the most common causes of syncope. The **underlying pathogenesis** is either a marked decrease in the intravascular volume or loss of the sympathetic tone necessary to maintain the actions of the vascular system. The most common causes of volume loss include gastrointestinal losses from vomiting or diarrhea, gastrointestinal bleeding, and excessive urinary losses, usually as the result of iatrogenic overzealous diuresis. The most common causes of sympathetic dysfunction include neuropathies due to diabetes and the use of β-blockers.

Specific manifestations include, for volume depletion, a source of the volume loss and an appropriate increase in heart rate when determining orthostatic parameters; and for autonomic dysfunction, an inappropriate lack of increase in heart rate.

II. Specific evaluation and management of syncope, by cause

A. Vasovagal causes

Make the clinical diagnosis and reassure the patient. The **natural history** of the disorder is uniformly benign.

B. Cardiac causes

The **specific evaluation and management** of cardiac syncope include that described in Box 1-4 and referral to a cardiologist. If the underlying cause is **bradycardia,** either cardiac or bradycardia due to carotid sinus hypersensitivity, a pacemaker is usually required. If the underlying cause is **supraventricular tachycardia,** treatment with an antidysrhythmic agent is indicated; if the underlying cause is **ventricular tachycardia,** electrophysiologic studies and potentially an automatic implantable cardiac defibrillator are indicated. Any **ischemic coronary arte-**

rial disease will require cardiac angiography and intervention.

The **natural history** of cardiac syncope shows a poor prognosis; therefore, evaluation and intervention must be inpatient and aggressive (Tables 1-11, 1-12, and 1-13).

C. **Orthostatic hypotension**

The **specific evaluation and management** of orthostatic syncope includes the steps listed in Box 1-4 and defining if the patient is volume depleted or has autonomic dysfunction. If the patient is **volume depleted,** replete with fluids. If IV repletion is necessary, normal saline is the fluid of choice. Furthermore, the underlying etiology of the volume loss should be defined and treated. Any diuretic therapy should be temporarily discontinued.

Autonomic dysfunction is more difficult to treat and includes the following simple measures:

1. Arising slowly or with assistance from a supine position.
2. Use of above-knee support stockings.
3. Use of a nonsteroidal anti-inflammatory agent, as these agents will cause volume retention and alleviate orthostatic hypotension.

III. **Consultation**

Problem	*Service*	*Time*
Any cardiac etiology	Cardiology	Required
Seizure disorder	Neurology	Urgent

IV. **Indications for admission:** Virtually all patients with syncope should be admitted. Exceptions are those who have had

(Text continues on page 30)

B O X   1 - 4

Overall Evaluation and Management of Syncope

Evaluation

1. **ABCs** as outlined by basic and advanced life support.
2. Perform a thorough **history,** looking for information on the activity or situation antecedent to the event. Further data include the use of any mood-altering agents, including ethanol; the use of medicinal agents; and any history of cardiac or seizure activity. Witnesses to the event may provide powerful

(continued)

historical data, including observation of any convulsive activity consistent with a seizure and the duration of the episode.

3. The **physical examination** includes looking for any signs of trauma resulting from the syncopal episode, and:
   a. **Vital signs,** including orthostatic blood pressure and pulse, looking for any evidence of intravascular volume depletion or any hemodynamically compromising tachydysrhythmia or bradydysrhythmia.
   b. **Cardiac examination,** looking for any significant murmurs and/or gallops. A systolic murmur at the base with decreased carotid pulsations is consistent with aortic stenosis or asymmetric septal hypertrophy (ASH). The murmur of ASH increases with valsalva. A diastolic murmur at the apex is consistent with mitral stenosis or an atrial myxoma. An S_3 gallop is consistent with left ventricular heart failure.
   c. **Neurologic examination,** looking for any new focal motor or sensory deficits, which might be consistent with a cerebrovascular accident or, in the setting of the postictal state, a Todd's paralysis. Focal deficits bespeak an intracranial focal etiology.
4. **12-lead ECG** with rhythm strip, looking for ischemic cardiac changes and/or AV nodal block.
5. **Telemetry** and/or **Holter monitoring**. These tests are used to monitor the patient's rhythm over a finite period of time. Telemetry entails monitoring while the patient is in the hospital. A Holter recording is a 24- or 48-hour recording of the patient's rhythm. To increase the specificity of this test, instruct the patient to record any symptoms and then correlate the symptoms with any rhythm disturbances.
6. **Laboratory** examinations
   a. Serum glucose (hypoglycemia).
   b. Serum electrolytes (baseline purposes).
   c. Serum BUN and creatinine. If both are elevated, with BUN greater than creatinine, the clinical picture is consistent with dehydration.
   d. Plasma levels of any antiseizure medication levels, if indicated.
   e. Hematocrit.

(continued)

7. If there is any murmur or any evidence of heart failure, **echocardiography** should be performed to look at the valves and myocardial wall.
8. If the patient has no carotid bruits and there is no other etiology noted, one can perform **carotid sinus massage,** which entails gentle massage of one of the carotid arteries and monitoring the blood pressure and rhythm strip. An abnormal response is hypotension, which may be due to or independent of a bradycardia.
9. If no cause is determined and there are no contraindications (e.g., aortic stenosis), a **symptom-limited stress test** looking for ischemia is indicated.
10. If there is any evidence that the patient has ventricular tachycardia (e.g., nonsustained ventricular tachycardia on Holter monitoring), **signal-averaged ECG** can be performed to look at the terminal aspect of the QRS complex. A normal test decreases the risk of sustained ventricular tachycardia; an abnormal test puts the patient at higher risk, and therefore further evaluation with **electrophysiologic studies is indicated.**
11. If no diagnosis has been made for the syncope using the above modalities, an **upright tilt table test** is indicated. This test is used to detect any autonomic dysfunction that might cause syncope. Further details of this test are beyond the scope of this text.
12. **No routine CT scans** of the head or electroencephalograms are indicated unless there is evidence from the history or physical examination of a seizure disorder or intracranial event.

Management

1. If the patient is intravascularly volume deplete, replete fluids either enterally or parenterally.
2. The specific management depends on the underlying cause (see text and references for specifics).

Referral

1. If a cardiac cause is suspected, referral to a cardiologist is indicated.
2. If a neurologic cause (e.g., seizure disorder) is suspected, referral to a neurologist is indicated.

T A B L E 1-11
Cardiac Dysrhythmias

Rhythm	ECG Manifestations	Physical Manifestations	Causes	Therapy
Atrial fibrillation	No discrete P-waves Narrow-complex QRS Irregularly irregular rhythm Ventricular response is usually fast	Irregularly irregular rhythm Hypotension Unstable angina pectoris Heart failure Any gallop ausculted must be an S₃; atrial fibrillation precludes the development of an S₄ gallop	Hyperthyroidism Valvular disease a) mitral b) aortic Hypertension with secondary cardiac damage Ischemia	Slow the rate with: a) Digoxin, 0.25 mg IV (see Table 1-12) b) Verapamil, 5 mg IV (see Table 1-12) If unstable, electrically cardiovert emergently, perform ACLS protocol (see Table 1-13) Once rate is controlled (i.e., <90 beats/min at rest): a) Determine the underlying etiology b) Continue digoxin 0.125–0.250 mg PO/day c) Consider anticoagulation; warfarin should be initiated to obtain an INR of 2.0–3.0 in any patient who is at risk for emboli (i.e., with poor left ventricular function, mitral stenosis, paroxysmal

	ECG findings	Clinical features	Associations	Treatment
(continued from previous row)				atrial fibrillation or desire to cardiovert the patient) d) All other patients should receive aspirin, 325 mg PO q.d. e) Concurrent use of a β-blocker or calcium channel blocker will further control the rate (see Table 1-12)
Atrial flutter	P-waves are large, best seen in lead II, and have a rate of 280–300 beats/min Narrow-complex QRS at a rate of 150 beats/min (2:1 conduction), 100 beats/min (3:1)	Hypotension Regular rhythm Palpitations Heart failure Unstable angina pectoris Syncope	Invariably there is a structural heart defect present, usually ASHD Other factors, those which precipitate atrial fibrillation exacerbate atrial flutter	Same as for atrial fibrillation, except: a) Always requires echocardiography and evaluation, after control of ventricular rate, for ASHD (e.g., a stress test) b) Anticoagulation is not necessary
Paroxysmal supraventricular tachycardia	Discrete P-waves Narrow-complex QRS complexes	Palpitations Hypotension Chest pain	Ethanol Caffeine Ischemic heart disease (ASHD)	a) Minimize ethanol and caffeine ingestion b) Same as for atrial fibrillation c) Anticoagulation not necessary

(continued)

T A B L E 1 - 1 1 (continued)

Rhythm	ECG Manifestations	Physical Manifestations	Causes	Therapy
Ventricular tachycardia	AV dissociation Wide QRS tachycardia Left axis deviation	Hypotension Sudden cardiac death Chest pain	ASHD, ischemia Hypokalemia Hypomagnesemia Hypoxemia Prolonged QTc syndromes as a result of medications (e.g., phenothiazines, tricyclic antidepressants), which predisposes patient to torsade du pointes	Therapy: a) ACLS protocol with emphasis on electrical cardioversion if the patient is unstable b) Lidocaine, 75 mg IV bolus and a 2 mg/min IV drip c) Correct any hypokalemia and/or hypomagnesemia d) Determine the underlying cause and attempt to reverse e) Admit and refer to a cardiologist for SA ECG and/or electrophysiologic study f) A further discussion of chronic antiventricular tachycardia agents is beyond the scope of the text

T A B L E 1 - 12
Medications for Tachydysrhythmias

Agent	Atrial Fibrillation	Atrial Flutter	Paroxysmal Supraventricular Tachycardia	Ventricular Tachycardia
Propranolol	Acute: 0.5–2.0 mg IV bolus, rate of bolus infusion not to exceed 1 mg/min Chronic: 10 mg PO q.i.d. to 40 mg PO q.i.d.	Acute: same as for atrial fibrillation Chronic: same	Acute: same as for atrial fibrillation Chronic: same	No indication
Esmolol	Acute: 500 μg/kg over 1 min IV, then 50–200 μg/kg/min IV drip Chronic: no indication	Acute: same as for atrial fibrillation Chronic: no indication	Acute: same as for atrial fibrillation Chronic: no indication	No indication
Verapamil	Acute: 0.075–0.15 mg/kg over 2 min IV; can repeat q.15 min × 2 Chronic: 80 mg PO t.i.d. to 120 mg PO t.i.d.	Acute: same as for atrial fibrillation Chronic: same	Acute: same as for atrial fibrillation Chronic: same	No indication
Diltiazem	Acute: 0.25–0.35 mg/kg over 2 min IV Chronic: 30 mg PO q.i.d. to 120 mg PO q.i.d.	Acute: same as for atrial fibrillation Chronic: same	Acute: same as for atrial fibrillation Chronic: same	No indication
Digoxin	Acute: 0.25 mg IV now, re-peat in 30 min × 1, then repeat q.6h. × 2 Chronic: 0.25–0.375 mg PO q. A.M.	Acute: same Chronic: same	Acute: same Chronic: same	No indication
Adenosine	Acute: 6.0 mg IV, can re-peat in 15 min × 1	Acute: same	Acute: same	No indication
Lidocaine	No indication	No indication	No indication	Acute: 75 mg IV bolus with a concurrent 2 mg/min IV drip

T A B L E 1 - 1 3
Cardioversion: Indications and Contraindications

Indications

Atrial fibrillation/flutter of recent onset (i.e., <3 days) with or without anticoagulation

Atrial fibrillation/flutter of any duration if anticoagulated with warfarin for >3 wk

No contraindications

Emergently if the patient is unstable

Contraindications to Elective Cardioversion

Any known or suspected intracardiac thrombus

TIA, recent CVA or cerebrovascular disease

Recent MI (relative contraindication)

Uncertain duration of adequate anticoagulation (i.e., >3 wk of warfarin with an INR of 2.0–3.0)

CHF (relative contraindication)

Electrolyte imbalance, especially hypokalemia

Digitalis toxicity

---

a vasovagal episode (fainting) or who have evidence of intravascular volume depletion that has resolved with fluid repletion.

Peripheral Vascular Disease of the Lower Extremities

The **anatomy** of the **peripheral vasculature** to the lower extremities is quite simple. The **arterial system** is a high-pressure system that supplies oxygen- and nutrient-rich blood to the lower extremities. The femoral artery enters the thigh immediately deep to the inguinal ligament and gives off several perforating branches into the thigh, including the profunda (deep) femoris artery. The femoral artery becomes the popliteal artery in the popliteal fossa. The popliteal artery then divides into the anterior and posterior tibial arteries and the anterior and posterior peroneal arteries. The anterior tibial artery gives off the dorsalis pedis artery. The clinically palpable arteries include:

1. The **femoral artery:** Palpable and auscultable at the level of the inguinal ligament.
2. The **popliteal artery:** Palpable and auscultable in the popliteal fossa.
3. The **dorsalis pedis artery:** Palpable on the proximal medial dorsal aspect of the foot.
4. The **posterior tibialis artery:** Palpable on the posterior aspect of the medial malleolus.

T A B L E 1 - 1 4
Differential Diagnosis of Syncope

Cardiac Causes

Structural
    Inflow track obstruction (e.g., atrial myxoma or mitral stenosis)
    Outflow track obstruction (e.g., aortic stenosis or ASH)
Dysrhythmia
    Tachyarrhythmia (e.g., ventricular tachycardia or atrial fibrillation)
    Bradyarrhythmia (e.g., third-degree AV nodal block—Adams–Stokes
      syndrome)
Anginal equivalent

Carotid Sinus Hypersensitivity

Vasodepressor type, which manifests with nonbradycardic hypotension
Cardio-inhibitory type, which manifests with bradycardic hypotension
Mixed type

Orthostatic Hypotension

Intravascular volume depletion (e.g., vomiting, diarrhea, overuse
   of diuretics)
Autonomic dysfunction

Situational Syncope

Post-tussive
Postmicturition
Defecation

Neurologic Causes

Vertebrobasilar insufficiency
Subclavian steal syndrome

Metabolic Causes

Hypoglycemia

The **venous system** parallels the arterial system, but with more
individual variation. The venous system is a low-pressure system
that returns oxygen-poor and waste-containing blood back to the
inferior vena cava. A major contribution to venous return is provided by extrinsic compression by the lower extremity musculature.

The venous system can be divided into the **deep** and **superficial**
venous systems. The **deep venous system** accounts for more than
90% of the venous drainage. The deep system includes the **anterior** and **posterior peroneal veins** and the **anterior** and **posterior
tibialis veins** of the **calf**, all of which drain into the **popliteal vein.**
The popliteal vein then drains into the **superficial femoral vein,**
which then drains into the **inferior vena cava.** The **profunda
(deep) femoral vein** drains the thigh into the femoral vein.

The **superficial venous system** drains less than 10% of the blood from the lower **extremities.** The system **consists of the greater (medial) and lesser (lateral)** saphenous veins.

The overall manifestations of and approaches to lower extremity vascular problems are quite diverse and are best categorized by the underlying pathogenesis, i.e., according to whether the arterial or venous system is predominantly affected.

I. Manifestations of lower extremity vascular disease

A. Arterial disease

The **specific manifestations** of arterial vascular disorders in the lower extremities are all attributable to **ischemia** in the affected lower extremity. These include **claudication,** that is, the development of pain, often crampy in nature, upon exercise of the lower extremity (e.g., while walking). There can be, and often are, **bruits** over the femoral artery; **decreased pulses** in the popliteal, dorsal pedis, and posterior tibialis arteries in the affected lower extremity; and a cool extremity with an **increased capillary refill time.** Capillary refill is measured by palpating over the distal toe, blanching the skin, and observing the amount of time for it to return to its baseline pink color.

Risk factors for the development of lower extremity arterial disease include hypertension, diabetes mellitus, smoking, hyperlipoproteinemia, and obesity.

The **natural history** is one of progression to symptomatic claudication, a manifestation that can severely limit the patient's activities; ulcers in the skin; cellulitis; and gangrene.

B. Venous disease

Many problems can develop in the low-pressure venous system. The vast majority of these problems are benign and cosmetic in nature; however, some entities, if untreated, are potentially mortal.

1. Varicosities. The **specific manifestations** of varicose veins include the presence of tortuous, dilated, enlarged, nontender veins within the skin of the lower extremities. Usually the process affects both lower extremities. The lesions are usually asymptomatic.

Risk factors for the development of varicosities include obesity, inactivity, wearing tight clothes, and wearing girdles.

The **natural history** is benign, with occasionally an episode of superficial thrombophlebitis.

2. Venous stasis. The **specific manifestations** of venous stasis include bilateral lower extremity edema that may be worse in the evenings and resolves overnight when the patient sleeps in a recumbent position. There often are concurrent lower extremity varicosities.

The **risk factors** are quite similar to those described in the development of varicose veins. However, one additional risk factor plays a role in development: damage to the **venous valves,** most commonly as the result of a past episode of DVT (the postphlebitic syndrome).

The **natural history** is usually benign, but complications can develop. These complications include changes in the overlying skin, such as increased pigment and skin breakdown, and therefore an increased risk of **cellulitis.** The risk of cellulitis is particularly high in patients who have a concurrent risk factor (i.e., neuropathy secondary to diabetes mellitus, or arterial insufficiency).

3. **Superficial thrombophlebitis.** The **specific manifestations** include an acute onset of pain, swelling, erythema, and warmth in one of the lower extremities. The patient often has a palpable cord, which represents the thrombosed vein itself. These manifestations are quite similar to those of DVT.

   Risk factors for the development of superficial thrombophlebitis include varicosities, trauma to the area, the placement of IV catheters, and, as with deep venous thrombophlebitis, immobilization and hypercoagulable states.

   The **natural history** of this entity is quite benign, with **no risk** of systemic embolization.

4. **Deep venous thrombophlebitis.** The **specific manifestations** include an acute onset of pain, swelling, erythema, and warmth in one of the lower extremities. There can be various degrees of warmth, redness, tenderness, and swelling in the affected lower extremity. **Risk factors** for the development of DVT include hypercoagulable states, inflammation, and immobilization.

   The **natural history** of DVT depends on the location of the thrombosis, either **distal** (inferior to the popliteal space) or **proximal** (in and superior to the popliteal space). **Distal thrombus** rarely embolizes to the pulmonary bed, whereas **proximal thrombus** is at **high risk for embolizing** to the pulmonary bed with resultant morbidity and mortality. Because distal thrombus can, over time, **propagate proximally,** repeated imaging is necessary to follow the thrombus.

II. Specific evaluation and management
A. Arterial disease
The **specific evaluation and management** include that described in Box 1-5, and if the distal pulses are nonpalpable, determining the ABI to assess the degree of obstruc-

B O X 1 - 5

Overall Evaluation and Management of Lower Extremity Vascular Disease

Evaluation

1. Take a history, focusing on:
   a. **Claudication,** i.e., the development of pain in one or both lower extremities upon exercise, indicative of decreased arterial flow.
   b. **Risk factors** for the development of atherosclerotic disease:
      i. Diabetes mellitus
      ii. Hypertension
      iii. Cigarette **smoking**
      iv. Hyperlipoproteinemia
      v. Family history
      vi. Obesity
   c. Any history of arterial or venous thrombotic events.
   d. The time of **onset** of lower extremity swelling and whether it is unilateral or bilateral.
   e. Concurrent symptoms, including pain in the affected lower extremity.
   f. **Risk factors** for the development of venous thrombotic disease:
      i. Recent immobilization
      ii. Any inflammation in one or both lower extremity(ies), including any infectious process
      iii. Hypercoagulable states, as manifested by a history of deep venous thrombosis; this might indicate a deficiency in one of the normally present proteins of anticoagulation (e.g., protein C, protein S, antithrombin III), or the reversible hypercoagulable state of pregnancy
2. Perform a **physical examination,** including:
   a. **Ausculting** for bruits over the femoral artery.
   b. **Palpating** for pulses over the popliteal artery, dorsalis pedis artery, and posterior tibialis artery.
      If the **pulses are nonpalpable,** perform a **Doppler flow** study of the lower extremity arteries. This examination determines the ratio of flow in the lower extremity arteries relative to flow in the arteries of the upper extremity (arterial blood ratio,

(continued)

B O X 1 - 5 *(continued)*

ABI). The ratio is normally 1; any ratio **less than 0.5** is indicative of significant obstructive lower extremity arterial disease.

If there is any evidence of **swelling or edema** in the lower extremities, determine whether there is any **asymmetry** by measuring calf and thigh **circumferences.**

c. Looking for **concurrent signs of inflammation,** i.e., redness (*rubor*), tenderness, warmth (*calor*), and any areas of skin breakdown.

Management

Based on the history and physical examination results, determine whether the process is predominantly **arterial or venous.**

1. If the process is **arterial,** check for and modify any risk factors in the development of atherosclerotic disease; initiate aspirin, 325 mg PO/day (unless contraindicated); and refer the patient to vascular surgery (see text).
2. If the process is **venous** and **asymmetric,** rule out deep venous thrombosis via imaging techniques (see text and Table 1-15). If deep venous thrombosis in the proximal venous system is diagnosed, admission and the initiation of heparin are mandated.

Referral

Referral to a vascular surgeon is necessary for any patient with lower extremity arterial disease or DVT.

tion to arterial flow. If the patient has a history of **arterial thrombosis at other sites** (i.e., cerebrovascular accident, upper extremity ischemia) or is in the rhythm of atrial fibrillation, perform echocardiography to look for intracardiac thrombus.

The **specific management** depends on the underlying pathogenesis.

1. If the **underlying pathogenesis** is atherosclerotic disease, the risk factors for the development of atherosclerotic disease must be modified, aspirin in the dose of 325 mg/day PO should be initiated, and a referral to a vascular surgeon for arterial bypass surgery should be made.

T A B L E 1-15
Imaging Techniques for the Lower Extremity Venous System

Test	Procedure Description	Results/Sensitivity/Specificity
Compression ultrasound	Segments of the proximal deep venous system are imaged on ultrasound; direct pressure is applied to the veins by the examiner: If compressible, indicative of no luminal defects; therefore, no thrombus. If not compressible, consistent with thrombus.	Proximal: Sensitivity: 89% Specificity: 97%
Doppler ultrasound	The Doppler probe measures flow within the vessel itself. Spontaneous flow and augmented (i.e., by compressing the vessels distal to the probe level) flow are measured. If flow in the vessel is not compromised and if there is an increase in flow upon augmentation, no thrombus is present. A decrease in flow and a decrease in augmented flow are consistent with thrombus.	Proximal: Sensitivity: 84% Specificity: 87%
Impedance plethysmography	This procedure is based on the facts that proximal thrombus will decrease the flow of blood from the distal bed and that the blood flow can be measured by measuring the impedance to the flow of AC current through an extremity. The procedure is performed by placing a blood pressure cuff around the proximal thigh and applying 50 mm Hg pressure. The flow will slowly decrease as measured by the impedance. When a plateau is reached, the cuff is deflated with, in the **normal setting**, a rapid flow from the distal to proximal systems as reflected by a marked and rapid decrease in impedance. If **proximal thrombus** is present, there is minimal flow into the proximal system and therefore a blunting of the normal rapid change in impedance.	Proximal: Sensitivity: 96%–100% Specificity: 94%
Contrast venography	Intravenous contrast dye is injected into the venous system of the lower extremity via a foot vein. This invasive procedure remains the reference standard to which all other procedures are compared. It can result in phlebitis and even anaphylaxis and is **no longer the first-line** procedure; essentially it is used for those cases in which DVT is suspected even with a negative noninvasive imaging study.	Proximal: Sensitivity: 95% Specificity: 95%

2. If the patient has any evidence that the **underlying pathogenesis** is one of arterial thrombotic events (i.e., the patient is in atrial fibrillation, or has a dilated cardiomyopathy, or has thrombus in the ventricle demonstrated with echocardiography), admit the patient and provide **anticoagulation** on a long-term basis with **warfarin.** The target International Normalized Ratio (INR) is 2.0–3.0, except in patients with a prosthetic heart valve, in whom the target INR is 3.0–4.2. Referral to vascular surgery is also indicated in the acute setting, as surgical removal of the thrombus may be of acute benefit.

B. **Venous disease**
   1. **Varicosities.** The **specific evaluation and management** include making the clinical diagnosis by performing a thorough history and physical examination (see Box 1-5) and preventing further progression of the process. The patient should be instructed to lose weight, wear loose-fitting clothes, not to cross the legs, to increase exercise, and not to wear girdles. The use of **above-knee elastic hose** is of benefit in prevention. If the varicosities are of significant concern to the patient, referral to a vascular or general surgeon for sclerotherapy is indicated.
   2. **Venous stasis.** The **specific evaluation and management** of venous stasis include making the clinical diagnosis by performing a thorough history and physical examination as described in Box 1-5 and preventing further progression of the disease. The patient should be instructed to lose weight, wear loose-fitting clothes, not to cross the legs, to increase exercise, and not to wear girdles. The use of **above-knee elastic hose** and **elevating the lower extremities** when sitting are also of benefit in prevention. There is **no indication** for diuretic therapy in a patient with edema due to venous stasis. Any cellulitis should be aggressively treated (see section on Bacterial Skin Infections, Chapter 6, page 313).
   3. **Superficial thrombophlebitis.** The **specific evaluation and management** of superficial thrombophlebitis include that described in Box 1-5 and ruling out any concurrent DVT via the imaging techniques described in Table 1-15. Specific management includes rest, lower extremity elevation, initiation of a nonsteroidal inflammatory agent (see Table 7-1, Musculoskeletal Disorders, page 363), and the application of local heat.
   4. **Deep venous thrombosis.** The **specific evaluation and management** of DVT include making the diagnosis and defining the thrombus as being distal or proximal,

by using the information detailed in Box 1-5 and Table 1-15. The specifics in management include:

a. Superficial thrombophlebitis

Evaluation and management are described in 3, above.

b. Conclusively distal DVT

Manage the patient conservatively with leg elevation and initiation of a nonsteroidal anti-inflammatory agent. A noninvasive imaging study (see Table 1-15) should be repeated in 3–5 days. If there is any **propagation of the thrombus proximally,** it must be treated as a proximal DVT.

c. Proximal DVT

The thrombus is at high risk for embolizing. For all intents and purposes, thrombosis in the deep venous system is the **same** disease process as pulmonary thromboembolic disease.

Specific management includes admission for anticoagulation, acutely with **heparin** 5,000–10,000 unit bolus IV and a 1,300 unit/hr drip to maintain a PTT of 60–80 sec, and initiation of **warfarin.** A **ventilation–perfusion** scan can be of diagnostic benefit in that several studies have demonstrated a high coincidence of pulmonary thromboembolism even in patients who have no pulmonary symptoms. Warfarin must be continued for a total of 3 months with a **target INR range of 2.0–3.0.** If DVT recurs or pulmonary thromboembolism develops, initiate long-term (lifelong) anticoagulation with warfarin.

An exciting new modality in the treatment of DVT and pulmonary thromboembolic disease will be **low molecular weight heparin,** which can be administered subcutaneously and on a daily basis. This agent will probably become available in the United States in 1993–1994 and may significantly affect the management of DVT. Many low-risk patients with DVT may be able to be managed as outpatients in the future using this modality.

III. Consultation

Problem	Service	Time
Recurrent venous disease	Hematology	Elective
Arterial thrombotic disease	Hematology	Required
Arterial thrombotic disease	Vascular surgery	Urgent
Intermittent claudication	Vascular surgery	Required
Varicosities	Vascular surgery	Elective

IV. **Indications for admission:** Development of a significant cellulitis, gangrene, acute arterial thrombosis, and all cases of proximal DVT.

Bibliography

Hyperlipidemia

Dyslipoproteinemia Education Program: Clinician's Manual. Gotto AM, ed. Science Press Limited, London, 1991.

Grundy SM, Denke MA: Dietary influences on serum lipids and lipoproteins. J Lipid Res 1990;31:1149–1172.

Grundy SM, et al: The place of HDL in cholesterol management. Arch Intern Med 1989;149:505–510.

Manson M, et al: The primary prevention of myocardial infarction. N Engl J Med 1992;326:1406–1416.

Report of the National Educational Program Expert Panel on Detection, Evaluation, and Treatment of High Blood Cholesterol in Adults. Arch Intern Med 1988;148:36–71.

Chest Pain

Abrams J: A reappraisal of nitrate therapy. JAMA 1988;259:396–401.

Bingle JF, Mayhew HE: Outpatient management of coronary artery disease. Am Fam Physician 1987;36:191–200.

Campeau L: Grading of angina pectoris (letter). Circulation 1976;54:522–523.

Diamond GA, Forrester JS: Analysis of probability as an aid in the clinical diagnosis of coronary artery disease. N Engl J Med 1979;300:1350–1358.

Evans CH, Karunaratne HB: Exercise stress testing for the family physician: Part I. Performing the test. Am Fam Physician 1992;45:121–132.

Goldman L, Lee TH: Noninvasive tests for diagnosing the presence and extent of coronary artery disease. J Gen Intern Med 1986;1:258–264.

Kotler TS, Diamond GA: Exercise thallium-201 scintigraphy in the diagnosis and prognosis of coronary artery disease. Ann Intern Med 1990;113:684–702.

Lewis HD, et al: Protective effects of aspirin against acute myocardial infarction and death in men with unstable angina pectoris. N Engl J Med 1983;309:396–403.

Physicians' Health Study Research Group: Final report on the Aspirin Component of the Ongoing Physicians' Health Study. N Engl J Med 1989;321:129–135.

Pryor DB, et al: Estimating the likelihood of significant coronary artery disease. Am J Med 1983;75:771–780.

Veterans Administration Cooperative Group: Comparison of medical and surgical treatment for unstable angina pectoris. N Engl J Med 1987;316:977–984.

Heart Failure

The Captopril-Digoxin Multicenter Research Group: Comparative effects of therapy with captopril and digoxin in patients with mild and moderate heart failure. JAMA 1988;259:539–544.

Chia-Sen Lee D, et al: Heart failure in outpatients. N Engl J Med 1982;306:699–705.

The Criteria Committee of the New York Heart Association: Nomenclature and Criteria for Diagnosis of Diseases of the Heart and Great Vessels, 8th ed. New York Heart Association/Little, Brown & Company. New York, 1979.

Deedwania PC: Angiotensin-converting enzyme inhibitors in congestive heart failure. Arch Intern Med 1990;150:1798–1804.

Harizi RC, et al: Diastolic function of the heart in clinical cardiology. Arch Intern Med 1988;148:99–108.

Packer M, et al: Comparison of captopril and enalapril in patients with severe chronic heart failure. N Engl J Med 1986;315:847–853.

Packer M, et al: Influence of renal function on the hemodynamic and clinical responses to long-term captopril therapy in severe chronic heart failure. Ann Intern Med 1986;104:147–154.

Pfeffer MA, et al: Effect of captopril on mortality and morbidity in patients with ventricular dysfunction after myocardial infarction. N Engl J Med 1992;327:669–677.

SOLVD Investigators: Effect of enalapril on mortality and development of heart failure in asymptomatic patients with reduced left ventricular ejection fractions. N Engl J Med 1992;327:685–691.

Cardiac Dysrhythmias

Brugada P, et al: A new approach to the differential diagnosis of a regular tachycardia with a wide QRS complex. Circulation 1991;83:1649–1659.

DiMarco JP, et al: Adenosine for paroxysmal supraventricular tachycardia: Dose ranging and comparison with verapamil. Ann Intern Med 1990; 113:104–110.

Kutalek SP, McCormick DJ: Classification of antiarrhythmic drugs. Am Fam Physician 1988;38:261–266.

The Stroke Prevention in Atrial Fibrillation Investigators: Predictors of thromboembolism in atrial fibrillation. Ann Intern Med 1992;116:1–5.

Wellens HJ, et al: The value of the electrocardiogram in the differential diagnosis of a tachycardia with a widened QRS complex. Am J Med 1978;64:27–33.

Syncope

Kapoor WN: Diagnostic evaluation of syncope. Am J Med 1991;90:91–106.

Peripheral Vascular Disease

Becker DM: Venous thromboembolism. J Gen Intern Med 1986;1:402–411.

Doyle DJ, et al: Adjusted subcutaneous heparin or continuous intravenous heparin in patients with acute deep vein thrombosis. Ann Intern Med 1987;107:441–445.

Huisman MV, et al: Management of clinically suspected acute venous thrombosis in outpatients with serial impedance plethysmography in a community hospital setting. Arch Intern Med 1989;149:511–513.

Hull RD, et al: Prophylaxis of venous thromboembolism: An overview. Chest 1986;89:374s–383s.

Levine MN, et al: Prevention of deep vein thombosis after elective hip surgery. Ann Intern Med 1991;114:545–551.

NIH Consensus Conference: Prevention of venous thrombosis and pulmonary embolism. JAMA 1986;256:744–749.

Pedersen OM, et al: Compression ultrasonography in hospitalized patients with suspected deep venous thrombosis. Arch Intern Med 1991;151: 2217–2220.

PIOPED Investigators: Value of the ventilation/perfusion scan in acute pulmonary embolism. JAMA 1990;263:2753–2759.

Wheeler HB: Diagnosis of deep vein thrombosis. Am J Surg 1985:7–13.

Wheeler HB, Anderson FA: Diagnostic approaches for deep vein thrombosis. Chest 1986;89:407S–412S.

Dale Berg, Ed. *Handbook
of Primary Care Medicine.*
Copyright © 1993 J. B.
Lippincott Company.

CHAPTER 2

Gastrointestinal Medicine

Abdominal Pain: Overall Approach

The **abdomen** is a large anatomical region that contains many
diverse structures, including those of the urinary system, the gastrointestinal system, and the reproductive system. Any dysfunction, trauma, or inflammation of any of these specific structures
can and will manifest with abdominal pain. In addition to intra-
abdominal structures, any structure adjacent to the abdomen can
result in referred abdominal pain.

There is as well considerable latitude in the **severity** of abdominal pain. Most abdominal pain is self-limited and benign, but in
certain cases abdominal pain can be a manifestation of a severe,
even life-threatening process. Therefore, the approach to the evaluation and management of abdominal pain must be thorough and
reproducible.

This section provides an overview of definitions, the differential diagnosis, evaluation, and management of abdominal pain,
followed by a **quadrant approach** to abdominal pain. Specific
common syndromes are discussed in subsequent sections.

I. **Definitions**

Definitions that are reproducible and workable are extremely
important in the assessment of abdominal pain. Some of the
most salient definitions include those listed below.

A. **Pain versus tenderness**

Pain is a **subjective** manifestation, whereas **tenderness** is
an **objective** finding which the examiner elicits. **Tenderness** is the reproduction of the pain symptomatology in
the course of performing an activity—usually **palpation**
or pressing on the symptomatic area.

B. Direct versus rebound tenderness

Direct tenderness is pain elicited by palpating over an area; **rebound tenderness** is pain elicited on rapid release of the palpation and is indicative of peritoneal irritation and/or inflammation.

C. Guarding

Guarding is the voluntary or involuntary contraction of all or portions of the abdominal wall. Whereas **voluntary guarding** can be a nonspecific manifestation, **involuntary guarding** is quite often associated with peritoneal irritation and therefore is more indicative of a pathologic process.

D. Acute abdomen

An **acute abdomen,** also known as a "surgical abdomen," denotes abdominal pain and associated peritoneal signs requiring **emergency** surgical intervention. Examples include appendicitis, bowel obstruction, and perforation of the GI tract.

II. Abdominal pain syndromes, by quadrant

Common abdominal pain syndromes and their characteristic features are described in Table 2-1. A more reproducible categorization is to stratify abdominal pain syndromes into four groups based on **location by abdominal quadrant.** The differential diagnosis of pain in each quadrant is distinct (Table 2-2), and thus allows the clinician to focus the evaluation and management on the more likely causes of pain at a given location.

A. Right upper quadrant

1. Anatomy

In the **right upper quadrant** are located the liver, the biliary tree, the gallbladder, and the right kidney. Dysfunction or inflammation of any of these structures can result in right upper quadrant pain. In addition, pain can also be referred from the stomach, pancreas, appendix, fallopian tubes, and ovaries. The specific differential diagnosis of etiologies is listed in Table 2-2.

2. Pain manifestations

Specific manifestations of pain in the right upper quadrant can include those listed in Box 2-1 and **Murphy's sign.** Murphy's sign is the presence of tenderness and the inability of the patient to inspire as a result of this tenderness when the clinician palpates the upper right quadrant. This sign, when present, is indicative of extrahepatic inflammation of the biliary tree. Furthermore, the **liver size** must be determined.

3. **Evaluation**
   The **specific evaluation** of right upper quadrant pain includes the steps listed in Box 2-1. Further tests include **liver function tests** (SGOT, SGPT, GGT, alkaline phosphatase, LDH, total bilirubin, direct bilirubin, albumin, and PT). If there is any abnormality in these tests, a **hepatitis A and B panel, amylase and lipase determinations** (both are elevated in acute pancreatitis), and **ultrasonography** (US) of the biliary tree are indicated.

   Biliary US should be used to determine the presence of cholelithiasis or choledocholithiasis, to demonstrate any hepatomegaly, and to examine the head of the pancreas for masses. Furthermore, the **diameter** of the **common bile duct** should be measured. The normal size is approximately 5 mm. Dilation of the duct system is consistent with obstruction. **Computed tomography** (CT) of the abdomen is indicated if the US examination is suboptimal, if there is any evidence of hepatomegaly or a pancreatic mass, or if the US study is negative and yet the suspicion for biliary tract disease is high.

4. **Management**
   The management of specific abdominal pain-producing entities is discussed in subsequent sections of this chapter.

B. **Left upper quadrant**
   1. **Anatomy**
      The left upper quadrant contains the spleen, the left kidney, the pancreas, and the stomach. Dysfunction or inflammation of any of these structures can result in left upper quadrant pain. In addition, pain can also be referred from the colon, small bowel, biliary tree, fallopian tubes, and ovaries. The specific differential diagnosis of etiologies is listed in Table 2-2.
   2. **Pain manifestations**
      The **specific manifestations** associated with pain in the left upper quadrant can include those listed in Box 2-1 or, if the cause is a peptic ulcer, a guaiac-positive stool.
   3. **Evaluation**
      The **specific evaluation** is as listed in Box 2-1. Additional tests may include determining amylase and lipase levels, each of which would be elevated in acute pancreatitis; urinalysis for detecting hematuria or pyuria; and, because dysfunction of the biliary tree can result in pain in this location, **liver function tests,** including SGOT, SGPT, GGT, alkaline phosphatase,

(*Text continues on page 50*)

T A B L E 2 - 1
Characteristics of Abdominal Pain Syndromes

Syndrome	Location	Exacerbating/ Alleviating Factors	Risk Factors	Associated Features
Peptic ulcer disease	Left upper quadrant; epigastric	Exacerbating: fasting, ethanol Alleviating: food, antacids	Ethanol Stress NSAIDs	Afebrile No leukocytosis UGI bleeding Perforation of ulcer
Pancreatitis	Left upper quadrant	Exacerbating: ethanol Alleviating: fasting	Ethanol Cholelithiasis Choledocholithiasis High triglycerides	Low-grade fever Leukocytosis without left shift Hypocalcemia Hypoxia Elevated amylase and lipase
Cholecystitis	Right upper quadrant	Exacerbating: fatty meals Alleviating: fasting	Obesity Female sex Use of oral contraceptives	Low-grade to spiking fever Normal to elevated WBC Murphy's sign present Elevated alkaline phosphatase and total bilirubin levels Icterus Bilirubinuria
Appendicitis	Right lower quadrant	Exacerbating: none Alleviating: extension of the thigh with flexion of the knee	None	Low-grade to spiking fever Leukocytosis with left shift Peritoneal signs present Rovsing's sign present

Diverticulitis	Left lower and/or right lower quadrant	Exacerbating: none Alleviating: none	Low-fiber diets Constipation Irritable bowel Straining upon bowel movements	Low-grade fever Mild leukocytosis Can have hematochezia if diverticulosis concurrently present If complications (i.e., perforation of the diverticulum, obstruction of the large bowel, abscess formation) occur, can have leukocytosis; peritoneal signs and fevers common
Pelvic inflammatory disease	Right or left lower quadrant pain	Exacerbating: none Alleviating: none	Past history of STD Multiple sexual partners	Low-grade to spiking fever Leukocytosis with left shift Purulent discharge from cervix and vagina Tender adnexal mass
Ruptured ectopic pregnancy	Right or left lower quadrant pain	Exacerbating: none Alleviating: none	Past history of PID Tubal ligation	Low-grade fever Leukocytosis without left shift Adnexal mass Orthostasis Positive pregnancy test No intrauterine products of conception visualized with pelvic US
Nephrolithiasis	Right or left upper quadrant pain	Exacerbating: none Alleviating: none	UTI with *Proteus* Hypercalcuria Abuse of vitamins C or D	Low-grade fever Leukocytosis without left shift Hematuria Flank pain, can be severe

T A B L E   2 - 2
Differential Diagnosis of Abdominal Pain

Right Upper Quadrant

Cholecystitis
Cholelithiasis
Hepatitis
Peptic ulcer disease
Pancreatitis
Pyelonephritis
Appendicitis (especially in pregnancy)
Fitz–Hugh–Curtis syndrome

Left Upper Quadrant

Peptic ulcer disease
Pancreatitis
Pyelonephritis
Splenic trauma/rupture
Pneumonitis
Angina pectoris
Pericarditis

Right and/or Left Lower Quadrant

Appendicitis
Diverticulitis
Nephrolithiasis
Pyelonephritis
Inflammatory bowel disease
Gastroenteritis
Ruptured ectopic pregnancy
Salpingitis
Ovarian cyst, especially if ruptured
Mittelschmerz (pain on day 14 of menstrual cycle, indicative of a normal ovulation)

B O X   2 - 1

Overall Evaluation and Management of Abdominal Pain

Evaluation

1. Obtain a thorough **history** of the pain.
   a. Determine **when** the pain started, its **location,** its **intensity,** what **makes it worse** (exacerbating factors), what **makes it better** (alleviating factors), and for **how long** it has been present (duration).
   b. Look for a **history** of any processes that can pro-
   (continued)

B O X 2 - 1 *(continued)*

duce pain. These processes include diverticulosis, urinary tract infections, cholelithiasis, choledocholithiasis, and nephrolithiasis.

c. Additional **historical data** of importance include the menstrual history in women, the sexual history, the use of medications ("recreational" and therapeutic), the use of ethanol, recent or distant history of trauma to the abdomen, and recent or distant history of abdominal surgery.

d. Document the presence or absence of **associated features** such as nausea, dysuria, pyuria, vomiting, diarrhea, constipation, fevers, loss of or decrease in flatus, hematemesis, or melena.

2. Perform a thorough **physical examination** to define any areas of **tenderness** and any associated, objective findings.

a. Determine the **presence and location** of direct tenderness, the presence and location of rebound tenderness, and whether guarding is present.

b. Determine **vital signs,** including **orthostatic parameters.** This information is important in determining volume status and whether fever is present.

c. Assess **bowel sound activity** and quality. If bowel sounds are **hypoactive,** the picture is usually consistent with ileus (the temporary loss of bowel activity). If bowel sounds are **hyperactive,** it can be as the result of a partial or complete small or large bowel obstruction.

d. Perform a **pelvic examination** in all women and a **scrotal and penile examination** in all men, looking for any discharge, tenderness, or masses in the scrotum, labia majora, or inguinal areas.

e. Perform a **rectal examination.** Note the color and guaiac response of the stool specimen. Melena (black, tarry stools) and hematochezia (red stools) are associated with GI bleeding, whereas a light, clay-colored stool is often associated with hepatic dysfunction and/or hepatic biliary obstruction.

f. If possible, perform **deep palpation** of the abdomen to determine the presence and quality of

(continued)

B O X 2 - 1 *(continued)*

    masses, i.e., whether they are pulsatile, tender, or contiguous with normal structures.

  g. Determine the **size of the liver** by the scratch test, percussion, and palpation. If the liver is enlarged, note the presence or absence of tenderness.

  h. Perform **percussion over the costovertebral angle.** Tenderness elicited by light percussion or palpation over the costovertebral angle is consistent with pyelonephritis or nephrolithiasis.

  i. Determine the presence of **abdominal distention** by observation and palpation of the abdomen. A distended abdomen without shifting dullness but with tympany to percussion is consistent with increased gas in the bowel and therefore with **obstruction.** A distended abdomen with shifting dullness and a hyporesonant (i.e., dull) percussion note is consistent with **ascites.**

  j. The clinician must perform **serial examinations,** as results will change as the underlying process evolves or resolves.

3. **Rule out pregnancy** with a urine pregnancy test in all women of childbearing age with an intact uterus.

4. Test the guaiac response of stools to rule out **occult bleeding.**

5. Obtain an **abdominal x-ray series** (rule out pregnancy before performing this study in women). The series consists of four views of the abdomen, including a cross-table lateral view. Particular attention should be focused on the following:

  a. The presence of **free air** (i.e., air outside the bowel itself), which is indicative of perforation (Fig. 2-1).

  b. Any areas of **distended bowel,** small or large. A distended bowel is consistent with obstruction or ileus. The small bowel can be differentiated from the large bowel in that the radiographic markings in the small bowel appear to extend across the width of the lumen (plicae semicircularis), whereas the radiographic markings in the large bowel appear not to extend across the entire lumen (haustra).

  c. The presence of **air–fluid levels** in the small bowel, which would be indicative of obstruction.

(continued)

B O X 2 - 1 *(continued)*

    d. The presence of **calcified areas within the gall-bladder,** indicative of cholelithiasis. However, less than 15% of stones in the gallbladder are calcified.

    e. The presence of **calcified areas within the renal pelvis,** indicative of nephrolithiasis. More than 90% of urinary tract stones are calcified.

    f. The presence of **calcifications in the area of the pancreas,** indicative of chronic pancreatitis.

    g. The presence of **large amounts of stool** in the large bowel.

    h. The **size of the large bowel** if the abdomen is distended. Specifically, if the cecum is more than 13 cm in diameter, there is an increased risk of perforation.

  6. The **KUB** (abdominal flat plate) study, while more convenient to obtain, is inferior to the abdominal series in demonstrating potential pathology.

  7. Withhold oral intake (**NPO**), at least initially.

  8. Provide **fluid repletion** and then maintenance. 0.9 normal saline is usually the most appropriate fluid, especially if vomiting is present.

  9. Perform **urinalysis** with microscopic examination to reveal any hematuria, crystals, or pyuria.

10. Contrast studies, such as an **air contrast barium enema examination** or an **upper gastrointestinal series** with barium, should be reserved for the patient who is stable, is experiencing subacute or chronic pain, and in whom there is little risk of perforation. An example is the patient with partial bowel obstruction who is stable. Contrast-enhanced studies may also be performed to evaluate for duodenal ulcer disease. If there is any suspicion of perforation, Gastrografin (meglumine diatrizoate) should be the contrast agent.

11. Based on the above, formulate a clinical diagnosis as to the **location,** by quadrant, and the **severity** of the pain. Further assessment and management will be based on these two clinical assessments.

Management

Specific management of abdominal pain-producing syndromes is given in subsequent sections of this chapter.

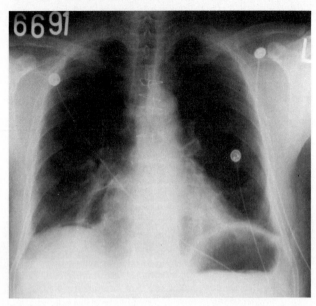

FIGURE 2-1
AP chest radiograph showing free air under the right hemidiaphragm in a patient with a perforated duodenal ulcer.

LDH, total bilirubin, direct bilirubin, albumin, and PT determinations. If there are any abnormalities in these tests, **US** of the biliary tree and pancreas can be considered.

US should be used to determine the presence of cholelithiasis, choledocholithiasis, or concurrent hepatomegaly, and to examine the head of the pancreas for masses. Furthermore, the **diameter of the common bile duct** should be measured. The normal diameter is approximately 5 mm. Dilation of the duct system is consistent with obstruction. CT of the abdomen is indicated if the US examination is suboptimal, if there is any evidence of hepatomegaly or a pancreatic mass, or if the US study is negative and yet the suspicion for a complication of pancreatitis is high (see section on Pancreatitis, page 57).

4. **Management**

The management of specific abdominal pain-producing entities is discussed in subsequent sections of this chapter.

C. Right and left lower quadrants

1. Anatomy

The right and left lower quadrants contain the ureters, the appendix (right side only), the colon, the fallopian tubes, and the ovaries. Dysfunction or inflammation of any of these structures can result in right upper quadrant pain. In addition, pain can be referred from the small bowel and kidneys. The specific differential diagnosis of etiologies is listed in Table 2-2.

2. Pain manifestations

The **specific manifestations** associated with pain in the lower quadrants can include those listed in Box 2-1.

3. Evaluation

The **evaluation** is as listed in Box 2-1. In addition, **US** of the kidneys and pelvis should be considered.

a. If nephrolithiasis is suspected clinically or if there is any renal dysfunction, US should be used to determine the presence of any ureteral obstruction, any nephrolithiasis, and to demonstrate the kidney size (normal is 12–13 cm in the longitudinal dimension).

b. If the clinical suspicion is of a pelvic mass or if the patient is pregnant, US should be used to determine the presence of any adnexal or uterine masses.

c. If diverticulosis or diverticulitis is suspected, CT of the pelvis can be performed to evaluate for any abscess formation.

4. Management

The management of specific abdominal pain-producing entities is discussed in subsequent sections of this chapter.

III. Consultation

Problem	*Service*	*Time*
Any acute abdomen	General surgery	Emergent
Adnexal mass, non-tender, negative pregnancy test	Obstetrics/ Gynecology	Urgent
Adnexal mass, tender, or positive pregnancy test	Obstetrics/ Gynecology	Urgent
Bowel obstruction	General surgery	Emergent

IV. Indications for admission:

Any evidence of an acute abdomen, any GI bleeding, any signs of infection or impending sepsis, any significant intravascular volume depletion, fever, bowel obstruction, biliary tree obstruction, worsening of pain or tenderness during serial examinations, or the presence of an adnexal mass.

Cholelithiasis and Choledocholithiasis (see Box 2-2)

The **anatomy** of the biliary tree is quite simple: it is a duct system that drains bile and secretions from the liver into the small intestine. The system has a reservoir, the gallbladder, attached to it via the relatively narrow-caliber cystic duct.

Biliary stones can be defined by their **location** within the biliary tree. In **cholelithiasis,** stones are located within the gallbladder itself. In **choledocholithiasis,** stones may be located anywhere within the biliary tree, from the intrahepatic ducts to the cystic duct to the common hepatic duct to the ampulla of Vater.

I. Pathogenesis

The **underlying pathogenesis** of stone formation, irrespective of location, is based on the fact that there are two different stone types, **cholesterol stones** and **bilirubin stones.**

A. Cholesterol stones

Cholesterol stones are by far the more common form of biliary tract stones. These stones result from supersaturation of cholesterol in the biliary contents; the cholesterol can precipitate with calcium and oxalate ions to form

---

B O X   2 - 2

Overall Evaluation and Management of Suspected Symptomatic Gallstone Disease

Evaluation

1. Take the history and perform a physical examination as described in Box 2-1 and above.
2. Obtain the **complete blood cell count** to look for any leukocytosis.
3. Perform **liver function tests** to determine the total bilirubin, direct bilirubin, alkaline phosphatase, GGT, SGOT, and SGPT levels. These determinations are made to look for **extrahepatic dysfunction or obstruction.** In extrahepatic processes, alkaline phosphatase and total bilirubin levels will be elevated to a greater degree than transaminase levels.

(continued)

B O X 2 - 2 (continued)

4. Obtain an **abdominal x-ray series** looking specifically for any radiopaque stones within the gallbladder or any concurrent manifestations—ileus, small bowel obstruction, perforation, etc. Only bilirubin stones are radiopaque.
5. Perform **US** of the biliary tree. Biliary tree US is pivotal: it defines the anatomy of the biliary tree, demonstrates any extrahepatic **biliary duct dilation,** and shows the location of stones in **cholelithiasis/choledocholithiasis.** The common bile duct diameter is normally 5 mm.
6. Other **imaging techniques** may be of value in certain patients and in defined settings.
   a. **Radionuclide imaging.** The PIPIDA scan entails injection of a radiolabeled derivative of a molecule that is normally excreted through the biliary tree. The rate of excretion of the molecule from the liver into the small intestine is measured. A **delay in the excretion time** of this molecule is consistent with an **obstructive process.** If the liver is severely damaged or if the obstruction is nearly complete, both as manifested by a significant increase in total bilirubin, the test will be essentially useless. Thus this specific evaluation tool is useful in diagnosing biliary obstruction if the total bilirubin is less than 10.0 mg/dL.
   b. **Oral cholecystography.** This classic test for cholecystitis is no longer commonly used; however, it remains a useful evaluative tool in the diagnosis of **acute cholecystitis.** The patient ingests an oral agent that is an organified iodinated molecule. This specific radiopaque molecule is concentrated within the biliary secretions and can, in the normal state, be visualized on abdominal radiographic series approximately 12–24 hours after ingestion. Nonvisualization of the gallbladder upon radiographic imaging at 24 hours is consistent with acute cholecystitis, either acalculous (without stones) or calculous (with stones).

Management

See text (**IV. Specific management**).

stones. Thus, the chemical composition of cholesterol stones includes a complex mixture of cholesterol and cholesterol salts.

Specific **risk factors** for the development of these stones include the following:

1. Use of oral contraceptives
2. Moderate to morbid obesity
3. Female sex
4. History of multiple pregnancies
5. Age over 40 years
6. Native American ancestry

B. Bilirubin stones

Bilirubin stones are relatively uncommon. They result from excess amounts of **conjugated bilirubin** within the biliary tree due to the catabolism of hemoglobin derivatives within the liver. As with cholesterol biliary stones, there are specific **risk factors** for their development. The most common risk factor is an antecedent, concurrent, or chronic **extravascular hemolytic process.** These stones are not uncommon in patients with **hereditary spherocytosis, SC hemoglobinopathy,** or **SS hemoglobinopathy.**

II. Natural history

The **natural history** of cholelithiasis can be clinically divided into three distinct subsets.

A. **Asymptomatic biliary stone disease**

The natural history of asymptomatic cholelithiasis discovered surreptitiously is quite benign. This conclusion is based on a retrospective autopsy study by Wenckert et al. in which the records of all patients with cholelithiasis found at autopsy were retrospectively reviewed for any evidence of symptoms attributable to gallstone disease. Very few (18%) had pain in life suggestive of biliary dysfunction.

B. **One episode of pain**

Symptomatic gallstone disease. Up to 50% of patients will have recurrence of pain or will develop complications of cholelithiasis. The complications include **ascending cholangitis, sepsis,** pancreatitis, biliary obstruction, and **death.**

C. **Recurrent episodes of pain**

Recurrently symptomatic gallstone disease. The vast majority of patients will develop significant, potentially life-threatening complications in the near future.

III. Manifestations

The **specific acute and chronic manifestations** of biliary stone disease depend more on the location of the stone than on the chemical composition of the stone. Although the vast majority of patients are asymptomatic, biliary stones can and do produce symptoms, especially when they develop or as they pass from the gallbladder through the biliary tree itself. If they are within the biliary tree, they cause manifestations of biliary obstruction (see Box 2-2, page 62).

A. Acute manifestations

Acute manifestations include the acute onset of right upper quadrant pain. The pain is usually sharp, exacerbated by the ingestion of fatty foods, and relieved when the patient is fasting. Pyrosis may be present, as may intermittent nausea and vomiting. The patient may report a yellow discoloration to the eyes and clay-colored stools, all results of obstruction to bile flow.

B. Examination findings

Upon **examination**, the patient may be febrile, icteric, tender to deep palpation over the right upper quadrant, have Murphy's sign (i.e., pain in the right upper quadrant when attempting to inspire while the examiner palpates over the right upper quadrant), a normal liver span, and a hypopigmented, guaiac-negative stool in the rectal vault.

IV. Specific management

The **specific management schemas** for gallstone disease are based on the natural history and are different for each subset.

A. Asymptomatic cholelithiasis

Because asymptomatic gallstones that are discovered incidentally on another evaluative test have a benign natural history, **intervention and therapy** entail observation.

1. The risk of elective surgery (cholecystectomy) far outweighs the risk of the asymptomatic cholelithiasis; therefore, conservative expectant therapy is indicated.

2. Watch the patient closely for the development of symptoms referable to biliary obstruction.

3. Risk factor modification includes losing weight and discontinuing oral contraceptives.

B. Symptomatic cholelithiasis/choledocholithiasis

Therapeutic intervention is based on the natural history of the disease.

1. Risk factor modification is necessary and includes weight loss and discontinuation of oral contraceptives.

2. Because of the natural history of the disease, the risks of recurrent symptoms and even complications are quite significant and far outweigh the risk of surgery. In these cases **surgical intervention** with chole-

cystectomy and biliary tree exploration, on an urgent or even emergency basis, is clearly indicated.

3. New modalities in the management of **acute cholelithiasis:**

   a. **Chenodeoxycholic acid.** Chenodeoxycholic acid decreases the synthesis of cholesterol within the hepatocytes and thus its overall excretion into the biliary tree. It is effective for noncalcified (i.e., radiolucent) cholesterol stones. Any calcified (radiopaque) stone, whether cholesterol or bilirubin, is refractory to this agent. The **dosage** is 250–750 mg PO q.d. for up to 2 years. There is a 25%–50% chance of **remission,** defined as either a total or partial resolution of the stones with complete resolution of symptoms. In patients who experience remission, long-term suppression therapy is indicated.

   Regardless of initial effectiveness, there is a high incidence of **recurrence. Side effects** are quite common and include an increase in LDL cholesterol, hepatotoxicity, and diarrhea, all of which can be dose-limiting. Thus, **this modality should be reserved** for specific patients who are at high risk for surgery, such as those who have had a recent myocardial infarction, the very aged, or those with severe pulmonary disease.

   b. **Laparoscopic cholecystectomy.** This novel surgical approach may be effective in high-risk patients with either cholesterol or bilirubin stones. The operation entails **laparoscopically directed exploration** of the gallbladder and biliary tree, removal of the gallbladder through the scope, and placement of a drainage tube (T-tube) **from the biliary tree to the skin.** This procedure has the advantage of **limiting the incision size** and therefore decreases the risk of traditional surgery.

V. **Complications of symptomatic cholecystitis**
   A. **Pancreatitis**

      Biliary stone disease is one of the most common causes of pancreatitis worldwide. This form of pancreatitis is reversed when the underlying cholelithiasis is treated via endoscopic retrograde cholangiopancreatography (ERCP) or by surgical intervention.

   B. **Ascending cholangitis**

      Ascending cholangitis is one of the most severe complications of cholelithiasis. The **underlying pathogenesis** includes the obstruction and pooling of biliary secretions within the biliary tract. Obstruction is a prerequisite for the development of an infection in the biliary tree. The infection begins distally and ascends the biliary tree, with resultant hepatic abscess formation and severe hepatic infection. The most common **pathogens** in ascending cholangitis include group D streptococci (i.e., the enterococci), the Enterobacteriaceae (e.g., *E. coli* and *Klebsiella* spp.), and the anaerobes (e.g., *Bacteroides* spp.).

The **specific management** of this life-threatening sequela of gallstone disease includes IV fluids, consultation with GI and **surgery,** and parenteral antibiotic administration to cover the above pathogens.

C. **Sepsis**

Sepsis is of special concern in patients with ascending cholangitis or a gangrenous gallbladder. Pathogens and management are the same as those described for ascending cholangitis (see above).

VI. **Consultation**

Problem	*Service*	*Time*
Symptomatic cholelithiasis	Surgery	Urgent
Complicated cholelithiasis		Emergent
Symptomatic cholelithiasis in patient who is high risk for surgery	GI	Urgent

VII. **Indications for admission:** Intravascular volume depletion, fever, intractable vomiting, any evidence of biliary obstruction, the development of acute pancreatitis, suspicion of ascending cholangitis.

Acute and Chronic Pancreatitis

The pancreas is located immediately posterior and inferior to the duodenum and therefore is mainly in the epigastric and left upper quadrant of the abdomen. It drains through the ducts of Wirsung and Santorini into the duodenum via the ampulla of Vater. The pancreas is both an **exocrine** and **endocrine** organ. The exocrine portion of the gland produces potent proteolytic enzymes, including trypsin and chymotrypsin, that are secreted into the small intestine via the ducts of Santorini and Wirsung and the ampulla of Vater. In the normal setting, these proteolytic enzymes from the exocrine pancreas digest the ingested proteins. The endocrine portion of the gland consists of islets of cells within the gland. The alpha islet cells produce glucagon, while the beta cells produce insulin. Both glucagon and insulin have profound effects on glucose utilization and, therefore, cellular function.

I. **Pathogenesis of pancreatitis**

The **underlying pathogenesis** is autodigestion of the gland itself by the abnormal release of the intrinsic proteolytic enzymes. If and when the pancreas is damaged, it releases and activates these enzymes within the gland itself, with resultant pancreatic damage, damage to the adjacent tissues, and, eventually, both exocrine and endocrine pancreatic insufficiency.

II. **Precipitants**

Precipitating agents in the pathogenesis of pancreatitis include significant **ethanol ingestion,** the most common cause in the United States; **choledocholithiasis** (stones in the biliary tree), the most common cause worldwide; a **duodenal ulcer** that penetrates through the posterior wall of the duodenum; **type I hyperlipidemia,** which is associated with recurrent pancreatitis; use of **thiazide diuretics;** chronic **hypercalcemia** of any cause; congenital (i.e., anatomic) dysfunction of the duct system; and **idiopathic** causes, which must be a diagnosis of exclusion, as the vast majority of cases of pancreatitis do have a discernible cause.

III. **Natural history**

Recurrent attacks of acute pancreatitis, with resultant partial destruction of the gland each time, eventually lead to insufficiency of the exocrine and endocrine functions of the gland. Reflecting this natural history, the following discussion is divided into acute pancreatitis and the chronic pancreatic insufficiency state.

IV. **Acute pancreatitis**

A. **Manifestations**

The **specific manifestations** of acute pancreatitis include the acute onset of epigastric and left upper quadrant pain that is usually greater after oral intake and is associated with nausea, vomiting, and orthostatic dizziness. Often the precipitant can be easily determined from the history (e.g., a recent binge with ethanol). **Examination** usually discloses intravascular volume depletion, diffusely hypoactive bowel sounds, deep and rebound tenderness in the epigastrium and left upper quadrant, and guaiac-negative stool in the rectal vault. Fever is not uncommon.

B. **Evaluation**

The **specific evaluation** of acute pancreatitis includes making the clinical diagnosis with the evaluation steps described in Box 2-1. Further specific evaluative tests include the following:

1. **Serum amylase determination.** The enzyme amylase, which is normally produced in the exocrine

pancreas, is abnormally **elevated** in acute pancreatitis. The **sensitivity** of this test is limited by the fact that in patients who have already had significant pancreatic destruction, amylase levels may not be elevated. The **specificity** is limited by the fact that dysfunction or diseases of other organs can cause amylase elevations, including renal insufficiency, diabetic ketoacidosis, inflammation or destruction of the salivary glands, or ischemia of the gut itself.

2. **Serum lipase determination.** The enzyme lipase, which is normally produced in the exocrine pancreas, is abnormally elevated in acute pancreatitis. This test has a higher **specificity** than serum amylase determination because lipase is produced almost exclusively within the pancreas. This test can confirm the diagnosis when clinical suspicion is present and the serum amylase test is equivocal.

3. **Abdominal US.** This imaging technique of the gallbladder, biliary tree, liver, and pancreas is a simple and reasonable cost-effective modality to visualize the structures and rule out any biliary obstruction and choledocholithiasis. If any abnormalities are demonstrated, **CT** of the area is indicated.

4. **Abdominal CT. Abdominal CT** is not routinely indicated in all cases. It is indicated when no etiology can be discerned after a thorough evaluation, when any complication is suspected, or if any abnormality is demonstrated on US.

C. **Management**

The **specific management** of acute pancreatitis in the acute setting includes the following measures:

1. **Resting the GI tract** by withholding oral intake. If the patient is NPO for greater than 3 days, initiate total parenteral nutrition until enteral feedings can be restarted.

2. **Providing fluids IV.** The clinician needs to replete any intravascular volume deficit and give maintenance fluids. Fluids should be dextrose 5% in 0.9 normal saline or, after the first several liters, dextrose 5% in lactated Ringer's solution.

3. If the patient has severe **nausea and vomiting, intermittent suction** via nasogastric tube is indicated. However, NG suction is not mandatory in all cases.

4. If ethanol is suspected as the etiology, concurrently manage as an acute ethanol ingestion.

5. **Stress ulcer prevention** with H_2-receptor blockers (e.g., ranitidine, 50 mg IV q.8h., or cimetidine, 300 mg IV q.6h.).

6. **Parameters** that need to be followed closely include

volume status, hematocrit, plasma calcium, arterial
oxygen tension, hepatic transaminases, renal function, and the development of a leukocytosis. A baseline abnormality or deterioration in any of these parameters, also referred to as **Ranson's criteria,** early
in the hospital course can be a harbinger of severe
pancreatitis and thus mandates more aggressive
management.

7. **Narcotic agents** are indicated for pain relief if pain
is present and severe. Meperidine (Demerol) can be
effective when given in appropriate and scheduled
dosing.
8. Watch for and aggressively manage any complications.
9. There is no evidence that empirical antibiotics are
of any benefit unless a complication is present.
10. If the stool is **guaiac positive** or if PUD is suspected,
esophagogastroduodenoscopy (EGD) to image the
stomach and duodenum to rule out any ulcer.
11. If **choledocholithiasis** is diagnosed, either surgical
or therapeutic intervention (ERCP) is indicated.
12. If **no etiology** has been demonstrated through the
evaluation listed above, ERCP should be considered
to directly image the ampulla of Vater and, with contrast, the biliary tree itself.

V. Chronic pancreatitis
A. Manifestations
The **manifestations** of this sequela of acute, especially
recurrent, pancreatitis reflect insufficiency of the exocrine and endocrine pancreas. Manifestations can be categorized into four different categories: those resulting
from another episode of acute pancreatitis, those resulting from exocrine pancreatic insufficiency, those resulting from endocrine pancreatic insufficiency, and
those that are idiopathic.

1. **Acute, recurrent pancreatitis.** This is similar to any
other acute pancreatitis episode.
2. **Exocrine insufficiency.** The deficiency in proteolytic
enzymes and lipase will decrease protein and fat/
lipid absorption. Thus, the manifestations can include **unintentional weight loss, diarrhea, steatorrhea** (i.e., loss of fat in the stool, as manifested by
greasy, frothy stools that are severely malodorous),
and fat-soluble vitamin malabsorption with the development of deficiencies in those vitamins. These
vitamins include **A, D, and K,** and deficiencies manifest as metabolic bone disease and coagulopathy
(i.e., an elevated prothrombin time).

3. **Endocrine insufficiency.** The development of insulin-dependent diabetes mellitus due to the destruction of alpha and beta cells in the islets of the pancreas. IDDM is usually quite labile because glucagon from the alpha cells is also deficient.
4. **Idiopathic.** The patient can and often does develop **chronic, severe, intractable abdominal pain** through an unclear yet probably noninflammatory mechanism.

B. **Evaluation**

The **evaluation** of chronic pancreatitis includes making the clinical diagnosis and performing evaluative tests, including a **Sudan stain** of the stool (positive if fat is present) and a **72-hour fecal fat test** to document steatorrhea. An **abdominal x-ray series** will demonstrate pancreatic calcifications, a sign of significant pancreatic insufficiency. Further evaluation should include determining calcium, PO_4, and albumin levels and, to screen for IDDM, a **fasting blood glucose level.** The **amylase level** and even the **lipase level** may be normal, for the gland is so destroyed that there is no longer a source of these marker enzymes.

C. **Management**

The **specific long-term management** includes the following elements:

1. **Provide narcotics** for pain control (codeine, oxycodone, morphine sulfate).
2. **Replace enzymes.** One of the best routes is via pancrealipase, an extract of porcine pancreatic enzymes (trypsin, lipase, and amylase), 500–2,000 mg PO 30 min before each meal. The size of the tablets is 250 mg.
3. **Discontinue all ethanol.**
4. **Initiate human insulin** as needed for control of glycemia.
5. **Provide nutritional support.**

VI. **Consultation**

Problem	Service	Time
Any complications	GI	Required
	Surgery	Elective
Choledocholithiasis	GI	Urgent
	Surgery	Urgent
Idiopathic	GI	Required

VII. **Indications for admission:** Intravascular volume depletion, acute pancreatitis, any evidence of a complication to the pancreatitis.

Peptic Ulcer Disease, Duodenal or Gastric

The anatomy of the upper stomach and duodenum is relatively simple but pivotal to an understanding of peptic ulcer disease. The stomach is immediately inferior to and connected with the esophagus. It consists of three anatomic portions—the **cardia,** which is superior, the **body,** which is the largest portion of the stomach, and the **pylorus,** the narrowing of the stomach as it becomes contiguous with the duodenum. The transition between the body and the pylorus is called the **antrum.** The pylorus empties into the relatively narrow C-shaped first portion of the small intestine, the duodenum. All of these structures are lined with mucosa consisting of simple columnar epithelium.

Peptic ulcer disease is defined as a breakdown in the overall integrity of the mucosa in the stomach or duodenum. Various classification schemes exist, based on different parameters:

1. Classification according to the **depth** of the ulcer defect. The lesion can range from an **erosion,** which is the superficial loss of mucosa, to an **ulcer,** which is deeper into the gastric or duodenal wall. Although any lesion in this spectrum can cause pain and hemorrhage, the deeper the defect, the greater is the risk of significant, severe complications.
2. Classification according to the **anatomic location** of the ulcer defect. The lesions usually are either mainly in the duodenum or mainly in the stomach.
3. Classification as **classic versus nonclassic peptic ulcer disease.** This classification scheme is most common and is used to organize the material in this section.

   I. **Classic versus nonclassic peptic ulcer disease**
      A. **Classic**
         Classic peptic ulcer disease usually affects and is **located** in the duodenum. The **epidemiology** of these lesions is different from that of nonsteroidal anti-inflammatory drug (NSAID)-induced ulcer lesions in that the population is younger and males have a much higher incidence than females.
         1. **Pathophysiology**
            The **underlying pathophysiology** of classic peptic ulcer disease is **excessive acid production.** The protective mucosal barrier of mucus and bicarbonate buffering agents in the stomach and duodenum is usually normal, but the abnormally high acid levels (i.e., low pH) can disrupt the integrity of this barrier. The parietal and chief cells of the gastric antrum indirectly and directly produce hydrogen ions to increase the acidity of the gastric content. These cells are directly influenced by local endocrine (i.e., **para-**

crine) and **neurotransmitter substances.** Any increase in paracrine substances, either **gastrin** or **histamine,** or an increase in **parasympathetic discharge** from the vagus nerve via the neurotransmitter **acetylcholine,** can and will increase gastric acid production.

2. **Risk factors**

   The most common **risk factor** for the development of classic peptic ulcer disease is **stress,** which can increase parasympathetic outflow via the vagus nerve, producing a secondary increase in histamine secretion and, therefore, acid production. Rarely, a **gastrinoma**—a rare tumor of the GI tract that secretes gastrin, resulting in a secondary increase in histamine secretion—can be the cause of severe, recurrent duodenal ulcers.

B. **Nonclassic**

   Nonclassic (NSAID-induced or ethanol-induced) peptic ulcer disease usually affects and is **located** in the stomach itself, although the duodenum can be concurrently involved. **Epidemiology**—This syndrome is more common in the elderly, in women, and in patients on chronic or multiple NSAIDs.

1. **Pathophysiology**

   The **underlying pathophysiology** of nonclassic peptic ulcer disease is based on an overall decrease in the effectiveness of the mucosal protective barrier of mucus and bicarbonate. Acid secretion and production are usually normal to low and thus are not a major factor in the pathogenesis of these NSAID-related ulcerations. NSAIDs, by virtue of their systemic inhibition of prostaglandin production, especially of the E group, are effective anti-inflammatory agents. However, **inhibition of prostaglandins** at the level of the gastroduodenal mucosa can cause the following abnormalities:

   a. Decrease in bicarbonate secretion from the mucosa

   b. Decrease in blood flow to the mucosa

   c. Decrease in mucus production

   All three of these abnormalities result in a significant decrease in the effectiveness of mucosal protective barrier and thus increase the risk of ulcer development. This pathophysiologic model has been extrapolated to **ethanol-induced** peptic ulcer disease. Ethanol can cause similar ulcers through an analogous mechanism of local prostaglandin inhibition.

   2. Risk factors
   Risk factors for the development of nonclassic peptic ulcer disease include the use of one or more
   NSAIDs, including aspirin. The chronic use or abuse
   of ethanol, especially if it is used concurrently with
   an NSAID, increases the risk. Cigarette smoking also
   increases the risk of this type of peptic ulcer disease.

II. Manifestations
   The **specific manifestations** of peptic ulcer disease are
   quite similar, regardless of the underlying pathophysiology. Symptoms usually include an acute onset of epigastric pain that is exacerbated by fasting and relieved by food
   or antacid ingestion. Other historical features include a history of peptic ulcer disease or similar manifestations in the
   past that spontaneously resolved.
   Nausea and vomiting are not uncommon. The specific
   manifestation of **postprandial vomiting** usually is a result
   of ulcer-induced swelling and obstruction, especially when
   the ulcer is in the pylorus. The patient can present with
   hematemesis ("coffee ground" emesis) or melena (black
   tarry stools), both indicative of significant bleeding. **Risk
   factors** for the development of peptic ulcer disease are often
   present.
   On **examination,** there often is tenderness to deep palpation in the epigastrium, usually without rebound; a guaiac-
   positive stool in the rectal vault; and, at times, signs and
   symptoms of intravascular volume depletion.

III. Specific management
   The **specific management** for all peptic ulcer disease includes the steps listed in Box 2-3 and the following interventions, which are based not only on the location of the ulcer
   but also on the presumptive pathophysiology.
A. Duodenal (classic) ulcers
   These lesions are acid-mediated, and therefore the central feature in therapy is to decrease acid production
   from the gastric antrum.
   1. Initiate **H_2-receptor antagonists:**
      a. Cimetidine, 400 mg PO q.i.d. for 6 weeks, or
      b. Ranitidine, 150 mg PO b.i.d. for 6 weeks. The
          parenteral form of ranitidine, 50 mg IV q.8h., can
          be used in the acute setting.
   2. **Antacids** (e.g., Mylanta II, 15 mL PO q.i.d.) can be
      prescribed PRN but have no effect on the natural
      course of the disease.
   3. If there is **no improvement** after 6 weeks of therapy,
      perform or repeat EGD to directly visualize the
      mucosa.

BOX 2-3

Overall Evaluation and Management of Peptic Ulcer Disease

Evaluation

1. Take a thorough **history** and perform a **physical examination** (see Abdominal Pain: Overall Approach, and as described above).
2. Determine **orthostatic vital sign parameters**.
3. Determine a baseline **complete blood cell count** to look for anemia.
4. Determine the **platelet count** and coagulation parameters (**aPTT, PT**) if there is any evidence of a coagulopathy.

Management

1. Instruct the patient to **discontinue all NSAIDs** and to **discontinue ethanol and cigarette smoking**.
2. If the patient is **severely symptomatic** or if there is **evidence of bleeding**, the clinician must:
   a. Admit the patient, preferably to an ICU.
   b. Place two peripheral large-bore (18-gauge or 16-gauge) IV catheters, each of 0.9 NS.
   c. Type and cross-match blood for packed RBCs.
   d. Emergently consult GI service to directly image the area with EGD.
   e. See section on Gastrointestinal Bleeding (page 104) for further details.
3. If the patient is **stable,** mildly symptomatic, **not acutely bleeding,** and **not anemic,** image the area radiographically with an **upper GI series** or consult a gastroenterologist for an EGD. If an upper GI series is performed and a **gastric ulcer** is demonstrated, EGD with biopsies of the ulcer crater is indicated to rule out a malignant gastric ulcer. If a **duodenal ulcer** is demonstrated, no biopsies or direct visualization are mandatory.

4. If disease **recurs** after complete resolution, check the **serum gastrin level.** This test is most specific and sensitive if performed before reinstituting H$_2$ blocker therapy. An elevated serum gastrin level may be indicative of a gastrinoma (Zollinger–Ellison syn-

drome), whereas a normal level essentially rules out this syndrome.

Further management of recurrent peptic ulcer disease includes:

a. The institution of a **standard course** of 6 weeks of an H_2-receptor blocker, followed by **long-term maintenance** therapy either with ranitidine, 150 mg PO q.h.s., or cimetidine, 400 mg PO q.h.s. The optimal duration of such maintenance therapy has not been studied but is usually years to lifelong.

b. Directing the patient to abstain from ethanol, cigarettes, and NSAIDs.

B. Gastric (nonclassic) ulcers (see Table 2-3)

These lesions occur as a result of dysfunction or lack of the normal mucosal barrier. Therefore, therapy is directed toward increasing the activity of this barrier.

1. Perform **EGD with biopsies** of the ulcer.

2. Use **H_2-receptor antagonists** for acute therapy as described above, in the same dosage but with a longer duration (8–10 weeks).

3. Sucralfate (Carafate) is also effective therapy acutely. This agent can reinforce the normal gastric mucosal barrier and, theoretically, increase prostaglandins on a mucosal level. The dose for acute therapy is 1 g PO q.i.d. for 8 weeks.

4. Instruct the patient to discontinue all NSAIDs, ethanol, and cigarette smoking.

5. Antacids for symptomatic relief are of use but do not change the natural history of the disease.

IV. Prevention

Prevention is of paramount importance. Preventative schemes include, at present, three specific components: **personal habit modification, NSAID use modification,** and evaluation of the patient for the potentially ulcerogenic bacterium, *Helicobacter pylori.*

A. Personal habit modification includes discontinuing ethanol ingestion and cigarette smoking, and minimizing stress.

B. No or limited use of NSAIDs is important in any patient at risk for the development of NSAID-induced gastropathy. These patients include older patients who are taking aspirin for other reasons, or patients who do not abstain from ethanol and cigarette smoking.

If NSAIDs are necessary and the patient has no active peptic ulcer disease, either **sucralfate,** 1 g PO q.i.d., or the prostaglandin analogue **misoprostol** (Cytotec), 100 µg PO t.i.d., should be administered concurrently. Either

T A B L E 2 - 3
Prevention of NSAID-Induced Gastropathy

1. Use other therapeutic modalities if possible, including:
   Physical therapy
   Intra-articular steroids
   Nonacetylated salicylates
   Acetaminophen
2. Limit NSAID therapy if possible.
3. Take the NSAID on a full stomach.
4. Discontinue cigarette smoking.
5. Limit ethanol ingestion.
6. The concurrent use of H_2-receptor antagonists has not proved effective in the prevention of this pathophysiologic entity.
7. The concurrent use of sucralfate *or* misoprostol is effective in the prevention of this pathophysiologic entity.
8. In the setting of prevention, sucralfate probably is the optimal pharmacologic agent, because of its efficacy and minimal side effects.

one of these agents is effective in preventing NSAID-induced peptic ulcer disease. Misoprostil induces abortions and is **contraindicated in women of childbearing age.** In addition, it induces significant diarrhea and is relatively expensive. For these reasons, sucralfate is currently the preferred agent.

C. **Screening** for and prophylaxis against the potentially ulcerogenic bacterium, ***Helicobacter pylori,*** may be of some effectiveness, especially in patients with recurrent ulcer disease. The screening should be undertaken only with consultation and follow-up with a gastroenterologist, for baseline and follow-up *H. pylori* cultures via EGD. This is a developing area in which recommendations for prophylactic intervention may rapidly change (see Bibliography).

V. **Complications**
   The complications of peptic ulcer disease can include the following, all of which require admission and surgical intervention:
   A. **Upper GI bleeding**
      The bleeding can be mild to exsanguinating and usually is a function of the depth and location of the ulcer crater. Specifically, a duodenal ulcer can erode anteriorly into the anterior gastroduodenal artery and cause massive, even exsanguinating hematemesis (see section on Gastrointestinal Bleeding, page 104).
   B. **Perforation of the gastric or duodenal wall**
      Any ulcer can extend through the entire wall and result in perforation. Perforation invariably has the associ-

ated comorbidities of peritonitis, acute abdomen, and even death (see section on Abdominal Pain: Overall Approach, page 41).

C. Pancreatitis

This complication occurs when a posterior duodenal ulcer erodes through the wall and into the head of the pancreas. It is usually associated with severe pain and signs of an acute abdomen (see section on Abdominal Pain: Overall Approach, page 41).

D. Obstruction

This complication is associated with recurrent peptic ulcer disease with inflammation and fibrotic changes. It is most commonly associated with distal gastric (i.e., antral) ulcer disease with resultant symptomatic pyloric narrowing.

VI. Consultation

Problem	Service	Time
Any complications	General surgery	Urgent/ emergent
Any complications	GI	Urgent/ emergent
Elevated gastrin level	Endocrinology	Elective

VII. Indications for admission: Development of any of the complications of peptic ulcer disease, i.e., obstruction, upper GI bleeding, perforation, intractable pain, severe nausea and vomiting requiring parenteral fluid repletion; or acute pancreatitis.

Anorectal Dysfunction

Although many patients are embarrassed by pain or problems in the anal area and thus attempt to self-treat or to minimize the problem, anorectal problems can cause significant discomfort, anxiety, and even morbidity.

The **anatomy** of the anorectal area is quite simple and is best described using the following anatomic definitions. The **anus** is the distalmost aspect of the GI tract. It is approximately 4 cm long and is divided into two components by the **dentate line** (also known as the pectinate line): a **distal component,** lined by stratified squamous epithelium, and a **proximal component,** lined by simple columnar epithelium. It is at the dentate line where the confluence of the distal ends of the columns of Morgagni occurs.

The **columns and crypts of Morgagni** are longitudinal columns of mucosa that are located in the **proximal anus** and fuse in a ring distally to form the anal papillae at the level of the dentate line. The crypts are the complementary invaginations of the columns of Morgagni.

B O X   2 - 4

***Overall Evaluation and Management of
Anorectal Disorders***

Evaluation

1. Perform a digital rectal examination.
2. Visualize the area internally with an anoscope.

Management

Management is described under specific entities in the
text.

I. **Specific anorectal pathologic entities** (see Box 2-4)
   A. **Hemorrhoids**

   Hemorrhoids are abnormally dilated veins within the venous network of the anus. These lesions can be minimally
   symptomatic or can, on a recurrent basis, cause severe
   pain and bleeding.

   Hemorrhoids are classified by **severity** and **location**.
   The classification by severity is:

First degree	Slight bleeding
Second degree	Prolapsed but easily reducible
Third degree	Prolapsed, nonreducible, usually recurrent

   The classification by **location**—either **external** or **internal**—is relative to the dentate line. The following discussion is organized according to this classification.
   1. **External hemorrhoids**
      a. An **external hemorrhoid** is any hemorrhoid **distal**
         to the dentate line. The **specific manifestations** in
         the **chronic setting** include purple-colored skin
         tags in the anal area that are nontender and non-
         bleeding but can result in mild soiling of under-
         pants and intermittent mild anal pruritus. These
         are old external hemorrhoids that have scarred
         and are now fibrosed asymptomatic lesions. In an
         acute exacerbation or **acute development** of ex-
         ternal hemorrhoids there is usually an acute onset
         of anal pruritus, which can be quite severe. Fur-
         thermore, there often is the presence of a pro-

lapsed mildly tender mass. Finally, underwear may be soiled by stool.

   b. The two **acute complications** of external hemorrhoids are **thrombosis** and **rupture.**

      i. **Thrombosed hemorrhoids** are exquisitely painful and tender, with concurrent bluish swelling of the hemorrhoid. Pain and induration develop acutely.

      ii. **Rupture** of an external hemorrhoid occurs concurrently or concomitantly with the development of thrombosis. When rupture occurs, a significant amount of bright red blood can be passed rectally; pain may also be relieved.

   c. **Risk factors** for the development or recurrence of external hemorrhoids include pregnancy, parturition, a history of straining during defecation, and occupations requiring sitting for prolonged periods of time.

   d. The **evaluation and management** of this entity include making the clinical diagnosis and performing anoscopy. **Acute management** entails application of a cold pack to the site for first hour, then warm sitz baths two to three times a day for 3–5 days. In addition, topical steroids (e.g., Anusol HC cream b.i.d. or Proctofoam b.i.d. to t.i.d.) are of benefit. A thrombosed hemorrhoid is easily excised by direct incision and drainage.

     Chronic management and prophylaxis includes the use of stool softeners or increased dietary fiber, exercise, and, if the condition is recurrent, possibly surgical removal or removal via **infrared coagulation** or **laser therapy.** Referral to gastroenterology in these cases is indicated on an elective basis.

2. Internal hemorrhoids

   a. **Internal hemorrhoids** are hemorrhoids that are **proximal** to the dentate line. The **specific manifestations** in the acute or chronic setting include bright red blood passed rectally, prolapse of a nontender mass through the anus, and virtually **no pain or tenderness.** The bleeding, which is intermittent, can be quite significant.

   b. The major **risk factor** for the development of internal hemorrhoids is hepatic portal venous hypertension. These lesions can be concurrent with external hemorrhoids.

   c. The **evaluation and management** include making the clinical diagnosis, performing anoscopy, and looking for other manifestations of portal venous hypertension (see section on End-Stage Hepatic Dysfunction). The specific management includes the local control of any bleeding, usually by applying direct pressure, and outpatient referral to gastroenterology.

B. **Fissure-in-ano**

Fissure-in-ano is the development of a superficial longitudinal laceration of the distal anus, usually as a result of trauma, usually while staining.

   1. **Specific manifestations** include an acute onset of severe pain in the anal area. The patient usually relates that the pain was precipitated by straining during a bowel movement and was exacerbated by each subsequent bowel movement. A small amount of bright red blood may be passed rectally.

   2. **Risk factors** for the development of fissure-in-ano include straining during bowel movements, constipation, and anal intercourse.

   3. The **evaluation and management** of this entity include making the clinical diagnosis and performing anoscopy. Acute management entails application of a cold pack to the site for first hour, then warm sitz baths two to three times a day for 3–5 days. Chronic management includes the use of stool softeners and increased dietary fiber, exercise, and abstinence from receptive anal intercourse. Referral to gastroenterology in recurrent cases is indicated on an elective basis.

C. **Fistula-in-ano**

A **fistula-in-ano** develops between the **anal lumen at the base of a crypt of Morgagni** (i.e., the papilla of Morgagni) and the perianal **skin.**

   1. **Specific manifestations** include the acute onset of pain in the anal or perineal area and a mass in the perineal area deep to the skin with associated discharge of liquid, at times purulent, material from an area immediately adjacent to the anus. This entity can develop into a **perirectal abscess.**

   2. **Risk factors** for the development of fistula-in-ano and the differential diagnosis of entities associated with this entity include Crohn's disease, carcinoma, lymphogranuloma venereum (LGV), past rectal irradiation, and immunocompromise. Fistula-in-ano or a perirectal abscess must always be considered in an immunocompromised patient with rectal or anal pain.

   3. The **evaluation and management** of this entity include making the clinical diagnosis and performing

anoscopy. The perirectal tissues are examined for any tender masses, which may be perirectal abscesses. The fistula is examined from the **internal side to the skin side.** Usually the fistula must be surgically closed. If an abscess is found in the adjacent tissues, it must be incised and drained, with the concurrent initiation of antibiotics to cover anaerobic and gram-negative bacillary bacteria. **Referral to surgery** is indicated.

D. Pinworm

Pinworm is a common helmintic parasite ("worm") that is noninvasive and benign, but quite contagious.

1. **Specific manifestations** include the onset of **severe anal pruritus** that is especially severe at night. Usually pinworm occurs in children, but adults can contract the infection from children.
2. **Risk factors** for the development of pinworm include having children in the family and poor hand-washing practices by family members.
3. The **evaluation and management** include making a clinical diagnosis from a thorough history and physical examination. As part of the examination a length of **Scotch Tape** is placed on the perianal skin, then removed, and helminths are sought in the residue on the tape. **Management** includes treating the patient and entire family with pyrantyl pamoate (Antiminth), 11 mg/kg of body weight. Before treatment one must document a **negative pregnancy test on all fertile family members,** as this agent is a teratogen.

II. Consultation

Problem	Service	Time
Hemorrhoids	GI (IRC/laser)	Elective
Fistula-in-ano	Surgery	Required
Perirectal abscess	Surgery	Urgent

III. Indications for admission:
Bleeding internal hemorrhoids in a patient with coagulopathy, or a perirectal abscess.

Dysphagia and Odynophagia

The basic **anatomy** of the oropharynx and esophagus is relatively simple. The **esophagus** is a tubelike structure that connects the posterior oral cavity (i.e., the **oropharynx**) with the stomach. It is approximately 25 cm long and is lined by stratified squamous epithelium.

I. Overall manifestations

Dysphagia is defined specifically as difficulty is swallowing. The patient usually reports that the bolus of food or liquid "gets caught" or "sticks" while swallowing. **Odynophagia** is defined specifically as pain upon swallowing. These two complaints can be interrelated or independent of each other.

Associated manifestations include postprandial vomiting, halitosis, a recent cerebrovascular accident, and a history of gastroesophageal reflux disease (GERD) or pyrosis. As it will be clearly demonstrated later in this discussion, it is of tremendous import for the clinician to query the patient regarding these associated features and if the dysphagia is to solids, liquids, or both.

A final feature is **weight loss.** If the process is so significant as to result in unintentional weight loss, it portends a more malignant process.

II. Differential diagnosis

As it is often quite difficult for the patient to identify the specific site of obstruction, the full differential diagnosis must be considered in every new case of dysphagia or odynophagia.

A. Diffuse esophageal spasm

1. **Manifestations**

   The **specific manifestations** of this fairly uncommon entity include odynophagia and dysphagia to liquids and solids from the outset of the disease. After onset, symptoms become chronic and progressively worsen over time.

2. **Pathogenesis**

   The **underlying pathogenesis** is a primary motor and/or neuronal dysfunction of the esophagus, with an overall diffuse marked increase in peristalsis within the **entire esophagus.**

3. **Evaluation**

   Evaluation of this entity entails making the clinical diagnosis from the history and physical examination results and performing an **upper GI radiographic study.** The **upper GI series** reveals an increase in diffuse peristaltic activity throughout the entire esophagus, a significant decrease in the bolus transit time from mouth to stomach, and no evidence of anatomic dysfunction. Further evaluation includes **manometry,** which confirms the above findings and shows an overall generalized increase in the amplitude and duration of peristaltic contractions within the entire esophagus. **Esophagogastroduodenoscopy (EGD),** if performed, will show the absence of intrinsic mucosal lesions in the esophagus.

4. **Management**

   The **specific management** includes expeditious referral to gastroenterology and the initiation of calcium channel blockers (e.g., nifedipine, 10–20 mg PO t.i.d.) to decrease the intensity of the peristaltic contractions.

B. Achalasia

1. Manifestations

The **specific manifestations** of this fairly uncommon entity include both odynophagia and dysphagia to liquids and solids from the outset of the disease. After onset, symptoms become chronic and progressively worsen over time. There is often concurrent associated postprandial vomiting.

2. Pathogenesis

The **underlying pathogenesis** is a primary neuronal defect with a localized loss of myenteric neurons about the distal esophagus. This results in the loss of normal lower esophageal sphincter relaxation. The most common underlying etiology worldwide, especially in South America, is Chagas' disease (South American trypanosomiasis).

3. Evaluation

Evaluation entails making the clinical diagnosis from the history and physical examination results and performing an **upper GI radiographic study.** The **upper GI study** demonstrates a dilated esophagus with narrowing of the distal esophageal area. The column of barium may be retained for significant periods of time. The esophagus exhibits severe tertiary contractions against the abnormally tight lower esophagus sphincter. Further evaluation includes **manometry,** which confirms the above findings and shows high-amplitude, repetitive tertiary contractions in the proximal esophagus. The baseline tone of the lower esophageal sphincter is extremely high overall. **EGD,** if performed, will show the absence of intrinsic mucosal lesions in the esophagus.

4. Management

The **specific management** includes expeditious referral to gastroenterology and the initiation of calcium channel blockers (e.g., nifedipine, 10–20 mg PO t.i.d.) to decrease the intensity of the peristaltic contractions.

C. Oropharyngeal dysfunction

1. Manifestations

The **specific manifestations** of this fairly uncommon entity include dysphagia to both liquids and solids from the outset, but minimal odynophagia. Once present, the manifestations are chronic but not progressive. **Associated manifestations** usually include dysarthria, dysphonia, and occasionally passage of the oral contents into the nose and nasopharynx upon swallowing. This usually occurs in an elderly patient with a significant past and present history of atherosclerotic disease and other neurologic evidence of cerebrovascular accidents.

2. **Pathogenesis**

   The **underlying pathogenesis** is related to a brain stem stroke with resultant dysfunction of and damage to the cranial nerves involved in mastication (chewing) and deglutination (swallowing). This is sometimes referred to as bulbar palsy.

3. **Evaluation**

   Evaluation entails making the clinical diagnosis from the history and physical examination findings and performing a **swallowing study.** This imaging study is of paramount importance in that it demonstrates the defect in the swallowing mechanism in real time. The swallowing study will also demonstrate any evidence of concurrent aspiration, which is important in preventing a common complication of this disorder, aspiration pneumonia. An **upper GI series** is not indicated if aspiration is demonstrated by the swallowing studies. **Manometry** of the esophagus is usually not necessary to make the diagnosis; however, if performed, the study reveals a dysfunctional upper esophagus and pharynx but a fairly normal middle and distal esophagus. **EGD** is usually not necessary unless concurrent GI indications are present. A complete neurologic examination and CT of the head are indicated as part of the baseline evaluation.

4. **Management**

   The **specific management** includes withholding oral intake of food and providing enteral feedings via a nasogastric or gastrostomy tube. Referral to a speech therapist with expertise in swallowing disorders should be made. Further management is as for other cerebrovascular accident syndromes (see Chapter 14).

D. **Anatomic disorders**

1. **Manifestations**

   The **specific manifestations** of anatomic lesions involving the esophagus include the subacute onset of progressive dysphagia, with dysphagia to solids evident before dysphagia to liquids, which may progress to total occlusion over time. When the occlusion is marked, the patient vomits within 5–10 minutes of swallowing food. **Odynophagia** is not a major component in any anatomic disorder. Usually the patient has a long history of cigarette smoking or ethanol ingestion, or a history of GERD. If the condition is quite symptomatic or if a malignant process is involved, there often is significant weight loss.

2. **Pathogenesis**

   The **underlying pathogenesis** involves direct anatomic constriction of the affected, usually **distal** portion of the esophagus. Entities that can produce such constriction include:

   a. **Peptic stricture:** fibrosis of the distal esophagus as a result of chronic inflammation due to GERD.

   b. **Squamous cell carcinoma:** the most common neoplastic stricture affecting the esophagus; it is clearly related to chronic ethanol ingestion or smoking.

   c. **Adenocarcinoma:** less common than squamous cell carcinoma; affects the distal esophagus and has been correlated with Barrett's esophagus.

   d. **Schatzki's ring:** a submucosal ring of tissue, usually in the mid- to distal esophagus; a rare and benign process.

   e. **Plummer–Vinson syndrome:** upper esophageal mucosal webs; a relatively rare anomaly. The webs have been associated with iron deficiency anemia and with squamous cell carcinoma of the upper esophagus.

   f. **Zenker's diverticulum:** posterior outpouching of the mid-esophagus, relatively uncommon. The pouch not only causes dysphagia but also significant postprandial regurgitation and **severe chronic halitosis.**

3. **Evaluation**

   Evaluation entails making the clinical diagnosis from the history and physical examination findings and performing an **upper GI radiographic study.** The upper GI study shows a nonspecific stricture in the distal esophagus and thus is of high sensitivity but relatively low specificity; however, Zenker's diverticulum is easily demonstrated on this study. **EGD** is requisite and is the most important study in the evaluation of a patient with a mechanical or anatomic lesion. This direct imaging study allows a histopathologic diagnosis to be made from the biopsy findings.

4. **Management**

   The **specific management** depends on the underlying pathology. Expedient **referral** to gastroenterology and surgery is necessary in all cases.

   a. **Benign stricture:** direct dilation and treatment of underlying reflex disease.

b. **Malignant strictures:** resection, palliative dilation, or palliative laser ablation, alone or in combination.

c. **Schatzki's ring:** direct dilation if symptomatic.

d. **Zenker's diverticulum:** resection if symptomatic.

E. **Esophagitis**

1. **Manifestations**

The **specific manifestations** of this fairly uncommon entity include a subacute to acute onset of symptoms, with odynophagia usually more marked than dysphagia. The highest incidence of this entity is in the immunocompromised population.

2. **Pathogenesis**

The **underlying pathogenesis** is inflammation of the esophageal mucosa with resultant odynophagia, dysphagia, and occasionally hematemesis. In immunosuppressed patients (AIDS), the most common causes include *Candida,* herpes simplex, and cytomegalovirus infections. Other potential though quite rare causes include tetracycline or vitamin C tablets stuck at the level of the distal esophagus with resultant ulceration of the adjacent mucosa. A final, quite common cause is gastroesophageal reflux (GERD).

3. **Evaluation**

Evaluation of esophagitis includes making the clinical diagnosis using the criteria listed in Box 2-5. A thorough search for risk factors for immunocompromise (HIV risk factors or chemotherapy) is required. An **upper GI study** is truly nonspecific and of little diagnostic utility if esophagitis is a high suspicion. **EGD** is the method of choice in the diagnosis of esophagitis. This procedure allows direct visualization and biopsy of the inflamed mucosa. Candidal, HSV, and CMV esophagitis can all be diagnosed from biopsy and cultures of the affected areas.

4. **Management**

The **specific management** includes discontinuing the offending medication and, if an infectious cause is suspected, initiating antibiotics in the following schedule:

a. *Candida:* Ketoconazole, 200 mg PO q. A.M. for 10 days

or

Nystatin, swish and swallow, 5 mL PO q.i.d.

or

Fluconazole, 200 mg PO q.d. for first day, then 100 mg PO q.d. for 10 days

b. **CMV:** Ganciclovir (DHPG) Intravenous

B O X 2 - 5

Overall Evaluation and Management of Dysphagia and Odynophagia

Evaluation

1. Take a thorough **history** and perform a **physical examination,** specifically querying the patient regarding the items listed under **Overall Manifestations.** In addition, ascertain whether the patient has any of the following:
   a. History of chronic smoking or ethanol abuse.
   b. History of immunocompromise (AIDS, chemotherapy).
   c. Any evidence of vesicular lesions in the oropharynx, common with herpes simplex, or thrush in the oropharynx, consistent with candidal infection.
   d. Examination of cranial nerves 9 and 10, testing the gag reflex and swallowing mechanism.
2. **Image** the oropharynx and esophagus.
   a. If there is evidence of a recent cerebrovascular accident or of swallowing weakness, perform a "swallow study." This test, which uses either barium or Gastrografin as the contrast agent, is performed under fluoroscopy to demonstrate the swallowing mechanism itself.
   b. If there is no evidence of vesicular lesions or of a poor gag reflex, the clinician may perform an upper GI radiographic study using barium or Gastrografin as the contrast agent to look for any functional or anatomic lesion in the esophagus.
   c. If there is evidence of vesicular lesions or any anatomic lesion, perform EGD for direct imaging and biopsy.

Management

The **specific management** of entities producing dysphagia or odynophagia is given in the text.

    c. Herpes simplex: Acyclovir, 5–10 mg/kg/24 hr IV in 8 hr dosing.

A **caveat** in therapy is that if the patient is immunosuppressed, has oral thrush, and develops symptoms consistent with esophagitis, it is reasonable to initiate **systemic therapy** (e.g., fluconazole or ketoconazole) against *Candida* empirically without performance of an EGD. If symptoms resolve, this is essentially a diagnostic and therapeutic trial, whereas if symptoms persist or worsen, EGD is mandated. Early and expedient consultation with gastroenterology and infectious disease experts is indicated, as is management of the underlying immunocompromised state. See the section on Infectious Diseases in Chapter 6 (page 321).

III. Consultation

Problem	Service	Time
Any esophageal motor disorder	GI (manometry)	Required
Any mechanical disorder	GI (EGD)	Urgent
Any esophagitis	GI (EGD)	Urgent
	ID	Required
Malignant stricture	Surgery	Urgent

IV. Indications for admission:
Any evidence of aspiration pneumonia, any evidence of esophageal rupture, any upper GI bleeding, any intractable vomiting, any evidence of malnutrition due to dysphagia or HSV esophagitis.

Diarrheal States: Acute, Recurrent, or Chronic

Diarrhea is a common problem worldwide. The approach to diarrhea entails making several basic distinctions, listed below.

1. **Volume of stool.** Stool volume is one of the most important features in describing and defining diarrheal states. Diarrhea is a manifestation of numerous underlying processes. Therefore, it is of utmost importance to set specific objective criteria, of which volume is the most reproducible and valuable. The number of stools and the qualitative consistency of the stool are of limited importance and are inferior to the volume of stool in terms of defining diarrhea. Diarrhea is defined as a **stool weight greater than 300 g/24 hr** on a low-fiber diet.

Once diarrhea is documented or suspected, the following qualifying clinical attributes are sought:

2. **Bloody versus nonbloody stool**
3. **Acute versus chronic condition.** By convention, any diar-

rhea less than or equal to 2 weeks in duration is acute, whereas any diarrheal state of more than 2 weeks' duration is chronic.

4. **Extraintestinal manifestations.** Extraintestinal manifestations are important for determining the cause of acute diarrheal states, and potentially more important for chronic diarrheal states. These manifestations can be a direct result of the diarrhea or its pathogenesis. Examples include intravascular volume depletion from water loss, macrocytic anemia from malabsorption of folate (vitamin B_{12}), and the extraintestinal manifestations of inflammatory bowel disease (uveitis, ankylosing spondylitis, sclerosing cholangitis).

5. **Immunocompromised versus immunocompetent host.** The approach to immunosuppressed patients, including those undergoing chemotherapy, those with AIDS, and those with other immunocompromised states, differs significantly from the approach to immunocompetent patients. The underlying causes, evaluative procedures, and management are different for the two populations.

6. **Locally acquired versus traveler's diarrhea.** Ascertain if the diarrhea began while the patient was in the local environment (at home) or during a trip to another location, either in the United States or elsewhere in the world.

I. **Diagnosis**

The **differential diagnosis** of diarrhea includes a number of extremely diverse entities. A general scheme for grouping the diarrheal syndromes is given below; this scheme follows the qualifying features described in the general discussion of diarrhea. **Acute diarrhea** is discussed in Tables 2-4 through 2-7 and **chronic diarrheal states** are summarized in Table 2-8.

A. **Acute, domestic (i.e., endemic to the United States) diarrhea, patient is immunocompetent (see Table 2-4).**

B. **Acute, nondomestic (i.e., not endemic to the United States) diarrhea, patient is immunocompetent (see Table 2-5).**

This form of diarrhea is often referred to colloquially as "traveler's diarrhea," "Montezuma's revenge," or "*Turista.*" It is a common problem in persons traveling outside of the United States and Canada, and it is best treated via **prevention.** Effective methods of prevention include drinking only bottled water or water that has been boiled at a temperature above 200°F for more than 10 minutes, and ingesting only completely cooked foods. This includes completely cooking any and all **fresh vegetables.** A useful regimen of **prophylaxis or therapy** includes the agents Pepto-Bismol, 60 mL PO q.i.d., and/or TMP-sulfa (Bactrim DS), PO every morning for the duration of the visit or of symptoms. Finally, the patient must be **educated** as to the sources of infection and effective preventive modalities. Antibiotics are required for *Entamoeba histolytica* and *Giardia lamblia* infections.

C. **Immunocompromised patient, acute or chronic diarrhea.** The **differential diagnosis** includes, in addition to any and all of the causes listed earlier, those described in Table 2-6.

D. **Drug-induced diarrhea**
  1. **Antibiotic-associated diarrhea**
    a. **Manifestations**
       The **specific manifestations** of this form of diarrhea include an onset of symptoms 2–10 days following initiation of antibiotics. The diarrhea can begin after completion of a course of antibiotics. Symptoms include a moderate amount of watery, nonbloody diarrhea with nausea, vomiting, and abdominal cramping, which may lead to modest intravascular volume depletion. The duration of symptoms and signs is variable but can extend until treatment is started.
    b. **Pathogenesis**
       The **underlying pathogenesis** is a *change* in the normal colonic flora or the inappropriate growth of *Clostridium difficile* as a side effect of a systemic antibiotic. *Clostridium difficile* is a gram-positive bacillus that can be present in small amounts in the normal colonic flora. Its growth is suppressed and held in check by the rest of the normal colonic bacterial flora. When this balance is disturbed, as when some of the other bacterial flora are suppressed by systemic antibiotics, *C. difficile* or other organisms can inappropriately dominate.
         i. *C. difficile* is enterotoxic to the GI mucosal cells, with resultant mucosal dysfunction.
         ii. Any and all **systemic antibiotics** can cause antibiotic-related diarrhea in general, and *C. difficile* colitis specifically.
         iii. A significant **complication** of this entity is the development of the ulcerative inflammatory colonic process, pseudomembranous colitis.
    c. **Evaluation**
       Evaluation includes making the clinical diagnosis and performing the overall evaluation and management as described in Box 2-6. A stool culture that yields *Clostridium difficile* and toxin clinches the diagnosis.

(Text continues on page 87)

T A B L E 2-4
Acute Domestic Diarrhea Syndromes

Organism	Manifestations/Mode of Transmission	Toxic Mechanism	Treatment
Viral agents (Norwalk agent, etc.)	Begins 6–12 hr after exposure Duration: 24–96 hr Nonbloody, watery diarrhea, usually with minimal concurrent vomiting except in children Transmitted by fecal-oral route	Enterotoxic to mucosal cells	Supportive (see Box 2-6)
Staphylococcus aureus food poisoning	Begins 2–6 hr after ingestion of food Duration: 18–24 hr Acute onset of large amounts of watery, nonbloody diarrhea; concurrent abdominal cramping and vomiting are common Acquired by ingestion of improperly stored prepared meats or custard-filled pastries	Enterotoxic to mucosal cells; gram-positive cocci	Supportive (see Box 2-6)
Clostridium perfringens food poisoning	Begins 8–20 hr after ingestion of food Duration: 12–24 hr Acute onset of large amounts of watery, nonbloody diarrhea; concurrent abdominal cramping and vomiting are common Acquired by ingestion of contaminated food from a buffet or smorgasbord, often food that has been steamed	Enterotoxic to mucosal cells; gram-positive rods	Supportive (see Box 2-6)

Salmonella spp. food poisoning	Begins 12–24 hr after ingestion of food Duration: 12–24 hr Acute onset of moderate to large amounts of nonbloody diarrhea; can progress to bloody diarrhea in a minority of cases; concurrent abdominal cramping and vomiting are common Acquired by ingestion of contaminated food, poorly cooked poultry or eggs, or foods washed in water contaminated with this organism	Enterotoxic to mucosal cells; gram-negative rods	Supportive (see Box 2-6)
Shigella spp.	Begins 12–30 hr after exposure Duration: 3–7 days Acute onset of moderate to large amounts of bloody diarrhea; concurrent abdominal cramping and vomiting are very common Transmitted by fecal–oral route; endemic in areas of poor sanitation	Enteroinvasive to the mucosa; gram-negative rods	See Box 2-6 and initiate antibiotics (Table 2-7)
Camphylobacter jejuni	Begins 3–5 days after exposure Duration: 3–7 days Acute onset of moderate amounts of bloody diarrhea Transmitted by fecal–oral route; can be spread from a household pet, which can act as a reservoir for infection Highest incidence occurs in summer and early fall	Enteroinvasive to the mucosa; gram-negative rods, "sea gull wing" shaped	See Box 2-6 and initiate antibiotics (Table 2-7)

T A B L E   2 - 5
Acute, Nondomestic Diarrhea

Organism	Manifestations/Mode of Transmission	Toxic Mechanism	Treatment
E. coli	Begins 8–18 hr after ingestion of contaminated food or water Duration: 24–48 hr Acute onset of moderate to large amounts of nonbloody diarrhea; concurrent abdominal cramping and vomiting are common Transmitted by fecal–oral route; spread by contaminated water or incompletely cooked food that was cleaned in contaminated water	Enterotoxic to the mucosa; gram-negative rods	See Box 2-6 and text
Shigella spp.	See text and Table 2-4		
Salmonella spp.	See text and Table 2-4		
Entamoeba histolytica	Begins 12–24 hr after ingestion of contaminated food or water Duration: 3–7 days Acute onset of large amounts of bloody diarrhea; concurrent abdominal cramping and vomiting are common Indirect hemagglutinin assay (IHA) on the patient's serum will reveal antibodies against E. histolytica. A titer >1:128 is positive	Enteroinvasive to the mucosa; parasitic infection	See Box 2-6 and initiate antibiotics (Table 2-7)

Organism	Clinical Features	Pathophysiology	Treatment
Giardia lamblia	Begins 24–72 hr after ingestion of contaminated food or water Duration: 3–7 days Subacute onset of mildly bloody, mucus-containing diarrhea Concurrent mild nausea and abdominal cramping are common Transmitted by fecal–oral route and by ingestion of contaminated ground water. Outbreaks have been described in St. Petersburg, Russia and the Rocky Mountain states of North America Patients at highest risk are those with an IgA deficiency Highest incidence occurs in summer and early fall	Unknown; highest concentration in the distal duodenum and proximal jejunum	See Box 2-6 and initiate antibiotics (Table 2-7)
Vibrio cholerae	Begins 8–24 hr after ingestion of contaminated food or water Duration: 3–5 days Acute onset of large amounts of nonbloody diarrhea; concurrent abdominal cramping and vomiting are very common Transmitted by fecal–oral route, via ingestion of contaminated water, improperly cooked foods washed with contaminated water, or contaminated seafood (e.g., sushi, salmon, oysters)	Enterotoxic to the mucosa; gram-negative rods	See Box 2-6 and initiate antibiotics (Table 2-7)

T A B L E 2 - 6
Immunocompromised Patient, Chronic Diarrheal Etiologies

Organism	Manifestations/Mode of Transmission	Toxic Mechanism/Organism	Treatment
HIV-related enteropathy	Insidious onset, recurrent Large amounts of watery, nonbloody diarrhea; mild to moderate concurrent nausea and vomiting Transmission is discussed in Chapter 6	Direct infection of mucosal cells and neuronal cells in GI system; enterotoxic	Supportive (see Box 2-6)
Cryptosporidium spp.	Recurrent episodes Variable amounts of watery, nonbloody diarrhea; the quantity can be massive—up to 8 L/day Transmitted by fecal-oral route in immunocompromised patients, either by ingestion of contaminated water or by direct oral-anal contact	Enterotoxic to mucosal cells; protozoan parasite	Supportive (see Box 2-6) and initiate antibiotics (Table 2-7)
Isospora belli	Recurrent episodes Variable amounts of watery, nonbloody diarrhea; the quantity can be massive—up to 8 L/day Transmitted by fecal-oral route in immunocompromised patients, either by ingestion of contaminated water or by direct oral-anal contact	Enterotoxic to mucosal cells; protozoan parasite	Supportive (see Box 2-6) and initiate antibiotics (Table 2-7)
Mycobacterium avium-intracellulare	Recurrent episodes Variable amounts of watery, nonbloody diarrhea; the quantity can be massive—up to 8 L/day Transmitted by fecal-oral route in immunocompromised patients, either by ingestion of contaminated water or by direct oral-anal contact	Enterotoxic to mucosal cells; protozoan parasite	Supportive (see Box 2-6) and initiate antibiotics (Table 2-7)

T A B L E 2 - 7
Antibiotic Treatment of Specific Infectious Diarrheal States

Organism	Antibiotic
Shigella spp.	Ampicillin, 500 mg PO q.i.d. for 7–10 days *or* TMP–sulfa (Bactrim DS) one tablet PO b.i.d. for 7–10 days
Campylobacter jejuni	Erythromycin, 500 mg PO q.i.d. for 7–10 days
Clostridium difficile	*Metronidazole, 500 mg PO q.i.d. for 7 days Vancomycin, 500 mg PO q.i.d. for 7–10 days *Adjunctive therapy:* Cholestyramine, one packet PO t.i.d. for 5–7 days
Entamoeba histolytica	*Metronidazole, 750 mg PO q.d. for 7 days **and** *Diiodohydroxyquin, 650 mg PO t.i.d. for 21 days
Giardia lamblia	*Quinacrine, 100 mg PO t.i.d. for 5–7 days *or* *Metronidazole, 250 mg PO t.i.d. for 5–7 days
Cryptosporidium spp.	*Spiramycin, Infectious Diseases consult
Isospora belli	TMP–sulfa (Bactrim DS), one tablet PO b.i.d. **and** Infectious Diseases consult
Traveler's diarrhea	Pepto-Bismol, 60 mL PO q.i.d. *and/or* TMP–sulfa (Bactrim DS), one tablet PO q. A.M. for 5–7 days

*Contraindicated in pregnancy.

d. **Management**

The **specific management** includes supportive therapy and, if possible, limiting the duration of systemic antibiotics (usually not possible). The clinician must concurrently initiate and administer **antibiotics by mouth.** Two antibiotics effective in the treatment of antibiotic-related diarrhea are **vancomycin,** 500 mg PO q.i.d. for 7–10 days, or **metronidazole,** 500 mg PO q.i.d. for 7–10 days (metronidazole is contraindicated in pregnancy). A further modality is to administer **cholestyramine,** two packets t.i.d. orally for a duration of 3–5 days. This agent decreases the diarrhea by

---

B O X   2 - 6

Overall Evaluation and Management of Diarrhea

Evaluation

1. Take a thorough **history,** with specific note of the qualifying features listed in the text in the introductory discussion of diarrhea.
2. Perform a **physical examination,** looking specifically for orthostatic changes, fever, and any abdominal findings, all of which portend a more acute and potentially malignant course necessitating a more aggressive evaluation. The physical examination includes a **rectal examination** to directly visualize the stool, to guaiac test the stool for occult blood, and to palpate the rectal mucosa for lesions.
3. If an infectious cause of the diarrhea is suspected (e.g., post-antibiotic use, the patient is febrile, the diarrhea is bloody), place the patient on **enteric precautions.**
4. Perform **stool studies** on a freshly collected sample as soon as possible. These studies include:
   a. **Gram stain,** looking for white blood cells, which are normally not present in the stool, or
   b. **Loeffler's methylene blue stain,** looking for white blood cells, which are normally not present in the stool.
   c. **Microscopic examination** of fresh stool for **ova and parasites.** The clinician must inform the laboratory if any unique protozoa are suspected.
   d. **Bacterial cultures** for enteric pathogens, i.e., *Salmonella, Shigella,* and *Campylobacter.* Cultures are mandatory if there is any evidence of concurrent leukocytes or blood in the stool, or if the patient is febrile.
5. Obtain **blood cultures** if the patient is febrile. Any of the enteric pathogens can invade the bowel, and therefore bacteremia is potentially a sequela.
6. Determine serum electrolyte, BUN, and creatinine levels as part of the baseline evaluation.
7. Assay for *Clostridium difficile* toxin, and culture the stool. This is mandatory if the patient is taking or has recently completed a course of antibiotics.

(continued)

B O X 2 - 6 *(continued)*

8. Determine the complete blood cell count with differential, for baseline purposes and to document any leukocytosis.

9. If there is evidence of intravascular volume depletion, **rehydrate** the patient either intravenously or orally.
   a. **Intravenous rehydration:** dextrose 5% in 0.9 normal saline is the fluid of choice and can easily be given in the outpatient setting.
   b. **Oral rehydration:** if indicated or attempted, use glucose + sodium + water solutions such as Pedialyte or Gatorade.

10. Alkalinize a sample of the stool with NaOH. If the stool turns pink, it is indicative of phenolphthalein use or abuse. Phenolphthalein is a commonly used over-the-counter laxative and cathartic agent; it is the active ingredient in Ex-Lax.

11. Perform a Sudan stain for fat in the stool. This is a good screening test for steatorrhea, i.e., fat malabsorption.

12. Consider **colonoscopy** or **flexible proctosigmoidoscopy** with biopsies of the mucosa **if** the stool is bloody, the patient is febrile, the diarrhea is severe, the diarrhea represents an acute exacerbation of a chronic diarrheal state, or the patient is immunocompromised.

13. **Initiate antidiarrheal agents** on the following schedule:
    a. Kaopectate, 15–30 mL PO q.4–6h. PRN,
       or
    b. Pepto-Bismol (bismuth subsalicylate), 15–30 mL PO q.4–6h. PRN,
       and/or
    c. Lomotil (diphenoxylate plus atropine), 2.5 mg PO q.4–6h. PRN.
       NOTE: Use extreme caution when using narcotic-type antidiarrheal agents in infectious or inflammatory bowel diarrhea.

14. **Use antibiotics cautiously.** In general, there are very few indications for antibiotics, even in infectious diarrhea. See Table 2-4.

decreasing the quantity of toxin in the lumen of the colon.

2. Diarrhea due to other agents

a. Manifestations

The **specific manifestations** of this type of diarrhea include the onset of watery diarrhea while the patient is taking a specific agent. Many forms of diarrhea, both acute and chronic, can result from or be exacerbated by medications which the patient is taking, either prescribed or over-the-counter. Therefore, in all cases of significant diarrhea, the history of medication use—prescribed, illicit, or OTC—must be obtained. The duration is usually quite dependent on the duration of use of the agent.

b. Pathogenesis

The **underlying pathogenesis** is usually either an osmotic-type diarrhea or one resulting from intestinal hypermobility. **Osmotic** diarrheal entities result from an abnormal increase in the water content of the stool. This can be due to many different, quite diverse agents, from the overuse of dietary fiber products, from lactulose, and from the use of magnesium-containing antacids. **Hypermobility** diarrhea is a result of increased peristalsis and therefore decreased transit time of the stool in the colon. The faster the transit time, the less water is absorbed from the stool, and therefore the more fluid is the stool. Hypermobility diarrhea can be due to overindulgence in caffeinated beverages, excessive ethanol use, and the use of phenolphthalein or other laxatives, cathartics, or stool softeners. There is a significant amount of overlap between these two mechanisms.

c. Evaluation and management

The **specific evaluation and management** include making the clinical diagnosis and performing the overall evaluation and management as described in Box 2-6. Invariably, withdrawing the agent and/or modifying the habits of the patient will result in resolution of the diarrhea in 1–3 days. If there is no resolution, other causes need to be explored.

II. Chronic diarrheal states

Refer to Table 2-8.

III. **Consultation**

Problem	*Service*	*Time*
Typhoid fever	Infectious diseases	Emergent
Immuno-compromised patient with diarrhea	Infectious diseases	Urgent
Chronic diarrhea	Gastroenterology	Required
Acute, bloody diarrhea	Gastroenterology	Urgent

IV. **Indications for admission:** Severe intravascular volume depletion, any evidence or suspicion of an acute abdomen, any fevers or manifestations of septicemia, any lower GI bleeding with a decrease in the hematocrit.

End-Stage Hepatic Dysfunction

End-stage hepatic dysfunction is a syndrome that results from the **permanent loss** of liver tissue and therefore of liver function. The manifestations and prognosis are virtually the same, irrespective of the underlying cause, and therefore this diagnosis supplants those previous diagnoses. The classic, virtually synonymous term is **cirrhosis.**

The **physiologic functions** of the liver include but are not limited to the following:

1. **Protein anabolism.** The liver produces proteins, including many of the coagulation factors (i.e., factors II, V, VII, IX, and X). The liver also produces **albumin,** a major determinant in the maintenance of intravascular colloid oncotic pressure and thus of keeping fluids within the intravascular system.

2. **Draining of venous blood from the GI tract.** Venous blood is drained from the GI tract via the hepatic portal system. Blood rich with nutrients is absorbed in the small intestine and delivered to the liver, where the nutrients are processed into usable substrates for energy and anabolism.

3. **Detoxification.** The liver helps maintain the physiologic milieu by detoxifying the body fluids of toxic substances.

I. **Manifestations of hepatic insufficiency** (see Box 2-7)

The **overall manifestations** of hepatic insufficiency are directly related to a want of the normal physiologic functions performed exclusively by the liver. Problems that can and will develop include coagulopathy, ascites, edema, portal hypertension with potential for bleeding, and mental status changes (i.e., encephalopathy as a result of toxin accumula-

(*Text continues on page 96*)

T A B L E   2 - 8
Features of Chronic Diarrheal Syndromes

Syndrome	Mechanism	Clinical Features	Diagnostic Tests/Treatment
Irritable bowel syndrome	Undefined motility disorder of the GI tract	Afebrile Mucous diarrhea alternating with periods of constipation No weight loss	Diagnosis of exclusion Treatment: a) Fiber (Metamucil) b) Reassurance
Diabetic enteropathy	Autonomic neuron dysfunction/destruction with an overall decrease in motility and, potentially, bacterial overgrowth	Nocturnal diarrhea Postprandial vomiting Malabsorption, especially of fats Concurrent other autonomic dysfunction	Diagnosis of exclusion in a diabetic patient Treatment: a) Prevention b) Lomotil PRN
Carbohydrate malabsorption	Either as a result of a decrease in the absorptive brush border, and/or as a relative or absolute deficiency in disaccharidases (most commonly lactase)	Bloating Increased flatus Diarrhea Exacerbated by ingestion of specific disaccharide (e.g., lactose)	Resolution of symptoms on a diet low in the offending sugar (e.g., a no-dairy-product diet: decrease lactose); this is both diagnostic and therapeutic H_2 breath test: Excessive H_2 production by bacteria in the colon if undigested disaccharide (lactose, etc.) is present; hydrogen is measured in air exhaled by the patient Treatment: Modify diet to exclude offending sugar

Fat malabsorption	A decrease in bile salts, pancreatic enzymes, and/or ileal surface area DDX: a) small bowel disorder, or b) pancreatic insufficiency	Steatorrhea Malodorous stools Greasy stools Vitamin K deficiency Vitamin A and D deficiencies	72-hour collection of stool for fecal fat on a 100-g fat diet KUB: to look for pancreatic calcifications, indicative of chronic pancreatitis Treatment: a) If small bowel, find and treat the underlying cause b) If pancreatic insufficiency, pancreatic enzyme replacement (e.g., Pancrease, 2 packets before meals)
Dumping syndrome	A motility disorder that can occur after gastrectomy	Postprandial: Diaphoresis Diarrhea Tachycardia	Clinical diagnosis Treatment: Frequent small meals
Zollinger–Ellison syndrome	Hypersecretion of gastrin due to a gastrinoma, resulting in hypersecretion of acid and GI hypermotility	Watery diarrhea Recurrent gastric and/or duodenal ulcers	Gastric acid measurements Serum gastrin levels (off of H$_2$ blockers) Treatment: a) H$_2$-receptor blockers (e.g., ranitidine, 150 mg/day PO) or b) H-K ATPase inhibitors (omeprazole, 40 mg PO q. day) c) Surgical resection d) Somatostatin

(continued)

T A B L E 2 - 8
Features of Chronic Diarrheal Syndromes (continued)

Syndrome	Mechanism	Clinical Features	Diagnostic Tests/Treatment
Carcinoid	An intestinal or extraintestinal tumor producing bradykinins, prostaglandins, and/or serotonin	Watery diarrhea If a primary bronchial carcinoid and/or if hepatic metastases are present, a syndrome occurs of: Pulmonic valve stenosis Flushing of skin Watery diarrhea Bronchospasm	24-hour urine collection for 5-HIAA (catabolite of serotonin) Chest radiography CT scan of liver Treatment (beyond scope of text): Somatostatin Treat tumor
Crohn's disease	Unknown	Fevers Bloody diarrhea Transmural lesions Involvement throughout GI tract	Colonoscopy with biopsies UGI with small bowel follow-through Treatment: a) Sulfasalazine, 2–4 g PO q.d. (500-mg tablets)

		Malabsorption Sacroiliitis Uveitis Pyoderma gangrenosum Erythema nodosum Fistulas/strictures	b) Acute flares: steroids c) Limit surgical procedures d) No clear efficacy of metronidazole
Ulcerative colitis	Unknown	Fevers Bloody diarrhea Mucosal lesions Proctitis/colitis Weight loss Increased risk of colon carcinoma	Colonoscopy with biopsy Treatment: a) Sulfasalazine, 2–4 g PO q.d. b) For acute flares and/or severe disease: steroids (prednisone, 60 mg PO q.d., or methylprednisone, 80 mg IV q.8h.) c) Hydrocortisone enema, 50–100 mg retention enema q.h.s., especially effective in the treatment of proctitis d) Opiate agents can be used with caution in patients with chronic findings (Lomomtil), 10 mg PO q.6–8h., or loperamide (Imodium), 2–4 mg PO q.6–8h.) e) Surgical intervention

BOX 2-7

Overall Evaluation and Management of Hepatic Insufficiency

Evaluation

1. Follow on a regular basis, such as every 3–6 months, the following parameters:
   a. SGOT and total bilirubin.
   b. Prothrombin time (PT) and albumin, to monitor the synthetic function of the liver.
   c. CBC count, to monitor for anemia and thrombocytopenia.
   d. Electrolytes, BUN, creatinine, and glucose.
2. Determine the Child–Turcotte class of the patient (see Table 2-9).

Management

1. Instruct the patient to **discontinue all ethanol use.**
2. Administer the Pneumovax polyvalent vaccine at the time of presentation.
3. All hepatotoxic agents are contraindicated (e.g., ethanol, acetaminophen).
4. Instruct the patient to avoid the use of agents catabolized in the liver, such as benzodiazepines and acetaminophen. If use is necessary, the agents should be used with great caution and, if possible, close monitoring of plasma levels.
5. The patient should take a multivitamin pill orally once daily.
6. Administer an influenza vaccine every fall.
7. Salicylates are contraindicated, especially if there is any evidence of a coagulopathy.

tion in the blood and CNS). The manifestations, pathogenesis, evaluation, and management of each of these problems are discussed subsequently.

Other examination findings include **icterus,** both scleral and skin; a **small liver,** i.e., a span of less than 6 cm; **palmar erythema,** i.e., a diffuse redness of the palms and soles; and **spider angiomas,** i.e., red spiderlike lesions on the skin of the upper trunk and arms, which are thought to be a result of excess estrogens. Of interest, these lesions occur only in the distribution of the superior vena cava. Finally, males may exhibit **decreased testicular volume** and **impotence,** along

T A B L E 2 - 9
Child-Turcotte Classification

Parameter	Class		
	A	B	C
Serum bilirubin (mg/dL)	<2.0	2.0–3.0	>3.0
Serum albumin (g/dL)	>3.5	3.0–3.5	<3.0
Ascites	None	Easily managed	Refractory
Encephalopathy	Absent	Mild	Severe
Nutritional status	Good	Fair	Poor

with **bilateral gynecomastia,** all as a result of excess estrogens.

II. **Complications of hepatic insufficiency**
   Specific complications include the following:
   A. **Coagulopathy**
      1. **Manifestations**
         The **specific manifestations** of coagulopathy include a subacute onset of easy bruisability, purpura, recurrent ecchymoses, epistaxis, and gingival bleeding. The patient may report uncontrolled bleeding after minor trauma.
      2. **Pathogenesis**
         The **underlying pathogenesis** involves a deficiency in the coagulation factors produced by the liver. These coagulation factors include II, V, VII, IX, and X, i.e., those of the **extrinsic coagulation** cascade. This arm of the coagulation cascade is measured using the **prothrombin test.** These factors, with the exception of factor V, are also vitamin K dependent, and therefore vitamin K deficiency can manifest with similar findings. **Vitamin K deficiency** is often present concurrent with the liver disease and thus needs to be ruled out in the evaluation.
      3. **Evaluation**
         Evaluation entails determining PT, aPTT, platelet count, and ruling out any concurrent process that may exacerbate the bleeding disorder. Examples of reversible exacerbating factors include the use of salicylates, a deficiency in vitamin K, and a consumptive coagulopathy (DIC). For example, an isolated **elevation of PT** can reflect either vitamin deficiency or liver disease.
      4. **Management**
         The **specific management** includes proscribing the use of aspirin and attempting to correct the elevated

PT with vitamin K. The dose of vitamin K is 10 mg subcutaneously once daily for 3 days, then orally, or 10 mg PO once daily from the outset. If a surgical procedure is planned, fresh frozen plasma (FFP) should be administered prior to the procedure to attempt to normalize the elevated PT, or, at minimum, to decrease it to **less than 15 seconds** during the procedure.

B. Variceal bleeding

1. Manifestations

The **specific manifestations,** in addition to those accompanying any other upper GI bleeding (see section on Gastrointestinal Bleeding, page 104), include other findings of **portal hypertension,** among them **distended superficial abdominal veins,** including the specific sign of caput medusae (i.e., distended cutaneous veins radiating from the umbilicus); **internal hemorrhoids;** guaiac-positive stools; hematemesis; melena; and hematochezia. The patient may be intravascularly volume depleted and hemodynamically unstable at the time of presentation. Variceal bleeding must always be considered in the differential diagnosis of GI bleeding in any patient with **hepatic dysfunction.**

2. Pathogenesis

The **underlying pathogenesis** involves hypertension in the portal venous system, which results in significant congestion and dilation of the veins in the portal system—the veins of the GI tract. The dilated portal veins usually form in the distal esophagus but can form anywhere in the GI tract. They are easily traumatized and therefore bleed quite easily, with resultant massive GI hemorrhages.

3. Evaluation

Evaluation entails making the clinical diagnosis and emergency management of active bleeding.

4. Management

Emergency consultation with gastroenterology for emergency EGD is indicated for potential sclerotherapy of the varices. Further treatment may include the initiation of vasopressin, 0.1–0.5 units/min IV, and, if the bleeding is massive and uncontrollable, placement of a Sengstaken–Blakemore tube. This last-ditch effort entails placing through the mouth a triple- or quadruple-lumen tube with an inflatable distal area that is used to tamponade any varices in the distal esophagus. Before placement of the tube, the airway must be protected with endotracheal intubation.

5. **Chronic therapy and prophylaxis**

   The **chronic therapy and prophylaxis** of variceal bleeding, especially esophageal variceal bleeding, includes the following:

   a. Checking the hematocrit frequently.

   b. Instructing the patient to watch for the development of melena.

   c. **Sclerotherapy** as a prophylactic modality by the gastroenterology service is probably effective in decreasing the number of upper GI bleeding episodes but has not been demonstrated to prolong life. In fact, one recent study demonstrated an increased mortality in the group receiving prophylactic variceal sclerotherapy. Therefore, it is **not at present a recommended procedure.**

   d. Some recent studies have demonstrated a positive effect of **β-blockers** (e.g., propranolol, 10–20 mg PO t.i.d.) in decreasing the magnitude of portal hypertension, thus potentially decreasing the risk of variceal development and bleeding. β-blockers can only be used in patients without contraindications to them, and frequent follow-up is necessary to monitor blood pressure and vital signs.

   e. **Surgical placement of a splenorenal (Warren) shunt** should be considered, especially in young patients of Child class of A or B (see Table 2-9). This procedure shunts blood from the portal to the systemic venous circulation, thus bypassing the liver and decreasing portal hypertension. Shunt placement decreases the risk of recurrence of upper GI hemorrhage due to varices but **has not increased the life expectancy** of patients. This is also an invasive procedure with inherent morbidity, an increased incidence of encephalopathy, an increased risk of infection, and even mortality. Therefore, it should be reserved for selected patients.

C. **Encephalopathy**

   1. **Manifestations**

      The **specific manifestations** of this not uncommon sequela of hepatic insufficiency include **asterixis,** i.e., bilateral involuntary flapping of the hands at the wrist when the patient is instructed to actively extend the hands; **confusion** (delirium); and **lethargy.**

   2. **Pathogenesis**

      The **underlying pathogenesis** is an increase in the level of nitrogenous wastes in the bloodstream, which in turn results in deterioration of brain function. A marker for this process is the serum ammonia level, which is elevated in encephalopathy but is **not directly correlated** with the degree of encephalopathy. Usually the encephalopathy is exacerbated by ingestion of proteinaceous foodstuffs, constipation, GI bleeding, intravascular volume depletion, and sepsis.

3. **Evaluation**

   Evaluation entails making the clinical diagnosis and, at the outset, determining the **serum NH$_4$ level**. In addition, any concurrent process that might cause mental status changes must be ruled out, and underlying, precipitating, or exacerbating factors must be sought and treated.

4. **Management**

   The **specific management** in the acute setting includes the initiation of lactulose and/or neomycin. **Lactulose** is a complex carbohydrate that increases colonic motility and results in diarrhea. The dose for lactulose is 15–30 mL PO q.4–12h. **Neomycin** is a nonabsorbable antibiotic that works well in the acute setting, especially when used with lactulose. This antibiotic is thought to be bactericidal for many of the bacterial flora that produce diarrhea and also decrease nitrogenous waste production by the bacteria in the distal small bowel and colon. The dose for neomycin is 500–1,000 mg PO b.i.d. The dose is titrated to symptoms and the number of bowel movements per day. The optimum number of bowel movements is two or three per day. Finally, central to management is **limiting protein consumption** to 40 g/day. To meet this goal, a dietary consultation is highly recommended.

D. **Ascites**

   1. **Manifestations**

      The **specific manifestations** of this quite common sequela of hepatic insufficiency reflect **excess fluid** within the peritoneal cavity. The patient will relate that the pants feel tight or that the waist size of clothing has been increased to accommodate the increased abdominal girth. There is often concurrent edema in **dependent areas** (feet if ambulatory, back if bedridden) of the body. Examination often discloses **abdominal distention,** a **shifting dullness** in the distended abdomen, and a **fluid wave.** Unless infection exists concurrently, there usually is **no tenderness to deep or rebound palpation.** Ascites can spontaneously become infected, usually with bacteria that are normally present in the GI tract; thus, one must always be concerned that this has occurred when a

T A B L E   2 - 1 0
Differential Diagnosis of Ascites

Transudative
  Right ventricular failure
  Constrictive pericarditis
  Venous occlusion
    Budd–Chiari syndrome
    Veno-occlusive disease (especially after irradiation to the liver bed)
  Hypoalbuminemia states
    Cirrhosis—decreased anabolism of proteins from the liver
    Nephrotic syndrome—loss of protein in the urine
    Kwashiorkor—profound protein malnutrition

Exudative
  Peritonitis
  Tuberculosis
  Pancreatitis
  Peritoneal carcinomatosis
  Pseudomyxoma peritonei (after rupture of mucus-secreting tumor)
  Hepatocellular carcinoma

Chylous
  Chronic inflammation of the peritoneal membrane
  Lymphoproliferative disorders

patient has concurrent pain or tenderness or an increase in the quantity of peritoneal fluid.

2. **Pathogenesis**

   The **underlying pathogenesis** of ascites is multifactorial but includes underlying **portal hypertension** with congestion of fluids in the portal system and concurrent moderate to profound **hypoalbuminemia,** all of which result in edema and leakage of fluids into the peritoneal cavity. In addition to these mechanisms, a **secondary hyperaldosteronism** develops, resulting in further sodium and water retention. The **differential diagnosis** of ascites is listed in Table 2-10.

3. **Evaluation**

   Evaluation entails making the clinical diagnosis. If there is any question as to its presence, abdominal ultrasound will clearly demonstrate it. Because ascites can become infected and result in potentially mortal infections and because other conditions can exacerbate ascites, **all new cases of ascites and all patients with an increase in ascites or any abdominal tenderness to palpation mandate paracentesis.** The evaluative studies that should be performed on the ascitic fluid are listed in Table 2-11.

T A B L E   2 - 1 1
Diagnostic Examinations of Ascites

1. Albumin gradient: Calculate gradient via:

   Serum albumin–Ascitic fluid albumin

   If the gradient is greater than 1.1 g/dL, this is consistent with an underlying pathogenesis of portal hypertension. If the gradient is less than 1.1 g/dL, this is consistent with an underlying pathogenesis not related to portal hypertension, e.g., bacterial or carcinomatous peritonitis.
2. Total protein, ascitic fluid:

   If <3.0 g/dL: transudate
   If >3.0 g/dL: exudate
3. Cell count in the ascitic fluid: If the total WBC count exceeds 500/mm³ or the total polymorphonuclear cell counts exceeds 200/mm³, the result should be interpreted and must be treated as bacterial peritonitis.
4. Amylase: If elevated, rule out pancreatic pseudocyst and pancreatic ascites.
5. Gram stain.
6. AFB smear.
7. Cultures of the ascitic fluid.
8. Triglycerides, especially if the fluid appears milklike, to rule out chylous ascites.
9. Cytology, if neoplastic process is suspected.

4. **Management**

   The **specific management** of ascites is divided into acute and chronic management.

   a. **Acute management** is necessary if the ascites is infected or is causing distress for the patient, especially if it is causing respiratory compromise.

      i. If there is any evidence of **peritonitis,** acute administration of antibiotics is mandatory. Regimens to cover the most common organismal causes—i.e., the gram-negative bacilli, anaerobes, and Group D streptococci—include:

         Ampicillin, 2 g q.4–6h. IV
            +
         Clindamycin, 900 mg IV q.8h.
            +
         Aminoglycoside, IV
            or
         Unasyn, 3.0 g IV q.6h.

      ii. If there is a large quantity of ascites resulting in respiratory compromise, one can **acutely**

remove the fluid. A highly effective modality is to perform **high-volume paracentesis** (HVP). This is accomplished by removing 3–4 L of fluid in the standard manner and concurrently repleting the intravascular fluid potentially lost with 12.5–25 g of salt-poor albumin (25% SPA) IV. Concurrent with any HVP therapy, the initiation of diuretics for chronic therapy is indicated. Two different diuretics can be of clinical use.

    (a) Potassium-sparing diuretics are very effective in that they decrease aldosterone levels and thereby reverse secondary hyperaldosteronism, one of the basic pathophysiologic mechanisms leading to ascites. The initial dose is spironolactone 25 mg PO t.i.d., which can be slowly increased to a maximum of 300 mg PO in a 24-hour period.

    (b) Loop diuretics (e.g. furosemide 20 mg PO q.d.) are excellent as adjunctive therapy to the potassium-sparing diuretics and may, especially if given early in the course of therapy, effect a more productive diuresis.

  b. Chronic therapy is for patients who have already received acute intervention or who have an asymptomatic transudative fluid. The specific management includes monitoring for the development of subacute bacterial peritonitis, effectively treating the underlying condition if possible, and titrating **diuretics** (potassium-sparing or loop diuretics) to minimize the ascites without causing hyperkalemia or intravascular volume depletion. Instruct the patient to modify the diet to **limit salt intake.** It is essential to attempt to restrict the patient to a diet containing less than 2 g of sodium per day. The dietary service should be consulted to aid in this instruction.

    i. A final and important point: certain parameters must be monitored closely when treating ascites using diuretics, with or without HVP. These parameters include **intravascular volume status,** serum potassium levels, urine output, urine sodium levels, and renal function. If any signs of intravascular volume depletion develop, even if there is a large quantity of ascites remaining, HVP should be interrupted and the diuretics decreased or even temporarily discontinued. The specific useful signs of intravascular volume depletion include orthostatic changes, increased BUN, decreased urine output, and a urine Na of less than 10 mEq/dL.

E. **Hepatorenal syndrome**

Hepatorenal syndrome is the development of **renal failure** as a result of or concurrent with severe hepatic dysfunction. The process is usually precipitated by intravascular volume depletion, either as a result of upper GI hemorrhage or of overzealous diuresis. The renal failure is irreversible, and once present, this syndrome has a grave prognosis. The best method of treatment is prevention. Renal consultation should be obtained.

III. **Prognosis**

The overall prognosis for patients with end-stage liver disease is quite bleak. Even with abstinence from ethanol and other hepatotoxic agents and with supportive care, the 2-year survival rate is **less than 50%.** Some hope in the treatment of this disorder has arisen from transplants, but this modality, at least in its present form and for the immediate future, will be of benefit for only a small minority of patients. The potential for transplantation should be explored in all patients, and referral to gastroenterology for this purpose should be performed.

The **Child-Turcotte classification scheme** for hepatic dysfunction is given in Table 2-9. A study by Christensen et al. demonstrated a correlation with overall prognosis: as the class goes from A to B to C, the life expectancy dramatically drops from years to months.

IV. **Consultation**

Problem	Service	Time
Variceal bleeding	GI	Urgent/emergent
Variceal bleeding	Surgery	Urgent/emergent
Consideration of shunt		Elective
For low-salt diet and low-protein diet	Dietary	Elective

V. **Indications for admission:** Fever, upper GI bleeding, new or exacerbation of encephalopathy, intravascular volume depletion, presence or clinical suspicion of spontaneous bacterial peritonitis, or massive ascites that restricts respiratory function.

Gastrointestinal Bleeding

The **overall manifestations** of GI bleeding are quite variable and are related to the site, duration, acuity, and intensity of the bleeding. They include **hematemesis** (coffee-ground-type emesis, if the site is in the upper GI area) and **melena** (black, tarry stools) as a result of blood passing through the GI tract and into the stool. Black stools may result from upper GI bleeding, lower GI bleeding (i.e., from the colon, especially if the transit time across the colon is long), the use of $FeSO_4$, or the use of bismuth subsalicylate (Pepto-Bismol). A further manifestation is **hematochezia**—bright red blood passed rectally—which may be indicative of a lower GI source or of a massive upper GI hemorrhage.

Other manifestations may include intravascular volume depletion with accompanying symptoms and signs, a pale skin and conjunctivae, guaiac-positive stool (the guaiac test is negative in black stool due to $FeSO_4$ or bismuth), and epigastric pain or tenderness. The patient may have a history of peptic ulcer disease, of hepatic disease with or without varices, of recent ethanol use, or of recent NSAID use.

Other, **nongastrointestinal sites of bleeding** can occasionally manifest with melena or what is presumed to be hematemesis. The most common of these conditions are epistaxis and hemoptysis. At the outset, the clinician must attempt to differentiate these causes from the history and physical examination findings.

I. Differential diagnosis

The **differential diagnosis** of GI bleeding is quite long, and one of the easiest methods of remembering the various possible entities is to divide them into sites proximal to the ligament of Treitz (i.e., upper GI) and sites distal to the ligament of Treitz. The ligament of Treitz is in the duodenum.

A. Upper gastrointestinal bleeding

The differential diagnosis from the ligament of Treitz proximally includes the following entities:

1. **Duodenal ulcer** (see section on Peptic Ulcer Disease, page 62)
2. **Gastric ulcer** (see section on Peptic Ulcer Disease, page 62)
3. **Hemorrhagic gastritis**
   a. **Manifestations**
      The **specific manifestations** include the development of epigastric pain that is worse with fasting and relieved by food intake. There is often an antecedent history of recurrent epigastric pain and melena prior to the development of the hematemesis. Associated with these manifestations can be the development of postprandial vomiting as a result of pyloric obstruction, a not uncommon gastric ulcer sequela. Of interest is the fact that there often is a past history of peptic ulcer disease.
   b. **Pathogenesis**
      The **underlying pathogenesis** is a diffuse, often marked, nonspecific superficial breakdown of the

gastric mucosa with the resultant development of diffuse **erosions.** This may, but not necessarily will, become associated with ulcer development. **Risk factors** for development include NSAID-induced gastropathy and ethanol use.

c. **Evaluation**

The specific evaluation and management of this entity includes that described in Box 2-8 and performing EGD on an emergency basis. EGD will demonstrate erosions and ulcers in the stomach. Biopsies of any ulcer present are indicated to rule out any underlying malignant neoplastic disease.

d. **Management**

The **specific management** includes the initiation of **H_2-receptor antagonists** in regimens and doses which are the same as for duodenal ulcers, and/or **sucralfate (Carafate),** 1 g PO q.i.d., either for a total duration of 6 weeks. In the acute stage, all NSAIDs and aspirin should be discontinued. In all cases referral to gastroenterology should be performed.

If after the acute event has resolved and the patient clearly requires an NSAID or aspirin, it can be restarted with caution and with the **prophylactic** concurrent administration of sucralfate, 1 g PO b.i.d., or misoprostol, 200 μg PO once a day (**contraindicated in pregnancy**). Furthermore, the patient should be instructed to discontinue all ethanol ingestion, especially in the acute setting.

4. **Gastric malignancies**

a. **Manifestations**

The **specific manifestations** of this relatively uncommon entity include weight loss, early satiety, and, if the underlying lesion is a lymphoma, some or all of the B symptoms. B symptoms include fevers, drenching night sweats, and unintentional weight loss.

b. **Pathogenesis**

The **underlying pathogenesis** of this entity is that it is the result of a primary adenocarcinoma or non-Hodgkin's lymphoma within the stomach wall itself. The **risk factors** for the development of gastric adenocarcinoma include gastric polyps and a family history of gastric carcinoma.

c. **Evaluation**

Evaluation of this entity entails making the clinical diagnosis via the overall approach described in Box 2-8. Any gastric ulcer mandates a biopsy.

B O X 2 - 8

***Overall Evaluation and Management of
Gastrointestinal Bleeding***

Evaluation

1. Evaluate ABCs and perform ACLS protocol as necessary.
2. Take the history and perform a physical examination, looking for the features described in the introductory section.
3. Determine the **complete blood cell count** with differential to determine the degree of anemia present at the time of presentation.
4. **Type and cross-match blood** for 4 units of packed red blood cells so that the blood is ready when needed for transfusion.
5. Determine the **platelet count** and coagulation parameters, including PT and aPTT, at baseline to rule out any exacerbating or concurrent coagulopathy.
6. Determine electrolytes, BUN, creatinine, and glucose levels as part of the baseline evaluation.
7. Obtain a 12-lead ECG as part of the baseline evaluation.
8. **Liver function tests,** including albumin, are important, for if there is any evidence of hepatic dysfunction, one must include variceal bleeding in the differential diagnosis.

Management

1. Place the patient on NPO orders at the outset in all cases.
2. Discontinue all NSAIDs for the short and intermediate term, as these agents can be the underlying cause of the bleeding.
3. Establish IV access with two large-bore IVs (18 gauge or greater) or a central venous catheter so that large volumes of blood or fluids can be easily administered.
4. Initiate IV fluids (normal saline or dextrose 5% in 0.9 normal saline) at 250–300 mL/hr, or faster if clinically indicated.

(continued)

B O X 2 - 8 (continued)

5. Correct any coagulopathies with platelet and fresh frozen plasma infusions to keep the platelet count above 50,000 and the PT below 15 seconds.
6. **Transfuse** packed RBCs to keep the hematocrit above 30%.
7. Administer H_2-receptor blockers (e.g., cimetidine, 300 mg IV q.6h., or ranitidine, 50 mg IV q.8h.).
8. Consultation with gastroenterology and surgery is mandatory.
9. Admission to an ICU usually indicated.
10. After initial stabilization, direct invasive imaging by **EGD,** if an upper GI source is suspected, or by **colonoscopy,** if a lower GI source is suspected, is indicated.
11. See each diagnosis for specific considerations and/or management schemae.

---

  d. **Management**
   The **specific management** is beyond the scope of this text, but referral to surgery and oncology is clearly indicated in an expedient fashion.
5. **Mallory–Weiss tears**
  a. **Manifestations**
   The **specific manifestations** include an antecedent history of severe vomiting. The initial emesis consists of normal gastric contents, i.e., fluids/food particles, which with repetitive vomiting and retching becomes **hematemesis.**
  b. **Pathogenesis**
   The **underlying pathogenesis** is a longitudinal tear in the mucosa of the distal esophagus and proximal gastric cardia. The majority of the tear is on the gastric side. The tear is invariably the result of the severe vomiting and retching. Due to this fact, a specific **risk factor** is bulimia, a state in which a patient induces recurrent vomiting after a food binge for the purposes of intentional weight loss. The underlying esophageal mucosa is usually normal before and, with healing, after the episode.
  c. **Evaluation**
   Evaluation entails making the clinical diagnosis via the overall approach described in Box 2-8 and

performing EGD. EGD will reveal the longitudinal mucosal tear.

   d. Management

The **specific management** includes a 6-week course of H_2 antagonists. If there is a component of bulimia, referral to psychiatry is indicated.

6. Esophageal varices

   a. Manifestations

The **specific manifestations** include the development of hematemesis and/or melena in a patient with an antecedent history of **hepatic dysfunction.** The concurrent manifestations of hepatic disease include but are not limited to ascites, gynecomastia, decreased testicular size, encephalopathy, portal hypertension, increased venous pattern on the abdominal wall, and internal hemorrhoids.

   b. Pathogenesis

The **underlying pathogenesis** is one of the development of abnormally enlarged veins of the portal system in the distal esophagus as a result of chronic portal hypertension. These thin-walled vessels are easily traumatized and easily bleed.

   c. Evaluation and management

The **specific evaluation and management** include making the clinical diagnosis using the overall approach described in Box 2-8 and emergency admission (see section on End-Stage Hepatic Dysfunction, page 91).

B. Lower gastrointestinal bleeding

The differential diagnosis includes the following entities:

1. Diverticular disease

   a. Manifestations

The **specific manifestations** include the acute to subacute onset of modest to significant amounts of bright red blood passed rectally (**hematochezia**). The patient will quite often have a past history of recurrent, self-limited, lower quadrant abdominal pain or hematochezia. The patient often has a long history of mild to moderate constipation and straining upon defecation over the past years to decades. There are no upper GI findings, no nausea, vomiting, or hematemesis. Furthermore, in diverticulosis there is minimal to no abdominal pain or tenderness.

   b. Pathogenesis

The **underlying pathogenesis** is that diverticuli are small, acquired herniations of the colonic mucosa through the wall of the colon. These can and do occur anywhere in the large intestine but most commonly will develop in the sigmoid and, occasionally, in the cecal areas of the colon. The **risk factors** in the development of diverticuli include increasing age and constipation with the recurrent need to strain, i.e., Valsalva maneuver, upon having bowel movements. There are two different, but interrelated, clinical syndromes associated with diverticuli, diverticulitis and diverticulosis.

    i. Diverticulitis. The diverticuli become inflamed with resultant pain, direct tenderness, and even some rebound tenderness. The natural history of this is usually self-limited, but systemic bacteremia, perforation of the bowel wall, and abscess formation can be sequelae of this form.

    ii. Diverticulosis. The diverticuli irritate and/or erode into adjacent vessels and result in bleeding. There is minimal inflammation, thus minimal pain and tenderness. The usual natural history is one of self-limited bleeding, but occasionally the bleeding can be quite massive.

c. Evaluation

Evaluation includes making the clinical diagnosis using the overall approach as described in Box 2-8. Colonoscopy is usually indicated in diverticulosis to rule out other pathologic entities.

d. Management

The **specific management** includes making the diagnosis and observing the patient for any anemia and/or any sequelae of diverticuli, and increasing the fiber in the patient's diet to decrease any constipation. The proscription of nuts, popcorn, and seeded berries is of no known benefit and thus is unnecessary.

If bleeding is severe and/or recurrent and/or if there is any evidence of the sequelae of diverticulitis, resection of the affected segment of colon is indicated. Thus gastroenterology and surgery consultations can be, and are, of diagnostic and therapeutic benefit, especially in recurrent cases.

2. Angiodysplasia

a. Manifestations

The **specific manifestations** include the acute onset of hematochezia without any other abdominal findings. This usually occurs in elderly patients who can be, and often are, otherwise relatively healthy. If in a younger patient, occasionally there can be evidence of angiomas on the skin and in the nasal and oral mucosa.

b. **Pathogenesis**

The **underlying pathogenesis** is one of the development of arteriovenous malformations within the mucosa of the bowel. These lesions are quite fragile and therefore easily bleed with minimal trauma. These lesions, which invariably are multiple, can increase in number and size with increasing age. Furthermore, a small number of patients have a genetic predisposition for the development of these AVM lesions. The most common and classic predisposing syndrome is the hereditary telangiectasia syndrome, i.e., the **Osler–Weber–Rendu syndrome.**

c. **Evaluation and management**

The **specific evaluation and management** includes making the clinical diagnosis. Furthermore, colonoscopy is indicated for diagnosis and to rule out any concurrent lesions. Colonoscopy, furthermore, is often a therapeutic modality as direct cautery can be performed on the specific AVM lesions.

3. **Colon polyps/adenocarcinoma**

a. **Manifestations**

The **specific manifestations** include the presence of intermittent hematochezia and/or melena. There virtually never are any associated upper GI manifestations. Furthermore, the bleeding can be minor and intermittent and, as such, not observed by the patient. There often is an overall paucity of manifestations until the lesion is quite advanced, at which time constipation and even obstipation can be present in addition to unintentional weight loss and/or increased fatigability as a result of iron deficiency anemia.

b. **Pathogenesis**

The **underlying pathogenesis** is one of the development of neoplastic growths in and of the colonic mucosa. The **differential diagnosis** includes benign and malignant neoplastic lesions. The **benign lesions** include the **premalignant** villous and pedunculated adenomas and the **nonpremalignant** hyperplastic polyps, whereas the **malignant lesion** is colon adenocarcinoma itself. The **risk factors** for development of polyps and colon carcinoma include a family history of colon polyps or of polyposis syndromes and/or a personal past history of polyps.

c. **Evaluation and management**

The **specific evaluation and management** include making the clinical diagnosis using the overall approach as described in Box 2-8. Furthermore, **colonoscopy with biopsy** of any and all polyps is required. If adenocarcinoma, surgical intervention is usually indicated, please refer to the section on Colon Carcinoma in Chapter 5 (page 296) for further discussion. Referral to a general surgeon is clearly indicated.

4. **Ischemic bowel**

a. **Manifestations**

The **specific manifestations** include the acute onset of bloody diarrhea associated with abdominal pain which is, early in its course, worse subjectively than objectively. There often is an antecedent episode of hypotension due to another reason, e.g., cardiac, intravascular volume depletion. Furthermore, the patient is invariably quite elderly and has significant atherosclerotic disease.

b. **Pathogenesis**

The **underlying pathogenesis** is the actual necrosis of the bowel wall as a result of hypoperfusion to the bowel, either from an embolism to the artery or after a period of profound hypotension with resultant loss of perfusion. The **natural history** of this is the inevitable rupture of the affected viscus with its resultant severe and **mortal sequelae.**

c. **Evaluation**

Evaluation includes making the clinical diagnosis using the overall approach as described in Box 2-8 and performing an abdominal series. The abdominal series will usually reveal any free air present from a perforation of the ischemic viscus. Colonoscopy should be performed and will reveal, if the large bowel is involved, **friable necrotic mucosa.**

d. **Management**

The **specific management,** once diagnosed and/or suspected, includes admission and emergent consultation with general surgical colleagues. Even with aggressive intervention, the overall prognosis is poor to grave.

5. **Hemorrhoids** (see the section on Anorectal Disorders, page 68)

Caveat: In patients over the age of 50 years, the bleed-

ing may be completely as the result of the hemorrhoids but given the risk that a concurrent etiology
might be present in this age group, **invasive imaging
is clearly indicated,** i.e., flexible proctosigmoidoscopy and air contrast barium enema or a full colonoscopy.
6. **Bloody diarrhea** (see section on Diarrheal States:
Acute, Recurrent, or Chronic, page 79)

II. Consultation

Problem	Service	Time
Any GI bleed requiring admission	Surgery	Urgent
	GI	Emergent
Acute abdomen	Surgery	Emergent
Adenocarcinoma in stomach/colon	Surgery	Urgent
Any evidence of ruptured viscus	Surgery	Emergent
Bloody diarrhea	GI	Urgent/emergent
Epigastric pain with normal HCT/guaiac-positive stools	GI	Required

III. Indications for admission:
Intravascular volume depletion,
melena, significant hematochezia, hypotension, any evidence
of peritoneal signs or the clinical suspicion of an acute abdomen, any anemia requiring transfusion, or the development
or exacerbation of angina pectoris.

Hepatitis

Hepatitis is nonspecific inflammation of the liver. The inflammation can lead to various acute and chronic manifestations and
sequelae, which may be potentially life-threatening of themselves.

I. Pathogenesis
The liver detoxifies **internally produced, biological (usually
catabolic) agents** and **ingested agents,** either biochemical,
chemical, or biological, that are toxic to human cells. In the
process of detoxification, the liver itself can be damaged.
Damage occurs as a result of a **direct effect of the toxin** on
the hepatocytes or as a result of the **inflammatory infiltrate**
that usually develops concurrently with the toxin-related insult. These two mechanisms produce hepatocyte dysfunction
and even acute hepatocyte necrosis.

II. Acute manifestations
The overall **acute manifestations** of hepatitis, irrespective of
cause, include an acute to subacute onset of mild to moderate

nausea, vomiting, and malaise. The patient often describes **clay-colored stools;** the light or clay color occurs as a result of an abnormally decreased secretion of bile into the GI tract with a resultant decrease in pigment in the stool itself. Patients often relate a sensation of **abdominal fullness,** especially in the right upper quadrant, as a result of hepatomegaly. The patient may also have **severe pruritus** as a result of the elevated bilirubin level. Pruritus can be so severe as to be the presenting complaint of the patient. Finally, the patient may relate a history, in the recent or distant past, of **transfusions** of blood or blood products, the **ingestion** of toxic agents (e.g., ethanol or acetaminophen), or the use of **intravenous drugs.**

Examination invariably discloses **icterus** that is especially prominent in the sclerae, mucous membranes, and skin. The icterus occurs as a result of an increase in bilirubin within the body due to a decrease in normal secretion or excretion from the liver. Icterus is usually correlated with a serum bilirubin level above 3.0 mg/dL. Right upper quadrant tenderness with **hepatomegaly** is often present. The normal liver span is 6–12 cm in width and has a smooth, nontender edge on palpation; in acute hepatitis the liver is enlarged and tender. A further manifestation is **darkened urine** as a result of excretion of urobilinogen and bilirubin in the urine instead of in the biliary tree or GI tract. The increased urobilinogen is associated with an increase in plasma conjugated bilirubin, whereas the increased bilirubin in the urine is associated with an increase in the unconjugated bilirubin in the plasma.

III. Hepatitis entities
A. Ethanol-related hepatitis
1. Manifestations
The **specific manifestations** of ethanol abuse, a common cause of acute hepatitis in the United States, include those described in the overall discussion above. Associated manifestations include gynecomastia, palmar erythema, spider angiomas, testicular atrophy, and Dupytren's contracture of the digits. Dupytren's contractures are bilateral acquired flexion contractures of the digits as the result of idiopathic fibrosis of the palmar fascia.

2. Pathogenesis
The **underlying pathogenesis** entails direct hepatocyte damage by ethanol, which results in fatty changes in the liver itself. The inflammatory response is modest and thus plays a negligible role in the overall pathogenesis.

3. **Evaluation**

   Evaluation entails making the clinical diagnosis according to the steps listed in Box 2-9. Whereas all of the **transaminase enzymes** can be and often are elevated in ethanol-related hepatitis, the classic pattern is GGT $\geqslant$ AST (SGOT) > ALT (SGPT). If the acute hepatitis is severe, there can be a concurrent significant increase in the bilirubin with resultant icterus.

4. **Management**

   The **specific management** of ethanol-induced hepatitis includes the steps listed in Box 2-9 and monitoring the patient for the development of withdrawal from ethanol—**delirium tremens.** Furthermore, it is of paramount importance to monitor the patient's **nutritional status** closely as many of these patients are malnourished and can develop symptomatic refeeding hypophosphatemia. An additional note is the potential initiation of **therapeutic steroids** in the setting of severe acute ethanol-related hepatitis. A recent study has demonstrated an overall better outcome in patients with severe ethanol-induced hepatitis who received steroids, relative to the control group. **Severe** was defined as an increased PT, increased bilirubin, severe transaminase elevations, and encephalopathy. The dose of steroids is either prednisone, 40–60 mg PO once daily for 3–7 days, or methylprednisone, 40 mg IV q.8h. for 4–7 days. Finally, consultation with an **addictionologist** should be made in an expedient fashion. Refer to the section on Substance Abuse Syndromes in Chapter 15 (page 748).

B. **Acetaminophen-related hepatitis**

   1. **Manifestations**

      The **specific manifestations** of this entity, which is a not uncommon cause of acute hepatitis in the United States, include those described in the overall discussion above. Acetaminophen can cause significant and severe hepatitis after ingestion of large quantities, either accidentally or in a suicide attempt. The specific manifestations of hepatic damage usually occur 36–48 hours after the ingestion.

   2. **Pathogenesis**

      The **underlying pathogenesis** involves the production of toxic catabolites. In therapeutic doses and in the normal state, acetaminophen is catabolized by the liver into several inactive components that are excreted into the biliary system. The usual pathway produces a catabolite that is conjugated with sulfate

B O X 2 - 9

Overall Evaluation and Management of Suspected Hepatitis

Evaluation

1. Take a thorough **history** and perform a **physical examination** based on the above discussion and that described under Abdominal Pain: Overall Approach.
2. Determine **liver function parameters,** including SGOT, SGPT, LDH, GGT, alkaline phosphatase, total bilirubin, and direct bilirubin. In acute hepatitis, all of these parameters may be elevated, but the transaminase levels (i.e., SGOT, SGPT, and GGT) are all elevated to a greater degree than the alkaline phosphatase and total and direct bilirubin levels.
3. Determine **serum albumin level** and **prothrombin time.** Although they are normal in most cases of acute hepatitis, a decreased albumin level or an elevated PT can occur as a result of superimposed chronic hepatic dysfunction and may portend a more malignant course.
4. Further tests to aid in evaluating the **underlying cause** include determining **ethanol** and **acetaminophen** levels and a **hepatitis A and B panel.**
5. Perform **urinalysis** to test for the presence of bilirubin or urobilinogen in the urine.
6. Consider **imaging studies.** US of the liver and biliary tree demonstrates liver size and any concurrent obstructive findings.
7. If there is any evidence of ethanol abuse, administer 100 mg of **thiamine** PO or IM to prevent the development of Wernicke's encephalopathy.

Acute Management

1. Instruct the patient on **safe sexual practices** (use of condoms, abstinence, etc.).
2. Encourage **good nutrition:** Encourage intake of fluids PO or, if the patient is intravascularly depleted and vomiting, parenterally.
3. Instruct the patient to **discontinue any agents** that may exacerbate the hepatitis or the hepatic dysfunction (i.e., ethanol, oral contraceptives, acetamino-

(continued)

B O X   2 - 9 *(continued)*

phen) and, if possible, other agents that are potentially hepatotoxic, such as the phenothiazines.
4. If the **pruritus** is severe, initiate cholestyramine, 2
   packets PO q.12h. PRN for itching.
5. If a viral cause is suspected or documented, notify
   the Public Health Service.
6. If the patient is CMV negative and if transfusions of
   blood or blood products are necessary, the trans-
   fused substances should, if possible, be CMV negative.
7. **Monitor** liver function test results, glucose, and PT
   closely **longitudinally,** as any decrease in glucose or
   increase in PT is a harbinger of a fulminant, quite
   malignant clinical course.

or glucuronide and is uniformly nontoxic. However,
when a large amount of acetaminophen is ingested
and in need of excretion, an **alternative pathway**
must be used. This alternative pathway involves the
cytochrome P450 system and produces a catabolite
that is a highly toxic **oxidizing agent** and damages
the hepatocytes.

In **normal hepatocytes** there is a concurrent safety
mechanism to inactivate any oxidizing agents. This
agent is the reducing agent **glutathione,** which will
inactivate any oxidizing agent in general and the
toxic catabolite of acetaminophen specifically. Glutathione occurs in limited quantity within the hepatocyte, and in large acetaminophen ingestions the supply is exhausted.

Risk factors for acetaminophen hepatotoxicity include:
a. Anything that activates the P450 system (e.g., ethanol, barbiturates), thereby increasing the production of the toxic catabolite.
b. Chronic ethanol ingestion, which decreases the
   stores of the reducing agent glutathione.
c. Large doses of acetaminophen taken over a short
   period of time.
As with ethanol, the effect is **direct hepatotoxicity.**
The inflammatory response is modest.

3. Evaluation
   Evaluation entails making the clinical diagnosis according to the steps described in Box 2-9. It is of

tremendous importance to ascertain the **quantity of acetaminophen** taken, the **specific time** it was taken, and the **acetaminophen level** at the present time. By knowing the two parameters, acetaminophen level and time since ingestion, one can determine the risk for acute hepatotoxicity. Plasma acetaminophen levels of greater than 200 μg/mL at 4 hours, 100 μg/mL at 8 hours or 50 μg/mL at 12 hours are highly correlated with hepatotoxicity.

4. **Management**

The **specific management** includes, in addition to that described in Box 2-9, management for any **ingestion** (i.e., effective emptying of the gastric contents, either by **Ipecac** or **gastric lavage,** followed by charcoal, 50 g given enterally, which decreases absorption). If the level of acetaminophen is in the toxic range, the immediate initiation of *N*-acetylcysteine (Mucomyst) enterally is mandated. A loading dose of 140 mg/kg PO or per nasogastric tube is followed by a maintenance dose of 70 mg/kg q.4h. PO or by nasogastric tube for 17 doses. This agent decreases toxicity by acting as a **reducing agent** for the toxic catabolites of acetaminophen. A further therapeutic intervention is the initiation of H_2-**receptor antagonists.** These agents decrease the activity of the cytochrome P450 system and thus decrease the production of the toxic catabolite. In all cases, admission and referral to gastroenterology and to psychiatry are indicated.

C. **Viral hepatitis A**

1. **Manifestations**

The **specific manifestations** of this type of hepatitis in addition to those described in the section on Acute Manifestations (page 113) are based on the biology, pathogenesis, and natural history of the virus itself.

The **organism** that causes this quite common form of hepatitis is an **RNA virus** that is transmitted by the fecal–oral route. Epidemics can occur in areas of poor sanitation or by infected patients intimately interacting with others.

The **natural history** includes an **incubation period** (duration of time from exposure to onset of manifestations) **of 2–6 weeks.** The present usually has a 1- to 2-week prodrome of nausea and vomiting, followed by several weeks of mild right upper quadrant pain and mild jaundice. The disease is virtually always self-limited and thus without major acute or long-term complications. It may be asymptomatic.

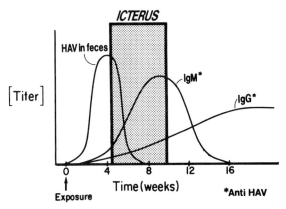

F I G U R E 2 - 2
Hepatitis A serology panel.

2. Evaluation

Evaluation includes making the clinical diagnosis and performing the tests listed in Box 2-9. The **hepatitis A IgM serology** will be positive (Fig. 2-2).

3. Management

The **management** of this self-limiting disorder is as listed in Box 2-9 and consists mainly of **support** and reporting the case to the Public Health Service. The patient should **not** be allowed to work in any occupation involving **contact with foodstuffs** until the hepatitis has resolved.

D. Viral hepatitis B

1. Manifestations

The **specific manifestations** of viral hepatitis B, in addition to those described in the section on Acute Manifestations (page 113) are based on the biology, pathogenesis, and natural history of the virus itself.

The **organism** that causes this quite common form of hepatitis is a **DNA virus** that is transmitted in blood and body fluids. Specific **risk factors** include IV drug abuse, blood transfusions with contaminated blood, and promiscuous sexual habits.

The **natural history** of this entity include an **incubation period** that is quite long and variable, lasting **6–20 weeks** after exposure to the agent. The patient usually has a prodrome of nausea, vomiting, urticaria, and arthralgias that can last for 2–3 weeks, followed by **significant icterus.** The icterus can be quite

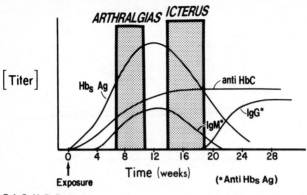

FIGURE 2-3
Hepatitis B serology panel.

severe and associated with pruritus and tender hepatomegaly. This form of viral hepatitis, unlike hepatitis A, can have several severe and potentially mortal complications (see **4. Potential sequelae**).

2. **Evaluation**
   Evaluation includes making the clinical diagnosis as described in Box 2-9. The **hepatitis B surface antigen serology assay** will be positive (Fig. 2-3).

3. **Management**
   The **management** of this self-limited disorder is as listed in Box 2-9 and consists of supportive care, watching for any sequelae, and prophylaxis of contacts.

4. **Potential sequelae of viral hepatitis B**
   a. **Fulminant hepatitis.** This severe and usually fatal sequela can occur during the acute infection or as a "flare" in patients with chronic active hepatitis B infection. This complication occurs in less than 5% of cases but is quite dramatic when it does occur. The patient usually has tremendous increases in transaminases, encephalopathy, coagulopathy, and, most ominously, hypoglycemia. Mortality can be as high as 80%. The **underlying pathogenesis** of this massive necrosis of the liver is thought to be concurrent infection with the delta agent, an RNA virus that parasitizes the DNA hepatitis B virus. Whereas hepatitis B is the highest risk of developing fulminant hepatitis, any type can have a fulminant course.

b. **Chronic active hepatitis.** This development occurs in 2% of all cases of hepatitis B. It can also occur in hepatitis C and other non-A, non-B hepatitides. The patient remains HBsAg-positive for an extended, indefinite period of time and has **chronic significant elevations of the hepatic transaminases.** A **liver biopsy** is required for definitive diagnosis and to completely differentiate this condition from chronic persistent hepatitis. The biopsy will demonstrate a **diffuse mononuclear infiltrate** that extends from the entire lobule and has associated bridging across the entire lobule and concurrent "piecemeal" necrosis of the hepatic tissue.

c. **Chronic persistent hepatitis.** This condition occurs in 5%–10% of all cases of hepatitis B. The patient remains HBsAg-positive for an extended, indefinite period of time but has **no resultant elevations of transaminases.** This condition has a better prognosis than chronic active hepatitis and should be differentiated from it. Because there is a significant amount of clinical overlap between these two sequelae, **liver biopsy** is indicated. Biopsy demonstrates a mononuclear infiltrate in the periportal area but not extending across the entire lobule, and virtually never with any necrosis.

d. **Cirrhosis.** This is the end result of any chronic, severe insult to the liver, irrespective of the cause. Although this diagnosis can usually be made clinically (see section on End-Stage Hepatic Dysfunction, page 91), it truly can only be diagnosed from liver biopsy results. In patients with chronic active hepatitis, the incidence of cirrhosis is 40%, whereas in chronic persistent hepatitis it is much lower, approximately 5%–10%.

e. **Primary hepatocellular carcinoma.** This sequela may occur in association with any chronic or recurrent hepatic insult but it most commonly occurs as a result of chronic infections with HBV.

The **evaluation and management** of these complications usually requires consultation with gastroenterology, preferably with a hepatologist. Often a **liver biopsy** is indicated, and empirical initiation of **α-interferon** can be considered (see section on End-Stage Hepatic Dysfunction, page 91, for a discussion of cirrhosis).

5. **Prophylaxis for contacts of index patient**
   a. **Gamma-globulin IM,** at presentation,
      and

b. **Hepatitis B vaccine:**
    Engerix-B (recombinant), 20 μg IM at 0, 1, and 6 months,
        or
    Recombivax HB, 10 μg IM at 0, 1, and 6 months.
    Hepatitis vaccine should be administered **prophylactically** in the doses and regimens described above to people who are not infected but who are at **high risk for exposure,** such as health care workers, close associates (family members) of IV drug abusers, noninfected IV drug abusers, and noninfected promiscuous people.

IV. Consultation

Problem	Service	Time
Any complication	GI	Urgent/emergent
Any viral hepatitis	Public Health	Required
Overdose in a suicide attempt	Psychiatry	Required

V. Indications for admission: Hypoglycemia, a coagulopathy, any suspicion of an ingestion or suicide attempt, or any evidence of intravascular volume depletion. The majority of patients can be treated as outpatients. Jaundice is not, in and of itself, an indication for admission.

Hernia

Hernias, colloquially referred to as "ruptures," are quite common. The vast majority are discovered and brought to the attention of the patient during a routine physical examination or are known by the patient, who has had it as a stable entity for years and has no specific complaints regarding it. The classic and most useful definition of a hernia is **an abnormal protrusion through an abnormal anatomic defect,** irrespective of the contents of the hernial sac. Hernias can be classified by severity and by location. Each of these classifications is discussed below.

I. **Clinical classification by severity (reducible, incarcerated, strangulated)**
    A. **Reducible hernia**
        A reducible hernia is easily and freely movable through the anatomic defect.
        1. **Manifestations**
            The **specific manifestations** include a nontender mass that occasionally goes away but will return, especially after a Valsalva maneuver. The vast majority of hernias are of this class and are quite asymptom-

atic and invariably found, occasionally to the surprise of the patient, on a routine physical examination.

2. Evaluation and management

The **specific evaluation and management** of this entity include making the clinical diagnosis and documenting the location of the hernia via physical examination. Referral to a general surgeon for **elective herniorrhaphy** should be made.

B. Incarcerated hernia

An incarcerated hernia is one that does not return to normal position spontaneously or with external manipulation.

1. Manifestations

The **specific manifestations** include a nontender soft mass in the inguinal, femoral, or abdominal areas that does not resolve with gentle external manipulation. Often, but not always, the patient will know that the mass is present.

2. Evaluation and management

The **evaluation and management** of this entity include making the clinical diagnosis and documenting the location of the hernia by physical examination. **No attempt to forcibly manually reduce the hernia should be made.** A referral to a general surgeon for **herniorrhaphy on an urgent basis** is indicated, as well as instructing the patient to return immediately if the mass becomes tender.

C. Strangulated hernia

A strangulated hernia is an incarcerated hernia that has developed concurrent edema with resultant ischemia to the structures within the hernial sac.

1. Manifestations

The **specific manifestations** include a tender mass that is nonreducible, fever, diffuse abdominal tenderness, and signs of small or large bowel obstruction (decreased flatus; high-pitched, "tinkling" bowel sounds, vomiting; nausea; and distention of the abdomen).

2. Evaluation and management

The **specific evaluation and management** of this entity include making the clinical diagnosis and documenting the location of the hernia by physical examination. **No attempt to forcibly manually reduce the hernia should be made.** Refer to a general surgeon for **herniorrhaphy on an emergent basis.** The patient must be made NPO, intravenous fluids of normal saline or dextrose 5% with normal saline initiated, and preoperative laboratory examination including CBC with differential, electrolytes, BUN, creatinine, glucose, PT, PTT, platelets, liver function tests, and urinalysis should be obtained. The patient should be typed and screened for blood and have an **abdominal series** performed to look for any signs of perforation (i.e., free air), or any signs of obstruction of the small or large bowel (i.e., multiple air–fluid levels). **Time is of the essence,** as expedient surgical intervention can reverse this potentially life-threatening condition.

II. Classification by anatomic location

Although the locations and mechanism of development are different, each of these can be reducible, incarcerated, or strangulated and in need of elective, urgent, or emergency surgical intervention, respectively. Only the anatomy is described here. Readers are referred to surgical textbooks for specifics on herniorrhaphy procedures.

A. Inguinal hernias

Inguinal hernias occur as the result of a congenital or acquired defect in the connective tissue supporting the inguinal area. There are two types, indirect and direct inguinal hernias.

1. **Indirect.** The anatomic defect is **congenital.** The hernia itself passes through the internal abdominal inguinal ring along the spermatic cord and exits the abdomen through the external inguinal ring. The hernial sac can extend into the scrotum or labium majora. This hernia is much more common in males than in females.

2. **Direct.** The anatomic defect is **acquired.** The hernia itself passes through the posterior inguinal wall immediately medial to the inferior epigastric vessels, i.e., through Hasselbach's triangle. This hernia is more common in males than in females. It is also the hernia that is least likely to incarcerate and thus strangulate.

   Risk factors for development include trauma, **recurrent Valsalva maneuvers** (e.g., lifting heavy objects, straining during bowel movement, and straining to urinate), dysfunctional connective tissue as a result of malnutrition or chronic steroid use. Because this is an acquired lesion, the clinician must determine the underlying mechanism of its occurrence. Therefore, an occupational history is required, as are an evaluation of the colon to rule out any lesion that may cause constipation (e.g., colon adenocarcinoma) and an evaluation of the distal urinary tract to rule out any lesion that may cause obstruction (e.g., prostatic hypertrophy).

B. **Femoral hernias**

In femoral hernias the anatomic defect is in the fascia deep to the inguinal ligament. The hernia sac passes out of the abdominal cavity and into the anterior thigh via abnormally passing through the femoral canal, immediately posterior to the inguinal ligament. It is more common in females than in males. Because the defect is usually small, it can easily become incarcerated and strangulated.

C. **Incisional hernias**

Incisional hernias occur in the site of a previous surgical or traumatic scar, usually in elderly people or those in whom wound healing is poor (e.g., patients taking steroids or those with diabetes mellitus). These hernias can be quite large but rarely will incarcerate because of the large defect size.

D. **Umbilical hernias**

The anatomic defect is in the umbilical ring. These hernias can be either congenital or acquired. **Congenital hernias** usually resolve by age 2 years; if the hernia does not resolve it should be repaired in an expedient manner because congenital umbilical hernias that do not resolve spontaneously have a very high incidence of incarceration and strangulation. **Acquired umbilical hernias** usually occur as a result of chronic increases in intraabdominal pressure, usually as the result of ascites.

III. **Consultation**

Problem	Service	Time
Reducible hernia	General surgery	Elective
Incarcerated hernia	General surgery	Urgent
Strangulated hernia	General surgery	Emergent

IV. **Indications for admission:** Strangulated hernia. Most nonemergent herniorrhaphies can be performed as ambulatory surgery procedures.

Pyrosis and Gastroesophageal Reflux Disease

The **anatomy** of the junction between the esophagus and the stomach is relatively simple. The esophagus, a long, relatively straight and narrow tube normally lined by stratified squamous epithelium, enters into the superior aspect of the stomach, a saclike structure normally lined by simple columnar epithelium. The transition between the mucosa of these two structures is marked by a discrete intraluminal mucosal line, the Z-line.

Both of these structures contribute differently to the overall goal of **food digestion.** The esophagus acts as a conduit for food and fluids to reach the stomach. It has a relatively **normal pH.** The stomach has a major function in the direct digestion of food, and integral to this digestion is an **acidic pH.** In the normal state, the low pH contents of the stomach rarely, if ever, enter the esophagus.

Certain **physiologic mechanisms** keep the low pH contents of the stomach from refluxing into the esophagus. The most important of these is the **lower esophageal sphincter (LES),** a collection of smooth muscle in the wall of the distal esophagus that constricts the luminal size of the distal esophagus in the immediate postprandial state. If the stomach contents do enter the esophagus, the **mucosa** of the esophagus will become damaged. The stratified squamous epithelium changes to a simple columnar epithelium in a process called **metaplasia.**

I. Pathophysiology

The **underlying pathophysiology** in the development of gastroesophageal reflux disease (GERD) and recurrent pyrosis may be an abnormal hypofunctioning of the LES sphincter or chronic increases in intra-abdominal pressure.

A. Abnormal hypofunctioning of the LES

This occurs as the result of the use of nicotine, ethanol-based anticholinergic medications, estrogen agents, or chocolate ingestion.

B. A chronic increase in intra-abdominal pressure

This usually occurs as the result of a significant infradiaphragmatic process, such as ascites, abdominal masses, and pregnancy.

C. Hiatal hernia

It has long been postulated that a **hiatal hernia,** i.e., the abnormal slippage of the stomach through the diaphragm, plays a role in the pathogenesis of pyrosis. This is controversial, and presently a hiatal hernia is thought to play, at most, a minor role in its development.

II. Natural history and sequelae

The **natural history** of this disorder is one of chronic, recurrent symptomatic episodes that can lead to significant sequelae. Some of the most common **sequelae** are described below.

A. Bronchospasm

A not infrequent but under-recognized complication of GERD is the development of reactive airway disease as a result of reflux and inhalation of gastric juices, especially when the patient is recumbent. The patient usually presents with a cough or shortness of breath at night, and in the evaluation no other cause is demonstrable. The pathogenesis of this sequela involves **extrinsic broncho-spasm.** Pulmonary function tests are invariably quite normal. When the GERD is effectively managed, symptoms resolve completely.

B. Barrett's esophagus

This specific complication is usually quite asymptomatic. This process is one in which the chronic reflux of low pH gastric fluids induces **metaplasia** of the distal esophageal mucosa from its normal stratified squamous epithelium to columnar cell epithelium, which is quite similar to gastric mucosa. This metaplasia has been indicated as a potential risk factor in the development of distal esophageal adenocarcinoma. Therefore, once Barrett's esophagus has been confirmed by EGD and biopsy, long-term follow-up is indicated.

C. Esophageal stricture

The distal esophagus can become strictured as a result of the chronic recurrent inflammation and irritation of the mucosa and deeper tissues by GERD.

III. Evaluation

Evaluation of this disorder includes making the clinical diagnosis based on the features listed in Box 2-10. Often esophagogastroduodenoscopy **EGD** is of clinical utility. Whereas EGD is not indicated in all cases, it should be performed in patients with symptoms that do not respond to 6 weeks of standard therapy, or if any abnormalities are demonstrated on an upper GI study, or if there are significant associated symptoms and signs (e.g., hematemesis or odynophagia), or if the process is recurrent. This direct imaging technique allows the clinician to view the mucosa and biopsy any affected areas. If there is any evidence of cough at night or of concurrent wheezing, **pulmonary function tests** should be performed. A final evaluative tool is the **Bernstein test.** A small-caliber nasogastric tube is placed in the distal esophagus. Water and 0.1N HCl are instilled. If symptoms of pyrosis are reproduced with the acid instillation, the picture is consistent with GERD.

IV. Management

The **specific management,** in addition to that described in Box 2-10, includes the initiation of **metoclopramide** (Reglan), a dopamine agonist that aids in gastric emptying through the pylorus and increases LES pressure, resulting in a decrease in GERD symptoms. This medication should be reserved for patients who have failed standard therapy and thus usually have undergone EGD to rule out other pathology.

B O X   2 - 1 0 *(continued)*

***Overall Evaluation and Management of Pyrosis and
Suspected GERD***

Evaluation

1. The **history and physical examination** are of paramount importance in this diagnosis. Salient features
   include:
   a. A burning sensation in the middle of the chest,
      which may mimic angina pectoris.
   b. Dyspnea at night, especially when the patient is ly-
      ing flat; probably a result of reflux-mediated bron-
      chospasm.
   c. Exacerbation of the pyrosis symptoms when the
      patient is lying flat and occasionally after inges-
      tion of spicy foods.
   d. Relief of symptoms with standing or use of ant-
      acids.
   e. Regurgitation of solid and liquid foodstuff.
   f. Sour, acid taste in the mouth.
   g. Halitosis.
   h. "Water brash"—a significant, reflex increase in
      oral saliva usually precipitated by food or an epi-
      sode of pyrosis.
   i. It is quite rare to have significant odynophagia or
      dysphagia associated with GERD unless as a mani-
      festation of the underlying pathologic entity.
   j. Wheezes and evidence of bronchospasm during
      the attack.
2. **Examine** the patient for evidence of abdominal distention and, if present, for a fluid wave, tympany,
   and an enlarged uterus with heartbeats (a gravid
   uterus).
3. Perform **radiographic imaging.** An upper GI series
   can be of benefit in assessment, especially if real-
   time imaging under fluoroscopy demonstrates reflux. Other findings of note include any esophageal
   stricture, any associated peptic ulcer disease, and,
   potentially of import, a hiatal hernia.

Management

1. Educating the patient to dietary modifications (i.e.,
   decrease fats in the diet, decrease weight if obese,

   (continued)

B O X   2 - 1 0

and decrease ethanol and caffeine ingestion, either of which can decrease LES function).
2. Instruct the patient to keep the head of the bed more than 15 degrees from horizontal (not just the pillow, the entire bed head).
3. Discourage the oral intake of food or fluids within 1 hour of bedtime.
4. Prescribe use of antacids at bedtime (e.g., Mylanta II liquid, 15–30 mL PO q.h.s.).
5. Prescribe H_2 blockers at bedtime (e.g., cimetidine, 800 mg PO q.h.s., or ranitidine, 300 mg PO q.h.s.

V. Consultation

Problem	Service	Time
Recurrent GERD	GI	Elective
Chronic GERD (unresponsive)	GI	Elective
Associated symptoms	GI	Required
Abnormalities on upper GI series	GI	Required

VI. Indications for admission: None.

Vomiting

Vomiting is an involuntary process in which the stomach empties its contents to the external environment via the mouth. The bolus of vomitus or emesis is transported from the stomach to the mouth via **reverse peristalsis** in the esophagus. Vomiting usually is a manifestation of another overall medical problem, acute or chronic, but it can be, in and of itself, a problem that needs to be evaluated and managed.

I. Diagnosis
The **differential diagnosis** is quite expansive and includes, but is not limited to, the entities described below.
A. Viral gastroenteritis
1. Manifestations
The **specific manifestations** of vomiting due to viral gastroenteritis include mild to moderate nausea and

vomiting and the associated symptoms and signs of myalgias, low-grade fever, malaise, arthralgias, and nonbloody diarrhea.

2. **Pathogenesis**

   The **underlying pathogenesis** involves a viral infection of the GI tract, usually with an enterovirus or other RNA viral agent. The natural history is that it is acute and self-limited. The majority of patients will self-treat and never present to a physician.

3. **Evaluation and management**

   Evaluation and management include making the clinical diagnosis and supporting the patient as described in Box 2-11.

B. **Medications**

1. **Manifestations**

   The **specific manifestations** of vomiting related to medications include an acute onset of vomiting after the initiation of a specific medication, such as chemotherapeutic agents. This form of vomiting can be severe and can lead to significant intravascular volume depletion.

2. **Pathogenesis**

   The **underlying pathogenesis** is usually an activation of the vomiting center in the brain stem. The **natural history** is that it is acute and self-limited but can be so severe as to cause intravascular volume depletion.

3. **Evaluation and management**

   Evaluation and management include making the clinical diagnosis and supporting the patient as described in Box 2-11. If possible, offending medications should be discontinued. This is a form which, especially if related to chemotherapeutic agents, often requires volume depletion and use of the more potent regimens listed in Table 2-12.

C. **Small bowel obstruction**

1. **Manifestations**

   The **specific manifestations** include an acute onset of nausea and vomiting, intravascular volume depletion, abdominal pain and tenderness, high-pitched, "tinkling" bowel sounds, and decreased flatus. The vomiting can become bilious (green) and then even feculent (malodorous and brown).

2. **Pathogenesis**

   The **underlying pathogenesis** involves a partial or complete obstruction of the small bowel as a result of hernia, adhesions, volvulus, or intussusception. The **natural history** is one in which the vomiting is often intractable and thus requires invasive interven-

---

B O X 2 - 1 1

Overall Evaluation and Management of Vomiting

Evaluation

1. Take a thorough **history** and perform a **physical examination,** looking for any associated abdominal pain, medication use, chest pain, diarrhea, nausea, hematemesis, melena, or hematochezia as clues to the cause of the vomiting. Two specific kinds of vomiting are defined further here:
    a. **Feculent**—Foul-smelling, dark emesis, usually as a result of distal bowel obstruction.
    b. **Hematemesis**—Red, guaiac-positive emesis and/ or emesis with "coffee ground," guaiac-positive material present; usually a result of upper GI bleeding.
2. Determine orthostatic vital signs (i.e., vital signs observed with the patient supine and standing) to assess and document the volume status of the patient.
3. If the patient is orthostatic, determine electrolyte, BUN, creatinine, and glucose levels. Vomiting will cause a loss of chloride, sodium, and potassium, and thus one should expect a **hypochloremic hyponatremic, hypokalemic, metabolic alkalosis.**
4. A **urine pregnancy test** in all fertile females is indicated, as vomiting—"morning sickness"—is quite common.

Management

1. Replace fluid and electrolyte deficits with **normal saline,** and replace any losses of potassium and magnesium.
2. Initiate antinausea agents (see Table 2-12) and specifically treat any underlying cause of the vomiting.

tion, although, especially in partial obstruction, the obstruction may resolve and symptoms improve markedly.

3. **Evaluation and management**
   The **evaluation and management** include making the clinical diagnosis and supporting the patient as de-

TABLE 2-12
Antinausea/Antiemetic Regimens

Agent	Dosage	Side Effects
Prochlorperazine (Compazine)	10 mg PO q.4–6h. PRN, *or* 10–20 mg IM q.4–6h. PRN	Sedation, extrapyramidal manifestations, hypotension
Thiethylperazine (Torecan)	10 mg PO q.4–6h. PRN, *or* 10 mg IM q.4–6h. PRN	Sedation
Droperidol	5–10 mg IM q.4h. PRN *or* 1.0–2.0 mg IV q.4h. PRN	Sedation, orthostatic hypotension
Combination of: Lorazepam (Ativan)	0.5 mg–1.0 mg PO or IM or IV q.6h. PRN	Sedation
Metoclopramide (Reglan)	10 mg PO or IM or IV q.6h. PRN	Sedation, extrapyramidal manifestations (especially in young patients)
Diphenhydramine (Benadryl)	25 mg PO or IM or IV q.4–6h. PRN	Sedation; used to prevent the extrapyramidal side effects of metoclopramide

scribed in Box 2-11. Further evaluation includes obtaining an **abdominal x-ray** looking for air–fluid levels, a finding virtually diagnostic of small bowel obstruction. A baseline CBC count with differential should also be determined. The patient should be made **NPO,** placed on nasogastric suction, and referred to a general surgeon emergently. Admission to the inpatient service is indicated.

D. **Pyloric obstruction, functional or anatomic**
   1. **Manifestations**
      The **specific manifestations** include an acute or subacute onset of nausea and vomiting, modest intravascular volume depletion, epigastric pain, and a succussion splash. The succussion splash is splash sensation/sound upon sitting up fast after ingesting fluids. It may be present in healthy people for up to 15 minutes postprandially, but if it is present for a longer period postprandially, it is a marker for ob-

struction at the gastric pylorus. Quite often the vomiting is postprandial.

2. **Pathogenesis**

The **underlying pathogenesis** involves either a **functional defect,** such as a neuronal dysfunction, usually as a result of diabetes mellitus, or an **anatomic defect,** such as stricture due to peptic ulcer disease. The **natural history** is one in which symptoms recur or become chronic. If the obstruction is due to a functional process, symptoms will wax and wane, but if the obstruction is due to an anatomic process, the symptoms will progressively worsen.

3. **Evaluation and management**

The **evaluation and management** include making the clinical diagnosis and supporting the patient using the regimen described in Box 2-11. An imaging study such as an upper GI survey is indicated to look for any anatomic defects. If it is performed fluoroscopically, any functional defects can also be visualized.

   a. **Functional pyloric obstruction** (no anatomic defects are found but the patient remains symptomatic)—Perform a radionuclide swallowing study to document poor or abnormal gastric emptying. Treatment for this entity is difficult but should include frequent small meals and a trial of metoclopramide (Reglan), 10 mg PO q.i.d. Referral to gastroenterology and/or endocrinology is indicated on an as-needed basis.

   b. **Structural pyloric obstruction** (an anatomic defect is found)—EGD with biopsies is indicated to make the diagnosis. Referral to gastroenterology is clearly indicated in an expedient fashion.

E. **Diabetic ketoacidosis**

1. **Manifestations**

The **specific manifestations** include an acute onset of nausea and vomiting and modest to severe intravascular volume depletion in a patient with a history of diabetes mellitus, usually insulin-dependent. On examination the patient has ketones on his breath and may have the classic, deep, rapid breathing pattern (Kussmaul's respirations) consistent with a metabolic acidosis.

2. **Pathogenesis**

The **underlying pathogenesis** is unclear in a patient with impending or active ketoacidosis from insulinopenic diabetes. The **natural history** is one in which there is acute onset that resolves completely with effective treatment of the diabetic ketoacidosis.

3. Evaluation and management
The **specific evaluation and management** include making the clinical diagnosis and supporting the patient using the regimen described in Box 2-11, and effectively treating the DKA.

F. Acute ethanolism

1. Manifestations
The **specific manifestations** include an acute onset of nausea and vomiting and modest intravascular volume depletion in a patient with a recent history of an ethanol binge. The patient often has the concurrent findings of a "**hangover**," i.e., headache, malaise, and fatigue. The patient invariably knows the diagnosis himself and has had similar episodes after ethanol binges in the past.

2. Natural history
The condition is acute and self-limited.

3. Evaluation and management
The **evaluation and management** include making the clinical diagnosis and supporting the patient using the regimen described in Box 2-11, and administering thiamine, 100 mg IM or IV or PO.

G. Bulimia

1. Manifestations
The **specific manifestations** include recurrent vomiting induced by the patient to lose weight. The patient often has the associated manifestations of a cachectic appearance, secondary amenorrhea, and caries or loss of tooth enamel due to the recurrent self-induced vomiting.

2. Pathogenesis
The **underlying pathogenesis** is a psychiatric disorder characterized by a dysfunctional self-image. It is not uncommon for the patient to abuse other agents, including diuretics and laxatives, and to have concurrent anorexia nervosa. **Natural history:** Chronic and/or recurrent.

3. Evaluation and management
The **specific evaluation and management** include making the clinical diagnosis and supporting the patient using the regimen described in Box 2-11. In addition, the clinician must assess the patient's nutritional status and refer expediently to a psychiatrist.

H. Vomiting due to other causes
Other causes of vomiting include angina pectoris, pancreatitis, gastritis, hepatitis, urinary tract infection, pyelonephritis, pregnancy, pelvic inflammatory disease, and vascular headaches (migraine).

II. Consultation

Problem	Service	Time
Bulimia	Psychiatry	Urgent
Small bowel obstruction	Surgery	Urgent/emergent
Hematemesis	Surgery	Emergent
Pyloric obstruction	Surgery	Required
Pregnancy	OB/GYN	Urgent
PID	OB/GYN	Emergent
Angina pectoris	Cardiology	Emergent
Pyloric obstruction	GI	Urgent

III. **Indications for admission:** Profound intravascular volume depletion, the suspicion of angina or acute coronary syndrome, small bowel obstruction or pyloric obstruction, any upper GI bleeding, peritoneal signs, evidence of pyelonephritis, pregnancy with severe vomiting (hyperemesis gravidarum), and diabetic ketoacidosis.

—D.D.B.

Bibliography

Abdominal Pain, General Approach

Adelman A: Abdominal pain in the primary care setting. J Fam Pract 1987;25:27–32.

Almy T, Howell DA: Diverticular disease of the colon. N Engl J Med 1980;302:324.

Brewer RJ, et al: Abdominal pain. Am J Surg 1976;131:219–223.

Dueholm S, et al: Laboratory aids in the diagnosis of acute appendicitis. Dis Colon Rectum 1989;32:855–859.

Edwards MW, et al: Audit of abdominal pain in general practice. J R Coll Gen Practitioners 1985;35:235–238.

Roth J: Diagnosis and management of colonic diverticulitis. Contemp Gastroenterol 1988;1:7–16.

Staniland JR, et al: Clinical presentation of acute abdomen: Study of 600 patients. Br Med J 1972;3:393–398.

Diarrhea

Blacklow NR, Greenberg HB: Viral gastroenteritis. N Engl J Med 1991;325:252–264.

Canۇey JR: Infectious diarrhea. Am J Med 1985;78:65–71.

DuPont HL: Nonfluid therapy and selected chemoprophylaxis of acute diarrhea. Am J Med 1985;78:81–90.

DuPont HL, et al: Prevention of traveler's diarrhea by the tablet formulation of bismuth subsalicylate. JAMA 1987;257:1347–1350.

Fischer MC, Agger WA: Cryptosporidiosis. Am Fam Pract 1987;36:201–204.

Gerding DN, et al: *Clostridium difficile*-associated diarrhea and colitis in adults. Arch Intern Med 1986;146:95–100.

Gitnick G: Inflammatory bowel diseases: Classification and cancer risk. Am Fam Pract 1989;39:216–220.

Guerrant RL, Bobak DA: Bacterial and protozoal gastroenteritis. N Engl J Med 1991;325:327–340.

Mekhjian HS, et al: Clinical features and natural history of Crohn's disease. Gastroenterology 1979;77:898–906.

Monson TP: Pediatric viral gastroenteritis. Am Fam Pract 1986;34:95–99.

Nelson JD: Etiology and epidemiology of diarrheal diseases in the United States. Am J Med 1985;78:76–80.

Peppercorn MA: Advances in drug therapy for inflammatory bowel disease. Ann Intern Med 1990;112:50–60.

Singleton JW, et al: A trial of sulfasalazine as adjunctive therapy in Crohn's disease. Gastroenterology 1979;77:887–897.

Steffen R, et al: Epidemiology of diarrhea in travelers. JAMA 1983;249:1176–1180.

Teasley DG, et al: Prospective randomized trial of metronidazole versus vancomycin for *Clostridium difficile*-associated diarrhea and colitis. Lancet 1983;2:1043–1046.

Cholelithiasis

Glenn F: Acute acalculous cholecystitis. Ann Surg 1979;189:458–465.

Marton KI, Doubilet P: How to image the gallbladder in suspected cholecystitis. Ann Intern Med 1988;109:722–729.

Welch CE, Malt RA: Surgery of the stomach, gallbladder, and bile ducts. N Engl J Med 1987;316:999–1008.

Wenckert A, Robertson B: The natural history of gallstone disease. Gastroenterology 1966;50:376–381.

Pancreatitis

Fan ST, et al: Early treatment of acute biliary pancreatitis by endoscopic papillotomy. N Engl J Med 1993;328:228–232.

Geokas MC, et al: Acute pancreatitis. Ann Intern Med 1985;103:86–100.

McPhee M: Treatment of acute pancreatitis. Hosp Pract 1985;1:83–90.

Ranson JHC, et al: Prognostic signs and the role of operative management in acute pancreatitis. Surg Gynecol Obstet 1974;139:69–80.

Hepatitis

CDC: Update on hepatitis B prevention. Ann Intern Med 1987;107:353–357.

Chopra S, Griffin PH: Laboratory tests and diagnostic procedures in evaluation of liver disease. Am J Med 1985;79:221–230.

Corless JK, Middleton HM: Normal liver function. Arch Intern Med 1983;143:2291–2287.

Farci P, et al: A long-term study of hepatitis C virus replication in non-A, non-B hepatitis. N Engl J Med 1991;325:98–104.

Kolts BE, Spindel E: Chronic active hepatitis. Am Fam Pract 1984;29:228–243.

Koretz RL: Chronic hepatitis. Am Fam Pract 1989;39:197–202.

Krugman S, et al: Viral hepatitis B: Studies on natural history and prevention re-examined. N Engl J Med 1979;300:101.

McKenna JP, et al: Abnormal liver function tests in asymptomatic patients. Am Fam Pract 1989;39:117–126.

Maddrey WC: Hepatic effects of acetaminophen. J Clin Gastroenterol 1987;9:180–185.

Murray BJ: The hepatitis B carrier state. Am Fam Pract 1986;33:127–133.

Osmon DR, et al: Viral hepatitis. Arch Intern Med 1987;147:1235–1240.

Rumack OH, Matthew H: Acetaminophen poisoning and toxicity. Pediatrics 1975;55:871–876.

Zarro VJ: Acetaminophen overdose. Am Fam Pract 1987;35:235–237.

Peptic Ulcer Disease

Agrawal NM, et al: Misoprostol compared with sucralfate in the prevention of nonsteroidal anti-inflammatory drug-induced gastric ulcer. Ann Intern Med 1991;115:195–200.

Dooley CP, Cohen H: The clinical significance of *Campylobacter pylori*. Ann Intern Med 1988;108:70–79.

Feldman M, Burton ME: Histamine-2 receptor antagonists. N Engl J Med 1990;323:1671–1680.

Feldman M, Burton ME: Histamine-2 receptor antagonists. N Engl J Med 1990;323:1749–1755.

Gough KR, et al: Ranitidine versus cimetidine in prevention of duodenal ulcer relapse. Lancet 1984;2:659–662.

Griffin MR, et al: Nonsteroidal anti-inflammatory drug use and increased risk for peptic ulcer disease in elderly persons. Ann Intern Med 1991; 114:257–262.

Gugler R: Current diagnosis and selection of patients for treatment of peptic ulcer disease. Dig Dis Sci 1985;30:30–35.

Maton PN: Omeprazole. N Engl J Med 1991;324:965–975.

Ohning G, Soll A: Medical treatment of peptic ulcer disease. Am Fam Pract 1989;39:257–270.

Roth SH, Bennett RE: Nonsteroidal antiinflammatory drug gastropathy. Arch Intern Med 1987;147:2093–2100.

Schiller LR, Firdtran JS: Ulcer complications during short-term therapy of duodenal ulcer with active agents and placebo. Gastroenterology 1986; 90:478–481.

Soll AH, et al: Nonsteroidal anti-inflammatory drugs and peptic ulcer disease. Ann Intern Med 1991;114:307–319.

Strum WB: Prevention of duodenal ulcer recurrence. Ann Intern Med 1986;105:757–761.

Gastrointestinal Bleeding

Geelhoed GW: Gastrointestinal bleeding. Am Fam Pract 1984;29:115–125.

Graham DY, Schwartz JT: The spectrum of Mallory–Weiss tears. Medicine 1977;57:307–318.

Johnson RE, Velozzi CJ: Colonic angiodysplasia and blood loss. Am Fam Pract 1985;32:93–102.

Larson DE, Farnell MB: Upper gastrointestinal hemorrhage. Mayo Clin Proc 1983;58:371–387.

Pascal JP, et al: Propranolol in the prevention of first upper gastrointestinal tract hemorrhage in patients with cirrhosis of the liver and esophageal varices. N Engl J Med 1987;317:356–361.

Sauerbruch T, et al: Prophylactic sclerotherapy before the first episode of variceal hemorrhage in patients with cirrhosis. N Engl J Med 1988;319: 8–15.

Sutton FM: Upper gastrointestinal bleeding in patients with esophageal varices. Am J Med 1987;83:273–275.

Wilcox CM, Truss CD: Gastrointestinal bleeding in patients receiving long-term anticoagulant therapy. Am J Med 1988;84:683–690.

Anorectal Disorders

Goldstein SD: Anal fissures and fistulas. Postgrad Med 1987;82:86–92.

Leff E: Hemorrhoids. Postgrad Med 1987;82:95–100.

Moore KT: The outpatient treatment of fissure-in-ano. Br J Clin Pract 1975;
29:181–182.

Parks AG: Pathogenesis and treatment of fistula-in-ano. Br Med J 1961;1:
463–469.

Smith LE, et al: Operative hemorrhoidectomy versus cryoreduction. Dis
Colon Rectum 1979;22:10–16.

Thomson WH: The nature of hemorrhoids. Br J Surg 1975;62:542–552.

Dysphagia/Odynophagia

Bonacini M, et al: The causes of esophageal symptoms in human immunodeficiency virus infection. Arch Intern Med 1991;151:1567–1572.

Dabaghi R, Scott L: Evaluation of esophageal diseases. Am Fam Pract
1986;33:119–129.

Heit HA, et al: Palliative dilation for dysphagia in esophageal carcinoma.
Ann Intern Med 1978;89:629–631.

Katz PO, et al: Esophageal testing of patients with noncardiac chest pain
or dysphagia. Ann Intern Med 1987;106:593–597.

Ott DJ, et al: Radiological evaluation of dysphagia. JAMA 1986;256:2718–
2721.

End-Stage Liver Disease

Busuttil RW, et al: Liver transplantation today. Ann Intern Med 1986;104:
377–389.

Christensen E, et al: Prognostic value of Child–Turcotte criteria in medically treated cirrhosis. Hepatology 1984;4:430–435.

Hoyumpa AM, et al: Hepatic encephalopathy. Gastroenterology 1979;76:
184.

Powell WJ, Klatskin G: Duration of survival in patients with Laennec's
cirrhosis. Am J Med 1968;44:406.

Rector WG: Drug therapy for portal hypertension. Ann Intern Med 1986;
105:96–107.

Runyon BA, et al: The serum-ascites albumin gradient is superior to
exudate-transudate concept in the differential diagnosis of ascites.
Ann Intern Med 1992;117:215–220.

Shear L, et al: Compartmentalization of ascites and edema in patients with
hepatic cirrhosis. N Engl J Med 1970;282:1391.

Vomiting

Drugs for relief of nausea and vomiting. Med Lett 1974;16:46.

Hanson JS, et al: The diagnosis and management of nausea and vomiting:
A review. Am J Gastroenterol 1985;80:210.

Malagelda JR, Camilllieri I: Unexplained vomiting: A diagnostic challenge.
Ann Intern Med 1984;101:211.

Hernias

Dunphy JE, Botsford TW: Physical examination of the surgical patient, in
An Introduction to Clinical Surgery, 4th ed, p 117. Philadelphia,
WB Saunders, 1975

Pyrosis/GERD

Adelman AM: Management of dyspepsia. Am Fam Pract 1987;35:222–230.

Barish CF, et al: Respiratory complications of gastroesophageal reflux. Arch Intern Med 1988;145:1882–1888.

Bozymski EM, et al: Barrett's esophagus. Ann Intern Med 1982;97:103–107.

Kitchin LI, Castell DO: Rationale and efficacy of conservative therapy for gastroesophageal reflux disease. Arch Intern Med 1991;151:448–454.

Lieberman DA: Medical therapy for chronic reflux esophagitis. Arch Intern Med 1987;147:1717–1720.

Lieberman DA, Keeffe EB: Treatment of severe reflux esophagitis with cimetidine and metoclopramide. Ann Intern Med 1986;104:21–26.

—D.D.B.

Dale Berg, Ed. *Handbook of Primary Care Medicine.* Copyright © 1993 J. B. Lippincott Company.

CHAPTER 3

Renal Disorders and Hypertension

Hematuria

The filtering efficiency of the kidneys is tremendous. The entire volume of blood is continuously and effectively filtered in the glomeruli. The **effectiveness** of the filter is matched only by its **specificity.** This is clearly demonstrated by the fact that only negligible amounts of albumin, plasma proteins, and cellular elements are lost in the urine. The specificity, however, is not 100%, even in the normal setting. It has been demonstrated that in the normal setting less than 1,000 RBCs are lost in the urine per minute, an essentially negligible loss. This loss is below the level of clinical detection by either the dipstick method or microscopic analysis.

Therefore, any blood loss greater than **approximately 1,000 RBCs/min** is, by definition, the pathologic problem **hematuria.** There are two categories of clinical hematuria, microscopic and gross.

1. **Microscopic hematuria.** This is an abnormal loss of RBCs in the urine that remains undetectable by visual examination of the urine. The loss of RBCs is in excess of >1000 RBCs/min. The problem is detected by the dipstick analysis or by microscopic evaluation of the urine sample. The hematuria is unknown to the patient.
2. **Gross hematuria.** Red- or brown-colored urine, usually of acute onset. It may be the chief presenting complaint. Usually gross or macroscopic hematuria is >1,000,000 RBCs lost per minute.

   Other conditions can cause significant brown or red discoloration to the urine. These conditions include **bilirubinuria, myoglobinuria,** and **medication-induced discoloration,** particularly that induced by rifampin. The dipstick test and microscopic urinalysis will differentiate these conditions from gross hematuria.

I. Differential diagnosis

The **differential diagnosis** of red- or brown-colored urine includes the following entities. The most common causes, especially of painful hematuria, are infections of the urinary tract and nephrolithiasis.

A. Coagulopathy

1. **Manifestations**

   The **specific manifestations** include microscopic and/or macroscopic hematuria with the acute to subacute onset of nonpalpable purpura, multiple petechiae, GI bleeding, easy bruising, menorrhagia, or recurrent epistaxis. Usually no urinary tract symptoms are present.

2. **Pathogenesis**

   The **underlying pathogenesis** is a defect of coagulation. Thrombocytopenia, elevations in PT or PTT, and any consumptive or hypoproductive coagulopathy can manifest with microscopic or macroscopic hematuria. Usually the hematuria is a small component of the overall constellation of presenting signs and symptoms.

3. **Evaluation and management**

   The **specific evaluation and management** of hematuria due to a coagulopathy include making the clinical diagnosis using the evaluative tools described in Box 3-1 and managing the underlying coagulopathy. Expedient referral to hematology is indicated. (See the section on excessive bleeding states in Chapter 5, page 275.)

   NOTE: A coagulopathy will **unmask any concurrent primary urinary tract lesion** and therefore should not be accepted as the cause of hematuria until a complete evaluation has been performed.

B. Urinary tract infection, bacterial

1. **Manifestations**

   The **specific manifestations** usually include dysuria, pyuria, and hesitancy. The patient may have flank pain and tenderness in the costovertebral angle, especially if pyelonephritis is present concurrently. Other associated manifestations include nausea, vomiting, and fever. If prostatitis is present, the prostate will be enlarged, boggy, and tender.

2. **Pathogenesis**

   The **underlying pathogenesis** is a bacterial urinary tract infection which progresses from the urethra

B O X 3 - 1

Overall Evaluation of Hematuria, Microscopic and Gross

Evaluation

1. Take a thorough **history** and perform a **physical examination,** including a prostate examination in males, looking for tenderness or enlargement, and a pelvic examination in females, looking for menstrual flow or cervical tenderness.
2. Obtain a urine specimen for **urinalysis** by dipstick and microscopic analysis. This test is **mandatory.** Specific methods of urine collection are described in Table 3-1.
3. If an **infectious etiology** is suspected as evidenced by prostate tenderness, pyuria concurrent with hematuria, or a positive nitrite or positive leukocyte esterase assay, send urine for culture and sensitivity testing and treat the patient with antibiotics. (See discussion in the text and in the section on Pyuria Syndromes, page 172.)
4. If **nephritic sediment** is present (i.e., hematuria, RBC casts, proteinuria, and fat oval bodies), the following laboratory tests are indicated to evaluate the patient for an underlying vasculitis, glomerulonephritis.
   a. Antinuclear antibody (ANA) assay.
   b. Anti-dsDNA assay.
   c. Antistreptolysin O (ASO) titer.
   d. CH_{50} of serum.
   e. C_3 and C_4 levels in serum.
5. If **no specific cause** of the problem is evident from the above tests or if the problem is **recurrent,** perform the following studies:
   a. Urine culture and sensitivity tests.
   b. Urine myoglobin test. Myoglobin, a breakdown product of muscle, may produce a dark discoloration of urine.
   c. CBC count with differential, looking for any concurrent anemia.
   d. Platelet count, PT, and aPTT, looking for evidence of a concurrent or antecedent coagulopathy.
   e. Chest radiography, PA and lateral views, looking

(continued)

B O X 3 - 1 (continued)

> for any granulomatous disease suggestive of my-
> cobacterial disease or Wegener's granulomatosis.
> f. PPD test with controls applied to the skin, looking
>   for exposure to mycobacterial disease.
> g. Urine cytology. To optimize the sensitivity of this
>   test, use the first urine sample of the morning.
> h. Acid-fast bacilli (AFB) smear and culture of urine.
>   To optimize the sensitivity of these tests, use the
>   first urine sample of the morning.
> i. Serum electrolytes, BUN, and creatinine, for base-
>   line purposes.
> j. Ultrasound of the kidneys to demonstrate any re-
>   nal parenchymal lesions, nephrolithiasis, or ob-
>   struction.
> k. CT of the kidneys if any abnormality is present on
>   the renal US study.
> l. Referral to genitourinary surgeons for **cystoscopy,**
>   i.e., the direct imaging and, if needed, biopsy of
>   the mucosa of the urinary tract.

proximally to the kidneys. (See section on Pyuria
Syndromes, page 172, for further discussion.)

3. **Evaluation and management**

   The **specific evaluation and management** of hematuria due to a bacterial urinary tract infection include making the clinical diagnosis using the evaluative tools described in Box 3-1, sending the urine
   for culture, initiating antibiotics to treat the most
   likely infections, and determining the underlying
   reason for the development of the bacterial urinary
   tract infection. **Antibiotic regimens** can include
   TMP–sulfa drugs (Bactrim DS), 1 tablet PO b.i.d.
   for 7 days, or amoxicillin, 500 mg PO q.i.d. for 7
   days, or Ciprofloxacin, 500 mg PO b.i.d. for 7 days.
   Check the culture and sensitivity results to make
   certain that the pathogen is sensitive to the antibiotic regimen used. (See section on Pyuria Syndromes, page 172, for further details.)

C. **Urinary tract infection, mycobacterial**

   1. **Manifestations**

      The patient is invariably asymptomatic, and thus,
      this is a true form of **painless hematuria.** Query the

T A B L E 3 - 1
Methods of Collecting Urine for Analysis

"Clean Catch" Sample: The patient, after cleaning the urethral orifice with an antiseptic solution such as an alcohol wipe, urinates. A sample of urine is collected midway through the stream.

Advantages
    Noninvasive
    Efficient
    Easy to perform
    Minimal patient discomfort and embarrassment

Disadvantages
    Sample is easily contaminated with extra-urinary fluids such as vaginal secretions, menstrual blood, and, in the uncircumcised man, smegma.

Urinary Bladder Catheterization (i.e., straight catheterization): A narrow-gauge soft rubber catheter is inserted by sterile technique into the urinary bladder via the urethra.

Advantages
    Yields uncontaminated specimen
    Optimal sensitivity and specificity of culture results
    Method can be used to determine residual volume if partial distal obstruction is suspected (e.g., in benign prostatic hypertrophy): instruct the patient to void completely, then perform straight catheterization; normally there will be <30 mL of urine; >30–50 mL is evidence of partial obstruction

Disadvantages
    Invasive
    Causes patient discomfort
    Can give a false positive indication of microscopic hematuria due to catheter-related trauma of the urethra

patient for any exposure to mycobacterial disease, any risk factors for development, and, if the patient has had a mycobacterial disease, what therapy was administered.

2. **Pathogenesis**

The **underlying pathogenesis** of this fairly rare cause of hematuria is of an infection of the kidney by *Mycobacterium hominis*. Usually the infection is hematogenously spread from another site, usually pulmonary.

3. **Evaluation and management**

The **specific evaluation and management** of hematuria due to a mycobacterial urinary tract infection include making the clinical diagnosis using the evaluative tools described in Box 3-1 and treating the underlying infection. Obtain a morning urine specimen for AFB smear and culture. Perform PPD skin tests, unless the skin PPD was reactive in the past. Referral to GU and infectious disease experts is indicated. (See section on Mycobacterial Diseases in Chapter 4 for further details.)

D. Trauma

　1. Manifestations

　　Except for manifestations attributable to trauma to the back or flank, there are few associated manifestations. Trauma may cause **painless hematuria.**

　2. Pathogenesis

　　The **underlying pathogenesis** is significant trauma to the kidneys or urinary bladder with resultant damage to these structures. The most dramatic event is trauma-induced rupture of the kidney.

　3. Evaluation and management

　　The **specific evaluation and management** of hematuria due to trauma include making the clinical diagnosis using the evaluative tools described in Box 3-1 and immediate referral to GU.

E. Transitional cell carcinoma of the bladder

　1. Manifestations

　　Transitional cell carcinoma of the bladder is invariably asymptomatic in its early, curable stage. This results in painless microscopic hematuria.

　2. Pathogenesis

　　The **underlying pathogenesis** is a primary malignant neoplasm in the mucosa of the urinary bladder.

　3. Evaluation and management

　　The **specific evaluation and management** of hematuria due to transitional cell carcinoma of the bladder include making the clinical diagnosis using the evaluative tools described in Box 3-1 and immediate referral to GU. A morning urine specimen for cytology, looking for malignant cells shed in the urine, should be obtained at the outset. The first morning specimen has remained in the bladder overnight, which increases the sensitivity of the examination.

F. Adenocarcinoma (clear cell carcinoma) of the kidney

　1. Manifestations

　　Adenocarcinoma of the kidney is invariably asymptomatic in its early, curable stage. This results in **painless microscopic hematuria.**

　2. Pathogenesis

　　The **underlying pathogenesis** is a primary malignant neoplasm in the renal parenchyma.

　3. Evaluation and management

　　The **specific evaluation and management** of hematuria due to adenocarcinoma of the kidney include making the clinical diagnosis using the evaluative tools described in Box 3-1 and immediate referral to GU. A morning urine specimen for **cytology,** looking for malignant cells shed in the urine, should be obtained at the outset. The first morning specimen has remained in the bladder overnight, which increases the sensitivity of the examination.

G. Berger's disease

1. **Manifestations**

   The **specific manifestations** of this not uncommon cause of microscopic painless hematuria in adults are few. In fact, it is invariably asymptomatic.

2. **Pathogenesis**

   The **underlying pathogenesis** is an IgA nephropathy, which is quite benign and rarely progresses to any renal dysfunction.

3. **Evaluation and management**

   The **specific evaluation and management** of hematuria due to Berger's disease include making the clinical diagnosis using the evaluative tools described in Box 3-1 and serum protein electrophoresis. The IgA titer will be elevated in Henoch–Schönlein purpura and Berger's disease, but Berger's disease will not have any of the extrarenal manifestations of Henoch–Schönlein purpura. Referral to nephrology is encouraged, but once the diagnosis is confirmed, reassurance and observation are the interventions required.

H. Henoch–Schönlein syndrome

1. **Manifestations**

   The **specific manifestations** include the development of nonpalpable purpura on the lower extremities with no evidence of concurrent or antecedent coagulopathy; arthralgias; painless microscopic or gross hematuria; and an increased risk of intussusception of the distal small bowel (ileum). The incidence is highest in children and young adults.

2. **Pathogenesis**

   The **underlying pathogenesis** of this systemic disease is not completely known but probably is autoimmune in nature. **Natural history:** The disease is usually **self-limited.**

3. **Evaluation and management**

   The **specific evaluation and management** of hematuria due to Henoch–Schönlein syndrome include making the clinical diagnosis using the evaluative tools described in Box 3-1 and serum protein electrophoresis. The IgA titer will be elevated in Henoch–Schönlein purpura and Berger's disease, but Berger's disease will not have any of the extrarenal manifestations of Henoch–Schönlein purpura. Referral to nephrology, initiation of salicylates (aspirin, 325 g q.6h.), and observing for sequelae are indicated.

I. **Medications**

Although many different medications can cause a discoloration to the urine, few will result in true hematuria. The medication most commonly described as causing microscopic or macroscopic hematuria is the chemotherapeutic and alkylating agent cyclophosphamide (Cytoxan).

1. **Manifestations**

The **specific manifestations** can include massive hematuria with a decrease in hematocrit and the potential for hemodynamic instability.

2. **Pathogenesis**

The **underlying pathogenesis** is direct irritation of the bladder mucosa by an agent or its catabolites.

3. **Evaluation and management**

The **evaluation and management** of medication-induced hematuria include making the clinical diagnosis using the evaluative tools described in Box 3-1 and referral to nephrology. The best treatment method is prevention. Specific modalities of prevention of the cyclophosphamide-induced hemorrhagic cystis include maintaining a urine output of greater than 100 mL/hr and the concurrent administration of the agent MESNA. MESNA is an agent that binds to and inactivates the active catabolites of cyclophosphamide in the urine, thereby preventing urinary bladder mucosal damage.

J. **Nephrolithiasis**

Nephrolithiasis causes painful hematuria and is discussed later in this chapter (page 159).

II. **Consultation**

Problem	Service	Time
Nephritic sediment	Renal	Urgent
Acute renal failure	Renal	Emergent
Nephrolithiasis	Renal	Elective
Recurrent prostatitis	GU	Elective
Unexplained hematuria	GU	Urgent
Any positive cytology	GU	Urgent

III. **Indications for admission:** Massive hematuria, evidence of pyelonephritis, any concurrent acute renal failure, or any evidence of obstruction.

Hypertension

Hypertension is a disease process of significant import for health care in the United States and the industrial nations of the world. It is quite **prevalent** in the United States and is also virtually **asymptomatic** until it manifests with morbid, even mortal sequelae. Because it is prevalent and asymptomatic early in its course, because the sequelae of untreated hypertension are significant, and because early and chronic treatment has been demonstrated to prevent the morbid and mortal sequelae, hypertension is a disease for which screening is beneficial. Fortunately, **effective screening techniques** are available. The best is a **blood pressure check** at the physician's office or at a clinic or a health fair every 6 months.

I. **Overall manifestations**

The **overall manifestations** of renal hypertension are few **early** in the course of the disease. The patient may present to a primary care physician after having an elevated blood pressure reading at a screening location or in the physician's office. Table 3-2 lists diagnostic criteria published by the Joint National Commission on the Detection, Evaluation, and Treatment of High Blood Pressure. Unless the patient presents with a hypertensive urgency or emergency, the blood pressure must be measured at **three different times** over a period of 1 to 2 weeks to confirm the diagnosis.

II. **Pathogenesis**

The **underlying pathogenesis** is a chronic increase in systolic and diastolic arterial blood pressure. The arterial tree

T A B L E   3 - 2
Categories of Hypertension

Diastolic Pressure

<85 mm Hg	Normal
85–89 mm Hg	High normal
90–104 mm Hg	Mild hypertension
105–114 mm Hg	Moderate hypertension
>115 mm Hg	Severe hypertension

Systolic Pressure (when the diastolic pressure is <90 mm Hg)

<140 mm Hg	Normal
140–160 mm Hg	Isolated borderline systolic hypertension
>160 mm Hg	Isolated systolic hypertension

(Modified from the Joint National Committee on the Detection, Evaluation, and Treatment of High Blood Pressure. 1988 Report. Arch Intern Med 1988;148:1023.)

can be thought of as a plumbing system in which the heart is the pump, the blood is the water, and the arteries are the pipes. Blood pressure is the product of the cardiac output (i.e., the pump function) and the total peripheral resistance of the arterial bed (i.e., the overall decrease in caliber of the pipes). Therefore, blood pressure can be increased by an increase in cardiac output or by an increase in arterial resistance to flow. Two different **categories of mechanisms** are known in the pathogenesis of hypertension, **primary** and **secondary.**

A. **Primary or idiopathic arterial hypertension** is the result of either an increase in cardiac output or an increase in the total peripheral resistance. The exact mechanism is unknown. The vast majority of patients with hypertension have primary hypertension.

B. **Secondary arterial hypertension** occurs as a result of a known, definable, and potentially curable underlying cause. A mechanism of secondary hypertension can be demonstrated in a small but significant minority of patients, about 10%–15%. Secondary causes include disorders of the endocrine, renal, and vascular systems. Table 3-3 lists specific causes of secondary hypertension.

   1. The **endocrine** lesions that can result in hypertension include hypercortisolism, hyperaldosteronism, pheochromocytoma, and hypothyroidism.

      a. **Hypercortisolism,** either iatrogenic or as the result of adrenal hyperplasia or adrenal hyperfunction with increased levels of glucocorticoids, results in hypertension with concurrent hypokalemia. Other specific manifestations of this cause of secondary hypertension include truncal obesity, hyperglycemia, and an increased incidence of cutaneous fungal infections.

T A B L E 3 - 3
Some Causes of Secondary Hypertension

1. Hypercortisolism
   a. Cushing's disease
   b. Cushing's syndrome
   c. Iatrogenic
2. Primary hyperaldosteronism (Conn's syndrome)
3. Renal arterial stenosis
4. Pheochromocytoma
5. Coarctation of the aorta
6. Hypothyroidism
7. Renal failure

b. **Hyperaldosteronism,** or Conn's disease, is hyperplasia or adenoma of the zona glomerulosa of the adrenal gland with increased levels of mineralocorticoids. This results in hypertension with concurrent hypokalemia.

c. **Pheochromocytoma** is the hyperplasia or adenoma of the adrenal medulla or of a sympathetic ganglion with increased levels of the catecholamines, either epinephrine or norepinephrine. Other specific manifestations include supraventricular or ventricular tachycardia, hypertension, paradoxical orthostatic hypotension, and hypokalemia.

d. **Hypothyroidism** is the decrease in thyroid hormone with resultant manifestations of thyroid hormone deficiency, cold, decreased energy, constipation, and hypertension (see section on thyroid dysfunctional states in Chapter 9, page 541).

2. The **renal lesions** that may result in hypertension include any significant renal failure or renal arterial stenosis.

a. **Renal failure** results in hypertension via multiple mechanisms, including chronic volume overload and the potential development of secondary hyperaldosteronism. Other specific manifestations include those described in the section on Renal Dysfunction, page 181.

b. **Renal arterial stenosis** occurs as a result of either atherosclerosis or fibromuscular hyperplasia. In arterial stenosis, a decrease in perfusion of the kidneys results in an increase in aldosterone and renin, with resultant hypertension and hypokalemia. Specific manifestations include an abdominal bruit.

3. The **vascular etiology** of hypertension is **coarctation of the aorta.** This is a rare entity which manifests with unilateral upper extremity hypertension with concurrent relative hypotension in other **extremities.**

III. Natural history

If untreated, hypertension will result in damage to any and potentially all areas of the arterial system. To continue the analogy with a closed plumbing system, the chronic elevation of fluid pressure (i.e., arterial pressure elevation) damages not only the pipes (the arteries), the pump (the heart), but also any filter system (the kidneys). These sequelae, which usually occur only after a long history of uncon-

trolled hypertension and also referred to as **"target organ"
damage,** include the following:

A. **Cardiac dysfunction.** There is abnormal hypertrophy of
the left ventricle in patients with longstanding uncontrolled hypertension. The hypertrophy causes a problem with filling of the ventricle and thus causes diastolic heart failure. Over time, the ventricle evolves
from hypertrophy to dilation and frank systolic heart
failure.

B. **Renal failure,** invariably antedated by proteinuria.

C. **Cerebrovascular accidents** as a result of hemorrhage in
the intracranial space or thrombotic infarctions.

D. Damage to the **thoracic and abdominal aorta,** with resultant **dissection** or **aneurysm formation.**

E. **Acceleration of atherosclerotic disease.** This acceleration of atherosclerotic disease is of tremendous import:
along with cigarette smoking, diabetes mellitus, obesity,
and hypercholesterolemia, it is a major risk factor in the
development of atherosclerotic heart disease and cerebrovascular atherosclerotic disease.

IV. **Manifestations of late hypertension**
The **specific manifestations of late, uncontrolled hypertension** reflect the natural history of the disease and the known
areas of target organ damage.

A. **Cardiac manifestations** include cardiomegaly, a fourth
heart sound, and, if heart failure is present, orthopnea,
paroxysmal nocturnal dyspnea, bipedal edema, dyspnea on exertion, a third heart sound, and crackles in
the lung fields. Furthermore, the entity can manifest
with the findings of ischemic heart disease, either angina pectoris or an acute coronary syndrome such as
a myocardial infarction (see section on Chest Pain in
Chapter 1, page 3).

B. **Renal manifestations** include pedal edema, anasarca,
and an exacerbation of symptoms of heart failure (see
section on Renal Dysfunction, page 181).

C. **Other manifestations** include a cerebrovascular accident; a palpable, pulsatile abdominal mass, indicative
of an abdominal aortic aneurysm; and retinopathy on
funduscopy.

V. **Management**
The **overall management** of hypertension entails documenting its presence, documenting any sequelae, and
screening for and evaluating any secondary cause (see
Boxes 3-2 and 3-3). The **specific management** includes the
following basic concepts:

A. Use **nonmedical management** as first-line therapy for

BOX 3-2

Overall Evaluation of Newly Diagnosed Renal Hypertension

1. **Make certain that the episode is not a hypertensive emergency or urgency.**
2. Take a thorough **history** and perform a **physical examination,** looking for a **history of diabetes mellitus,** the age of first elevated blood pressure, any concurrent medication use, the quantity of ethanol ingested, and any symptoms referable to target organ damage. The **physical examination** includes determining the blood pressure in both arms to look for coarctation of the aorta; a cardiac examination for PMI displacement and a third or fourth heart sound; an extremity examination for edema; an abdominal examination for pulsatile or nonpulsatile masses or bruits; and a funduscopic examination to look for any microvascular disease. **Funduscopy is mandatory.**
3. Determine electrolyte, BUN, and creatinine levels for baseline purposes and to look for any concurrent hypokalemia, hyperglycemia, or renal dysfunction.
4. Perform urinalysis with microscopic examination to look for proteinuria or a nephritic sediment.
5. Determine calcium, phosphorus, and albumin levels as part of baseline evaluation.
6. Obtain a **12-lead ECG** for baseline purposes and to look for any evidence of left ventricular hypertrophy.
7. Obtain **chest radiographs** in PA and lateral views to look for any left ventricular hypertrophy.
8. If there is any evidence of heart failure or of LV hypertrophy on the ECG, obtain an echocardiogram to determine the size and wall motion activity of the left ventricle.
9. If there is any evidence of a pulsatile mass in the abdomen, image the abdomen with CT or US to define the probable abdominal aortic aneurysm.
10. Evaluation for secondary hypertension should be performed only in patients who are at risk or who have specific markers that make a secondary etiol-

(continued)

B O X   3 - 2 (continued)

ogy more likely (see Box 3-3 for the evaluation of
secondary hypertension). Patients in whom an evaluation for secondary hypertension should be performed include:
a. Those with **concurrent hypokalemia** or **hypomag-
   nesemia.**
b. Those with a **renal bruit.**
c. Those with an **onset** at age <25 years or >65
   years.
d. Those with orthostatic manifestations or concurrent tachydysrhythmias.
e. Those with disease **difficult to control.**

B O X   3 - 3

Evaluation of Suspected Secondary Hypertension

1. If **hypercortisolism** is suspected:
   a. Perform a 24-hour urine collection for free cortisol
      and creatinine. The urinary cortisol will be ele-
      vated in hypercortisolism.
2. If **renal arterial stenosis** is suspected:
   a. Image the kidneys with US to determine their
      size.
   b. Perform angiography of the renal arteries, looking
      for stenosis of the renal artery.
3. If **pheochromocytoma** is suspected:
   a. Perform a 24-hour collection for fractionated cate-
      cholamines, metanephrines, and creatinine. The
      catecholamines and/or metanephrines will be ele-
      vated in pheochromocytoma.
4. If **Conn's syndrome** is suspected:
   a. Determine plasma renin activity (PRA) and
      plasma aldosterone level. If the aldosterone/PRA
      ratio is >20, the result is consistent with Conn's
      syndrome.

mild to moderate hypertension. This includes limiting salt intake, weight reduction if the patient is obese, and prescription of an exercise program.

B. If and when pharmacologic intervention is required, use agents that optimize compliance, such as those with **minimal side effects;** that can be taken in a **once daily regimen;** and that are effective as **monotherapy.**

C. **Modify other risk factors** for the development of atherosclerotic heart disease to minimize the risk factor profile. This is even more important given the fact that some of the antihypertensive agents (listed in Table 3-4), while decreasing blood pressure, actually worsen the risk factor of hypercholesterolemia via increasing LDL or decreasing HDL cholesterol levels.

D. If **other disease processes are present,** attempt to use agents which will treat that disease and the hypertension concurrently. Examples include:

1. Hypertension with **concurrent angina pectoris.** Treatment can include nitrates and/or β-blockers (if not contraindicated) and/or calcium channel blockers.

2. Hypertension with **concurrent left ventricular failure.** An angiotensin-converting enzyme (ACE) inhibitor is strongly indicated to decrease afterload.

3. Hypertension with **concurrent diabetes mellitus.** An ACE inhibitor is strongly indicated, as recent data indicate that an ACE inhibitor may slow or even prevent the development of nephropathy in hypertensive diabetics.

4. The agents that fit the **best profile** today (i.e., have minimal side effects, have a long duration of action resulting in once daily dosing, and provide effective control of hypertension without exacerbating other risk factors for atherosclerotic disease) are **calcium channel blockers** or **ACE inhibitors.** An agent from either one of these categories should be initiated and titrated to establish a normal arterial blood pressure or to maximal dosage. If maximal dosage is reached without effective arterial pressure control, another agent can be added and increased, again titrated to the normal blood pressure range. Table 3-4 lists commonly used antihypertensive agents.

VI. Hypertensive emergencies

A **hypertensive emergency** is defined as an acute syndrome directly attributable to the hypertension that will, if the hypertension is not emergently treated, result in severe morbidity or mortality. The patient is hypertensive, usually

T A B L E 3 - 4
Antihypertensives

Dosages are given in ranges. In general, start with a low dose and gradually increase it.

Nonpharmacologic Therapy

Institute a 2-g sodium diet
Encourage weight loss, if patient is obese
Prescribe **regular exercise**
Minimize the use of NSAIDs, as these agents will cause fluid retention and exacerbate the hypertension
Minimize other risk factors for atherosclerotic disease. Measures include:
    smoking cessation
    weight loss
    control of diabetes mellitus
    control of hyperlipidemia

Diuretic Agents

Hydrochlorothiazide
    Dose: 25–50 mg/day PO
Dyazide (triamterene 50 mg, hydrochlorothiazide 25 mg)
    Dose: 1 tablet/day PO
Maxide (triamterene 75 mg, hydrochlorothiazide 50 mg)
    Dose: ½ to 1 tablet/day PO
Potential **side effects of thiazide diuretics**
    Decreased intravascular volume
    Increased renin
    Hypocationemia
    Hyperuricemia
    Increased LDL, increased VLDL (HDL unchanged)
Potential **side effect of triamterene**
    Hyperkalemia, especially in patients with type IV renal tubular acidosis (patients with concurrent diabetes mellitus often have this type of tubular dysfunction)

β-Blockers

Metoprolol (Lopressor)
    Dose: 50–100 mg PO b.i.d.
    Tablet size: 50 mg
    β_1 selective
Atenolol (Tenormin)
    Dose: 50–100 mg/day PO
    Tablet size: 50 mg
    β_1 selective
Contraindications to use of β-blockers
    Heart failure
    Second-degree or greater AV nodal block
    Intermittent claudication
    Reversible airway disease
Potential **side effects** of β-blockers
    Exacerbation of preexisting heart failure
    Exacerbation of AV nodal block

(continued)

T A B L E   3 - 4 (continued)

Exacerbation of intermittent claudication
Exacerbation of reversible airway disease
Development of impotence
A decrease in HDL lipoproteins

Angiotensin-Converting Enzyme (ACE) Inhibitors

Captopril
  Dose: 6.25–25 mg PO q.8–12h.
  Tablet size: 25 mg
Enalapril
  Dose: 2.5–10 mg/day PO
  Tablet size: 2.5–5 mg
Lisinopril
  Dose: 2.5–10 mg/day PO
  Tablet size: 5 mg
Side effects of ACE inhibitors
  Proteinuria
  Angioedema (deep tissue swelling)
  Lupus-like syndrome
  Hyperkalemia
  Leukopenia
  Bronchospasm, nocturnal cough
  Exacerbation of renal failure

Calcium Channel Blockers

Verapamil
  Dose: 40–80 mg PO t.i.d.
  Tablet size: 80 mg
  Sustained release form:
  Dose: 120–240 mg/day PO
  Tablet size: 120 mg and 240 mg
Diltiazem
  Dose: 30–120 mg PO t.i.d. to q.i.d.
  Tablet size: 30 mg and 60 mg
  Sustained release form:
  Dose: 60 mg PO b.i.d.
  Tablet size: 60 mg
Nifedipine
  Dose: 10–20 mg PO b.i.d. to t.i.d.
  Tablet size: 10 mg
  Sustained release form:
  Dose: 30–60 mg PO q. A.M.
  Tablet size: 30 mg
Mechanism of action (MOA)
  Calcium channel blocking agents act via three major mechanisms:
  suppression of the AV node, vasodilation of the arterial bed with re-
  sultant afterload reduction, and a negative ionotropic effect (i.e., a
  decrease in the cardiac output). Each of these agents has a differ-
  ent intensity of effect on these mechanisms.

but not always has a diastolic blood pressure above 120 mm Hg, and has one or more of the syndromes listed under **A.**

A. **Specific syndromes** precipitated by hypertension, thus defining a hypertensive emergency, include:
   1. Left ventricular heart failure.
   2. Cerebrovascular accident.
   3. Dissecting thoracic aortic aneurysm.
   4. Eclampsia.
   5. Acute renal failure.
   6. Papilledema on funduscopic examination.
   7. Hypertensive encephalopathy.

B. The **specific evaluation and management** of hypertensive emergencies include making the clinical diagnosis, performing the ACLS protocol as indicated, performing the overall evaluation as described in Box 3-2, and initiating emergent, therapeutic intervention. The agent of choice is **sodium nitroprusside** (see Table 3-5 for dosing). Place an arterial line, and strive for a blood pressure of 180–200/95–105 mm Hg in the first 4–6 hours. Then slowly decrease the elevated blood pressure to normal in 24–36 hours.
   1. Once the patient has stabilized, add an oral agent that will be used on a long-term outpatient basis and gradually withdraw the nitroprusside. These steps are performed in the hospital, invariably in the ICU, and are included here for the reader's edification.
   2. Eclampsia is managed differently, with admission, emergent referral to obstetrics, and the initiation of magnesium and/or hydralazine.

VII. **Hypertensive urgencies**
   In **hypertensive urgencies** the diastolic blood pressure is significantly elevated but there are **no acute syndromes or findings** present that are directly attributable to or precipitated by the elevated blood pressure. Thus an urgency is more of an **asymptomatic severe hypertension,** i.e., a numerical diagnosis. An urgency is one in which the diastolic blood pressure is greater than 115 mm Hg.
   A. The **specific evaluation and management** of hypertensive urgencies include making the clinical diagnosis, performing the overall evaluation as described in Box 3-2, and making certain that there are no findings that would make the blood pressure elevation a hypertensive emergency.
      1. The **acute goal** is to decrease the blood pressure to 180–190/95–105 mm Hg in the first several hours. Then place the patient on an oral agent that will be

T A B L E 3-5
Agents Used in the Management of Hypertensive Emergencies and Urgencies

Agent	Indications	Dosage	Side Effects
Sodium nitroprusside (Nipride)	All hypertensive emergencies except eclampsia	0.5 µg/kg/min IV initially, titrate dosage (increase/adjust) by increments of 0.5 µg/kg/min to target blood pressure (see text); maximum dosage is 8.0 µg/kg/min Concurrent use of intra-arterial catheter is recommended IV loop diuretics, 20 mg furosemide IV, usually needed at or soon after initiation of nitroprusside Advantage: Extremely short half-life, which allows clinician to rapidly titrate dose to target blood pressure; if overshoot, can rapidly adjust dosage down	Hypotension Fluid retention Headache Thiocyanate toxicity if used >3–5 days
Hydralazine	Eclampsia	**Loading dose:** 50 mg IV **Maintenance dose:** 5–20 mg IV q. 30 min, titrate to target blood pressure (see text) **Deliver fetus**	Hypotension Tachycardia
Nifedipine (Procardia)	Urgency	10 mg PO or sublingually; can repeat dose in 30–40 min; titrate to target blood pressure (see text) Can initiate chronic oral therapy with this agent as soon as target blood pressure is reached	Hypotension
Nitroglycerin ointment (Nitropaste)	Urgency	Apply 0.5–1 inch of paste to skin; titrate to target blood pressure (see text); can easily control—if overshoot, just wipe off Best in emergency room (ER), especially in patients with concurrent atherosclerotic heart disease	Hypotension Headache

continued for the long-term control of the hypertension.

2. In the acute setting, do not decrease the blood pressure to normal, as this can result in **syncope** or a **cerebrovascular event.**

3. A **model for therapy** is to use nifedipine, 10 mg PO or sublingually, and then initiate treatment with nifedipine, 10 mg PO t.i.d., with blood pressure measured daily until stabilized, then weekly, and with the medication adjusted following the principles discussed under **V. Management,** until the patient is normotensive.

4. A hypertensive urgency may be managed on an outpatient basis, especially if the blood pressure responds to therapy and the patient is **compliant with therapy and keeps appointments.**

VIII. Consultation

Problem	Service	Time
Any renal failure	Renal	Urgent
Renal artery stenosis	Renal	Urgent
Conn's disease	Endocrine	Urgent
Hypercortisolism	Endocrine	Urgent
Pheochromocytoma	Endocrine	Urgent

IX. **Indications for admission:** All hypertensive emergencies and all hypertensive urgencies that are refractory to acute intervention.

Nephrolithiasis

The presence of calculi (stones) in the urinary tract is a medical problem that is quite prevalent in the United States, affecting between 4% and 8% of the population at some time during life. The stones may be in the upper tract (nephrolithiasis) and/or in the lower urinary tract (cystolithiasis).

I. Overall manifestations

The **overall manifestations** of urinary tract stones include the acute onset of unilateral flank pain that is invariably quite severe. The pain originates in the flank and radiates into the ipsilateral labium majora or scrotum. There may be associated nausea, anorexia, vomiting, dysuria, and gross hematuria. The patient may have a history of urinary tract infections or of crystal arthropathies, especially gout. Also, because there is a high recurrence rate for any type of urinary tract calculus, there often is a history of nephrolithiasis. Although the majority of patients have symptoms, many quite severe, the stones can be asymptomatic and thus found incidentally, during the workup for microscopic hematuria or recurrent pyuria.

II. Types of stones

Although virtually all urinary stones have the same manifestations and acutely require the same overall evaluation and management, there are several types of urinary stones, each with different physical properties, a unique pathogenesis, a unique natural history, and specific features in long-term management (Table 3-6).

A. Calcium stones

Calcium stones are by far the **most common crystal stones** that result in symptomatic nephrolithiasis. There are two subtypes of calcium stones—calcium oxalate, which causes 40% of all stones, and calcium phosphate–oxalate, which causes 40% of all stones in the renal system. Any of the calcium-containing stones are **radiopaque** and thus are easily visualized on standard radiographic imaging.

1. Pathogenesis

The **underlying pathogenesis** in virtually all cases is an increase in levels of calcium in the urine. The **differential diagnosis** and the unique pathogenetic features resulting in the development of calcium-based calculi include:

a. **Primary hyperparathyroidism.** This is hypersecretion of parathormone (PTH) from the parathyroid glands, either as a result of a parathyroid adenoma or of parathyroid hyperplasia. The **mechanism** is an elevated PTH causing a secondary hypercalciuria, which increases the risk of calcium stone development in the renal system.

b. **Increased GI load and/or absorption of calcium.** This is the chronic ingestion of large quantities of calcium, usually in the form of calcium carbonate antacids, with or without a concurrent increase in the amount of vitamin D ingested, by a patient with normally functioning kidneys. The normally functioning renal tubules handle the overall increased calcium load by excreting more, with resultant hypercalciuria. This increases the risk of calcium stone development in the renal system. Of interest is the recent report that modest calcium ingestion in patients without a history of nephrolithiasis is effective in the *primary* prevention of calcium nephrolithiasis.

TABLE 3-6
Nephrolithiasis

Stone Type	Urine pH	Radiographic Appearance	Sex Ratio
Calcium	Alkaline (>7)	Radiopaque	Men > women (most common type in both)
Urate (purine)	Acidic (<7)	Radiolucent	Men > women
Struvite	Alkaline (>7)	Radiopaque	Women > men
Cystine	Variable	Radiopaque	Equal

c. **Renal tubular dysfunction,** usually **type I (distal)** is an uncommon etiology. The **mechanism** is one of tubular dysfunction causing an inappropriate loss of calcium in the urine and a concurrent decrease in the normal amount of citrate within the urine. Citrate normally will chelate calcium in the urine, thus decreasing the risk of calculus formation. Thus a significant hypercalciuria results, which increases the risk of calcium stone development in the renal system.

d. **Hyperoxaluria.** This is most common in patients who frequent health food stores and ingest large doses of water-soluble **vitamin C.** These patients may ingest 1–4 g of vitamin C per day. The **mechanism** is one in which there is an increase in oxalate in the urine. The presence of this anion in the urine results in an increased risk for the development of **calcium oxalate** calculi. Other causes of hyperoxaluria include inflammatory bowel disease, intestinal bypass surgery, and hereditary hyperoxaluria.

2. **Evaluation and management**

   The **specific evaluation and management** of calcium stones within the urinary tract include making the clinical diagnosis and acutely treating as described in Box 3-4. Specific evaluative tools include:

   a. Obtaining 24-hour urine collections to measure calcium. Normal is <300 mg/24 hr. If >300 mg/24 hr, the chance is greater that the stone is indeed calcium related.

   b. If renal tubular acidosis is suspected (i.e., the patient has a non-anion gap metabolic acidosis and an inappropriately alkaline urine), obtain a 24-hour urine collection to measure citrate. Normal urinary citrate is >250 mg/24 hr. Thus, <250 mg is indirect evidence not only of calcium nephrolithiasis, but also of a concurrent distal RTA.

   c. If hyperparathyroidism is suspected, determine the serum PTH-N-terminal (intact).

3. **Chronic management**

   Chronic management and secondary prevention of calcium nephrolithiasis include:

   a. Recommending a low calcium diet. This is a controversial point in that it may increase the risk of osteoporosis in **at-risk populations** (e.g., ethanol abusers, postmenopausal females), and

B O X 3 - 4

Overall Evaluation and Management of Nephrolithiasis

Evaluation

1. Take a thorough **history** directed toward uncovering past urinary tract infections, arthritides, diet of the patient, medication and vitamin use, or a family history of renal calculi.
2. Perform a **physical examination,** especially looking for costovertebral angle tenderness and fever.
3. Perform urinalysis with microscopic analysis, looking especially for any crystals.
4. Determine urine pH, as it can aid in predicting the type of stone present. An alkaline pH is associated with struvite calculi.
5. Determine serum electrolyte levels for baseline purposes.
6. Determine serum uric acid level, especially if the patient has gout or is at risk for uric acid nephrolithiasis.
7. Perform **renal ultrasound.** This is an important imaging technique to ascertain:
   a. The presence of a stone.
   b. The size of the stone.
   c. The size of the kidneys.
   d. The presence or absence of ureteral obstruction. The advantages of US over standard radiographic imaging are several: (1) there is no radiation exposure; therefore, the study can be safely performed in pregnant women; (2) one can directly image all stones, including radiolucent uric acid stones; (3) one can directly image the size of the ureters and therefore detect early renal obstruction.
8. Determine serum calcium, PO_4, albumin, and magnesium levels for baseline purposes and to screen for hyperparathyroidism.
9. Determine CBC count with differential for baseline purposes.
10. **Strain all urine.** 80% of first stones will pass.
11. **Send the stone for chemical structure analysis.**
12. Perform spot tests for urine calcium and creatinine, and calculate the ratio of calcium to creatinine.
    a. Normal: <0.1.

(continued)

B O X 3 - 4 *(continued)*

> b. Hypercalciuria: >0.3. Hypercalciuria is a risk fac-
>   tor for the development of calcium stones.
>
> *Management*
>
> 1. If the patient is acutely ill and vomiting, place on
>   NPO orders.
> 2. Replete any fluid deficit, then maintain IV fluids
>   with 0.9 normal saline.
> 3. **Provide analgesics.** Acutely, patients usually need
>   narcotic analgesia. The following regimens can be
>   used:
>   a. Meperidine (Demerol), 50 mg, plus Vistaril, 25
>   mg IM, q.3–4h. PRN.
>   b. Morphine sulfate, 2–3 mg IV q.2–3h. Occasion-
>   ally a morphine sulfate drip, 1–3 mg/hr IV, is
>   necessary for acute management.
> 4. Monitor fluid input and output closely. Maintain a
>   urine output of at least 100 ml/hr to aid in flushing
>   the stone out.
> 5. If pyuria is present and the urine is alkaline, treat
>   the urinary tract infection with ampicillin and an
>   aminoglycoside, covering for *Proteus mirabilis* (see
>   section on Pyuria Syndromes, page 172).
>
> *Referral*
>
> 1. Obtain a renal consultation.
> 2. If the stone is large (>5 mm in diameter) or if ob-
>   struction is present, consult urology urgently or
>   emergently.

therefore should be used judiciously in such
groups.
  b. Initiation of a thiazide diuretic, e.g., hydrochlo-
     rothiazide, 25 mg/day PO, which acts on the re-
     nal tubules to decrease the calcium in the urine.
  c. Attempting to discontinue or limit the adminis-
     tration of agents that can exacerbate the patho-
     genesis of these stones (e.g., loop diuretics and
     vitamin C).
  d. Recommending that the patient increase oral

fluid intake to increase urine output and thus decrease the risk of stasis and crystal formation.
    e. If RTA is the underlying cause, referral to nephrology and the initiation of potassium citrate, 1 mEq/kg/day PO, are indicated.
    f. If hyperparathyroidism is diagnosed, referral to an endocrinologist is indicated, as well as referral to nephrology for treatment of recurrent stones or any evidence of renal tubular dysfunction.
B. **Uric acid stones**
    Uric acid stones are **relatively uncommon.** This crystal type makes up approximately 5%–10% of all urinary calculi. They are the only stones that are **radiolucent** and thus invisible on standard radiographic imaging techniques.
    1. **Pathogenesis**
        The **underlying pathogenesis** in virtually all cases is increased uric acid in the urine. The **differential diagnosis** and unique pathogenetic features of uric acid–based calculi include:
        a. **Tophaceous gout.** This is a specific form of gout in which the patient has a long history of severe, recurrent, untreated gouty arthritis. The total body stores of uric acid are extremely elevated. The uric acid is deposited in the soft tissues, resulting in formation of indurated, nontender lesions, i.e., **tophi.** As an outcome of these elevated purine and urate stores in the body, there invariably is concurrent hyperuricosuria and therefore an increased risk of uric acid stone formation.
        b. Deficiency in **hypoxanthine–guanine phosphoribosyl transferase (HGPT).** The partial or complete deficiency of this ubiquitous enzyme results in a decreased ability of the cells to catabolize purines, with resultant chronically extremely elevated uric acid levels in the serum and the urine and, therefore, an increased risk of uric acid stone formation. Complete deficiency may manifest as the Lesch–Nyhan syndrome.
        c. **Medication side effect.** Several medications, including salicylates in high doses and probenicid, will effect a decrease in uric acid in the body and in the serum by increasing the tubular excretion of uric acid and increasing the risk of uric acid nephrolithiasis. Thus, when prescribing high-dose aspirin or probenicid, one must know of this potential side effect.

2. **Evaluation and management**

   The **specific evaluation and management** of uric acid stones in the urinary tract include making the clinical diagnosis and acutely treating as described in Box 3-4. Specific evaluative tools include:

   a. Obtaining a 24-hour urine collection to determine uric acid. The normal value is <700 mg/24 hr. Thus >700 mg/24 hr increases the probability that the stone is indeed uric acid.

3. **Chronic management**

   The specifics in the **chronic management** and **prevention** of uric acid nephrolithiasis, once the diagnosis is made, include initiating allopurinol, 300 mg PO once daily. This agent, which should be used chronically, decreases the overall serum and urinary uric acid levels by inhibiting the enzyme, xanthine oxidase. Other steps include alkalinizing the urine with oral $NaHCO_3$, and discontinuing probenicid or high-dose aspirin.

C. **Struvite stones**

   This crystal type, referred to as triple phosphate, with a chemical composition of $NH_4Mg(PO_3)3:(6\ H_2O)$, accounts for approximately 5%–10% of all urinary calculi. These calculi are uniformly radiopaque and thus are easily demonstrated by standard radiographic techniques. The stones are usually quite large and can cause ureteral obstruction.

   1. **Pathogenesis**

      The **underlying pathogenesis** is recurrent infection with urea-splitting organisms, most commonly *Proteus* or *Morganella* spp. These organisms contain the enzyme urease, which effectively breaks down urea and causes an alkaline urine and NH_4 in the urine. These two processes—i.e., alkalosis and increased urinary NH_4—increase the risk of formation of triple-phosphate crystals and thus of struvite, also known as "staghorn" calculi. These calculi are foreign bodies and, once present, increase the risk of future urinary tract infections, which in turn leads to further growth of the calculi.

   2. **Evaluation and management**

      The **specific evaluation and management** of struvite stones within the urinary tract include making the clinical diagnosis and acutely treating as described in Box 3-4. Invariably, the diagnosis is clinically evident at the time of presentation. **Specific acute management** includes obtaining urine culture and sensitivity and the empirical initiation of antibiotics. Regimens can include amoxicillin, 500 mg PO q.i.d. for 7–10 days, or, if inpatient management is required, ampicillin and an aminoglycoside or ampicillin–sulbactam (Unasyn). Expedient referral to urology for stone removal, either surgically or by lithotripsy, is indicated.

   3. **Chronic management**
   The specifics in the **chronic management** and **prevention** of struvite stones include effective removal of the stones and aggressively treating the underlying urinary tract infections. Follow-up with urology is mandatory.

D. **Cystine stones**
   These stones are quite uncommon and usually occur as a result of a congenital process. Approximately 0.5% of all calculi are cystine stones. The stones are **radiopaque** and thus easily visualized on radiographic imaging.

   1. **Pathogenesis**
   The **underlying pathogenesis** is an increase in the urinary levels of cystine. The most common etiology is **hereditary cystinuria,** inherited as an autosomal recessive trait.

   2. **Evaluation and management**
   The **specific evaluation and management** of cystine stones in the urinary tract include making the clinical diagnosis and acutely treating as described in Box 3-4. Further evaluation includes querying the patient regarding a family history of stones affecting both sexes and screening for it in the patient and in family members by performing a **nitroprusside test on the urine.** Specific management includes referral to a nephrology consultant and is beyond the scope of this text.

III. **Consultation**

Problem	*Service*	*Time*
Obstruction	GU	Emergent/ urgent
Large calculus (>5 mm)	GU	Urgent
Recurrent calculi	Renal	Elective
Hyperparathyroidism	Endocrinology	Elective

IV. **Indications for admission:** Any evidence of ureteral obstruction, pyelonephritis, septicemia, severe pain, or intravascular volume depletion.

Proteinuria

One of the most important and central functions of the kidneys is to filter the blood. The filtering activity is performed by the glomeruli. This filtration is efficient and quite specific in that only low molecular weight substances are filtered out of the blood. The specificity is such that medium and large molecular weight molecules, such as albumin and plasma proteins and all cellular components, are uniformly not filtered out of the blood. Although the filter system is efficient and specific there is, even in the normal setting, the potential for some loss of scant amounts of albumin and protein. Moreover, the cells of the urinary tract distal to the glomeruli can produce small amounts of protein, including the protective immunoglobulin IgA, which eventually is lost in the urine. Therefore, in healthy people a very small amount of protein may be lost in the urine. This protein loss does not exceed 150 mg/24 hr and is below the detection threshold of the test for proteinuria most commonly employed, the urine dipstick analysis.

I. **Definition**
   Proteinuria, by definition, is the loss of an excessive quantity of protein in the urine. The patient may have significant manifestations directly due to the loss of protein and albumin, as well as manifestations indirectly associated with the underlying disease process. Any quantity of protein which is greater than normal, i.e., 150 mg/day in the urine, is by definition proteinuria. Therefore even a trace of protein on the dipstick is considered proteinuria.

II. **Nephrotic range proteinuria**
   This is a large amount of protein lost in the urine—by definition, >2 g/24 hr. The classic **nephrotic syndrome** is the quintessential but nonspecific example of this type of protein loss. This classic syndrome consists of hypoalbuminemia, hypercholesterolemia, and >2 g of protein lost in the urine per 24 hours.
   A **spot urine protein–creatinine ratio >3.5** is quite sensitive and specific for nephrotic range proteinuria, thus giving the clinician a simple and inexpensive evaluative tool with which to document proteinuria. This evaluative tool should replace the older, more expensive, and less convenient 24-hour urine collection for protein and creatinine determination.
   A. **Manifestations**
      The **specific manifestations** of nephrotic range proteinuria include those **related to the nephrosis itself** and those **related to the underlying etiology** of the nephrotic range proteinuria. The manifestations specific to the nephrotic range proteinuria include the development of

edema, first dependent then diffuse, leading to anasarca and biventricular heart failure. Further findings include the onset of frothy or foamy urine without other urinary symptoms, as a result of albumin in the urine, or xanthelasma as a result of the secondary hypercholesterolemia present.

B. **Differential diagnosis**

The **differential diagnosis** includes membranous glomerulonephritis (GNP); minimal change GNP; SLE, especially if mesangial or membranous GNP is present; primary or secondary amyloidosis; diabetes mellitus; uncontrolled hypertension; exposure to heavy metals; and monoclonal gammopathies, including multiple myeloma. The pathogenesis of proteinuria in each of these entities is different but beyond the scope of this textbook.

The most common causes of nephrotic range proteinuria in the United States today are **hypertension** and **diabetes mellitus.**

C. **Evaluation and management**

The **specific evaluation and management** of this disorder include making the clinical diagnosis using the evaluative tools described in Box 3-5 performing specific tests to determine the underlying cause and concurrent sequelae. These tests include **US of the kidneys** to reveal the size of the kidneys. If the disease process is acute, the kidney size is usually normal, whereas if the process is chronic, the kidney size is small.

1. If a vasculitis or glomerulonephritis is suspected, the ESR and antinuclear antibody (ANA) titer should be determined; both would be abnormally elevated. Referral to nephrology to consider a renal biopsy and to consider the initiation of steroid treatment is indicated.

2. If the SSA assay is positive, urine protein electrophoresis on a 24-hour collection of urine should be performed. It will demonstrate what specifically the protein is, kappa or lambda light chains, or albumin. Furthermore, serum protein electrophoresis should be performed.

3. A fasting glucose and examination of the retinas looking for hypertensive or diabetic changes should be performed. Furthermore, aggressive control of serum glucose and aggressive control of any hypertension needs to be done. If the patient has no renal failure yet, the drug classes of choice to control hypertension, especially in patients with concurrent diabetes mellitus, are ACE inhibitors and/or calcium channel blockers.

B O X 3 - 5

Overall Evaluation of Proteinuria

Evaluation

1. Take a thorough history and perform a physical examination, looking for any signs of chronic protein or albumin loss (e.g., peripheral edema, heart failure, ascites).
2. Repeat the dipstick analysis of the urine and perform a microscopic analysis of the urine, specifically looking for the concurrent findings of RBC casts, RBCs, WBCs, bacteria, and fat oval bodies, which are manifestations of a "nephritic" urinary sediment.
3. The **sulfosalicylic acid (SSA) test** should be performed on the urine specimen. This reagent is used to determine if Bence Jones proteins (light chains in a gammopathy) are present in the urine. Two drops of the SSA reagent are added to a small sample of urine. If light chains are present, a white precipitate forms. Light chains (Bence Jones proteins) are not revealed by the standard dipstick method.
4. Obtain spot levels of protein and creatinine in the urine, both in mg/dL. If the ratio of protein to creatinine is >**3.5,** it is consistent with nephrotic range proteinuria. This rapid test has virtually supplanted the 24-hour collection of urine for protein determination. **Alternatively,** the clinician can perform the traditional 24-hour urine collection for protein.
5. Determine serum electrolyte levels for baseline purposes.
6. Determine serum creatinine, BUN, and glucose levels; for baseline purposes and to document the degree of renal impairment.
7. Determine the serum albumin, calcium, and phosphorus levels for baseline purposes and to document any hypoalbuminemia.
8. Determine the CBC count with differential for baseline purposes.
9. Categorize the proteinuria into nephrotic range proteinuria (>2 g/24 hr or a spot protein–creatinine ratio of >3.5) or non-nephrotic range proteinuria (<2 g/24 hr or a spot protein–creatinine ratio of <3.5).

III. Non-nephrotic range proteinuria

This is a modest but abnormal amount of protein lost in the urine—<2 g of protein lost in 24 hours. A **spot urine protein–creatinine ratio** <3.5 is quite sensitive and specific for non-nephrotic range proteinuria, thus giving the clinician a simple and inexpensive evaluative tool with which to document proteinuria. This evaluative tool should replace the older, more expensive, and less convenient 24-hour urine collection for protein and creatinine determination.

A. Manifestations

The **specific manifestations** of non-nephrotic range proteinuria include the fact that it is virtually always asymptomatic unless it is due to a urinary tract infection, in which case the findings of dysuria, pyuria, and increased frequency are to be expected (see section on Pyuria Syndromes, page 172).

B. Differential diagnosis

The **differential diagnosis** includes urinary tract infections, fever, diabetes mellitus, hypertension, exercise, (especially if strenuous), and benign positional proteinuria (mild proteinuria that occurs when the patient is in an upright position but resolves when the patient is recumbent). The pathogenesis of proteinuria in each of these entities is different and beyond the scope of this textbook.

The most common causes of non-nephrotic range proteinuria in the United States today are **hypertension** and **diabetes mellitus.**

C. Evaluation and management

The **specific evaluation and management** of this disorder include making the clinical diagnosis using the evaluative tools described in Box 3-5 and performing specific evaluative tests, listed below.

1. If **diabetes mellitus** is suspected, determine the fasting blood glucose level. If it is above 140 mg/dL, the diagnosis of diabetes is confirmed; then look for any proliferative retinal changes consistent with microvascular diabetic disease. Treat aggressively (see section on Diabetes Mellitus in Chapter 9, page 515).

2. If **hypertension** is thought to be poorly controlled, obtain a 12-lead ECG to look for evidence of hypertension-induced left ventricular hypertrophy and perform a retinal examination. Treat aggressively (see section on Hypertension, page 148).

3. If **benign positional proteinuria** is suspected, obtain two urine collections, one during the day (~12 hours) and the other at night while the patient is

recumbent (~12 hours). The mild proteinuria should resolve when the patient is recumbent.

4. If **urinary tract infection** is found, treat as such (see section on Pyuria Syndromes, page 172).

5. If **no clear cause can be determined** or if the proteinuria is thought to result from hypertension or diabetes mellitus, consultation with a nephrologist, performing urinalysis, and monitoring serum electrolyte, BUN, and creatinine levels every 4–6 months all indicated. If the proteinuria progresses to the nephrotic range, perform the evaluations listed for that entity.

IV. **Consultation**

Problem	*Service*	*Time*
Nephrotic range	Nephrology	Urgent
Non-nephrotic range	Nephrology	Elective

V. **Indications for admission:** Any evidence of biventricular failure, especially if new onset, or of new-onset anasarca.

Pyuria Syndromes

Pyuria is the abnormal presence of leukocytes in the urine. The **overall manifestations** of pyuria include a diverse array of symptoms and signs, among them **dysuria** (pain or burning upon urination), an increased **frequency** of urination, a clear or **purulent discharge** from the urethral orifice, and the onset of **cloudy urine.** Further manifestations include pruritus of the vulva or distal glans, **hesitancy** (inability to generate a forceful urinary stream), and **dribbling** of urine after the completion of voiding.

Associated manifestations may include nausea, vomiting, urinary incontinence, and pain and tenderness in the suprapubic area. If **pyelonephritis** develops, there invariably will be unilateral pain and tenderness in the flank or costovertebral angle area.

The intensity of the overall manifestations can range from very severe to virtually asymptomatic. In fact, many cases of pyuria are completely asymptomatic and are only diagnosed by urinalysis. The reader is referred to a discussion of pyuria syndromes by Stamm et al. referenced in the Bibliography.

The sex of the patient plays a major role in the differential diagnosis and even in the evaluation and management of pyuria. Thus, one should approach pyuria in females differently from pyuria in males. The distal urinary tracts and adjacent reproductive structures are significantly different in females and males.

I. Pyuria in females

Pyuria, either asymptomatic or symptomatic, is quite common in females. Various reports indicate a 20%–40% chance that a pyuria syndrome will develop sometime during a female's lifetime.

A. Pathogenesis

The **underlying pathogenesis** of many pyuria syndromes in females is an infection that initially infects the distal urethra and, if not treated, **ascends the urinary tract** to the kidneys. Certain procedures and activities predispose to urinary tract infections. These risk factors include but are not limited to:

1. The presence of a Foley catheter.
2. Poor perineal hygiene or techniques of hygiene, such as wiping posterior to anterior, potentially infecting the urethra with fecal material.
3. Anal intercourse with subsequent vaginal intercourse.
4. Nephrolithiasis.

B. Subcategories

Two major subcategories are discussed, symptomatic pyuria without bacteria and symptomatic pyuria with bacteria.

1. **Symptomatic pyuria without bacteriuria**

   a. The **specific manifestations** include those listed in the introductory material of this section. They usually are mild to moderate in intensity and usually are only referable to the distal aspects of the urinary tract. Invariably, the number of WBCs/hpf is low, 5–10. On dipstick analysis, the **leukocyte esterase** (LE) in the urine is positive whereas the **nitrite** in the urine is negative. This is a not uncommon form of pyuria, especially in females. There are no bacteria demonstrated on urinalysis or urine culture.

   b. The **differential diagnosis** includes **extraurinary tract infections** (cervicitis, PID, vaginitis) and **primary urinary tract infections** with atypical bacteria, including *Chlamydia trachomatis* or *Mycobacterium hominis* (i.e., tuberculosis). Chlamydial infections are the most common of these causes.

   c. The **specific evaluation and management** of this category of pyuria in females include performing those examinations described in Box 3-6. If an **extraurinary source** is found, such as cervicitis or vaginitis, treat that entity. If the **source is the urinary tract** (i.e., no extraurinary

B O X 3 - 6

Overall Evaluation and Management of Pyuria Syndromes

Evaluation

1. Take a thorough **history** and perform a **physical examination.** In the history, emphasis should be placed on the manifestations described at the beginning of this section. The physical examination in **females** includes a pelvic examination looking for any areas of inflammation, discharge, or tenderness. In **males,** the GU tract must be examined with emphasis on the testes, penis, and prostate gland, again looking for tenderness or discharge. The prostate must be examined by rectal examination.
2. Obtain a sample of urine for **dipstick** and **microscopic urinalysis** (see Table 3-1 in the section on Hematuria, page 140, for effective methods of urine sample collection). The **dipstick analysis** is for nitrite and leukocyte esterase; the **microscopic analysis** is for leukocytes, WBC casts (Fig. 3-1), erythrocytes, and bacteria.
3. Send the urine for culture and sensitivity testing.
4. Further evaluation and management differ according to the sex of the patient, reflecting different anatomical organization.

source is demonstrated), the clinician can initiate antibiotics. Antibiotic regimens may include:

tetracycline, 500 mg PO q.i.d. for 7 days
or
doxycycline, 100 mg PO b.i.d. for 7 days
or
erythromycin, 250 mg PO q.i.d. for 7 days.

If the manifestations are recurrent, send a first morning urine specimen for AFB smear and culture and perform a skin PPD test. Education in good perineal hygiene is indicated in all patients. Referral to gynecology for suspected PID is indicated.

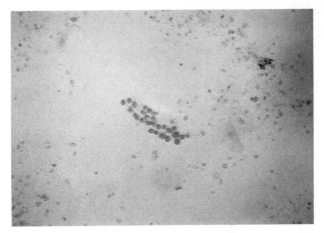

F I G U R E 3 - 1
White blood cell cast in a patient with a urinary tract infection.

2. **Symptomatic pyuria with bacteriuria**
   a. The **specific manifestations** of this not uncom-
      mon form of pyuria include those described in
      the introductory material of this section. The
      manifestations may range from mild to moderate
      to severe in intensity and may be referable to
      the distal and/or proximal aspects of the urinary
      tract. On **microscopic analysis** the number of
      WBCs/hpf is variable from low (5–10) to "too
      numerous to count." Also, the microscopic anal-
      ysis will reveal bacteria in the urine specimen.
      On **dipstick analysis** the **leukocyte esterase** (LE)
      in the urine is positive and the **nitrite** in the
      urine is positive if the infection is with a gram-
      negative organism, but the nitrite is negative if
      the infection is with a gram-positive organism.
      Culture of the urine will yield the etiologic or-
      ganism.
   b. The **differential diagnosis** includes **extra-
      urinary tract infections** (cervicitis, PID, vagini-
      tis) and **primary urinary tract infections** with
      gram-negative bacilli (i.e., the Enterobacteria-
      ceae), and the gram-positive cocci (i.e., *Staphy-
      lococcus saprophyticus* and the Group D strep-
      tococci).
      The most common examples of gram-negative

bacilli that result in urinary tract infections are
Proteus, E. coli, Pseudomonas, and *Morganella*
spp.

c. The **natural history** involves an infection that
begins in the lower tract (the urethra or urinary
bladder) and then ascends the tract to one or
both kidneys. Thus, potential sequelae and complications of urinary tract infections include **pyelonephritis** (infection of the kidney itself) and
abscess formation. Another potential complication is **nephrolithiasis,** especially struvite
stones, concurrent with *Proteus* infections. Finally, bacteremia and even septicemia can be
potential outcomes of urinary tract infections.
These complications manifest with fevers,
chills, flank pain, and, in cases of septicemia,
hemodynamic instability.

d. The **specific evaluation and management** of this
category of pyuria in females include performing the evaluative examinations listed in
Box 3-6. The urine pH is a useful tool in that an
alkaline pH indicates an infection with a urea-
splitting organism and thus an increased risk
for struvite nephrolithiasis. If an **extraurinary
source** is found (e.g., cervicitis or vaginitis),
treat that entity. If the **source is the urinary tract**
(i.e., no extraurinary source is demonstrated),
the clinician must initiate antibiotics.

The **specific antibiotic regimen** used should
reflect the clinical picture of the patient. If the
infection is limited to the lower tract and is
without sequelae, a single-dose regimen can be
used. If the patient is febrile and has flank pain,
findings suggestive of pyelonephritis or impending sepsis, parenteral agents are mandatory. Typical regimens, categorized according to
the clinical picture, are listed below:

For a first episode in the distal tract (i.e., the
urethra or urinary bladder):

amoxicillin, 3.0 g PO once,
> *or*

Bactrim DS, 2 tablets PO once,
> **and**

follow-up urinalysis in 7 days.

**If the patient has had recurrent UTIs or if
the single-dose regimen fails,** one must initiate
longer duration regimens:

amoxicillin, 500 mg PO t.i.d. for 10 days,
> or

Bactrim DS, 1 tablet PO b.i.d. for 7–10 days,
> or

Augmentin (ampicillin–clavulinic acid), 250 mg PO t.i.d. for 7–10 days,
> or

Ciprofloxacin, 250–500 mg PO b.i.d. for 7 days.

If the patient is febrile and ill-appearing, parenteral antibiotics are required from the outset. Regimens may include:

ampicillin, 2 g IV q.4–6h. with or without an aminoglycoside,
> or

piperacillin, 3 g IV q.4–6h. with or without an aminoglycoside.

Further evaluation is required if there are any recurrent infections of the urinary tract or if there have been any complications or sequelae of urinary tract infections, such as nephrolithiasis, renal dysfunction, or pyelonephritis. Further evaluation includes renal US and referral to GU for potential direct imaging with cystoscopy.

II. Pyuria in males

There are **three different categories** of pyuria in males: those of the urinary tract proper, the sexually transmitted purulent urethritides, and prostatitis. Each is discussed separately.

A. Categories

1. **Symptomatic pyuria, not sexually transmitted**
   a. The **specific manifestations** of this quite uncommon form of pyuria in males are described in the introductory material to this section. There are symptoms present in virtually all males who have pyuria. The **intensity** of the manifestations can be mild to moderate to severe and the manifestations may be referable to both the lower and upper urinary tract. On **microscopic analysis,** the number of WBCs/hpf is variable from low (5–10) to "too numerous to count." Also, the microscopic analysis will reveal bacteria in the urine specimen. On **dipstick analysis,** the **leukocyte esterase** (LE) in the urine is positive and the **nitrite** in the urine is positive if the infection is with a gram-negative organism, but the nitrite

is negative if the infection is with a gram-positive organism. Culture of the urine will yield the etiologic organism.

b. **Risk factors** that predispose to urinary tract infections in males include but are not limited to prostatic hypertrophy, nephrolithiasis, anal intercourse, straight catheterization, and Foley catheter placement.

c. The **differential diagnosis** includes **extra-urinary tract infections** (e.g., prostatitis or sexually transmitted purulent urethritis) and **primary urinary tract infections** with gram-negative bacilli (i.e., the Enterobacteriaceae), and the gram-positive cocci (i.e., *Staphylococcus saprophyticus* and the Group D streptococci). The most common gram-negative bacilli that result in urinary tract infections are *Proteus, E. coli, Pseudomonas,* and *Morganella* spp.

d. The **natural history** involves an infection that begins in the lower tract—the urethra or urinary bladder—and then ascends the tract to one or both kidneys. Thus, potential sequelae and complications of UTIs include **pyelonephritis** (infection of the kidney itself) and abscess formation. Another potential complication is **nephrolithiasis,** especially struvite stones concurrent with *Proteus* infections. Finally, bacteremia and even septicemia can be potential outcomes of urinary tract infections. These complications may manifest with fevers, chills, flank pain, and, in cases of septicemia, hemodynamic instability.

e. The **specific evaluation and management** of this category of pyuria in males include performing those examinations described in Box 3-6. The urine pH is a useful tool in that an alkaline pH indicates an infection with a urea-splitting organism and thus an increased risk for struvite nephrolithiasis. If an **extraurinary source** is found (e.g., prostatitis or sexually transmitted purulent urethritis), treat that entity. If the **source is the urinary tract** (i.e., no extraurinary source is demonstrated), the clinician must initiate antibiotics.

The **specific antibiotic regimen** used should reflect the clinical picture of the patient. If infection is limited to the lower tract and is without sequelae, an oral regimen may be used. If the patient is febrile and has flank pain, findings suggestive of pyelonephritis or impending sepsis, parenteral agents are mandatory. **Single-dose regimens for pyuria in males are contra-indicated.** Several regimens, categorized according to the clinical picture, are listed below:

If the patient has had acute or recurrent UTIs in the past, regimens include:

amoxicillin, 500 mg PO t.i.d. for 10 days,
> or

Bactrim DS, 1 tablet PO b.i.d. for 7–10 days,
> or

Augmentin (ampicillin–clavulinic acid), 250 mg PO t.i.d. for 7–10 days,
> or

Ciprofloxacin, 250–500 mg PO b.i.d. for 7 days.

If the patient is febrile and ill-appearing, parenteral antibiotics are required from the outset. Regimens may include:

ampicillin, 2 g IV q.4–6h. with or without an aminoglycoside,
> or

piperacillin, 3 g IV q.4–6h. with or without an aminoglycoside.

Further evaluation is mandatory in **all cases of UTI in males.** Expedient referral to GU and renal US are indicated. All cases of nonsexually transmitted pyurias must be thoroughly evaluated by a GU colleague.

2. **Sexually transmitted purulent urethritis.** This is the most common form of pyuria in males, and is usually clinically evident (see the section on Sexually Transmitted Diseases in Chapter 6, page 342).

3. **Prostatitis**

a. The **specific manifestations** of this fairly common etiology of pyuria in males are best described by categorizing prostatitis as either acute or chronic in duration. Chronic prostatitis is defined as symptoms present for more than 2 weeks.

   i. **Acute prostatitis.** Manifestations include an acute onset of perineal pain and, on examination, an enlarged, boggy feeling, and exquisitely tender prostate gland. Other manifestations include leukocytes, but rarely bacteria, on microscopic analysis of the urine, and, on dipstick analysis, a positive leukocyte esterase (LE) test but not necessarily a positive nitrite.

ii. **Chronic prostatitis.** There can be, but not necessarily is, an antecedent history of acute prostatitis with recurrent pain and discomfort in the groin and perineum. Often there are some associated urinary obstructive symptoms, including hesitancy, dribbling, and frequency. On examination the gland is, at most, mildly tender and moderately enlarged. Other manifestations include leukocytes, but rarely bacteria, on microscopic analysis of the urine, and, on dipstick analysis, a positive leukocyte esterase (LE) test but not necessarily a positive nitrite.

b. The **underlying pathogenesis** is inflammation, usually as the result of an infection, of the prostate gland. The prostate gland is located at the base of the penis and, in the pelvis, is immediately anterior to the rectum. The gland completely surrounds the urethra as it enters the penis, and thus causes manifestations of urinary tract obstruction when inflamed or enlarged. **Causative agents** in prostatitis, acute or chronic, include the gram-negative bacillary organisms (i.e., the Enterobacteriaceae) and *Chlamydia trachomatis*. Very rarely, *Mycobacterium* or *Blastomycetes* will result in chronic but never acute prostatitis.

c. The **specific evaluation and management** of this category of pyuria in males include performing those examinations described in Box 3-6. **Antibiotic regimens** include the following:

Acute prostatitis:

Bactrim DS, 1 tablet PO b.i.d. for 21 days,
   or
amoxicillin, 500 mg PO t.i.d. for 21 days,
   or
doxycycline, 100 mg PO b.i.d. for 21 days,
   or
Ciprofloxacin, 500 mg PO b.i.d. for 14–21 days.

Chronic prostatitis: The treatment is the same as for acute prostatitis but is of longer duration, i.e., 6 weeks. In addition, GU should be consulted.

III. **Consultation**

Problem	Service	Time
Recurrent infections	GU	Elective
First infection in males	GU	Required
Nephrolithiasis	GU	Elective
Chronic or recurrent prostatitis	GU	Elective
Benign prostatic hypertrophy	GU	Elective
Prostatic nodule	GU	Required

IV. **Indications for admission:** Pyelonephritis, inability to take adequate fluids by mouth, or any signs of impending sepsis.

Renal Dysfunction, Acute or Chronic

Acute renal failure is the sudden onset of **decreased renal function,** which has significant manifestations and sequelae. It may be a new episode or an exacerbation of chronic renal dysfunction. Any acute decrease in renal function, even if asymptomatic, is by definition acute renal failure and mandates an aggressive evaluation. Further underscoring the need for aggressive evaluation and management is the fact that although the differential diagnosis is quite large and diverse, many of the specific causes of acute renal failure are, especially early in their course, **quite reversible.**

Chronic renal failure may be the result of an episode of irreversible acute renal failure or of longstanding systemic disease.

I. **Physiologic functions of the normal kidneys**
   A. **Excretion of nitrogenous wastes**
      The kidneys filter the entire volume of blood on a repetitive, continuous basis. The blood is filtered through one of the active sites of the kidneys, the **glomeruli.** It is in the glomeruli that low molecular weight nitrogenous wastes, such as the catabolites of respiration, catabolism, and anabolism, are filtered from the plasma to be excreted in the urine. Although this effective filter removes the low molecular wastes from the blood, it does not filter out the formed cellular elements of the blood, the plasma proteins, or albumin. A physiologic measurement of kidney function is therefore the glomerular filtration rate (GFR), or the amount of blood filtered through the entire set of glomeruli in the renal cortices.
   B. **Intravascular volume homeostasis**
      Because the kidneys filter the blood continuously, a basic physiologic function of the kidneys is to maintain

volume status. This is maintained using the other active portion of the kidneys, the **renal tubules,** and is mainly under the direction of antidiuretic hormone (ADH) from the neurohypophysis and of mineralocorticoids from the adrenal cortices.

1. If the patient is **intravascularly volume depleted,** the neuroendocrine cells of the thirst center of the hypothalamus will secrete ADH through the neurohypophysis. **ADH** acts on and stimulates the collecting tubules of the kidneys to actively resorb free water from the urine. Furthermore, the glomeruli sense the decrease in volume being filtered and produce the hormone **angiotensin.** This hormone, produced by the juxtaglomerular (JG) cells of the kidneys, is activated in the lung parenchyma and stimulates the release of the mineralocorticoid, **aldosterone,** from the adrenal cortices. **Aldosterone** acts on the renal tubules to increase the resorption of water and sodium from the urine. All of these activities lead to appropriate retention of free water by the blood and **concentration** of the urine.

2. If the patient is **intravascularly volume overloaded,** the converse of the above processes occurs, with the secretion of ADH and aldosterone being minimal. Furthermore, as the result of more volume, quite often the GFR increases. All of these steps lead to an appropriate loss of free water from the blood and **dilution** of the urine.

C. **Endocrine function**

The kidneys can, through the hormone **erythropoietin,** stimulate erythropoiesis and thus act to maintain a normal level of hemoglobin and therefore oxygen-carrying capacity of the blood.

D. **Calcium homeostasis**

The kidneys are integral to calcium homeostasis. Under the direction and influence of **parathormone** (PTH), the renal tubules adjust the level of calcium in the urine and therefore in the serum. An increase in PTH results in decreased tubular secretion of calcium, i.e., retention of calcium in the serum; whereas a decrease in PTH results in increased excretion of calcium into the urine. Furthermore, the kidneys are the site of hydroxylation of 25-hydroxyvitamin D into its active component, 1,25-OH vitamin D. **1,25-OH vitamin D** is required for effective absorption of calcium from the GI tract.

E. **Phosphorus homeostasis**

The kidneys are integral to the homeostasis of phosphorus. Under the direction and influence of **PTH,** the renal tubules control the loss of phosphorus. An increase in

PTH results in increased excretion of phosphorus, while a decrease in PTH results in decreased phosphorus excretion.

F. **Acid–base homeostasis**

The renal tubules play a major role in maintaining the serum pH at a constant level of 7.4. The tubules control pH by adjusting the loss of hydrogen ions and HCO_3 ions. If there is an increase in fixed acids within the body, the tubules compensate by retaining HCO_3 and excreting H^+.

G. **Potassium homeostasis**

The kidneys, under the direct influence of **aldosterone,** maintain serum potassium levels at a constant physiologic level. The normal range of serum potassium is 3.8–5.0 mEq/dL. When the serum potassium level increases, there is an increase in aldosterone secretion by the zona glomerulosa of the adrenal cortices which acts upon the renal tubules to increase the excretion of potassium.

II. **Overall manifestations of renal failure**

A. **Edema**

Both pulmonary and peripheral edema are common. Clinically, edema manifests with a subacute to insidious onset of orthopnea, paroxysmal nocturnal dyspnea (PND), a third heart sound, dependent pitting edema (especially of the lower extremities), and pleural effusions. The **underlying pathogenesis** is based on:

a. An **overall decrease in GFR.** If the blood is not filtered, the excess volume cannot be removed by the kidneys. This is central to the pathogenesis.

b. An **abnormal loss of albumin** into the urine. Albumin is an osmotically active substance—that is, it takes water with it—and thus is a major factor in maintaining water in the intravascular tree. If albumin is lost and the patient develops hypoalbuminemia, water, which as a result of the decreased GFR cannot be efficiently excreted, transudes (is lost) into the extracellular tissues, with resulting edema.

B. **Oliguria**

Oliguria clinically manifests with the decrease in urine output to less than 30 mL/hr. This manifestation usually is not present until late in the course of disease. The **underlying pathogenesis** is a decrease in urine production due to an **overall decrease in the normal GFR.**

Even in relatively marked chronic renal failure, if the damage is predominantly to the tubules and relatively spares the glomeruli, the patient may be nonoliguric (i.e., with a normal urine output) or even polyuric (i.e., with an increased urine output).

C. **Anemia, normochromic normocytic**

The anemia is usually mild to moderate, but it can result in increased fatigability and a pale color to the nail beds and mucous membranes. Moreover, it can exacerbate any concurrent angina pectoris or heart failure. The **underlying pathogenesis** is a deficiency in the hormone erythropoietin, and therefore the reticulocyte count is low. An anemia usually is a manifestation of chronic rather than acute renal failure.

D. **Hypocalcemia**

Usually this will be quite asymptomatic as it rarely will be of a magnitude as to cause the classic findings of hypocalcemia, i.e., tetany, Trousseau's sign, Chvostek's sign, and/or seizures. The **underlying pathogenesis** is twofold, involving first the loss of renal tubular function and therefore response to PTH, and second a decrease in the hydroxylation of the inactive 25-OH vitamin D to the active 1,25-OH vitamin D. Through these mechanisms the serum calcium levels slowly but steadily **decrease.**

E. **Osteodystrophy**

This disorder closely resembles rickets. The patient develops an asymptomatic decrease in the mineral component of bone and bony structures. There is an increased risk for vertebral compression fractures and fractures of the long bones; quite often, a fracture is the sentinel manifestation of this disorder. The **underlying pathogenesis** is essentially twofold, involving first a **decrease in the hydroxylation of 25-OH vitamin D** with a resultant decrease in calcium absorption from the GI tract, and second the development of **secondary hyperparathyroidism** caused by the chronic hypocalcemia, which results in increased resorption of calcium from bone, with a resultant **osteodystrophy.** This entity has been termed "vitamin D–resistant rickets," but actually it responds to high doses of oral 1,25-OH vitamin D.

F. **Hyperphosphatemia**

Although usually asymptomatic until markedly elevated, the manifestations can include lethargy and increased fatigability. The underlying pathogenesis is a significant decrease in the GFR as the kidneys fail and a decrease in the ability of the kidney tubules to excrete phosphorus.

G. **Metabolic acidosis**

As the kidneys fail, there is a decreased ability of the renal tubules to excrete H^+ and fixed acids, resulting in a chronic, usually high anion gap, metabolic acidosis.

H. **Hyperkalemia**

Hyperkalemia usually is not a major problem until late in renal failure, when the patient becomes oliguric because the GFR has been markedly compromised. The underlying mechanism is a decrease in GFR and, concurrently, a decrease in tubular function and therefore ability to excrete potassium, even if aldosterone is markedly elevated. The hyperkalemia is further exacerbated by the metabolic acidosis that is usually concurrently present. (See the section on Hyperkalemia in Chapter 9, page 536.)

I. **Encephalopathy**

Encephalopathy manifests clinically with a diverse set of findings ranging from an insidious onset of lethargy to an acute onset of delirium. There often is asterixis, or "flap," present on examination. A harbinger is the development of **intractable hiccups,** or myoclonic jerks of the diaphragm. The **underlying pathogenesis** is an accumulation of nitrogen and other wastes of respiration and catabolism which, over a given threshold, will result in decreased function of the brain. Encephalopathy is more common in chronic than in acute renal failure. The **natural history** of uremic encephalopathy is grave; if no intervention is implemented, the mean survival time is less than 100 days.

J. **Coagulopathy**

Coagulopathy manifests clinically with the acute, subacute, and/or chronic onset of epistaxis, menorrhagia, easy bruisability, petechiae, and/or non-palpable purpura. The **underlying pathogenesis** is an abnormal elevation in nitrogenous wastes, which, over a certain threshold, causes significant dysfunction of the platelets. Coagulopathy is more common in chronic than in acute renal failure.

K. **Hypertension**

Hypertension is one of the most common manifestations of chronic renal failure. It results from and is exacerbated by the secondary hyperaldosteronism that develops in chronic renal failure. Hypertension is a risk factor for the development of other significant cardiovascular diseases and independently exacerbates and accelerates renal failure (see the section on Hypertension, page 148).

III. **Acute renal failure**

The causes of **acute renal failure** are quite diverse but relatively easy to recall if they are divided into **prerenal, renal,** and **postrenal subsets.** This classification is somewhat artificial, as there is some **overlap** between the subsets and acute renal dysfunction often is **multifactorial.**

A. **Prerenal**
1. **Manifestations**
   The **specific manifestations** include orthostatic blood pressure and volume changes (see Box 3-7), an overall decrease in urine output, and an increase in concentration of the urine. Also seen are dry mucous membranes, dry axillae, and skin "tenting." The patient is assessed to be **hypovolemic.** Finally, there invariably are manifestations of the underlying cause of the loss of intravascular volume. Both serum BUN and serum creatinine are increased; however, the elevation in serum BUN is relatively greater than the elevation in serum creatinine.
2. **Pathogenesis**
   The **underlying pathogenesis** of this very common cause of renal dysfunction is an overall decrease in fluid in the intravascular tree, a decrease in blood flow to the kidneys, and therefore a decrease in GFR. In other words, there is an effective decrease in the intravascular volume of the patient. **Specific states** that result in a significant decrease in renal perfusion include intravascular volume depletion, acute hemorrhage from any source, low output left ventricular failure, and inappropriate third spacing of fluids. Third spacing of fluids is a unique mechanism in that the patient has an overall increase in total body water, but the increase is mainly in third spaces (e.g., producing ascites or pleural effusions) and paradoxically results in a decrease in **effective** intravascular volume.
3. **Evaluation and management**
   Evaluation includes making the clinical diagnosis by performing the evaluations listed in Box 3-7 and looking for any evidence of concurrent GI hemorrhage by performing stool guaiacs.
4. **Management**
   Specific management includes administering fluids to the patient. The fluid of choice is 0.9 normal saline first and a repletion rate of more than 250–300 mL/hr for several hours. The goal is to replete $\frac{1}{2}$ of the total volume deficit in the first 12–18 hours and complete repletion in 24–30 hours. Use the baseline, pre-illness weight of the patient as a target for volume repletion and therefore euvolemia. Once euvolemia is achieved, administer maintenance fluids at 100–150 mL/hr until the underlying cause of the volume depletion has been effectively treated.

(*Text continues on page 190*)

B O X 3 - 7

Overall Evaluation and Management of Renal Dysfunction

Evaluation

1. Take a thorough **history** and perform a **physical examination** with emphasis on the manifestations of acute renal dysfunction (see text). In addition, the history focuses on medication use, recreational drug use, and a history of renal or hepatic dysfunction. A rectal examination to determine prostate size is mandatory.
2. **Assessment of the volume status** clinically is of utmost importance. This is best done by determining blood pressure and pulse parameters with the patient supine and standing (i.e., **orthostatic parameters**), by examining the **cardiopulmonary system,** and by **weighing** the patient. Using the results of these examinations, the clinician assesses the patient's volume status and places the patient into one of three intravascular volume groups: hypovolemic, euvolemic, and hypervolemic.
   a. **Hypovolemic**—Characterized by a decrease in blood pressure and/or an increased heart rate when the patient stands up and a decrease in the patient's weight from a pre-illness baseline weight.
   b. **Hypervolemic**—Examination of the cardiopulmonary system discloses rales, a third heart sound, increased jugular venous pulsations, and dependent pitting edema. The weight is invariably increased from a pre-illness baseline weight.
3. **Straight catheterization** of the urinary bladder to determine volume, relieve any retention or obstruction, and to obtain a specimen of urine for analysis. If the specimen is obtained in the postvoid state (i.e., immediately after the urinary bladder has been voluntarily emptied), any quantity >**50 mL is abnormal.**
4. **Ultrasonography of the kidneys** and bladder is indicated in all cases to ascertain the size of the kidneys and if obstruction (i.e., hydronephrosis) is present. Normally, the kidneys are approximately 12 cm

(continued)

B O X 3 - 7 *(continued)*

long. If the kidneys are small, the failure is essentially irreversible; if the kidneys are normal sized, the failure is more likely reversible.

5. **Perform urinalysis with microscopic examination.** Many clues to the cause of renal dysfunction are gleaned from the urinalysis. Urinalysis should be done by the primary care physician and, if needed, with the direct assistance of a nephrology consultant. **The importance of this examination cannot be overstressed.** Clinical clues include the following:

   a. **Pyuria** (>5 WBCs/hpf) indicates infection of the urinary tract (see section on Pyuria Syndromes, page 172).

   b. **Muddy brown casts,** i.e., broad-based casts with pigment within; indicate acute tubular necrosis.

   c. **Eosinophils** on urinalysis, specifically demonstrated on Wright's stain, indicate interstitial nephritis.

   d. **Red cell casts,** i.e., smaller casts composed of RBCs, indicate a glomerular etiology.

   e. **Fat oval bodies,** i.e., oval-shaped collections of fat, indicate a glomerular etiology.

   f. **Granular casts,** i.e., clear narrow casts. These are nonspecific findings and not necessarily pathologic.

   g. **White cell casts,** i.e., casts composed of polymorphonuclear cells, indicate an infection of the urinary tract.

6. **Wright's stain of urine** for eosinophils. If eosinophils are present, it is consistent with interstitial nephritis.

7. **Spot urine** for protein, creatinine, and sodium.

   a. The **spot urine protein–creatinine ratio** indicates whether significant proteinuria is present. A >3.5 indicates significant if not nephrotic range proteinuria (see section on Proteinuria, page 168).

   b. **Spot Na** can help differentiate certain forms of acute renal failure. The subsets include:
      Urine Na < 10 mEq/L:
      Prerenal ARF

(continued)

B O X   3 - 7 *(continued)*

> Hepatorenal syndrome
> Acute glomerulonephritis (GNP)
> **Urine Na > 10 mEq/L**
> Oliguric phase of acute tubular necrosis (ATN)
> Obstructive nephropathy
>
> 8. Send urine for culture and sensitivity testing if any pyuria is demonstrated.
> 9. Determine serum electrolytes for baseline purposes.
> 10. Determine serum creatinine and BUN levels for baseline purposes.
> 11. Determine albumin, PO_4, Ca, and CPK levels, determine ESR, and perform a drug screen at the time of presentation.
> 12. If possible, discontinue all nephrotoxic agents. Adjust dosages of all agents that are excreted through the renal system, and if possible, follow the serum levels of these drugs. Examples of this category of agents are digoxin, aminoglycoside antibiotics, and penicillin antibiotics.
> 13. **Differentiate acute from chronic renal failure:** see Table 3-7.

T A B L E 3 - 7
Clinical Differentiation of Acute from Chronic Renal Failure

Size of the kidneys on ultrasound	
Normal:	Acute
Small:	Chronic
Anemia	
Absent:	Acute
Present:	Chronic
Phosphorus	
Normal:	Acute
Elevated:	Chronic
Calcium	
Normal:	Acute
Low:	Chronic

    a. One must always follow weight, orthostatic parameters, creatinine, urine output, K, PO_4, Mg, and BUN levels on a frequent basis. Observe the patient for any signs of volume overload or heart failure. If these signs appear, decrease the rate of fluid input.

    b. Acutely, a consultation with nephrology is strongly recommended for all patients unless the renal dysfunction is mild, is due to a known and documented etiology, and rapidly reverses.

B. Renal

1. Manifestations

The **specific manifestations** include those described under **II. Overall manifestations,** but the patient is clinically euvolemic. Furthermore, there are manifestations specific to the underlying condition causing the renal failure, such as arthralgias, serositis in SLE, and hemoptysis in Wegener's granulomatosis.

2. Pathogenesis

The **underlying pathogenesis** of this category of renal failure is direct damage to the kidneys themselves. Specific conditions that can result in renal damage may be subgrouped into **tubular** or **glomerular** types.

    a. Tubular damage or dysfunction results from one of two mechanisms:

        i. An episode of **renal ischemia** due to profound hypotension, or

        ii. Direct damage to the tubules by nephrotoxic agents, including IV contrast agents, aminoglycoside antibiotics, *cis*-platinum chemotherapy, NSAIDs, and a vast array of other agents.

    b. Glomerular damage or dysfunction results from many discrete entities. Classic or common entities are described below.

        i. Post-streptococcal glomerulonephritis, or glomerulonephritis that closely follows a suspected or documented streptococcal infection, usually a pharyngitis. This is a complement-fixing proliferative type of glomerulonephritis that is invariably reversible with supportive care.

        ii. Vasculitides, including systemic lupus erythematosus, polyarteritis nodosum, and Wegener's granulomatosis (see the section on Polyarticular Arthritis in Chapter 7, page 432, for a discussion of SLE). **Wegener's**

granulomatosis is a necrotizing vasculitis that manifests with rapidly progressive GNP, sinusitis with nasal and sinus mucosal lesions, and hemoptysis due to necrotizing pulmonary lesions. **Polyarteritis nodosum** is a vasculitis of medium-sized arteries that may rapidly develop into progressive GNP.

iii. **Thrombotic thrombocytopenic purpura/hemolytic uremic syndrome (TTP/HUS).** This syndrome consists of the **pentad** of microangiopathic hemolytic anemia, thrombocytopenia, fever, mental status changes, and acute renal failure.

iv. The **hepatorenal syndrome,** i.e., the development of acute renal dysfunction in the face of severe (Child's C) hepatic failure. This is a grave and irreversible form of acute renal failure.

v. **Hypertension**—Uncontrolled hypertension can cause acute, subacute, or chronic renal failure as a result of significant glomerular damage.

3. **Evaluation**

   Evaluation includes making the clinical diagnosis by performing the evaluation listed in Box 3-7 and looking for the underlying cause. The patient is usually euvolemic. Specific evaluative tools should include, if a vasculitis or GNP is suspected, serum levels of ANA, RF, ESR, CH_{50}, C_3, C_4, and anticytoplasmic antibody. The ANA, RF, and ESR often will be, in general, elevated, whereas often the complement levels will be decreased. The anticytoplasmic antibody may be quite specific for Wegener's granulomatosis. If there is any evidence of concurrent hepatic dysfunction, obtain liver function tests, including total bilirubin, SGOT, SGPT, GGT, alkaline phosphatase, PT, and albumin (see the section on Polyarticular Arthritis in Chapter 7 for specifics on ANA assays).

4. **Management**

   Specific management includes making the clinical diagnosis and following the parameters of weight, creatinine, urine output, K, PO_4, Mg, and BUN on a frequent basis. Acutely, a nephrology consult is strongly recommended for all patients. Hemodialysis or peritoneal dialysis should be initiated if severe (see Table 3-8). Consultation with a dietician to modify diet to decrease potassium, sodium, and fixed acids (i.e., proteins) is also clearly indicated.

T A B L E   3 - 8
Indications for Emergency Dialysis

1. Volume overload that is resistant to aggressive diuretic therapy and is symptomatic
2. Hyperkalemia that is resistant to aggressive standard treatment (see the section on Hyperkalemia in Chapter 9, page 536)
3. Severe, refractory acidosis
4. Uremic encephalopathy
5. Uremia-induced pericardial friction rub
6. Uncontrollable bleeding due to uremia causing platelet dysfunction
7. Severe rhabdomyolysis
8. Dialyzable toxin or an overdose of agent that is dialyzable (e.g., theophylline)

Specifics in management are beyond the scope of this text.

C. **Postrenal**
   1. **Manifestations**
      The **specific manifestations** include, in addition to those described in the overall manifestations section, a recent onset of a urinary tract infection and manifestations of urinary obstruction. These associated manifestations can include hesitancy, dribbling, urgency, and frequent small quantity urination episodes.
   2. **Pathogenesis**
      The **underlying pathogenesis** is obstruction to the flow of urine between the kidneys and the external environment. The kidneys are functioning appropriately. The differential diagnosis includes **multiple renal calculi** (see the section on Nephrolithiasis, page 159). A second cause is **urinary bladder obstruction** with retention of urine as a result of benign prostatic hypertrophy, prostate adenocarcinoma, or the use of anticholinergic agents. A third cause is retroperitoneal lesions, including lymphoproliferative disorders, fibrosis, or sarcomas, causing bilateral ureteral obstruction. A final, uncommon cause of obstruction is iatrogenic, such as an obstructed Foley catheter.
   3. **Evaluation**
      Evaluation includes making the clinical diagnosis by performing the overall evaluation listed in Box 3-7 and looking for the underlying etiology. The patient is usually euvolemic but may be hypervolemic.

4. **Management**

   Specific management includes the placement (or replacement) of a Foley catheter and emergent referral to a urologist for evaluation and placement of internal or external drainage stents. A nephrology consult is strongly recommended for all patients, as significant electrolyte disturbances and polyuria may develop after acute relief of the obstruction. This polyuric phase occurs as a result of nephrogenic diabetes insipidus after the acute relief of obstruction. The polyuric phase is treated supportively with repletion of the excessive urine output with 0.45 normal saline.

IV. **Chronic renal failure**

The causes of chronic renal failure include irreversible or **recurrent acute renal failure** and **systemic diseases.**

A. **Causes—renal subgroup**

   The most common conditions giving rise to **acute renal failure that progresses to chronic renal failure** are in the "renal" subgroup, that is, the vasculitides and many of the glomerulonephritides. Most prerenal, postrenal, and drug-related causes of acute renal failure will not progress to chronic renal failure if they are effectively treated.

B. **Causes—systemic diseases**

   Systemic diseases are the most common conditions leading to chronic renal dysfunction in the United States today. These diseases include diabetes mellitus and hypertension.

   1. **Diabetes mellitus.** Uncontrolled diabetes mellitus, especially with concurrent hypertension, will result in glomerular damage. This is more commonly subacute to chronic renal failure.

   2. **Hypertension.** Uncontrolled hypertension may cause acute, subacute, or chronic renal failure as a result of significant glomerular damage.

B. **Evaluation and management**

   The **specific evaluation and management** of chronic renal failure include making the clinical diagnosis and performing the tests described in Box 3-7. Other tools are described below.

   1. **Reciprocal creatinine line.** To determine whether any component of acute renal failure is exacerbating the chronic dysfunction, the clinician should attempt to obtain several creatinine levels from the past and plot the reciprocals of the serum creatinine values against time. One can then easily determine the slope of the line. The clinician then plots the most recent 1/creatinine value. If the most recent

reciprocal creatinine value is in the same line—that is, if the slope of the line is unchanged—the creatinine elevation is due to a natural progression of the chronic failure, whereas if the value changes the slope of the line, there is a concurrent acute process occurring.

2. Long-term monitoring of the patient's vital signs, K, BUN, creatinine, general urine output, PO_4, and CO_2 every 2 to 4 weeks. Monitor drug levels, Ca, and hemoglobin every 8–12 weeks.

3. Define and treat any concurrent cause of acute renal failure.

4. Administer the pneumococcal vaccine (Pneumovax) at the time of presentation and provide yearly influenza vaccinations.

5. **Aggressively control hypertension.** The goal is to completely normalize the blood pressure. An effective regimen includes a calcium channel blocker with a loop diuretic. The loop diuretic is especially useful to treat any evidence of fluid retention, either due to the renal failure or as a result of the calcium channel blocker. The dose of loop diuretic often is very large. A rule of thumb is to start with furosemide (Lasix), 20 mg PO, and double the dose every 5–7 days until an effective diuretic dose is found. It is not uncommon to require 160–200 mg of Lasix or 4–5 mg of bumetanide (Bumex) every day.

6. **Dietary modifications.** The diet that should be recommended and described to the patient is 1 g of salt (NaCl), 1,500 mL fluid restriction, and low protein (0.5 g/kg/day). This diet is required in patients with oliguric renal failure who are not on dialysis. If the patient is nonoliguric, sodium and fluid restrictions can be liberalized significantly.

7. Administer **vitamin D 1,25-OH, 50,000 units/day PO;** $CaCO_3$, 600 mg PO b.i.d., and $NaHCO_3$, dosed to keep the serum $CO_2 > 15$ mEq/dL. The usual dose is 500 mg PO once or twice a day.

8. If hiccups are bothersome or recurrent, administer thorazine, 25 mg PO q.6–8h. PRN, or prochlorperazine, 5–10 mg PO q.i.d. PRN.

9. If recurrent bleeding due to uremia-induced platelet dysfunction is present, DDAVP can be used (see discussion above).

10. **Kayexalate,** 15–30 g PO b.i.d., is effective in the chronic management of hyperkalemia in patients not yet on hemodialysis or CAPD. If there is an acute increase in serum potassium, one must treat emergently (see **II. Overall manifestations. H. Hyperkalemia**).

11. **Erythropoietin** is now available as a therapeutic agent. It is effective in increasing the hemoglobin in patients with renal failure–induced anemia. The target is to keep hematocrit in the mid-30s.

12. $Al(OH)_3$ antacids (e.g., Amphogel, 15–30 mL PO t.i.d. to q.i.d. with meals) bind the phosphorus in food. Aluminum-containing antacids should not be used on a *chronic* basis as they can exacerbate metabolic bone disease.

13. **CAPD/HD:** The patient must be prepared for the need for dialysis, either hemodialysis using a surgically constructed arteriovenous fistula or peritoneal dialysis using a peritoneal catheter (see Table 3-8). The patient should have dialysis initiated when the **creatinine time is** <**10 mL/min.** Specifics are beyond text.

14. Consider the patient for **renal transplantation.** This is an issue which the primary care physician should discuss with the patient. The patient should be informed that renal transplants are effective and that none of the above treatments nor being on dialysis is a contraindication to transplant. The patient should discuss this with family members, and any first-degree relatives should be typed for blood and tissue as potential donors. Cytomegalovirus (CMV) titers of the patient should be obtained at baseline. If negative, the patient should receive, if transfusions are ever required, CMV-negative blood.

V. Prevention

This is one of the most critical areas in which the primary care physician or ambulatory care physician can have a major impact. Because many cases of ARF are **iatrogenic,** it is of great importance to follow the renal function of patients placed on potentially nephrotoxic agents, such as NSAIDs or ACE inhibitors. Levels of agents that can be nephrotoxic, such as aminoglycoside antibiotics or lithium, should be determined regularly. Finally, when IV contrast media are used for radiographic imaging studies in patients at high risk for contrast-induced tubular damage (i.e., the elderly, any patients with diabetes mellitus, and any patients with a monoclonal gammopathy), the following preventive measures should be undertaken.

Minimize the dose of contrast agent.

Make certain the patient is euvolemic at the time of contrast-enhanced imaging.

After injection of the contrast agent, administer mannitol,

12.5–25 g IV, to cause a forced diuresis and aid in excreting the agent, thereby minimizing potential tubular damage.

VI. Consultation

Problem	Service	Time
All	Dietary	Elective
If dialysis is indicated	Renal	Emergent
All	Renal	Urgent/emergent
Complete obstruction	GU	Emergent
BPH with partial obstruction	GU	Urgent
Chronic renal failure	Transplant	Elective

VII. Indications for admission: Urgent or emergent need for dialysis, significant hyperkalemia, significant volume overload, hemodynamic instability, or acute tubular necrosis.

Bibliography

Hematuria

Mohr DN, et al: Asymptomatic microhematuria and urologic disease. JAMA 1986;256:224–229.

Restrepo NC, Carey PO: Evaluating hematuria in adults. Am Fam Pract 1989;40:149–156.

Sutton JM: Evaluation of hematuria in adults. JAMA 1990;263:2475–2480.

Thompson C: Hematuria: A clinical approach. Am Fam Pract 1986;33:194–200.

Renal Hypertension

Buck C, et al: The prognosis of hypertension according to age at onset. Hypertension 1987;147:820.

Croog SH, et al: Sexual symptoms in hypertensive patients. Arch Intern Med 1988;148:788–794.

Ferguson RK, Vlasses PH: Hypertensive emergencies and urgencies. JAMA 1986;255:1607–1613.

Frolich ED, et al: Recommendations for human blood pressure determinations by sphygmomanometers. Hypertension 1988;11:209A.

Hommel E, et al: Effect of captopril on kidney function in insulin-dependent diabetic patients with nephropathy. Br Med J 1986;293:467–470.

Hypertension in diabetes mellitus. Arch Intern Med 1987;147:830–842.

Joint National Committee on Detection, Evaluation, and Treatment of High Blood Pressure. Arch Intern Med 1988;148:1023–1038.

Kaplan NM: Non-drug treatment of hypertension. Ann Intern Med 1985;102:359–373.

Kaplan NM, et al: A differing view of treatment of hypertension in patients with diabetes mellitus. Arch Intern Med 1987;147:1160–1162.

Pacheco JP, et al: Monotherapy of mild hypertension with nifedipine. Am J Med 1986;81(suppl 6A):20–24.

Sinclair AM, et al: Secondary hypertension in a blood pressure clinic. Arch Intern Med 1987;147:1289–1293.

Wikstrand J: Primary prevention with metoprolol in patients with hypertension. JAMA 1988;259:1976–1982.

Williams GH: Converting-enzyme inhibitors in the treatment of hypertension. N Engl J Med 1988;319:1517.

Nephrolithiasis

Jacobson EJ, Fuchs G: Nephrolithiasis. Am Fam Pract 1989;39:233–244.

O'Brien WM, et al: New approaches to the treatment of renal calculi. Am Fam Pract 1987;36:181–194.

Pak CY, et al: Ambulatory evaluation of nephrolithiasis. Am J Med 1980; 69:19–29.

Uribarri J, et al: The first kidney stone. Ann Intern Med 1989;111:10006–10009.

Proteinuria

Bernard DB, et al: Extrarenal complications of the nephrotic syndrome. Kidney Int 1988;33:1184–1202.

Levey AS, et al: Idiopathic nephrotic syndrome. Ann Intern Med 1987;107: 697–713.

Schwab SJ, et al: Quantitation of proteinuria by use of protein-to-creatinine ratios in single urine samples. Arch Intern Med 1987;147:943–944.

Stewart DW, et al: Evaluation of proteinuria. Am Fam Pract 1984;29: 218–225.

Pyuria Syndromes

Fihn SD, et al: Trimethoprim-sulfamethoxazole for acute dysuria in women: A single dose or ten day course. Ann Intern Med 1988;108: 350–357.

Hoffman SA, Moellering RC: The enterococcus: Putting the bug into our ears. Ann Intern Med 1987;106:757–761.

Hooten TM, et al: Erythromycin for persistent or recurrent nongonococcal urethritis. Ann Intern Med 1990;113:21–26.

Komaroff AL: Urinalysis and urine culture in women with dysuria. Ann Intern Med 1986;104:212–218.

Pels, et al: Dipstick urinalysis screening of asymptomatic adults for urinary tract disorders: II. Bacteriuria. JAMA 1989;262:1221–1224.

Stamm WE, et al: Acute renal infection in women: Treatment with trimethoprim-sulfamethoxazole or ampicillin for two or six weeks. Ann Intern Med 1987;106:341–345.

Zweig S: Urinary tract infections in the elderly. Am Fam Pract 1987;35: 123–130.

Renal Dysfunction, Acute or Chronic

Clive DM, Stoff JS: Renal syndromes associated with nonsteroidal antiinflammatory drugs. N Engl J Med 1984;310:563–572.

Eschbach JW, et al: Recombinant human erythropoietin in anemic patients with end-stage renal disease. Ann Intern Med 1989;111:992–1000.

Fine RN, et al: Renal transplantation update. Ann Intern Med 1984;100:246.

Fraser CL, Arieff AI: Nervous system complications in uremia. Ann Intern Med 1988;109:143–153.

Goldstein MB: Acute renal failure. Med Clin North Am 1983;67:1325–1341.

Madaio MP, Harrington JT: The diagnosis of acute glomerulonephritis. N Engl J Med 1983;309:1299–1302.

Mooradian AD, Morley JE: Endocrine dysfunction in chronic renal failure. Arch Intern Med 1984;144:351–353.

Moore J, Maher JF: Management of chronic renal failure. Am Fam Pract 1984;30:204–213.

Myers BD, Moran SM: Hemodynamically mediated acute renal failure. N Engl J Med 1986;314:97–105.

Porush JG: New concepts in acute renal failure. Am Fam Pract 1986;33:109–118.

—D.D.B.

Dale Berg, Ed. *Handbook
of Primary Care Medicine.*
Copyright © 1993 J. B.
Lippincott Company.

CHAPTER 4

Pulmonary Diseases

Asthma

Asthma is a common disease that affects all age groups. It has its
greatest incidence in the younger population, but it can begin in
patients in their eighth and ninth decades. Furthermore, it can be
concurrent with, but independent of, chronic obstructive pulmonary disease (COPD) and other cardiopulmonary problems.
Asthma is similar to COPD in that it is a chronic recurrent pulmonary disease with bronchoconstriction and leads to morbid, even
mortal events, but it is **quite different** from COPD in that it involves a pathogenic mechanism in which the bronchoconstriction
is **reversible.**

I. **Pathogenesis of asthma**

The **pathogenesis** of asthma is based on reversible **bronchoconstriction** that occurs as a result of the **release of histamine** and other short- and intermediate-acting mediators
(leukotrienes) from **mast cells** and other inflammatory cells
that have been activated by an **allergen–IgE complex.** This
results in the acute and significant contraction of smooth
muscle fibers within the airways, with resultant markedly
increased airway resistance. Among the large number of **allergens** that can precipitate such a pathogenic response are
pollens, dusts, and, via an analogous mechanism with the
same reversible results, exercise.

A. **Anaphylaxis**

Asthma and other processes that are mediated by IgE
result not only in acute **bronchoconstriction** but also in
other acute and life-threatening states, such as anaphylaxis, **hypotension, urticaria, angioedema of the face
and pharyngeal tissues,** and even **death.** Therefore, in
addition to the bronchoconstriction, the clinician must
watch for and be able to manage effectively any episode

T A B L E   4 - 1
Acute Emergent Management of Anaphylaxis

1. Evaluate and maintain ABCs using the techniques of basic and advanced life support.
2. Administer epinephrine aqueous, 1:1000, 0.3 mL IM or SC. May repeat the dose 2 times.
3. Establish IV access; if patient is hypotensive, give a 500-mL bolus of .9 normal saline.
4. If the anaphylaxis is due to a skin test or an insect bite on an extremity, apply a tourniquet to an area 2–4 cm proximal to the bite or test site.
5. Administer diphenhydramine (Benadryl), 50–75 mg IM or IV or PO q.6–8h. This should be continued for 48–72 hours after the acute event to prevent another anaphylactic event from the same allergen.
6. Administer Solumedrol, 80 mg by IV bolus.
7. Administer cimetidine, 400 mg by IV bolus.
8. Clean the site of the bite.
9. Prescribe a topical β_2 agonist (e.g., albuterol) by hand-held nebulizer for any bronchospasm.

of anaphylaxis in any patient with asthma. The acute management of anaphylaxis is described in Table 4-1.

II. Overall manifestations

The **overall manifestations** of asthma are quite diverse in terms of **type** and **severity** of symptoms and signs. Patients often present with symptoms of an acute attack; at other times the problem of wheezing, shortness of breath, and cough at various times during the year or associated with certain activities becomes evident only after a thorough review of systems.

A. If the patient is having an **acute attack,** the symptoms and signs include tachypnea, tachycardia, dyspnea upon exertion, cough, diffuse wheezing in inspiration and expiration, and, in severely symptomatic patients, cyanosis, stridor, and hypotension. The patient invariably has had similar episodes in the past.

B. In patients who are **not acutely symptomatic** there is usually a paucity of clinical findings; however, one can increase the sensitivity of the auscultatory pulmonary examination by auscultating the lungs during maximal and forced expiration.

C. The patient should be queried for specific **precipitating factors,** including seasonal occurrence, exposure to pet hair, and exercise. This information will indicate what **specific allergens** are involved. If the condition is **seasonal,** pollen or mold are the probable allergens; if **pet-related,** animal dander is the most likely allergen;

B O X 4 - 1

Overall Evaluation and Management of Asthma

Evaluation

1. Evaluate and maintain **ABCs**—*a*irway, *b*reathing, and *c*ardiac maintenance—using basic and advanced life support protocols, as needed.
2. Consider **chest radiography** in PA and lateral views to look for any infiltrate.
3. Obtain a sputum specimen for **gram stain** to look for PMNs or organisms, indicative of an infectious precipitating event.
4. Consider determining the **complete blood cell count** with differential, looking for a leukocytosis. If an eosinophilia is present, it is quite consistent with atopic-related bronchospasm.
5. Determine **oxygen saturation** using a noninvasive finger monitor. If the oxygen saturation is <92% on room air, determine **arterial blood gas values** while the patient is breathing room air. ABG values are sought to document any hypoxemia or hypoventilation, which manifest with a decreased Pao_2 and an elevated $Paco_2$. An **elevated $Paco_2$** is a risk marker for respiratory decompensation.
6. Take a thorough **history** and perform a **physical examination.**

Management

1. The acute emergency management of anaphylaxis is described in Table 4-1.
2. Administer **epinephrine** 1:1000, 0.3 mL subcutaneously. This agent is a potent β_2-receptor agonist that bronchodilates optimally and effectively.
3. β_2-**receptor agonists** are excellent first-line modalities in the treatment of asthma. Specific agents include **albuterol** (Proventil), 2.5 mL in 3 mL normal saline, administered by hand-held nebulizer, or **metoproterenol** (Alupent), 0.3 mL in 3 mL normal saline, administered by hand-held nebulizer. Either is very effective.
4. Provide **oxygen** by nasal canula, face mask, or, if necessary, mechanical ventilation to maintain Pao_2 above 60 mm Hg or O_2 saturation above 90%.

(continued)

B O X   4 - 1 (continued)

> 5. **Steroids** are effective and **indicated** in the manage-
>   ment of bronchospastic disease. For acute treat-
>   ments, agents include methylprednisolone (Solumed-
>   rol), 80 mg IV q.8h., or prednisone, 60 mg PO once
>   daily. The steroids, once initiated, should have a
>   dose taper. A specific model for tapering steroids is
>   given in Table 4-2.

if associated with **exercise,** the underlying cause is
exercise-induced bronchospastic disease. Moreover, a
history of **other allergies,** including "hay fever" and
atopic dermatitis, is not uncommon.

III. **Evaluation and management** (see Box 4-1)
   The **long-term evaluation and management** of reversible airways disease consist of first, preventing or minimizing the
   periods of asthma, and second, minimizing, treating, and
   preventing any concurrent exacerbating cardiopulmonary
   problems. Efforts to meet these long-term goals can be initiated during and immediately after the acute asthmatic or
   anaphylactic event has been reversed.

T A B L E   4 - 2
Model for Tapering Steroids

Treat acutely: Methylprednisolone, 80 mg IV q.8h. or prednisone, 60
mg PO q. A.M. Continue until the desired effect has been achieved, then
the protocol for tapering is begun.

Weaning days 1–3:	60 mg prednisone
Weaning days 4–6:	50 mg prednisone
Weaning days 7–9:	40 mg prednisone
Weaning days 10–12:	30 mg prednisone
Weaning days 13–15:	20 mg prednisone
Weaning days 16–18:	10 mg prednisone
Discontinue	

Notes:
1. Titrate to the symptoms and signs. If symptoms increase, slow the
   taper or increase the dose and start again.
2. Invariably in severe cases a slower taper is required.
3. If unable to wean, document the symptoms that occur at that level
   and attempt to minimize dose to lowest level.
4. Dosing of steroids for asthma should be on a daily basis.

T A B L E   4 - 3
Pulmonary Function Tests

Pulmonary function tests are routinely performed to aid in the diagnosis of pulmonary dysfunction. These tests should be performed after the clinician has formulated a clinical opinion of what the patient has and should be performed when the patient is at his baseline performance status. PFTs and classic findings in common pulmonary diseases are described below.

FEV₁ (forced expiratory volume in 1 second): The patient is instructed to maximally inspire, then maximally exhale. The volume in the first second of expiration is measured. If this is decreased from normal for that age group, the finding is consistent with **airway obstruction.**

FVC (forced vital capacity): The patient is instructed to inspire maximally, then, using maximal force in minimal time, exhale all of the air. The entire volume of air is measured. If this is decreased from normal for the patient's age group, the finding is consistent with a **restrictive disease** process.

FEV₁/FVC: This calculated ratio is normally **.80.** If it is less than .80, the finding is consistent with **airway obstruction.**

Residual volume: The volume of air remaining in the lungs after the completion of maximal expiration. It is the dead-space air. The value cannot be directly measured; but it is calculated using the following equation:

$$RV = FRC - ERV,$$

where FRC is forced respiratory capacity and ERV is expiratory residual volume. Normal is 1,200 mL. A **decrease** in residual volume is consistent with **restrictive disease.** An **increase** in residual volume is consistent with **obstructive disease.**

DLco (diffusing capacity): This is a measurement of the ability of the alveolar membrane unit to **perform gas exchange.** It is measured using carbon monoxide. If **decreased,** it is indicative of either a decrease in the number of alveoli (e.g., emphysema), or an increased alveolar–arterial gradient ($A-ao_2$) as a result of left ventricular failure, pulmonary thromboembolic disease, or interstitial lung disease.

Arterial blood gas values

A. **Pulmonary function tests** aid in defining the specific type of obstructive airways disease. Pulmonary function tests are described in Table 4-3; typical findings in various disease categories are summarized in Table 4-4.

   1. If the test reveals obstructive disease, it must be immediately repeated after a topical β_2 agonist is administered. If the obstruction resolves, it is reversible and thus essentially diagnostic of asthma.

   2. If the PFT results are **equivocal,** the patient is undiagnosed and asymptomatic, and the clinical suspicion is moderate to high, a challenge with the cholinergic agent **methacholine** can be performed to increase the sensitivity of PFTs for asthma.

B. Determine the precipitating agents or events, and then advise the patient to **avoid** them. This should be done via a meticulous history and skin tests performed under the direction of an allergist (see the section on Rhinitis, Chapter 12, page 635, for specifics).

C. Patient and family must **discontinue smoking**.

D. **Chronic pharmacologic intervention** is best divided into two groups of patients, mildly symptomatic and significantly symptomatic.

    1. If the attacks are **mild and infrequent,** β_2-receptor agonist inhaler (Alupent or Proventil) can be prescribed, to be administered through a metered-dose inhaler, two puffs q.i.d. on a **PRN** basis.

    2. If the symptoms are **recurrent or severe,** the patient should be placed on **scheduled β_2 agonists** delivered by metered-dose inhaler, two puffs q.i.d., and **topical steroid inhalers,** beclomethasone, delivered by metered-dose inhaler, two puffs q.i.d. As described in the section on Chronic Obstructive Lung Disease, the β_2 agent should be taken 3–5 minutes before the topical steroid.

        a. If the patient is still symptomatic, systemic steroids are indicated. The goal is to use the lowest possible daily oral dose and weaning off when indicated. The topical steroid will usually aid in the weaning process.

E. Topical anticholinergic agents, oral methylxanthines, and oral β_2 agents are of little use in the management of reversible airway disorders; at most they are adjuvants. A qualification to this statement comes from an NIH consensus group, which recommends adjuvant theophylline therapy in patients with **severe** asthma.

F. If the symptoms are **exercise-induced,** the patient should be instructed to exercise in an environment with a **warm ambient temperature.** The patient should also be instructed not to go from a warm ambient temperature to exercise in the cold. The use of either a β_2 **agonist** delivered by metered-dose inhaler or **cromolyn sodium,** two puffs inhaled, either at the initiation of exercise, is effective in **preventing** the development of this form of bronchospastic disease.

IV. Consultation

Problem	Service	Time
All atopic-related asthma	Allergy	Elective
Severe asthma	Pulmonary	Urgent

V. Indications for admission: Any evidence of anaphylaxis, or any concurrent angina pectoris, left ventricular failure, or

T A B L E 4 - 4
Classic PFT Findings in Various Diseases

Disease Type	FEV₁	FVC	FEV₁/FVC	DLco	RV
Chronic bronchitis	Decreased	Normal to increased	Decreased	Normal	Normal
Emphysema	Decreased	Normal to increased	Decreased	Decreased	Increased
Asthma	Decreased	Normal to increased	Decreased	Normal	Normal
Interstitial diseases	Normal	Decreased to normal	Decreased to normal	Decreased	Normal

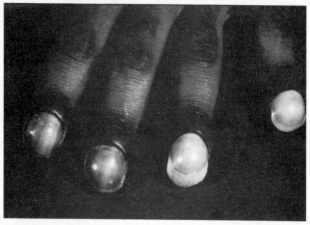

FIGURE 4-1
Clubbing.

pneumonia; the patient is not improving or is deteriorating after initial therapy.

Clubbing

Clubbing is a subtle yet significant sign that, when demonstrated on physical examination, becomes a specific problem with its own differential diagnosis and evaluation. This sign (or problem) is rarely symptomatic and rarely a presenting complaint, but as an acquired finding, it is potentially a harbinger of an underlying malignant neoplastic or other pathologic process.

The **definition** of clubbing has existed since the time of Hippocrates and is quite specific. It includes two components, both of which must be present to make the diagnosis.

1. The **angle** between the nail plate and the proximal nail fold is **inappropriately obtuse.** The normal angle is ~160 degrees. An angle of 160–180 degrees is abnormal and consistent with clubbing.
2. There is an abnormal **sponginess** at the base of the **nail plate on its bed.** (Figs. 4-1 and 4-2).

   I. Differential diagnosis
      The **differential diagnosis** of clubbing is quite diverse and is best categorized using the dichotomous variables of con-

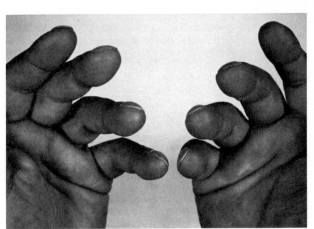

F I G U R E 4 - 2
Clubbing.

genital versus acquired processes and unilateral versus bilateral processes.

A. **Congenital clubbing** implies an underlying congenital cardiac problem, such as tetralogy of Fallot, or any chronic **right-to-left shunt.**

B. **Unilateral, acquired clubbing** usually implies relative ischemia to that extremity, such as that which occurs in thoracic outlet syndrome.

C. **Bilateral, acquired clubbing** is the most common form. The differential diagnosis includes the following:

1. Pulmonary neoplastic disease, especially non-small cell carcinomas.
2. Pulmonary granulomatous diseases, including chronic sarcoidosis, typical and atypical mycobacterial diseases.
3. Bronchiectasis.
4. Inflammatory bowel disease.
5. Rheumatoid arthritis.
6. Chronic, nonspecific hepatic dysfunction.

II. **Evaluation and management**

The **evaluation and management** of clubbing are based on a thorough history and physical examination directed toward findings that may be associated with causative processes. Instruct the family members and patient to discontinue smoking. Evaluative tests that may be indicated include chest radiography in PA and lateral views, PPD skin testing with controls, echocardiography if any valvular abnormality is ausculted on examination, and ESR and RF determinations. There is no specific therapy for clubbing because the condition is asymptomatic. The clinician therefore focuses on determining the underlying cause.

III. Consultation

Problem	*Service*	*Time*
Pulmonary nodule	Pulmonary	Urgent
Congenital valvular lesion	Cardiology	Urgent

IV. Indications for admission: Few, as this problem is asymptomatic. Admission is indicated only if the underlying process is causing severe symptoms.

Chronic Obstructive Lung Disease

Chronic obstructive pulmonary disease (COPD) comprises a large group of chronic disorders in which a major pathophysiologic component is non- or minimally reversible airways disease. This is a chronic, often progressive disorder in which obstruction develops within the bronchi and bronchioles, with or without associated destruction of alveolar tissue itself. The result is an increase in resistance to air flow during both inspiration and expiration, but to a greater degree during expiration.

I. Pathogenesis
The **underlying pathogenesis** of COPD is damage, thickening, or destruction of airway tissue that results in the chronic disease process. If the underlying pathogenetic mechanism is corrected, the disease stabilizes: there is **no further deterioration** but also **no improvement.** However, if the underlying pathogenetic mechanism is not reversed, there will be **continuation** of the damage. Thus it is of great importance to attempt to determine and modify the underlying causes early in the course of the disease in order to prevent further damage.

Although there is considerable overlap, the group of disorders can be divided into two large subsets, **emphysema** and **chronic bronchitis.**

A. **Emphysema** is predominantly the destruction of pulmonary tissue, predominantly alveoli, with resultant irreversible loss of gas-exchange surface and the formation of bullae, but only a mild to modest increase in airway resistance.

B. **Chronic bronchitis** is mainly a minimally reversible airways disease with resultant increased resistance to air
flow and, due to dysfunction of cilia within the airways,
a decrease in the ability of the lungs to mobilize secretions. This decrease in sputum clearance results in the
development of tenacious sputum and an increased risk
of pulmonary infections.

II. **Prevalence**
The **prevalence** of COPD in the United States is quite high,
particularly in middle-aged and elderly people. **Smoking
tobacco** or marijuana is a major risk factor in the development of COPD and a major reason for its high prevalence.
Even with public health education and legislative efforts to
decrease the use of tobacco, **30% of the population** still uses
tobacco on a regular basis. Furthermore, there is a disconcerting increase in the use of such products by young
people. Another risk factor for the development of COPD,
especially emphysema, is a deficiency in the enzyme α_1-
antitrypsin.

III. **Overall manifestations** (see Box 4-2)
The **overall manifestations** of COPD often will not occur
until quite **late in the disease course** or during an **acute
exacerbation** of the chronic process. Although there are
some overlapping features, the symptoms and signs will be
divided into those related to emphysema, chronic bronchitis, or acute exacerbations of COPD.
A. **Emphysema** in the chronic state manifests with diffuse hyperresonance, increased AP diameter of the
chest wall, decreased exercise tolerance, nonproductive
cough, and peripheral cyanosis.
B. **Chronic bronchitis** in the chronic state manifests with
cough productive of purulent sputum. By definition, the
cough must be one that occurs daily and is productive
of purulent sputum for more than 3 months per year
for 3 consecutive years. In addition to the cough, other
common findings include an increased AP diameter of
the chest wall, significant wheezes, especially at the end
of expiration, and potentially cyanosis.
C. An **acute exacerbation** of any of the chronic processes
includes an increase in cough from baseline, an increase
in the quantity of sputum, and/or a change in sputum
from white to yellow; fevers; chills; an increase in shortness of breath; an increase in wheezing; chest tightness;
and any symptoms and signs associated with the precipitating factor. Table 4-5 describes the various precipitating factors and their specific manifestations.

B O X 4 - 2

Overall Evaluation and Management of an Acute Exacerbation of COPD

Evaluation

1. Evaluate and maintain **ABCs**—*a*irway, *b*reathing, and *c*ardiac maintenance—via basic and advanced life support protocols, as indicated.
2. Determine the **underlying precipitating event** and the basic underlying major pathologic group (see Table 4-5).
3. Take a thorough **history,** including tobacco use in the past or present, and perform a **physical examination.**
4. Determine **arterial blood gas values** on room air if possible, looking for hypoxemia or any evidence of hypoventilation as manifested by a respiratory acidosis (i.e., an increased $Paco_2$). The new onset of an **elevated $Paco_2$** is a marker for impending respiratory failure.
5. **Laboratory examinations** include determining levels of theophylline, electrolytes, BUN, creatinine, and glucose, and a CBC with differential for baseline purposes.
6. Obtain **chest radiographs** in PA and lateral views and a **12-lead ECG** at the time of presentation to look for any evidence of an infiltrate, indicative of a pneumonitis, or any ischemic cardiac changes, respectively.
7. Perform baseline **spirometry** at the bedside or in the examination room. Peak expiratory flow is a baseline marker and is repeated as an objective marker for therapeutic improvement in the acute setting. The normal value of this **marker of airway resistance,** in which the number measured is inversely related to airway resistance, is greater than 300 mL. It is a crude objective measurement that is best used when interpreted within the clinical setting and for acute follow-up of therapeutic interventions.
8. Obtain a **sputum specimen** of any productive cough for gross observation and Gram stain. The presence of PMNs and organisms strongly suggests an infection as the precipitating event.

(continued)

B O X 4 - 2 *(continued)*

Management

1. Administer **oxygen** by nasal cannula, face mask, or other methods (including mechanical ventilation) to maintain arterial oxygen pressure above 60 mm Hg or O_2 saturation greater than or equal to 90%. Follow **Paco$_2$** closely after initiating oxygen therapy as O_2 can, in some cases, decrease the patient's ventilatory drive and result in respiratory failure.
2. The **acute management** of an acute exacerbation is tailored to the underlying specific precipitating cause, i.e., heart failure, pulmonary thromboembolic disease, bronchitis, or pneumonitis.
   a. If due to **left ventricular failure,** treat as such.
   b. If due to **pulmonary thromboembolic disease,** treat as such (see section on Pleuritic Chest Pain, Pulmonary Thromboembolic Disease, page 231).
   c. If an **infectious etiology** is suspected, either bronchitis or pneumonitis, and especially if purulent sputum is present, **antibiotics** are clearly indicated.

IV. **Pharmacologic agents**
   Agents of use in the management of an **acute exacerbation of COPD** include the following:
   A. **Beta-2 agonist inhalers** administered by hand-held nebulizer. Either albuterol (Proventil) or metoproterenol (Alupent) is quite effective.
      1. The **mechanism of action** is to increase cAMP in the smooth muscle cells of the bronchial tree via the stimulation of β-adrenergic receptors on those cells. The increase in cyclic AMP results in relaxation of these bronchi and therefore a decrease in the airway resistance.
      2. **Side effects** include the development of supraventricular tachycardias and muscle tremulousness.
      3. Recommended **regimens:**

         albuterol (Proventil), 2.5 mL in 3 mL of normal saline by hand-held nebulizer,
            or
         metoproterenol (Alupent), 0.3 mL in 3 mL of normal saline by hand-held nebulizer.

      These treatments can be repeated in 30–60 minutes.

T A B L E   4 - 5
Precipitating Factors in Acute Exacerbations of COPD

Process	Features
Left ventricular failure	Orthopnea Paroxysmal nocturnal dyspnea Dyspnea upon exertion Third heart sound Crackles, bibasilar Pulmonary vasculature redistribution and cardiomegaly on chest radiograph
Pulmonary thromboembolic disease	Pleuritic chest pain Dyspnea Asymmetric lower extremity swelling Tachypnea No acute change on chest radiograph
Acute bronchitis	Purulent sputum Low-grade fever Rhonchorous breath sounds Wheezing, diffuse Dyspnea No acute change on chest radiograph
Pneumonitis	Purulent sputum Fevers, often spiking to >102°F Lobar consolidation with bronchial breath sounds Infiltrate on chest radiograph

B. Antibiotics are of use in the management of acute exacerbations of COPD, even when given empirically.

1. The **mechanism of action** of these agents is to kill any bacteria acutely infecting the bronchial airways, thus decreasing secretion production in general and purulent sputum production in specific.

2. **Side effects** include diarrhea and the risk of anaphylaxis.

3. The **doses** and **regimens** depend on the suspected infection.

   a. If **pneumonitis,** refer to the section on Community-Acquired Pneumonitis, page 237.

   b. If **bronchitis** or for **empirical therapy,** initiate therapy with:

   TMP–sulfa (Bactrim DS) PO t.i.d.,
   or
   amoxicillin, 500 mg PO q.i.d.,
   or
   ciprofloxacin, 500 mg PO b.i.d.

Any of these regimens is effective against the most common bacterial pathogens in acute bronchitis, the gram-negative coccobacillus *Hemophilus influenzae* and the gram-positive coccus *Streptococcus pneumoniae*.

C. **Topical anticholinergic agents** are of benefit in the acute setting.

1. The **mechanism of action** of these agents, which include ipratropium bromide (Atrovent), is to relax smooth muscle and to decrease the quantity of secretions within the airways.

2. **Side effects** are rare but can include dry mouth and tachycardia.

3. **Dosage:**

   Atrovent, two puffs q.i.d. by metered-dose inhaler, given 5 minutes after β agonist inhalation therapy.

D. **Steroids** are indicated acutely if the patient remains symptomatic or has signs of obstruction after initiation of the above therapy, or if there is any component of atopic disease to the underlying process.

1. The **mechanism of action** of steroids is not completely clear but is probably multifactorial and includes inhibition of the release of inflammatory mediators (leukotrienes, histamines) that mediate the reversible component of the bronchoconstriction. These agents often take a longer period of time to be effective, and thus benefit from them is not immediate but occurs 12–24 hours after initiation.

2. **Side effects** include delirium and psychotic behavior, and, in the long term, immunosuppression, osteoporosis, and decreased would healing.

3. The **dosing** of steroids in the acute setting is:

   Solumedrol, 80 mg IV q.8h.,

   or

   prednisone, 40–60 mg PO q.d.

   Either regimen is continued for several (3–5) days, then tapered (see Table 4-2).

E. **Theophylline.** Before the development of other, more effective modalities, this agent was a mainstay of acute management of an exacerbation of COPD; this is no longer the case.

1. The **mechanism of action** of this agent is to increase cAMP by completely inhibiting the enzyme that degrades cAMP, phosphodiesterase, and, with the increased cAMP, to relax bronchiolar smooth muscle; furthermore, it has a mild diuretic effect.

2. **Side effects** include nausea, vomiting, tremor, restlessness, and tachycardia.

3. The **loading dose** is 5 mg/kg IV given over 15 minutes, followed by a maintenance dose of 0.5 mg/kg/hr IV. The loading dose should be administered only after the baseline theophylline level has been checked and documented to be below 4 mg/dL. If the patient has at presentation a theophylline level in the therapeutic range, place the patient on the maintenance dose only. The **therapeutic range** is 10–20 mg/dL.

V. Evaluation and management

The **intermediate** and **long-term evaluation** and **management** of these disorders, whether emphysema or chronic bronchitis predominates, include the following points. The major goals of management are prevention, patient education, and providing pharmacologic palliation on a long-term basis.

A. **Define the extent** of the COPD and determine whether there is any underlying reversible component to the process. This is best done through the history and physical examination and pulmonary function tests after the patient is at **baseline,** i.e., not during an acute exacerbation of the process (see Table 4-4 for pulmonary function test diagnostic criteria).

B. **Instruct** the patient and all family members to **discontinue smoking,** which will decrease the patient's exposure to direct and second-hand smoke.

C. **Vaccinations** include a one-time dose of Pneumovax (pneumococcal vaccine) and a yearly influenza immunization.

D. **Pharmacologic interventions** for the chronic management of COPD include the same types of agents as are used for acute exacerbations of COPD. Because this is not a reversible process, the agents used must assist the normally functioning pulmonary tissue, reverse any and all concurrent reversible bronchospastic disease, and minimize secretions.

1. **Inhalation agents** include the β_2 **agonists** Proventil (albuterol) or Alupent (metoproterenol) delivered by metered-dose inhaler, two puffs q.i.d.; the **topical anticholinergic** Atrovent (ipratropium sulfate) delivered by metered-dose inhaler, two puffs q.i.d.; and the **topical steroid** beclomethasone delivered by metered-dose inhaler, two puffs q.i.d. These topical/inhalation modalities are the cornerstone of chronic pharmacologic therapy.

a. The agents should be initiated and **used in the order in which they are listed here.** The β_2 agonist should be started first, then, if the patient remains symptomatic, the topical anticholinergic agent should be added, followed by the topical steroid. If two or all three of the agents are being used, the patient should be instructed to use the β_2 agonist by metered-dose inhaler first, wait 3–5 minutes, use the topical anticholinergic agent, wait 3–5 minutes, and then use the topical steroid.

b. Because all of the agents are delivered through a metered-dose inhaler, be sure the patient knows how to use this device.

2. **Chronic oral steroid use** should be reserved for patients with severely symptomatic disease that remains clinically significant even with optimal and maximal therapy. The daily dose should be as small as possible and titrated to the symptoms of dyspnea and wheezing.

3. **Chronic oral methylxanthines** such as theophylline can be of some adjuvant use, especially in patients who remain symptomatic on maximal topical therapy. The oral maintenance dose is usually 200–300 mg PO q.12h. of the long-acting theophylline preparation (e.g., Theodur). The therapeutic range is 10–20 mg/dL.

4. The use of **oral β_2 agents** in addition to or instead of topical β_2 agents results in more side effects than inhalation treatment alone and is of no clear advantage. Therefore, it is of little or no benefit even as an adjuvant modality.

5. **Low-flow chronic oxygen therapy** is a relatively high-cost modality that benefits only a subset of patients with COPD. These patients include patients with cor pulmonale (right ventricular failure), patients who have a PaO_2 below 55 mm Hg, and patients with sleep apnea. (The evaluation and management of sleep apnea is quite complex, requires the consultation of a pulmonary colleague, and is beyond the scope of this textbook). Table 4-6 lists specific indications for the home use of chronic oxygen therapy.

6. **Phlebotomy** to keep the hematocrit at or below 52% if secondary erythrocytosis is present is of acute and chronic benefit.

7. Instruct the patient to **initiate TMP–sulfa,** for which he or she has as a pre-written prescription, for 5–7 days at the **onset of any purulent sputum** changes.

T A B L E   4 - 6
Indications for Low-Flow Home Oxygen Therapy
(American Thoracic Society)

1. $Pao_2 < 55$ mm Hg on room air
2. O_2 saturation < 90% on room air
3. Exercise-induced or sleep-induced decrease in Pao_2 to <55 mm Hg
4. Primary pulmonary hypertension
5. Cor pulmonale

VI. **Consultation**

Problem	*Service*	*Time*
Severe COPD	Pulmonary	Elective
Any atopic component	Allergy	Elective
If heart failure is present	Cardiology	Urgent

VII. **Indications for admission:** Any patient who requires steroids in the acute setting; any patient who does not improve after two β_2 agonist treatments; or any patient with concurrent or concomitant unstable angina pectoris, pulmonary thromboembolic disease, left ventricular failure, or pneumonitis.

Hemoptysis (see Box 4-3)

The anatomy of the **airway system** is quite simple. It is essentially an inverted hollow tree in which the trunk is the **upper airway system,** consisting of the nasopharynx, mouth, oropharynx, hypopharynx, larynx, and trachea; and the branches compose the **lower airway system,** consisting of the bronchi, bronchioles, and alveoli. Although the anatomy is simple to describe, the component structures are quite diverse, and **any part** of it can bleed, resulting in hemoptysis. **Hemoptysis is the coughing up of blood.** Because the blood can come from any part of the respiratory tract, because the gastrointestinal tract is contiguous with the respiratory tract, and because patients themselves define hemoptysis in different ways, the problem of hemoptysis is quite diverse.

I. **Overall manifestations**

The **overall manifestations** of hemoptysis include the features of the hemoptysis itself and associated manifestations. Hemoptysis is best described in terms of quantity. If there is a scant amount of blood or whitish yellow sputum streaked with blood, it is called **mild hemoptysis,** whereas if there is a large quantity of gross blood, i.e., >200 mL (~1/2 cup) in a 24-hour period, it is called **massive hemoptysis.**

The **associated manifestations** can include a change in

B O X 4 - 3

Overall Evaluation and Management of Hemoptysis

Evaluation

1. Evaluate **ABCs** and institute basic and advanced life support modalities, as airway maintenance and ventilation are major concerns in patients with hemoptysis.
2. Take a thorough **history** and perform a **physical examination,** looking for features described under **I. Overall manifestations.** Query the patient regarding the source of the bleeding. Often the patient can localize the site of bleeding to the right or left lung, the upper airways, or the lower airways.
3. Examine the **mouth** for bleeding sites and the **nose** for epistaxis.
4. Obtain **chest radiographs** in PA and lateral views to look for infiltrates, nodules, and lesions.
5. Determine **PT, PTT,** and **platelet count,** looking for any evidence of coagulopathy such as an increased PT, an increased aPTT, or a decreased platelet count.
6. Determine the **complete blood cell count** with differential for baseline purposes.
7. Determine **arterial blood gas values** for baseline purposes and to diagnose any hypoxemia, which would be indicative of significant blood in the pulmonary tree.
8. Examine the **sputum directly visually** to ascertain what specifically the patient is expectorating.
9. Obtain a **Gram stain of the sputum,** looking for any PMNs and bacteria indicative of an infectious bronchitis or pneumonitis.
10. Send a sputum sample for **AFB smear** and culture. The presence of acid-fast bacilli is indicative of active mycobacterial disease. This procedure is unnecessary if the chest radiograph is normal.
11. Place the patient on **respiratory isolation** if mycobacterial disease is suspected.
12. Send a sputum sample for **cytology** to look for malignant cells, diagnostic of a malignant lesion in the respiratory tree.
13. Provide **oxygen supplementation** to keep $Pao_2 > 60$ mm Hg.

(continued)

B O X 4 - 3 (continued)

Management

If the bleeding is **mild,** determine its source and cause, and treat the underlying condition. If the bleeding is **massive,** the patient's condition can rapidly deteriorate, and thus emergent management is clearly indicated. A basic approach includes the following steps.

1. **Admit** the patient to a monitored bed, preferably in an ICU.
2. If the **lesion is localized** on the chest radiograph, the patient should keep the **ipsilateral** side inferior.
3. Correct any coagulopathy.
4. Provide cough suppression with codeine, 30 mg PO q.4–6h.
5. Obtain emergent consultation with cardiothoracic surgeons and pulmonologists for **rigid bronchoscopy.**

Further management is beyond the scope of this text.

---

the quantity or quality of sputum, tachypnea, dyspnea, chest pain, pleuritic chest pain, nausea, vomiting, hematemesis, and fevers. Because the GI tract is contiguous with the respiratory tract, the clinician must differentiate **hematemesis** from hemoptysis.

II. Differential diagnosis

The **differential diagnosis** of hemoptysis, the pathogenesis, the unique characteristics of each underlying state, and a brief summary of evaluation and management are given below and in Table 4-7.

A. Acute bronchitis

This is a common cause of hemoptysis. The **pathogenesis** is thought to be recurrent cough with irritation and breakdown of the airway mucosa with resultant bleeding. The usual pathogens that cause acute bronchitis include *Hemophilus influenzae, Branhamella catarrhalis,* and *Streptococcus* spp. **Specific manifestations** include mild hemoptysis with associated purulent sputum, low-grade fever, and occasional diffuse wheezes elicited on auscultation. **Evaluation and management** include Gram stain of the sputum, which reveals PMNs and the specific

T A B L E 4 - 7
Hemoptysis: Differential Diagnosis and Features

Etiology	Mild/Massive	Associated Features	Chest Radiograph	Evaluation and Management
Bronchitis	Mild	Cough, worse at night Purulent sputum Low-grade fever	Normal, or no change from baseline	Basic Cough suppression TMP–sulfa or amoxicillin for 7 days
Neoplastic lesion	Mild to massive	Weight loss Smoking history Cough	Solitary nodule Mass Can have cavity and/or infiltrate	Basic, and sputum cytology Bronchoscopy
Pulmonary infarction	Mild to massive	Pleuritic chest pain	Normal, or pleural-based infiltrate with effusion	Basic See section on Pleuritic Chest Pain, page 227 V/Q, venous Doppler studies Anticoagulate with heparin
Mycobacterial infections	Mild to massive	Reactive PPD Weight loss	Simon foci Ghon focus/complex	Basic Respiratory isolation INH/rifampin/ethambutol
Left ventricular failure	Mild	Orthopnea PND Dyspnea Third heart sound	Cardiomegaly Increased pulmonary vascular distribution	Basic Oxygen Loop diuretics Nitrates Digoxin

pathogen, and a chest radiograph, which usually is at baseline or "normal." Therapy is with cough suppressants and antibiotics, either TMP–sulfa (Bactrim DS, 1 tablet PO b.i.d.) or amoxicillin (500 mg PO t.i.d. for 7 days).

B. Neoplasia

This is a relatively uncommon but very important cause of hemoptysis. The usual **pathogenesis** is either erosion of the mucosa by the tumor with mild bleeding, or direct invasion of a vein or artery by the tumor with massive hemoptysis. Benign or malignant neoplasia, either non-small cell or small cell carcinoma, is often associated with hemoptysis. The **specific manifestations** usually include mild hemoptysis, but occasionally a neoplastic lesion can result in massive hemoptysis. The patient often is a user of tobacco and, if the disease is advanced, may have the associated features of unintentional weight loss, acquired bilateral clubbing, and constitutional symptoms. **Evaluation and management** include obtaining a chest radiograph, which invariably demonstrates the location of the primary lesion. Cytologic examination of the sputum often reveals malignant neoplastic cells (sensitivity < 50%); however, consultation with pulmonologists or interventional radiologists to biopsy the lesion may be required to make the diagnosis (see the section on Bronchogenic Carcinoma in Chapter 5 for specifics in management).

C. Pulmonary infarction

This is a quite uncommon cause of hemoptysis. The **pathogenesis** involves infarction of an area of lung tissue. This form of pulmonary thromboembolic disease results when an embolism occurs in an area of relative bronchial arterial hypoperfusion; thus, both sources of blood flow to the lung are impeded, resulting in infarction concurrent with the embolism. The **specific manifestations** include pleuritic chest pain, cough, low-grade fever, splinting, tachypnea, tachycardia, dyspnea, mild to massive hemoptysis, and signs of consolidation in the area involved. **Evaluation and management** include obtaining a chest radiograph, which is usually normal but may show a pleural-based infiltrate and pleural effusion on the ipsilateral side. The arterial blood gases reveal an increased A–aO$_2$ gradient (for further discussion see the section on Pleuritic Chest Pain, page 227).

D. Mycobacterial disease

The **pathogenesis** involves destruction of pulmonary tissue by reactivation of mycobacterial disease, usually by cavity formation. It can become massive if the cavity involves a pulmonary vein or artery or if there is the development of a dilated pulmonary artery in the wall of the cavity, the "aneurysm of Rasmussen." The **specific manifestations** include mild to moderate hemoptysis. Associated features may include unintentional weight loss, cough with purulent sputum production, and a history of mycobacterial disease exposure in the past. **Evaluation and management** include obtaining a chest radiograph, which will demonstrate the findings of mycobacterial disease, i.e., Ghon focus, Ghon complex, or Simon foci, or the classic finding of a cavity in the upper zone of the lung. Sputum should be sent for Gram stain and AFB smear and culture. The patient must be placed in respiratory isolation. (See section on Mycobacterial Diseases, page 248, for further discussion.)

E. **Left ventricular failure**

The underlying **pathogenesis** involves edema within the interstitial spaces of the lungs that, when severe, fills the alveoli and is coughed up. Although quite uncommon in the United States today, the entity mitral valve stenosis is the quintessential example of a lesion causing hemoptysis. The **specific manifestations** include very mild hemoptysis with a scant amount of blood in the sputum, resulting in pink, frothy sputum. Associated manifestations may include orthopnea, paroxysmal nocturnal dyspnea (PND), dyspnea upon exercise, dyspnea at rest, and a history of cardiac dysfunction or valvular disease, especially mitral stenosis. Signs may include a laterally displaced point of maximal impulse (PMI), a third heart sound, bibasilar crackles, and, if the condition is due to mitral valve stenosis, a diastolic murmur at the apex. **Evaluation and management** include obtaining a chest radiograph, which will reveal an increase in pulmonary vasculature, cardiomegaly, Kerley B lines, and pleural effusions (right > left). (See the section on Congestive Heart Failure in Chapter 1 for further discussion.)

F. **Coagulopathy**

The underlying **pathogenesis** is the inability to form clots even after mild trauma to the respiratory mucosa. The **specific manifestations** include mild hemoptysis and diffuse bleeding from many sites, as manifested by epistaxis, purpura, petechiae, menorrhagia, and hematuria. **Evaluation and management** are discussed extensively in the section on Excessive Bleeding Disorders in Chapter 5, page 275.

G. **Aspergilloma**

This is one of the most common causes of **massive** hemoptysis. The **pathogenesis** involves underlying emphysema with bullous disease, or a chronic cavitary process that secondarily becomes infected or colonized with *As-*

pergillus spp. *Aspergillus* can grow and form a fungus ball, or aspergilloma, within the bulla or cavity. The aspergilloma can then erode into or irritate the blood vessels adjacent to the cavity. The **specific manifestations** include massive hemoptysis in a patient with a history of any bullae or cavity-forming process, including emphysema or reactivation tuberculosis. **Evaluation and management** include obtaining a chest radiograph, which demonstrates a cavitary lesion with a mass inside. Therapy is directed toward removal of the lesion via lobectomy of the affected lobe.

H. **Bronchiectasis**

This cause of hemoptysis is relatively uncommon today. The **pathogenesis** arises from the bronchiectasis itself. Bronchiectasis is a chronic process secondary to partial obstruction of a bronchus, with chronic mild dilation of the bronchioles and bronchi distal to the partial obstruction and with resultant chronic infection. The trauma of recurrent cough and infection and inflammation results in mild hemoptysis. The quintessential example of an entity that results in bronchiectasis is cystic fibrosis. **Specific manifestations** include the presence of recurrent, intermittent, mild hemoptysis with chronic purulent sputum production and a severe cough. The patient often knows that he or she has the diagnosis and presents with the concern that the hemoptysis either recently started or has recently increased in quantity. **Evaluation and management** include obtaining a chest radiograph, which will demonstrate the classic findings of bronchiectasis, i.e., a chronic infiltrate with an associated area of dilated bronchi. Therapy is directed toward ruling out any concurrent lesions, including cystic fibrosis, and suppressing the chronic infection with long-term penicillin therapy PO. Consultation with pulmonologists is indicated.

III. **Consultation**

Problem	Service	Time
Any suspicion of neoplasia	Pulmonary	Urgent
Massive hemoptysis	Pulmonary	Emergent
Bronchiectasis	Pulmonary	Urgent
Massive hemoptysis	Cardiothoracic surgery	Emergent
Left ventricular failure	Cardiology	Urgent

IV. **Indications for admission:** Massive hemoptysis, heart failure, hemodynamic instability, or any evidence of respiratory compromise.

Pleural Effusions (see Box 4-4)

The **pleural space** is normally a potential space. It is, by definition, the area between the **visceral pleura**—a simple squamous epithelial lining directly applied to the lung—and the **parietal pleura**—a simple squamous epithelial lining applied to the inner surface of the chest wall. The pleural space in each hemithorax is essentially **independent** of the other in the normal state. The pleural space in the healthy, normal adult has <50 mL of transudative fluid in each hemithorax. Any quantity of fluid in excess of that amount in either hemithorax is termed a **pleural effusion.**

I. **Overall manifestations**

The **overall manifestations** of pleural effusions include **orthopnea,** especially if the effusions are bilateral; **trepopnea,** if the effusion is unilateral (the patient preferentially sleeps with the side ipsilateral to the effusion down); **dyspnea upon exertion;** nonproductive cough; and baseline dyspnea. Further **signs** over the area of effusion include localized **dullness to percussion** with concurrent **decreased breath sounds** and **decreased tactile fremitus** in the same area. There is often an area of bronchial breath sounds at the superior border of the area of decreased breath sounds. The bronchial breath sounds occur as a result of adjacent atelectasis of the lung tissue.

II. **Additional evaluation**

Further evaluation entails categorizing the pleural effusion as **transudative, exudative,** or **bloody.** Each category of pleural effusion has differentiating features, a specific differential diagnosis, and thus a different scheme of evaluation and management (see Tables 4-8 and 4-9).

A. **Transudative effusions: LDH of pleural fluid** <200 IU, **protein of pleural fluid** <3.0 g, ratio of LDH in pleural fluid to LDH in plasma <0.6, ratio of total protein in pleural fluid to total protein in plasma <0.5.

1. The **pathogenesis** of transudative effusions results from changes in the Starling forces that maintain fluid in the intravascular spaces, either an **increase in the hydrostatic pressure** (as in heart failure) and/or a **decreased albumin** (e.g., as a result of cirrhosis or nephrotic syndrome) (see Table 4-9).

2. The **evaluation and management** of transudative effusions entail treating the underlying pathologic process, which is virtually always clinically evident. No other evaluation of the fluid itself is necessary. **Therapeutic thoracentesis** of 500–1,000 mL of fluid is indicated only if the effusion is massive and the patient is quite symptomatic due to its size. Management of

---

B O X 4 - 4

Overall Evaluation of Pleural Effusions

Evaluation

1. Take a thorough **history** and perform a **physical examination,** looking for overall manifestations.
2. Obtain **chest radiographs** in PA, lateral, and **decubitus** views (Fig. 4-3). The **decubitus radiograph** is best obtained with the affected side down and is used to determine what quantity of fluid moves, or "layers out," with gravity. If >1 cm fluid layers out, then it is quite safe to perform thoracentesis. Any effusion that does not "layer out" or is <1 cm should be further localized by ultrasonography and thoracentesis performed under US guidance.
3. Perform **thoracentesis.** The tests used to evaluate **all** pleural effusions include the following:
   a. Gross appearance: clear, bloody, or purulent.
   b. Pleural fluid LDH.
   c. Plasma LDH (obtained within 24 hours of thoracentesis).
   d. Total protein content of pleural fluid.
   e. Total protein content of plasma (obtained within 24 hours of thoracentesis).
4. Categorize the fluid as **transudative** or **exudative,** based on the above parameters; see discussion in this section and Table 4-8.
5. Save some fluids in case the fluid is exudative. If it is, further tests are indicated.
6. Obtain a postthoracentesis chest radiograph to rule out any postprocedure **pneumothorax.**

---

left ventricular failure, cirrhosis, and nephrotic syndrome is described elsewhere in the book.

B. **Exudative effusions: LDH of pleural fluid >200** IU, **protein of pleural fluid >3 g,** ratio of LDH in pleural fluid to LDH in plasma >0.6, ratio of total protein in pleural fluid to total protein in plasma >0.5.

1. The **pathogenesis** of exudative effusions is more diverse and portends a more malignant course. The **differential diagnosis** is outlined in Table 4-9.
2. The **evaluation and management** are significantly more extensive than for transudative effusions. Labo-

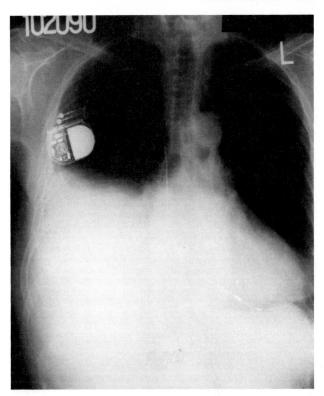

F I G U R E 4 - 3
Posteroanterior chest radiograph showing massive right pleural
effusion.

T A B L E 4 - 8
Light's Criteria for Transudative versus Exudative Effusions

Parameter Evaluated	Transudative	Exudative
LDH	<200 IU	>200 IU
Pleural fluid/plasma LDH ratio	<0.6	>0.6
Total protein	<3 g	>3 g
Pleural fluid/plasma protein ratio	<0.5	>0.5

T A B L E   4 - 9
Differential Diagnosis of Pleural Effusions

Transudative

Left ventricular failure
Cirrhosis
Nephrotic syndrome

Exudative

Parapneumonic
  Viral
  Bacterial
Pulmonary infarction
Mycobacterial
Rheumatoid
SLE
Lymphoproliferative
Malignant neoplastic
Pancreatitis

Bloody

Trauma
Malignant neoplasia
Mesothelioma
Pulmonary infarction

---

ratory tests on the pleural fluid itself include pH, Gram stain, cultures, cytology, AFB smear, glucose, amylase, cell count, and rheumatoid factor assay. Further **evaluation and management** depend on the results of these tests and are beyond the scope of this text.

  a. If there is **gross pus,** if Gram stain **demonstrates bacteria** (i.e., empyema), or if the pleural fluid **glucose is <20 mg/dL and pH is <7.0** (i.e., a **complicated parapneumonic effusion** as a result of a bacterial pneumonia), the clinician must involve pulmonologists or cardiothoracic surgeons for drainage procedures.

  b. If the effusion is parapneumonic but the glucose level is >20 mg/dL and the pH is >7.0 (i.e., an **uncomplicated parapneumonic effusion**), the clinician must watch closely and repeat the thoracentesis on alternate days until it has resolved, looking for a decrease in the pleural fluid glucose or pH, or the development of an empyema, any of which would necessitate the placement of a chest tube.

    c. If **malignant cytology** is present (i.e., malignant neoplastic effusion), consultations with oncologists and pulmonologists should be sought. Chest tube drainage is indicated if the effusion is massive and symptomatic.

C. **Bloody pleural effusions** are not uncommon and are virtually always exudative in nature. The diagnosis is quite evident at the time of thoracentesis.

    1. The **pathogenesis** of bloody effusions is diverse and portends a more malignant course. The **differential diagnosis** is outlined in Table 4-9.

    2. The **evaluation and management** of bloody effusions are significantly more extensive than for transudative effusions. Laboratory studies of the pleural fluid itself include pH, Gram stain, cultures, cytology, AFB smear, glucose, amylase, cell count, hematocrit, and rheumatoid factor assay. As with other pleural effusions, **therapy** must be tailored to the underlying process. Consultation with pulmonologists should be sought.

III. Consultation

Problem	*Service*	*Time*
Exudative effusion	Pulmonary	Urgent
Bloody effusion	Pulmonary	Urgent
Empyema	Cardiothoracic surgery	Urgent
Nephrotic syndrome	Renal	Urgent
Malignant effusion	Oncology	Urgent

IV. **Indications for admission:** Any evidence of respiratory compromise due to the effusion, or any evidence of an empyema or a complicated parapneumonic effusion.

Pleuritic Chest Pain

Pleuritic chest pain is defined as pain that is exacerbated by inspiration or expiration. It is often pain that is invariably referable or attributable to irritation of the pleura. The **pleura** is a simple squamous epithelium that is derived from mesoderm and lines the lungs and chest wall. The **visceral pleura** lines the lungs, whereas the **parietal pleura** lines the inside of the chest wall. Inflammation, disruption, or dysfunction of either the parietal or visceral pleura manifests with pleuritic-type chest pain. Although many processes can manifest with pleuritic-type chest pain, four of the most common or reversible specific syndromes are discussed here: pneumothorax, musculoskeletal chest pain, pneumonitis, and pulmonary thromboembolic disease.

I. Pneumothorax

Pneumothorax may cause a patient to present with pleuritic chest pain. There is the acquired disruption of the parietal or visceral pleural membrane with resultant leakage of atmospheric air into the pleural space. The pleuritic chest pain is always on the same side as the pneumothorax. There are two types of pneumothoraces, **simple** and **tension.**

A. A **simple pneumothorax** remains the same size acutely, then resolves with time. Simple pneumothoraces can be dangerous in and of themselves because they result in restriction of respiratory volume and may lead to significant respiratory compromise, or may develop into tension pneumothoraces. The **specific manifestations** include pleuritic-type chest pain, mild tachypnea, and decreased breath sounds in the lung ipsilateral to the pneumothorax. **Precipitating causes** of simple and tension pneumothoraces may be **iatrogenic** (e.g., thoracentesis or central line placement), **traumatic** (e.g., rib fracture or a penetrating wound to the chest), or **spontaneous,** usually in patients with risk factors (e.g., coughing fits, bullous disease, a history of pneumothoraces). **Evaluation and management** include that described in Box 4-5 and watching for the development of a tension pneumothorax.

B. A **tension pneumothorax** is one in which the process is severe and unchecked, with a significant and progressive inflow of air into the pleural space. The process invariably results in collapse of the ipsilateral lung and displacement of all thoracic structures to the contralateral hemithorax. A tension pneumothorax can be rapidly fatal if not diagnosed and treated acutely. The **specific manifestations** of a tension pneumothorax include pleuritic-type chest pain, decreased breath sounds, and hyperresonance, all **ipsilateral** to the pneumothorax. Additional manifestations include tachycardia, tachypnea, and a shift of the trachea and other mediastinal structures to the **contralateral side. Evaluation and management** of a tension pneumothorax include that described in Box 4-5 and emergency intervention. Intervention entails the insertion of a 14-gauge needle into the affected hemithorax, or, better, emergency chest tube placement either laterally or, for time efficiency, anteriorly. All tension pneumothoraces require chest tube placement and hospitalization with consultation with cardiothoracic surgeons. The pleuritic chest pain will resolve with resolution of the pneumothorax.

II. Musculoskeletal chest pain

This is the most common reason for pleuritic-type chest pain. In the vast majority of cases it is self-limited and

B O X 4 - 5

Overall Evaluation and Management of Pneumothorax

Evaluation

1. Evaluate and maintain **ABCs** using basic and advanced life support protocols.
2. Obtain **chest radiographs** in PA and lateral views to look for, diagnose, or confirm the presence of a pneumothorax (Fig. 4-4).
3. Determine **arterial blood gas values,** preferably with the patient breathing room air, as baseline. Any hypoxemia is of significant import.
4. Provide **supplemental oxygen** via nasal cannula or face mask to maintain Pao_2 above 60 mm Hg.
5. A **tension pneumothorax** or a **simple pneumothorax** that occupies **>20%** of the ipsilateral hemithorax requires immediate chest tube placement.
6. If the patient has a **simple pneumothorax** and it is **asymptomatic and <20%** of the hemithorax is affected, conservative treatment is indicated. Follow up with examinations and chest radiographs every 12–24 hours until the process has resolved.

benign, but it may be a harbinger of a more significant problem.

A. **Trauma** is the most common cause of musculoskeletal chest pain. The **specific manifestations** include antecedent blunt trauma with associated bruising, ecchymosis, splinting, and potentially one or more rib fractures. **Evaluation and management,** especially if the pain is significant, include rib films and chest radiographs in PA and lateral views. The chest radiographs are required to rule out any concurrent pneumothorax or hemothorax. If there are no associated or evident complications, NSAIDs (e.g., ibuprofen, 600–800 mg PO q.6h. PRN) or even a short course of a narcotic agent (e.g., Tylenol 3, one tablet PO q.4–6h. PRN) can be prescribed and are effective in affording analgesia. The application of tape to the chest wall is of little value. Follow-up should be as clinically needed.

B. **Tietze's syndrome** is a not uncommon cause of pleuritic musculoskeletal chest pain. This is nonspecific, usually trauma-related, costochondritis, i.e., inflammation of the

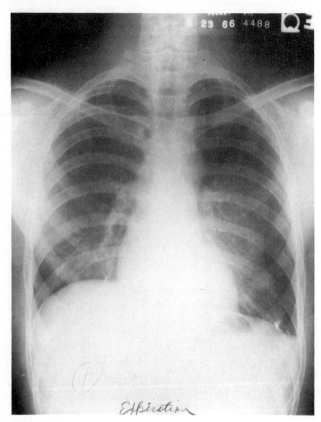

Expiration

F I G U R E   4 - 4
Anteroposterior chest radiograph taken in expiration and showing a large left pneumothorax.

joints between the ribs and the sternum. The **specific manifestations** include pain that is demonstrable and completely reproduced by palpation of the costochondrial joints. **Specific evaluation and management** include initiation of a NSAID or a narcotic-type agent.

C. **Nontraumatic rib fracture** can occur in a patient with severe recurrent cough or with lytic rib lesions; therefore, if a rib fracture occurs and there is no history of antecedent trauma, one must ask why it did occur. If a lytic lesion is present, **evaluation and management** with serum protein electrophoresis (SPEP), erythrocyte sedimentation rate (ESR), urine protein electrophoresis (UPEP), and bone biopsy are indicated as the most likely diagnosis is a **monoclonal gammopathy.**

III. Pneumonitis

This is a not uncommon cause of pleuritic chest pain. Inflammation of the lung parenchyma invariably leads to inflammation of the adjacent pleura, causing pleuritic-type chest pain. This is most evident in *Streptococcus pneumoniae* pneumonitis. (See section on Community-Acquired Pneumonitis for further discussion.)

IV. Pulmonary thromboembolic disease (PTE) (Box 4-6)

This is perhaps, with the exception of a tension pneumothorax, the most acutely ominous diagnosis which manifests with pleuritic-type chest pain. It is a relatively common disease process, especially in patients at high risk for the development of deep venous thrombosis.

A. The **pathogenesis** and **natural history** of this disorder are integral to its evaluation and management. This will be divided into two areas of discussion, the **sites** where **emboli originate** and the **risk factors** for their development.

   1. Emboli that reach the **pulmonary arteries** originate from some specific **site.**

      a. The **deep venous systems** of the **thighs** and **pelvis** are the most common sites of formation of thrombi that embolize to the pulmonary arteries. In fact, the vast majority (>95%) of emboli come from these sites.

      b. Another site of potential thrombus formation is the **deep system of the upper arm.** Although it is quite uncommon for an arm DVT to develop, once present, it may embolize to the pulmonary arteries.

      c. Another potential but quite rare site of venous thromboembolism is the **right ventricle.**

   2. It is **exceedingly rare** for a thrombus **isolated to the calf** (i.e., distal to the popliteal fossa) to embolize to the pulmonary artery unless it has already propagated (extended) into the popliteal fossa or even further proximally into the thigh.

B. **Risk factors** for the development of thrombi and therefore of thromboembolic events include, but are not limited to, **immobilization, concurrent carcinoma,** the recent **donation of plasma,** a **past history of thromboembolism,** a **family history of PTE** events, the use of

estrogens, and a congenital or acquired **hypercoagulable state.** Defined hypercoagulable states include **deficiencies** in natural anticoagulation factors such as antithrombin III, protein C, and protein S.

C. The **overall manifestations** of PTE disease include pleuritic-type chest pain, but this is a far from universal finding. Other symptoms and signs include tachypnea, dyspnea, hemoptysis, pleural friction rub, low-grade fever, and asymmetric swelling of the lower extremities. Pao_2 is decreased, as is $Paco_2$, all leading to an **increased A–ao_2 gradient. Chest radiographs** are usually at baseline, or normal; however, a pleural-based infiltrate can be present in severe pulmonary thromboembolism (Hampton's hump sign). Finally, the **ECG** usually shows sinus tachycardia; again, however, the classic pattern of a right axis deviation, S1, Q3, T3 pattern may be present.

D. Further **evaluation and management** are based on the **clinical suspicion for PTE** at the time of the initial assessment. This clinical suspicion is the cornerstone in the diagnosis and therapy of this condition. The three subsets are identified:

1. **High clinical suspicion.** Risk factors and baseline clinical evidence make PTE the likely cause of the pleuritic chest pain.

2. **Low clinical suspicion.** A condition other than PTE is known or is likely to be the cause of the pleuritic chest pain (e.g., angina pectoris, pneumothorax, pneumonitis, or musculoskeletal etiologies).

3. **Intermediate clinical suspicion.** Some features of PTE are present, but other diagnoses may be possible; thus, no clear-cut diagnosis emerges from the initial assessment. This occurs in the majority of cases. **Further diagnostic tests are necessary** to aid the clinician in making the diagnosis of PTE.

E. The **evaluation and management** for each subgroup are described below.

1. **High clinical suspicion.** Essentially the diagnosis is made. **Treatment should not be postponed** for any evaluative tools unless there is a relative or absolute contraindication to first-line, standard therapy, anticoagulation. (See Table 4-10 for contraindications to anticoagulation.)

   a. The patient should be **anticoagulated** with **heparin,** 5,000–10,000 units by IV bolus, followed by a maintenance dose of 1,300 units/hr IV. The aPTT should be checked 6 hours after the initiation of therapy. The **therapeutic goal is an aPTT of 60–80 seconds.** The bolus can be given in the clinician's office as arrangements are made for inpatient ad-

BOX 4-6

***Overall Evaluation and Management of Potential
Pulmonary Thromboembolic Disease***

Evaluation

1. Take a thorough **history** and perform a **physical examination,** documenting any past history of venous thromboembolic disease and the items described under **IV, C** (overall manifestations) in the text.
2. Assess the patient for **risk factors.**
3. Perform a **guaiac test on the stool** to document that the patient is not concurrently bleeding from a GI site, a contraindication to anticoagulation.
4. Determine **arterial blood gas values** for baseline purposes. Values suggestive of mild hyperventilation (i.e., a **decreased $Paco_2$**) and hypoxemia (i.e., a **decreased Pao_2**) are consistent with pulmonary thromboembolic disease. A normal arterial oxygen level, however, does not rule out PTE, as evidenced by the fact that 20% of patients with PTE have arterial oxygen levels above 80 mm Hg.
5. Obtain **chest radiographs** in PA and lateral views, looking for any infiltrates. The vast majority of patients with PTE disease will have normal chest radiographs.
6. Consider obtaining a **12-lead ECG** for baseline purposes. The vast majority of patients with PTE disease will have **sinus tachycardia** as the sole ECG manifestation.
7. Determine **aPTT** and **PT** for baseline purposes in the event that anticoagulation is indicated.
8. Determine the **complete blood cell count** with differential for baseline purposes in the event that anticoagulation is indicated.
9. Determine the **platelet count** for baseline purposes in the event that anticoagulation is indicated.
10. Further evaluation and management are based on the clinical suspicion for PTE as determined by the evaluation described above.

T A B L E 4 - 1 0
Contraindications to Anticoagulation

1. Heparin-induced thrombocytopenia (only heparin is contraindicated)
2. Intracranial hemorrhage within the preceding 6 weeks
3. Major GI or GU bleeding within the preceding 6 weeks
4. Major surgery in an area that is not compressible (e.g., a neurosurgical or intra-abdominal surgical procedure) within the preceding 6 weeks.

mission. The heparin is continued for a total of 5–7 days. Early in the course it is best to err on the high side, as the risk for PTE is greatest early in the course.

Mechanism of action of heparin: Heparin acts on the naturally occurring inhibitor of thrombin formation, **antithrombin III.** Heparin prevents further propagation and embolization of the thrombus and allows the intrinsic fibrinolytic pathway to lyse some of the thrombus.

b. After initiation of heparin and admission, a V/Q scan can be performed to confirm the diagnosis (see discussion below under **3. Intermediate clinical suspicion**).

c. The initiation of **warfarin** therapy is indicated, to begin the day after heparin is started. The **starting dose** of warfarin is 5–10 mg PO q.d., with a target PT of 16–18 seconds (control = 1.3–1.5 seconds). A more valid measure to target therapy is the international normalized ratio **(INR).** The **target INR** should be **2.0–3.0.** The warfarin is continued for a total of 3 months.

Mechanism of action of warfarin: Warfarin inhibits the activity of vitamin K–dependent coagulation factors, with a resultant anticoagulant effect.

d. If there is any **contraindication** to anticoagulation, a definitive diagnosis is required via pulmonary angiography and then **inferior vena caval interruption/filter placement.** Therefore, consultation with interventional radiologists for the pulmonary angiography and/or IVC placement is indicated.

2. **Low clinical suspicion.** Evaluation and management are directed toward the underlying suspected cause. The indications for admission and for consultations depend on the underlying clinical diagnosis and the stability of the patient. No further PTE-directed evaluation is necessary.

3. **Intermediate clinical suspicion.** The patient can be

evaluated acutely (within 1–3 hours as an outpatient, or if logistically impossible or if the patient is not stable, admitted for the same evaluation as an inpatient). If the patient is stable, efficient, effective, **acute outpatient evaluation** is optimal. This evaluation includes the following evaluative tools, which should be performed in the order listed.

a. **Ventilation/perfusion scan.** This radionuclide imaging study is performed in two distinct parts. In one part radiolabeled xenon gas is used to assess ventilation (V). In the other part technetium 99m–labeled albumin microaggregates are used to assess pulmonary arterial perfusion (Q). To increase the sensitivity and specificity of this test, a chest radiograph should be obtained at the time of the V/Q scan. These scans are read as (or should be **interpreted by the clinician** to be) one of the following:

   i. **High probability.** This scan has one or more subsegmental or larger V/Q mismatches. PTE is the diagnosis. **Treat as such.** No further PTE evaluation is necessary acutely. See Figs. 4-5 and 4-6.

   ii. **Normal.** PTE is essentially **ruled out** as the cause of symptoms. No further PTE evaluation is necessary acutely.

   iii. **Intermediate/indeterminate probability.** The scans are interpreted as "low probability." Most scans fall into this group. *Low* does not mean *no* probability. An intermediate or indeterminate scan **necessitates further evaluation.** This further evaluation includes:

b. Looking for the **site source of emboli**, specifically in the lower extremity system. If thrombus is demonstrated in the deep system, especially in the **proximal deep lower extremity venous system**—that is, in the area including and proximal to the popliteal fossa—the treatment is essentially the same as for PTE, and the diagnosis of PTE is strongly inferred. Modalities to image the lower extremity venous system, along with their clinical utility, include the following.

   i. **Impedance plethysmography (IPG).** Sensitive for proximal deep venous thrombosis (DVT), and one of the best tools for evaluating the venous system proximal to the popliteal fossa for thrombus.

   ii. **Venous duplex Doppler study.** A sensitive test for proximal DVT, and one of the best tools

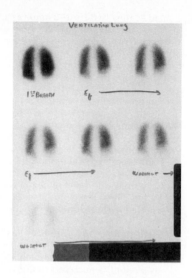

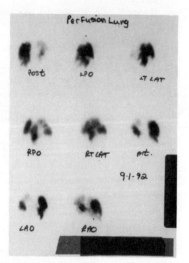

F I G U R E S   4 - 5   a n d   4 - 6
Ventilation–perfusion lung scans. The **ventilation** portion is completely unremarkable, with normal ventilation to all areas of the lungs. The **perfusion** portion is grossly abnormal, with several large perfusion defects, predominantly in the right lung.

for evaluating the venous channels proximal to the popliteal fossa for thrombus.

   iii. **Venography.** Entails injection of contrast material into the venous system of the lower extremity. The test is good for diagnosing the relatively benign distal thrombus, but it has only a **fair sensitivity** for the much more dangerous **proximal thrombus.** (See also the section on Peripheral Vascular Disease in Chapter 1, Table 1-15, page 36.)

  c. If results on the lower extremity examinations are equivocal perform **pulmonary angiography** to clarify the diagnosis. Consultation with pulmonologists and interventional radiologists is indicated at this time. If the angiogram is normal, PTE is ruled out; if the angiogram is positive, PTE is ruled in and therapy as discussed above should be initiated.

F. The **long-term follow-up and management** of patients with PTE include the following steps.

  1. The duration of warfarin for the **first episode of DVT or PTE is 3 months,** then warfarin is discontinued.

  2. If a **DVT or PTE recurs,** use the same regimen as for acute therapy, but warfarin is continued for **1–2 years** and may need to be continued **indefinitely.** A hematologist with specialty training in hypercoagulable states should evaluate the patient for a hypercoagulable state.

  3. If **PTE or DVT recurs** even though adequate anticoagulation has been provided, IVC interruption is indicated.

  4. The patient should **never use aspirin** concurrently with warfarin or heparin; other NSAIDs are relatively contraindicated for use concurrently with warfarin.

  5. Follow-up should be on a **frequent and regular basis,** usually every 2–4 weeks with a PT measurement.

  6. All **estrogens,** including oral contraceptive pills, **are contraindicated** for the remainder of the patient's life.

Community-Acquired Pneumonitis (see Box 4-7)

In the broadest sense, **pneumonitis** is the nonspecific inflammation of pulmonary parenchymal tissue. It is synonymous with the term **pneumonia.** Although a diverse set of pathogenetic mechanisms and causes exists for the development of inflammation of the pulmonary parenchymal tissue, only infectious agents (bacteria and viruses) in the local community are discussed here.

I. **Spectrum and pathogenesis**
   The **spectrum** and **pathogenesis** of infection-mediated lung disease can be generally overviewed using the models of **bronchitis, pneumonitis,** and **abscess formation.**
   A. **Bronchitis** is an infection-related inflammation limited to the trachea and bronchial airways.
   B. **Pneumonitis** is an infection-mediated inflammation of the pulmonary parenchyma with exudative material, including but not limited to PMNs and the pathogen itself, in the tissue itself, resulting in **alveolar pneumonitis** (i.e., material in the alveoli with resultant patchy or lobar infiltrates) or **interstitial pneumonitis** (i.e., material in the interstitium with resultant diffuse reticular or reticulonodular infiltrates).
   C. **Abscess formation**—any area of necrosis of lung tissue in an area of pneumonitis. This usually occurs in specific types of pneumonias. The most common organism types include **Gram-negative bacillary pneumonitis,** in which necrosis of the tissue occurs acutely with the development of multiple small cavities; **anaerobic pneumonias,** in which the necrosis is insidious and a single large cavity forms; and **reactive typical mycobacterial disease,** which is insidious and forms a single large cavity.

II. **Manifestations, differential diagnosis, evaluation, and management**
   The **manifestations, differential diagnosis, evaluation,** and **management** of community-acquired pneumonias are best approached by dividing the entities into two overall groups, **typical pneumonias** and **atypical pneumonias** (see Table 4-11).
   A. The **classic** or **typical forms** of community-acquired pneumonia manifest with cough productive of yellow–green, even blood-streaked sputum; dyspnea; pleuritic chest pain, often in the site adjacent to the pneumonia; fevers, often spiking to 104 °F; chills; and shaking rigors. The **chest examination** reveals signs of consolidation, including an area of **dullness to percussion** with concurrent **increased tactile fremitus,** and **increased breath sounds,** which are bronchial in nature.
      1. The **organisms** that cause classic or typical pneumonias are the bacterial pathogens *Streptococcus pneumoniae* and *Hemophilus influenzae.*
      2. **Sputum examination,** which is **mandatory** in all cases, will add significantly to the evaluation and management. A sputum from an *S. pneumoniae* infection will reveal polymorphonuclear cells and many **gram-positive diplococci** (positive = blue);

BOX 4-7

Overall Evaluation and Management of Pneumonias

Evaluation

1. Take a thorough **history** and perform a **physical examination,** with attention to the overall manifestations described in the text.
2. Determine the **complete blood cell count** with differential to look for any leukocytosis or a left shift, indicative of an infectious process.
3. Determine basic serum chemistry for baseline purposes.
4. Determine **arterial blood gas values** for baseline purposes. Any evidence of hypoxemia is indicative of a significant process.
5. Obtain **blood samples for culture** in all patients with pneumonia and fever. Culture results will indicate the bacterial pathogen in a significant minority of cases. Blood cultures yield the pathogen in 30%–40% of cases of *Streptococcus pneumoniae.*
6. Obtain **chest radiographs** in PA and lateral views as an integral component of the evaluation. Chest radiography complements the physical examination in localizing any infiltrate present (Fig. 4-7).
   a. **Lobar, consolidative infiltrates** are associated with *Streptococcus pneumoniae.*
   b. **Lobular, patchy infiltrates** are associated with *Hemophilus influenzae.*
   c. **Diffuse interstitial infiltrates** are associated with *Mycoplasma pneumoniae, Legionella,* or viruses.
7. **Sputum examination,** both gross and with Gram stain, is mandatory. Gross inspection will reveal any purulence, Gram stain will reveal any PMNs and the predominant organism present.
8. **Sputum cultures** should be done **only** on samples representative of the pulmonary infectious process, i.e., those with PMNs and organisms. If the specimen is saliva only (i.e., contains no PMNs and only squamous epithelial cells), **do not send** it for culture as the data obtained will be misleading.
9. Initiate **antibiotics** based on the Gram stain results, chest radiograph, and the clinical picture.

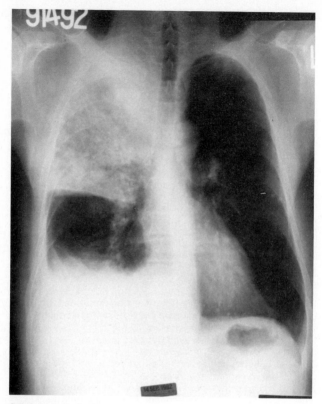

F I G U R E 4 - 7
Chest radiograph in PA view showing right upper lobe consolidation
with a concurrent parapneumonic effusion.

whereas *H. influenzae* infection will reveal polymorphonuclear cells and many **gram-negative coccobacilli** (negative = pink).
3. The **cornerstone** in management of typical pneumonias is the initiation of antibiotics based on the suspected organism.
   a. If ***Streptococcus pneumoniae*** is suspected, one of
      three regimens can be used:
      i. Penicillin G, 600,000 units q.4h. IV for 3–5
         days, followed by penicillin VK, 500 mg PO
         q.i.d. for 5 days, or

T A B L E 4-11
Community-Acquired Pneumonias

Organism	History	Gram Stain	Chest Radiograph	Treatment
Streptococcus pneumoniae	Spiking fevers Rigors Pleuritic chest pain Cough Red-tinged sputum	Many PMNs Gram-positive diplococci	Lobar infiltrate	Penicillin Erythromycin
Hemophilus influenzae	Spiking fevers Cough Yellow-green sputum	Many PMNs Gram-negative diplococci	Lobar infiltrate or, more commonly, a patchy infiltrate	Ampicillin Second-generation cephalosporin
Legionella spp.	Low-grade fevers Cough Scant sputum Diarrhea	Many PMNs No organisms	Diffuse, interstitial	Erythromycin
Mycoplasma spp.	Low-grade fevers Cough Scant sputum Otalgia, ear popping	Many PMNs No organisms	Diffuse, interstitial	Erythromycin
Viral agents	Low-grade fevers Cough Myalgias Arthralgias Scant sputum Nausea, vomiting Diarrhea Rhinorrhea	Occasional PMNs No organisms	Diffuse, interstitial	Amantadine if influenza A is suspected Supportive; monitor for complications, e.g., superinfection with *Staphylococcus aureus*

       ii. Penicillin VK, 500 PO q.i.d. for 10 days, or
      iii. Erythromycin, 500 mg PO or IV q.6h. for 10 days.

  b. If *Hemophilus influenzae* is suspected, one of the following regimens can be used:
       i. A second-generation cephalosporin, e.g., cefuroxime (Zinacef), 750–1,500 mg IV q.8h. for 5 days, followed by Ceftin, 500 mg PO q.i.d. for 5 days, or
      ii. Ceftin, 500 mg PO b.i.d. for 10 days, or
      iii. Augmentin (amoxicillin–clavulinate), 500 mg PO t.i.d. for 10 days, or
      iv. Ciprofloxacin, 500 mg PO b.i.d. for 7–10 days, **(contraindicated in pregnancy).**

B. The **nonclassic** or **atypical forms** of community-acquired pneumonias manifest with a low-grade fever; a hacking, nonproductive cough; dyspnea; rhinorrhea; and malaise. The **chest examination** usually reveals a slight tachypnea with diffuse crackles but rarely any signs of consolidation.

  1. The **organisms** that cause these classic or typical pneumonias are the bacterial and viral pathogens *Mycoplasma pneumoniae*, *Legionella pneumophila*, *Chlamydia psittaci* (psittacosis or "bird lover's pneumonia"), TWAR agent, and viruses, especially influenza A and B.

  2. The **sputum examination** is very important, but, because the cough is often nonproductive, sputum can be difficult to obtain. Gram stain will reveal polymorphonuclear cells but no organisms, for these pathogens do not stain with Gram stain.

  3. The **cornerstone** of management of atypical pneumonias is the initiation of antibiotics based on the suspected organism.
    a. Erythromycin, 500–1,000 mg IV q.6h. for 5 days, followed by erythromycin, 500 mg PO for 5 days, or
    b. Erythromycin for 10 days. Three different formulations are available. The PCE and EES forms, while more expensive, may have less associated abdominal cramps and nausea.
      i. Erythromycin stearate, 500 mg PO q.i.d.
      ii. PCE (polymer-coated erythromycin), 500 mg PO q.6–8h.
      iii. EES (erythromycin ethylsuccinate), 400 mg PO q.i.d.

  4. These pathogens, especially the RNA virus causing influenza B, cause a systemic infection that predisposes to **bacterial superinfection,** especially with

Staphylococcus aureus. The physician in the ambulatory care setting must remain current with the specific pathogens in the community. The incidences of the above pathogens change between different seasons (influenza B rarely occurs in summer, but can be in epidemic proportions in late winter) and between communities (psittacosis is uncommon in the United States but quite common in Great Britain owing to the increased prevalence of birds as pets in the United Kingdom).

C. **If the process cannot be defined as typical or atypical** or if the process has components of both, initiate **empirical therapy.**

    a. A **second-generation cephalosporin** (cefuroxime, 750 mg IV q.8h.) and **erythromycin** (500 mg IV or PO for 10 days) are indicated; or

    b. **Azithromycin,** 500 mg PO on day 1, then 250 mg PO q. A.M. for 4 subsequent days. This novel macrolide antibiotic is effective against *Streptococcus pneumoniae, Hemophilus influenzae,* and the atypical pathogens. It must be taken on an empty stomach for optimal effectiveness.

    c. If influenza A is in the community and is a potential diagnosis, **amantadine, 100 mg PO b.i.d. for 7 days,** can be added empirically to the regimen.

III. **Follow-up**

Follow-up will be discussed in the **acute, intermediate,** and **chronic settings.**

A. **Acute follow-up** includes monitoring the symptoms and signs and temperature curve, whether the patient is an inpatient or an outpatient. It is not uncommon for the patient to have a febrile spike within the first 24–36 hours after initiation of therapy, and unless other factors indicate a deteriorating condition, this single spike should not affect the overall management scheme.

B. **Intermediate-duration follow-up** should include, if the patient clinically improves and has no clinical complications, chest radiography repeated approximately 4–6 weeks after treatment. Pneumonias take 3–6 weeks to resolve radiographically. If there is any evidence of complications or recurrence of symptoms earlier, chest radiography is repeated at that time, with closer radiographic follow-up as necessary.

C. **Principles in chronic follow-up:** If this is the **second pneumonia,** or if **another pneumonia occurs,** the clinician needs to ascertain whether there are any underlying systemic risk factors for recurrent pneumonias, such as immunodeficiency, hypogammaglobulinemia, or splenic dysfunction. If the **recurrence is in same lobe,** the clinician needs to evaluate for an anatomic lesion in that area, such as a neoplastic lesion with bronchial obstruction.

IV. **Consultation**

Problem	*Service*	*Time*
Recurrent pneumonia	Pulmonary	Urgent/ bronchoscopy

V. **Indications for admission:** Most patients with active pneumonia need to be admitted for a short period of time for parenteral antibiotics. This is particularly true for the elderly population. Overall indications for admission include **hypoxemia;** a pneumonia that acutely exacerbates a chronic condition that itself is now symptomatic and requires therapy (e.g., **COPD** or **left ventricular failure**); a patient who is **malnourished** and needs nutritional supplementation to fight infection; a patient who is **noncompliant;** and any patient who is clinically ill with **impending septicemia** and cardiovascular or respiratory compromise.

Solitary Pulmonary Nodule

A **solitary pulmonary nodule** is usually discovered incidentally on a chest radiograph obtained for other reasons.

By **definition,** a **nodule** is a lesion less than 6 cm in diameter, whereas a **mass** is a lesion more than 6 cm in diameter. The definition of a solitary pulmonary nodule is quite specific and involves, in addition to size, the following qualifications, all of which must be met to make the diagnosis. The lesion is **single, round,** has **distinct margins,** is **non-pleural-based,** and is **without** any concurrent **mediastinal enlargement.** The lesion may or may not have intralesional calcifications.

I. **Overall manifestations**
Overall manifestations are minimal and, if present, are nonspecific. This is true even on retrospective questioning of the patient after the nodule is discovered. Although there is a paucity of manifestations at the time of presentation, the patient's medical and personal history should be amplified, as certain features in the history will aid the clinician in establishing a ranked differential diagnosis and, more important, will aid the clinician in overall evaluation and management.

A. **Smoking** of tobacco or marijuana as a habit is an important feature. There is clear and irrefutable evidence that smoking is a risk factor for the development of bronchogenic carcinoma.

T A B L E 4 - 1 2
Factors in Assessing the Risk of Malignancy of a Solitary Pulmonary Nodule

1. Age (<30 years or >30 years)
2. Rate of growth of lesion (no growth, doubling time < 1 month, doubling time > 1 month)
3. Presence or absence of calcifications in the nodule
4. Patient smokes or has ever habitually smoked tobacco products or marijuana

B. The patient's **geographic area of residence,** past and present, is important. Certain chronic infections that may manifest with a solitary pulmonary nodule are endemic to specific parts of the United States. As examples, histoplasmosis is endemic to the Ohio River valley and blastomycosis is endemic to the upper Midwest.

C. A history of **exposure to mycobacterial disease** must be sought. Mycobacterial lesions may rarely manifest as solitary pulmonary nodules.

D. **Old chest radiographs** are important and, if available, are mandatory and integral to the evaluation and management.

II. **Diagnosis**
   The **differential diagnosis** includes **bronchogenic carcinoma,** which usually is noncalcified; the residua of **primary mycobacterial disease,** which usually is calcified and called a Ghon focus; **histoplasmosis,** which usually is calcified and associated with other calcified lesions, especially in the spleen; **metastatic neoplastic disease,** which is invariably noncalcified and **multiple;** and **benign hamartoma,** which invariably is calcified. Other specific differentiating features of these entities are listed in Table 4-13.

III. **Evaluation and management**
   The **evaluation and management** of a solitary pulmonary nodule depend on the clinical suspicion of malignancy (Table 4-12). The clinician uses data gleaned from the history and physical examination and reviews, if at all possible, all old chest radiographs for comparison. If no old chest radiograph is available, one must assume the lesion is new.

   A. If the patient is at **low risk** for malignant neoplasm—that is, the patient is **<30 years old,** the lesion shows **no growth** or **rapid growth** (i.e., doubling time < 1 month) from baseline, the nodule contains **calcifications,** and the patient is a **nonsmoker**—management can be conser-

TABLE 4-13
Differentiating Features of Solitary Pulmonary Nodules

Lesion Type	Patient Age	Lesion's Rate of Growth	Smoking History	Calcification
Carcinoma—non-small cell	>30 yr	Doubling time > 1 mo.	Present	Absent
Carcinoma—small cell	>30 yr	Doubling time < 1 mo.	Present	Absent
Metastatic neoplasia	>30 yr	Doubling time < 1 mo.	Present or absent	Absent
Hamartoma	Irrelevant	No change	Absent	Present, popcorn distribution
Mycobacterial	Irrelevant	No change	Absent	Present throughout the lesion
Histoplasmosis	Irrelevant	No change	Absent	Present; ringed calcifications in the lesion

vative. A conservative approach includes the following steps.

1. Perform a **PPD skin test.**
2. **Repeat the chest radiograph** in 1–2 months. If there is no change in the lesion at that time, repeat the chest radiograph 2–4 months for two visits, to document the lack of change.

B. If the patient is at moderate to high risk—that is, the patient is >**30 years old,** the lesion shows **slow, steady growth,** the nodule contains **no calcifications,** and the patient is a past or current **smoker** (several or all factors present)—aggressive therapy is indicated. Furthermore, if the patient was at **low risk** but follow-up chest radiographs show that the nodule is **slowly increasing** in size, aggressive therapy is indicated. An aggressive approach includes the following measures.

1. **CT of the thorax** to look for concurrent lesions in the lungs or mediastinum.
2. **Pulmonary function tests.** These tests are indicated in all patients, because if FEV_1 is less than 1.5 L, the patient is virtually never a candidate for thoracic surgery, as removal of a lobe or entire lung would be fatal to the patient.
3. If there is **no evidence of metastatic disease** and **FEV_1 is >1.5 L,** obtain a consultation with **cardiothoracic surgery** to resect the pulmonary lobe for diagnosis and, in all likelihood, **curative therapy.** Preoperative bronchoscopy or needle biopsy would add little benefit if surgery is to be performed.
4. If complete resection is performed and the tumor is a **non-small cell carcinoma,** expectant management with repeated chest radiographs is indicated. If the lesion is a **small cell carcinoma,** adjuvant chemotherapy is indicated.

C. **Education** of the patient is of paramount importance. This is especially true if the patient has an FEV_1 preoperatively of <1.5 L. The primary care physician must inform the patient of the likely outcome of the disease with and without surgery and that, if the lesion is neoplastic, therapy will be palliative. The patient must be educated as to the outcomes, response rates, and potential side effects of various therapeutic modalities in the nonsurgical treatment of a solitary pulmonary nodule that is a malignant neoplastic lesion.

1. If the patient **desires no therapy,** diagnosis by bronchoscopy or invasive needle biopsy is **not indicated** until the patient becomes symptomatic. The reasoning is as follows: palliative treatment, invariably local irradiation, would start only when and if symptoms

begin; moreover, the diagnosis may be made by **sputum cytology** during subsequent follow-up, obviating the need for invasive testing.

2. If the patient **requests treatment,** the clinician should obtain sputum for cytology and then either refer to an invasive radiologist for fine needle biopsy of the lesion or to a pulmonologist for bronchoscopic examination of the lesion. If and when the diagnosis of a malignant neoplastic disease is made, referral to an oncologist or radiation oncologist for therapy is indicated. The response rates of non-small cell carcinoma to the chemotherapeutic agents used today is dishearteningly low. (For further discussion see the section on Bronchogenic Carcinoma in Chapter 5, page 289.)

IV. **Consultation**

Problem	Service	Time
If bronchoscopy is considered	Pulmonary	Elective
If needle biopsy is considered	Radiology	Elective
If SPN in high-risk patient	Cardiothoracic surgery	Urgent

V. **Indications for admission:** Admission is only indicated on a scheduled basis for a specific procedure that has been orchestrated by the primary care physician, or if the lesion causes a secondary postobstructive pneumonitis requiring palliative therapy.

Mycobacterial Diseases (see Box 4-8)

Typical mycobacterial disease, that due to the **acid-fast bacillus,** *Mycobacterium hominis,* has become significantly less common following the availability of effective antimycobacterial chemotherapeutic modalities and the initiation of preventive health strategies in the 1940s and 1950s. There has been, however, a significant and disconcerting increase in the incidence of this disease in the recent past. Several potential reasons for this increased incidence can be postulated.

1. A decreased sensitivity of primary care and all physicians to this specific diagnosis, because it was uncommon during their training.
2. Syndromes of **immunodeficiency** with predominantly cell-mediated deficiency (e.g., AIDS) increase the risk of mycobacterial disease development.
3. The inherent immunosuppression of anticancer chemothera-

peutic agents increases the risk of mycobacterial disease development.

4. Immunosuppression or immunocompromise is causing a significant increase in the incidence of the **atypical mycobacterial diseases,** especially those due to *M. kansasii* and *M. avium-intracellulare,* agents that a "normal" immune system adequately deals with.

I. **Natural history of typical mycobacterial disease**

The **natural history** of mycobacterial disease can be described using infection by *M. hominis* as a model. The agent is transmitted by air, invariably by aerosolized sputum from an infected patient. Once the mycobacterial agent is transmitted into the pulmonary tree of a new host individual, its natural history falls into three major and quite distinct temporal phases: **primary disease, a quiescent period,** and finally **reactivation disease.**

A. **Primary infection** is usually quite mild. Once the organism reaches the pulmonary airways, infection of the pulmonary tissue occurs. In the vast majority of cases, this is immediately followed by cell-mediated responses forming **granulomas,** usually of the **caseating** type. In the immunocompetent host, this stage of the infection is virtually always asymptomatic.

B. The **quiescent period** begins after the cell-mediated responses have controlled and neutralized the original infection. These cell-mediated responses will, over months, result in granulomas in the pulmonary tissue and the adjacent draining mediastinal lymph nodes. Virtually all of these granulomas **calcify** over a relatively short period of time. These calcified lesions manifest as **Ghon complexes** or a **Ghon focus** on chest radiographs.

1. A **Ghon focus** is a calcified granuloma in the lung adjacent to the mediastinum.

2. A **Ghon complex** is a calcified granuloma and adjacent calcified mediastinal lymph nodes.

Either or both of these findings are evidence and thus manifestations of past primary infection with *M. hominis,* i.e., the shadows of past, now quiescent mycobacterial infection. These lesions remain stable, **asymptomatic,** and quiescent for months, years, or even for the remainder of the lifetime of the patient. It is during the quiescent period that the majority of patients present, usually discovered by the primary care physician from a chest radiograph which was obtained for other reasons.

C. **Reactivation** occurs after a period of dormancy or quiescence. If the patient did not receive therapy or chemoprophylaxis during the primary or quiescent period, the infection may reactivate. Reactivation occurs in both

B O X 4 - 8

*Overall Evaluation and Management of
Mycobacterial Disease*

The following discussion pertains to typical mycobacterial disease. Atypical disease management is beyond the scope of this text.

Evaluation

1. Take a thorough **history** and perform a **physical examination.** The history focuses on any history of past purified protein derivative (PPD) reactivity, any history of exposure to mycobacterial disease, inoculation with bacille Calmette–Guérin (BCG) vaccine, and any history of or risk factors for immunocompromise (see Table 4-14).
2. Obtain **chest radiographs** in PA and lateral views. Obtain and review any old chest radiographs and use this data, along with PPD results and the history, to clinically assess whether the patient has typical or atypical disease and whether the disease is primary, quiescent, or reactivation disease.
3. **Respiratory isolation** of the patient is strongly indicated, especially if there is any sputum production or any cavitary lesions on the chest radiographs. Respiratory isolation is relatively simple: a mask must be worn either by patient or by people who come in contact with the patient.
4. Obtain **sputum** for examination on three consecutive mornings for Gram stain, **acid-fast bacilli (AFB)** smear, and culture.
5. Perform a **PPD test with controls** unless there is a history of reactivity or BCG inoculation in the past. This is due to the fact that once a patient is reactive, the PPD should not again be applied. The PPD test is described in Table 4-15.

Management

1. If the **sputum contains AFB** or the **suspicion** of disease is **high,** initiate therapy with triple or dual chemotherapy (see Table 4-16). Regimens require **more than one agent** because the mycobacterial agents

(continued)

B O X 4 - 8 (continued)

will develop resistance to one agent alone. The regimens include:
  a. 9 months of isoniazid (INH), 300 mg PO q. A.M., **and** rifampin, 600 mg PO q. A.M., *or*
  b. 1 month of INH, 300 mg PO q. A.M., and rifampin, 600 mg, PO q. A.M., **followed by** 8 months of INH, 900 mg PO q. A.M., **and** rifampin, 600 mg PO q. A.M. 2 times per week.
2. Obtain consultations with pulmonologists or infectious disease experts.
3. Report the case to the Public Health Service.
4. **Screen other family members** for disease. Screening includes a baseline PPD test, and, if the test is reactive, a chest radiograph. If exposed, INH chemoprophylaxis is indicated; if a family member has evidence of infection, treat as listed above (see Table 4-17).
5. Administer pyridoxine (vitamin B_6), 50 mg PO q. A.M., to prevent the side effects of INH.

lung apices and manifests on **chest radiographs** as **nodular infiltrates in the apices** adjacent to the pleural surfaces **(Simon foci)** and the development of **cavitary lesion(s)** in the upper lobe(s). Invariably the reactivation begins in the **posterior segment** of the upper lobe(s). The **clinical manifestations** include cough, sputum production, hemoptysis, fevers, and night sweats. This phase, especially when cavitary lesions are present, is a phase in which the disease is highly transmissible to other people. If the disease in this phase is left unchecked, it will progress over variable periods of time to cause necrosis

T A B L E 4 - 1 4
Groups at High Risk for the Development of Mycobacterial Diseases

1. Immunocompromised hosts
2. Recent immigrants to the United States from the tropics, especially from Southeast Asia
3. Untreated patients with reactive PPD skin tests (*not* including patients who received BCG in the past)
4. Patients with recent exposure to mycobacterial disease

TABLE 4-15
Skin Tests for Mycobacterial Diseases

Type	Indications	Contraindications	Mechanism	Reactive*
Purified protein derivative (PPD)	Demonstrate exposure to mycobacterial disease	Tested reactive in the past	Derivative of *M. hominis*	Immunocompromised: 5 mm induration; High risk group, non-immunocompromised: 10 mm; Nonimmunocompromised, non-high risk group: 15 mm induration
Trichophyton	Control, used to demonstrate active cell-mediated immunity	Tested reactive in the past	Derivative of this ubiquitous dermatophyte	10 mm induration
Mumps	Control, used to demonstrate active cell-mediated immunity	Tested reactive in the past	Derivative of this ubiquitous viral infection	10 mm induration

*Outcome of test measured at 48 hr.

T A B L E 4-16
Antimycobacterial Agents

Agent	Mechanism of Action	Dose	Side Effects
Isoniazid (INH)	Bactericidal	300 mg PO q.d.	Hepatitis Peripheral neuritis, which can be prevented with vitamin B_6, 50 mg PO q.d. Decreased seizure threshold
Rifampin	Bactericidal	600 mg PO q.d.	Hepatitis Thrombocytopenia Discoloration of all secretions to orange
Ethambutol	Bacteriostatic	25 mg/kg/day PO for 2 mo., then 15 mg/kg/day PO for 7–10 mo.	Optic neuritis; affects green–red vision
Streptomycin	Bactericidal	1 g IM for 60 days, then 1 g IM 2 times per week for 6 mo.	Vertigo Paresthesias Ototoxicity Nephrotoxicity
Pyrazinamide	Bactericidal	25 mg/kg/day in q.8h. dosing for 6–8 mo.	Arthralgias Hepatitis Hyperuricemia
Para-amino-salicylic acid (PAS)	Bacteriostatic	200 mg/kg/day PO in b.i.d. dosing for 10–12 mo.	Diarrhea Hemolysis, in G6PD deficiency

T A B L E 4 - 1 7
Indications for Isoniazid (INH) Chemoprophylaxis for
Mycobacterial Diseases (American Thoracic Society)

Dose: INH, 300 mg PO q. A.M. for 12 mo.

Administer to:

1. Household contacts of patients with typical mycobacterial disease, even if contacts are PPD negative. If the contact remains PPD negative with reactive controls at 3 months, can discontinue chemoprophylaxis.
2. Untreated PPD reactive patients more than 35 years old who have evidence of disease on old chest radiographs (Ghon foci, Simon foci).
3. PPD converters within the past 2 years of any age.
4. All untreated PPD reactive patients less than 35 years old.
5. Any untreated PPD reactive patients who develop any immunocompromise.

of the lung tissue, pleural diseases, systemic mycobacterial disease, and eventually death.

II. **Natural history of atypical mycobacterial disease**
The **natural history of atypical mycobacterial disease** is quite different from that of the typical disease. Although a comprehensive discussion is beyond the scope of this text, because the incidence of this disorder is markedly increasing, a brief discussion of the features of this infectious process is included.

   A. The most common causative **organisms** are *Mycobacterium kansasii* and *M. avium-intracellulare*. Neither of these organisms results in infection in an immunocompetent host with normal lung tissue.

   B. The **hosts** invariably are patients who are immunosuppressed, especially those with **cell-mediated immunity,** or who have significant pulmonary disease.

   C. The **primary disease** may be **miliary** or **indolent.**

   1. **Miliary disease** is an intense and severe process in which there is an acute dissemination of the mycobacterial infection throughout the lungs and potentially the body. The **acute manifestations of miliary tuberculosis** include chest pain, dyspnea, low-grade and spiking fevers, hypoxemia, respiratory compromise, and even death.

   2. **Indolent disease** is the other side of the spectrum. Infection with an atypical mycobacterial agent causes a slow, progressive disease with the development of diffuse nodular infiltrates in the mid- and upper lung fields. The **pathophysiology** of the insidious form, which is the most common form of atypical mycobac-

terial disease, results in destruction of lung tissue and decreased pulmonary function. The **clinical manifestations** of this type are minimal until late in the process; they include dyspnea, especially upon exertion, a nonproductive cough, and hypoxemia. The **evaluation and management** of atypical mycobacterial disease are beyond the scope of this text; however, **early consultation** with **pulmonary** and **infectious disease colleagues** for bronchoscopy and antimycobacterial chemotherapeutic initiation is clearly indicated. Often regimens will include four or five specific agents (see Table 4-15 for representative agents).

Bibliography

Asthma

Bochner B, Lichtenstein L: Anaphylaxis. N Engl J Med 1991;324:1785–1790.

Diagnosis and care of patients with chronic obstructive pulmonary disease (COPD) and asthma. Am Rev Respir Dis 1987;136:225–246.

Fiel B et al: Efficacy of short-term corticosteroid therapy in outpatient treatment of acute bronchial asthma. Am Med J 1983;75:259.

Gilbert R, Auchincloss H: The interpretation of the spirogram: How accurate is it for "obstruction"? Arch Intern Med 1985;145:1635–1639.

Kaliner MA: Inhaled corticosteroids for chronic asthma. Am Fam Pract 1990;42:1609–1616.

Littenberg B, Gluck E: A controlled trial of methylprednisolone in the emergency treatment of acute asthma. N Engl J Med 1986;314:150–152.

McFadden ER Jr: Clinical appraisal of the therapy of asthma: An idea whose time has come. Am Rev Respir Dis 1986;133:723.

Stein L, Cole R: Early administration of corticosteroids in emergency room treatment of acute asthma. Ann Intern Med 1990;112:822–827.

Williams MH: Beclomethasone diproprionate. Ann Intern Med 1981;95:464.

Clubbing

Hansen-Flaschen J, Nordberg J: Clubbing and hypertrophic osteoarthropathy. Clin Chest Med 1987;8:287–298.

Segumacher HR: Articular manifestations of hypertrophic pulmonary osteoarthropathy in bronchogenic carcinoma: A clinical and pathologic study. Arthritis Rheum 1976;19:629.

Siegal RC: From clubbing to collagen. West J Med 1981;134:352.

Chronic Obstructive Lung Disease

Anthonisen N, et al: Antibiotic therapy in exacerbations of chronic obstructive pulmonary disease. Ann Intern Med 1987;106:196–207.

Anthonisen NR: Long-term oxygen therapy. Ann Intern Med 1983;99:519.

Bertka K, Wunderink R: Outpatient management of COPD. Am Fam Pract 1988;37:265–280.

Fulmer J, et al: American College of Chest Physicians–National Heart, Lung and Blood Institute Conference on Oxygen Therapy. Arch Intern Med 1984;144:1645–1655.

Gilbert R, Auchincloss H: The interpretation of the spirogram: How accurate is it for "obstruction"? Arch Intern Med 1985;145:1635–1639.

Kanner RE, et al: Predictors of survival in subjects with airflow limitation. Am J Med 1983;74:249.

Lakshminarayan S: Ipratropium bromide in chronic bronchitis/emphysema. Am J Med 1986;81(S):76–80.

Pennock B, et al: Pulmonary function testing: What is normal? Arch Intern Med 1983;143:2123–2127.

Rice K, et al: Aminophylline for acute exacerbations of chronic obstructive pulmonary disease. Ann Intern Med 1987;107:305–309.

Standards for the diagnosis and care of patients with chronic obstructive pulmonary disease (COPD) and asthma. Am Rev Respir Dis 1987;136:225–246.

Tobin M: The use of bronchodilator aerosols. Arch Intern Med 1985;145:1659–1663.

Hemoptysis

Jackson C, et al: Role of fiberoptic bronchoscopy in patients with hemoptysis and a normal chest roentgenogram. Chest 1985;87:142–144.

Johnston H, Reisz G: Changing spectrum of hemoptysis. Arch Intern Med 1989;149:1666–1668.

O'Neil K, Lazarus A: Hemoptysis: Indications for bronchoscopy. Arch Intern Med 1991;151:171–174.

Pleural Effusions

Light R, et al: Pleural effusions: The diagnostic separation of transudates and exudates. Ann Intern Med 1972;77:507–513.

Light RW, Ball WC: Glucose and amylase in pleural effusion. JAMA 1973;225:259.

Light RW, et al: Cells and pleural fluid. Arch Intern Med 1973;132:854.

Peterman TA, Speicher CE: Evaluating pleural effusions. JAMA 1984;252:1051.

Pleuritic Chest Pain

Fulkerson WJ, et al: Diagnosis of pulmonary embolism. Arch Intern Med 1986;146:961–967.

Hirsh J: Heparin. N Engl J Med 1991;324:1565–1574.

Hirsh J: Oral anticoagulant drugs. N Engl J Med 1991;324:1865–1875.

Hoellerich V, et al: Diagnosing pulmonary embolism using clinical findings. 1986;146:1699–1704.

Hull RD, et al: Diagnostic value of ventilation-perfusion lung scanning in patients with suspected pulmonary embolism. Chest 1985;88:819–828.

Hull RD, et al: Optimal therapeutic level of heparin therapy in patients with venous thrombosis. Arch Intern Med 1992;152:1589–1595.

Hull RD, et al: Pulmonary embolism in outpatients with pleuritic chest pain. 1988;148:838–844.

Moser K: Venous thromboembolism. Am Rev Respir Dis 1990;141:235–249.

PIOPED Investigators: Value of the ventilation/perfusion scan in acute pulmonary embolism. 1990;263:2753–2759.

Pneumonitis

Chokshi S, et al: Aspiration pneumonia: A review. Am Fam Pract 1986;33:195–202.

Garibaldi RA: Epidemiology of community-acquired respiratory tract infections in adults. Am J Med 1985;78:32.

Gudiol F, et al: Clindamycin vs penicillin for anaerobic lung infections. Arch Intern Med 1990;150:2525–2529.

Levy M, et al: Community acquired pneumonias. Chest 1988;92:43–48.

Mayer RD: *Legionella* infections: A review of five years of research. Rev Infect Dis 1983;5:258.

McKellar P: Treatment of community acquired pneumonias. Am J Med 1985;79(S):25–31.

Prevention of influenza and pneumonia. Am Rev Respir Dis 1990;142:487–488.

Solitary Pulmonary Nodule

Lillington GA: Pulmonary nodules: Solitary and multiple. Clin Chest Med 1982;3:361.

Stoller J, et al: Solitary pulmonary nodule. Cleve Clin J Med 1988;55:68–74.

Toomes H, et al: The coin lesion of the lung: A review of 955 resected coin lesions. Cancer 1983;51:534.

Trunk G, et al: The management and evaluation of the solitary pulmonary nodule, Chest 1974;66:236–239.

Mycobacterial Diseases

American Thoracic Society: Treatment of tuberculosis and tuberculosis infection in adults and children. Am Rev Respir Dis 1986;134:355–363.

Centers for Disease Control: The use of preventive therapy for tuberculosis infection in the United States. MMWR 1990.

Dowling P: Return of tuberculosis: Screening and preventive therapy. Am Fam Pract 1991;43:457–467.

Dutt A, et al: Short-course chemotherapy for tuberculosis with mainly twice-weekly isoniazid and rifampin. Am J Med 1984;77:233–241.

—D.D.B.

Dale Berg, Ed. *Handbook
of Primary Care Medicine.*
Copyright © 1993 J. B.
Lippincott Company.

CHAPTER 5

Hematology/Oncology

Anemia

Anemia is an abnormally low number of erythrocytes.

Erythrocytes are non-nucleated cells that contain a unique protein called **hemoglobin.** Hemoglobin allows the erythrocyte to perform with alacrity its main function, the **delivery of oxygen to the tissues,** and is also the basis for the unique red color of these cells. All normal erythrocytes are produced in the bone marrow by normoblasts. The life span of a normal erythrocyte is approximately 120 days.

I. **Normal counts**

The number of erythrocytes can be measured with various tests, but the two most common and reproducible measures are the **hematocrit** and the **hemoglobin.** The **hematocrit** is the percent volume of cells in a given volume of blood; the **hemoglobin** is a direct measurement of this constituent and of the functional protein of erythrocytes. The normal range of the hematocrit and hemoglobin depend on the sex of the person:

> **Hematocrit**
> Men: 42%–52%
> Women: 40%–50%
> **Hemoglobin**
> Men: 14–18 g/dL
> Women: 13–16 g/dL

II. **Overall manifestations**

The **overall manifestations** of anemia include, but are not limited to, increased fatigability, a decrease in exercise tolerance, pale mucous membranes, pale conjunctivae, and high output heart failure with a hyperdynamic heart; related findings include systolic murmurs, a fourth heart sound, and even unstable angina pectoris. Additional symptoms and signs that are directly attributable to the underlying will be described in the discussion of various entities that can give rise to anemia.

Compensatory mechanisms. Although the patient may present with the above manifestations, it is not uncommon for a patient to be only mildly symptomatic or even asymptomatic in the face of a marked anemia. Patients with mild to moderate degrees of anemia on a chronic basis may be asymptomatic as a result of adaptation to the anemia. Adaptive mechanisms include an **increased extraction of oxygen** from the hemoglobin molecule, thereby shifting the **oxyhemoglobin dissociation curve to the left,** and an **increased cardiac index** as a result of an **increase in heart rate and stroke volume.** Patients who become symptomatic either have sustained an acute loss of blood, or have severe, chronic anemia, or have concurrent diseases that are exacerbated by the anemia and the decrease in oxygen delivery.

III. **Categories of anemia**

Using the data gleaned from the basic evaluation described in Box 5-1, the clinician assigns the anemia to one of three major categories, based on the size of the erythrocytes and the amount of hemoglobin in each erythrocyte. Although there is some overlap, each category has a different differential diagnosis, evaluation, and management outline. The three categories are **hypochromic microcytic** anemias, **macrocytic** anemias, and **normochromic normocytic** anemias. Underlying conditions and evaluative tools for each category are listed in Table 5-2.

IV. **Hypochromic microcytic anemia**

Hypochromic microcytic anemias are relatively common. The underlying conditions and specific tests for the further evaluation of these anemias are given in Table 5-2. The four specific forms of hypochromic microcytic anemia that are further discussed below are **iron deficiency anemia, anemia of chronic disease, thalassemia, and hemoglobinopathies.**

A. **Iron deficiency**

Iron deficiency is the most common cause of hypochromic microcytic anemia.

1. **Pathogenesis**

The underlying **pathogenesis** of iron deficiency anemia is a chronic loss of blood, and therefore iron, from any site in the body. Iron is requisite for the synthesis of hemoglobin; therefore, a deficiency in this cationic metal will result in the decreased production of erythrocytes and the onset of anemia. The

B O X 5 - 1

Overall Evaluation of Anemia

Evaluation

1. Take a thorough **history,** including the medication history, and perform a **physical examination.**
2. Perform **laboratory studies** to determine the characteristics of blood listed in Table 5-1.
3. Take a female patient's **menstrual history.**
4. Review the **peripheral blood smear** (see Figs. 5-1 through 5-6).
5. Determine electrolytes, BUN, and creatinine for baseline purposes.

---

most common origins of blood loss are from the **gastrointestinal tract** (most frequently from colon carcinoma and recurrent peptic ulcer disease) and, in a menstruating woman, **menstrual blood loss.**

2. Manifestations

   The **specific manifestations** of iron deficiency anemia include a guaiac-positive stool or excessive menstrual losses and **koilonychia** ("spoon nails") or **cheilosis** (skin cracking at the corners of the mouth).

3. Evaluation

   The **evaluation** includes performing iron studies. **Iron studies** are quite important in the evaluation. As the **serum iron** is decreased, the **total iron-binding**

   (Text continues on page 264)

T A B L E 5 - 1
Normal Values for Blood Parameters in the Evaluation of Anemia

Parameter	Normal Range
Mean corpuscular volume (MCV)	80–94 fL
Mean cell hemoglobin (MCH)	27–31 pg/cell
Red blood cell count	4.0–6.0 million
Reticulocyte count	1%–2%
Reticulocyte index (Reticulocyte count × (Hct./45%))	1.0–1.5
White blood cell count	5,000–10,500 cells/mm³
Platelet count	150,000–450,000/mm³
Stool guaiac	Negative

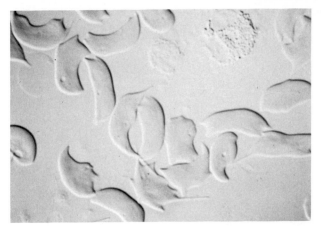

FIGURE 5-1
Peripheral smear as seen under a phase contrast microscope.
Drepanocytes (sickled erythrocytes) in an individual with sickle cell
disease (SS hemoglobin).

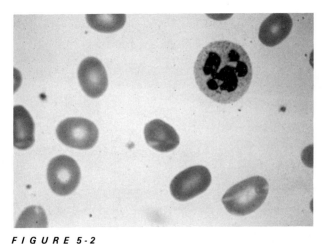

FIGURE 5-2
Peripheral smear showing profound macrocytic anemia in a patient
with vitamin B_{12} deficiency as a result of pernicious anemia. Note the
large erythrocytes, paucity of platelets, and a hypersegmented
polymorphonuclear cell.

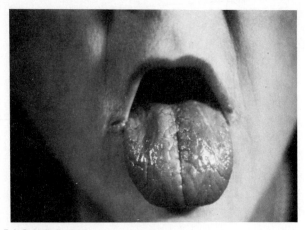

FIGURE 5-3
Atrophic glossitis in a patient with vitamin B$_{12}$ deficiency as a result of pernicious anemia. No loss of tongue papillae as indicated by the shiny and smooth tongue surface.

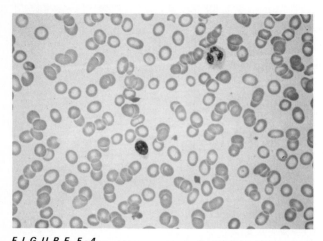

FIGURE 5-4
Peripheral smear showing rouleaux, i.e., abnormal stacking of erythrocytes. This individual had an IgG monoclonal gammopathy.

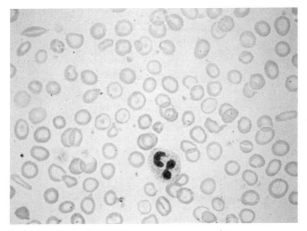

FIGURE 5-5
Peripheral smear from a patient with profound hypochromic microcytic anemia as a result of iron deficiency. Note marked decrease in pigment (hemoglobin) within the erythrocytes.

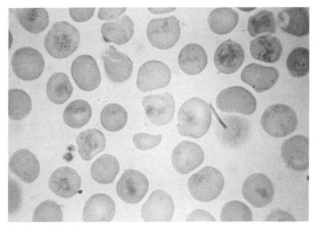

FIGURE 5-6
Wright's stain of peripheral smear from a patient with reticulocytosis.

T A B L E 5 - 2
Categories of Anemia

Type	Underlying Causes	Evaluation May Include
Hypochromic microcytic	Iron deficiency Anemia of chronic disease Thalassemia Plumbism (lead) Hypothyroidism	Serum iron TIBC Transferrin saturation Sickledex screen test RBC, elevated in thalassemia Hb electrophoresis Serum lead, in children Bone marrow (Prussian blue stain for iron stores)
Macrocytic	B_{12} deficiency Folate deficiency Hypothyroidism Ethanolism Reticulocytosis	LDH, total bilirubin B_{12} level Folate level Liver function tests History of chronic ethanol abuse T_3RU, T_4, and TSH Bone marrow examination Schilling test, if B_{12} level is low
Normochromic normocytic	Acute hemorrhage Chronic renal failure Acute hemolysis Aplastic anemia Monoclonal gammopathies	BUN, creatinine Coombs test Haptoglobin, LDH, and total bilirubin Serum free hemoglobin SPEP (serum protein electrophoresis) ESR (erythrocyte sedimentation rate) Glucose-6-phosphate dehydrogenase level; only in patients at risk and after the hemolysis has resolved Bone marrow examination

capacity (TIBC) is normal to increased, **transferrin saturation** is <30%, and **serum ferritin** is decreased. GI and uterine sources of blood loss need to be evaluated with a pregnancy test, pelvic examination, and/or imaging of the GI tract. Three different approaches to imaging the GI tract are available.

a. Flexible proctosigmoidoscopy, air contrast barium enema examination, and an upper GI series, or

b. Colonoscopy and an upper GI series, or

c. Colonoscopy and esophagogastroduodenoscopy.

4. **Management**

As evaluation proceeds, **iron replacement therapy** is indicated; $FeSO_4$, 325 mg PO t.i.d. for 2–3 months. A follow-up hematocrit determination and reticulocyte count in 2 weeks are indicated. Any GI lesion must be managed specific to its diagnosis and location. (See section on Gastrointestinal Bleeding in Chapter 2, page 104, for further discussion.)

B. **Anemia of chronic disease**

Any inflammatory process that is chronic or any significant chronic disease can result in mild to moderate anemia with hypochromic microcytic indices.

1. **Pathogenesis**

The underlying **pathogenesis** is a decreased production of erythrocytes due to a decreased ability of the bone marrow to produce erythrocytes. The material necessary for erythrocyte production is present, but the inflammatory process, via a not completely understood mechanism, depresses erythropoiesis.

2. **Manifestations**

The **specific manifestations** are attributable to the underlying chronic disease process.

3. **Evaluation**

The **evaluation** of this type of anemia includes determining iron indices, which will reveal a decreased serum iron level, decreased TIBC, a normal to elevated serum ferritin level, and a normal transferrin saturation.

4. **Management**

Treatment is focused on determining the underlying etiology and effectively managing that process. $FeSO_4$ replacement is not indicated.

C. **Thalassemia**

Thalassemia is a not uncommon cause for a decreased MCV and MCH, with or without a concurrent decrease in hematocrit and hemoglobin.

1. **Pathogenesis**

The underlying **pathogenesis** is a deficiency in either the alpha or beta components of the hemoglobin molecule. The normal hemoglobin molecule has two alpha and two beta chains. If the patient is **completely deficient** in alpha or beta chains, the condition is, respectively, alpha or beta thalassemia **major.** Alpha thalassemia major leads invariably to death in utero or early in life. Beta thalassemia major also results in a marked decrease in lifespan. Further discussion of thalassemia major is beyond the scope of this text. An **incomplete deficiency** in alpha or beta chains is termed alpha or beta thalassemia **minor.**

Alpha thalassemia, i.e., a deficiency in alpha chains, is common in people of Asian descent, whereas **beta thalassemia,** or a deficiency in beta chains, is common in people of African or Mediterranean descent. In alpha or beta thalassemia minor, there are no pathologic consequences of the decreased hematocrit and hemoglobin.

2. **Manifestations**

There are **no specific outward manifestations** of thalassemia minor, either alpha or beta. Most patients with thalassemia major die early in life.

3. **Evaluation and management**

The **evaluation and management** of thalassemia minor entail making the diagnosis and then reassuring the patient that the condition is "normal" for the patient. The iron studies are all normal, as are virtually all other tests, including a negative sickle cell screen (Sickledex). A hemoglobin electrophoresis in **beta thalassemia minor** will reveal an increased quantity of hemoglobin A_2. The only other clue to the diagnosis is that these patients invariably have an **elevated RBC count.** The management of thalassemia major is beyond the scope of this text; the diagnosis is made while the patient is a neonate. A hematologist should be consulted in all cases of thalassemia major.

D. **Hemoglobinopathies**

Hemoglobinopathy is a not uncommon cause of a decreased hematocrit and hemoglobin. The three most common hemoglobinopathies affect only select subgroups of the population, specifically African Americans.

1. **Pathogenesis**

The **underlying pathogenesis** of these disorders is a change in the functional structure of the hemoglobin molecule.

Hemoglobin is a complex protein. Any change in the primary structure of hemoglobin, such as a change in the order of amino acids in the protein, will result in significant changes in its function and usefulness. A change in one amino acid can decrease the life span of the molecule and thus of the erythrocyte. Moreover, a single amino acid change can significantly decrease the ability of the molecule, and thus the ability of the erythrocyte, to perform its life-sustaining functions of transporting oxygen to the tissues and carbon dioxide from the tissues.

The **sixth amino acid on the beta chain** is the site of common pathologic changes and as such is a de-

T A B L E 5 - 3
The Basis of Hemoglobin Electrophoresis

Type	Amino Acid at Position 6, Beta Chain	Isoelectric Point
A	Valine	7.2
S	Glutamic acid	7.0
C	Lysine	7.4

fining feature in the three most common types of adult hemoglobin: **A, S,** and **C** (see Table 5-3).

   a. Hemoglobin A: The normal hemoglobin molecule. The amino acid at beta position 6 is the uncharged valine. This neutral charge is required to maintain the normal structure.

   b. Hemoglobin S: Hemoglobin which, if homozygotic (**SS**), results in sickle cell disease, but if heterozygotic (**SA** or **SC**) results in either sickle cell trait (SA) or the disease of hemoglobin SC. The amino acid at beta position 6 is the negatively charged molecule, glutamic acid.

   c. Hemoglobin C: Hemoglobin which, if homozygotic (**CC**), results in death early in life, but if heterozygotic (**SC** or **AC**) results in either the disease of hemoglobin SC or the benign AC hemoglobin. The amino acid at the beta position is the positively charged molecule, lysine.

2. Manifestations and evaluation

   The **specific manifestations and evaluation** are based on the specific hemoglobinopathy. In all cases the overall evaluation as listed in Box 5-1 and hemoglobin electrophoresis are clearly indicated. The **Sickledex screen** is positive and **serum iron studies** are normal. Because the life span of these cells is decreased, there is a compensatory erythropoiesis, and therefore the **reticulocyte count** is invariably quite elevated, between 10% and 20%. The three most common hemoglobinopathies are **SC disease; SA, sickle cell trait;** and **SS, sickle cell disease.**

   a. SC disease is a fairly uncommon hemoglobinopathy in which 45% of the hemoglobin is S, 45% is C, and 10% is F. The **peripheral smear** reveals target cells and drepanocytes. The patient may have mild pain crises but is otherwise relatively asymptomatic. Also, unlike SS disease, autosplenectomy will rarely occur and thus splenomegaly is often evident.

b. **SA,** i.e., sickle cell **trait,** is a disease in which 40%–45% of the hemoglobin is S, 50% is the normal A, and 5% is F. This form is virtually always asymptomatic. The **peripheral smear** reveals virtually all of the erythrocytes to be normal, and anemia, if present, is quite mild. The spleen is normal in size.

c. **SS disease,** i.e., sickle cell **anemia,** is the classic and most severe form. Ninety to 95% of the hemoglobin is S, with a small proportion of hemoglobin F. The **peripheral smear** reveals drepanocytes (see Fig. 5-1). Because the patient has recurrent splenic infarctions early in life, or autosplenectomy, the spleen is never palpable in an adult. A classic manifestation of SS disease is the sickle cell **pain crisis.**

Pain crises occur when, for some reason, there is sludging of blood flow to specific areas of the body, resulting in relative ischemia. Precipitants include an antecedent viral infection or anything that can result in intravascular volume depletion. The patient presents with excruciating pain, usually deep and boring in nature, and may have findings of intravascular volume depletion. The pain is usually in the axial skeleton but can be in any location. Invariably the patient has had similar pain crises in the past.

3. Management

The **specific management** of sickle cell–related syndromes includes preventing crises and infections. Pain crises may be a significant manifestation of SS and at times SC disease. In addition, as the result of the rapid turnover of cells, the patient can become deficient in cofactors, especially folate, which may further exacerbate the anemia. Furthermore, there can be splenic dysfunction, which can result in an increased risk of infections. Box 5-2 lists specific modalities integral to the management of sickle cell–related syndromes.

a. The **acute management** of a **pain crisis** involves keeping the patient hydrated with IV fluids, supplying supplemental oxygen by nasal cannula, administering narcotic analgesia, and, in the majority of cases, admitting the patient. This is a major morbid problem and can result in many admissions to the hospital for management.

b. Other interventions that can be performed include **exchange transfusion** and the use of **hydroxyurea.**

B O X   5 - 2

Specific Management of Sickle Cell–Related Syndromes

Management

1. Administer Pneumovax at time of presentation in adults.
2. Provide yearly influenza B vaccination.
3. Provide folate supplementation, 5 mg PO q. A.M.
4. Instruct the patient to stop smoking.
5. Watch for and rapidly intervene in any pain crises.
6. Obtain a hematology consult for SS disease.
7. Determine the hematocrit and reticulocyte count every 6 months and with any change in the clinical condition of the patient.
8. Manage any acute crises, as described in text.

   i. In **exchange transfusion** a unit of the patient's blood is **removed** and **replaced** with a unit from a patient with hemoglobin A. The goal is to give the patient normally functioning erythrocytes. This can be performed before a surgical procedure or during a particularly severe pain crisis. This has the risks of hepatitis and AIDS transmission and should be reserved as a "last-ditch" effort.
   ii. Another exciting potentially beneficial agent is **hydroxyuria.** This must be used under the direction of a hematologist. This agent has been demonstrated to increase the level of **HbF,** fetal hemoglobin, thus decreasing the level of HbS and decreasing the intensity and frequency of pain crises. Obviously, this has a number of potentially significant side effects and should be reserved for severe cases.

4. **Crises, non-pain**
   In addition to pain crises, other crises can occur in sickle cell syndromes. These include the **aplastic, hyperhemolytic,** and **sequestration** crises. These are relatively rare, and thus only the aplastic crisis will be discussed here. The normal reticulocyte count in sickle cell anemia is 10%–20%; therefore, anything less than 10% may be indicative of impending aplas-

tic crisis. The most common reasons for **aplastic crises** include a deficiency in cofactors, especially folate, and a viral infection. The clinician must watch for the development of this crisis type.

V. **Macrocytic anemias**

In a macrocytic anemia the MCV of the erythrocytes is >94. Macrocytic anemias are not uncommon. The differential diagnosis includes processes that are eminently treatable and quite curable. The underlying causes and specific tests for the further evaluation of these anemias include those listed in Table 5-2. Two specific forms of macrocytic anemia are discussed below, **vitamin B$_{12}$ deficiency** and **folate deficiency.**

A. **Vitamin B$_{12}$ deficiency**

A deficiency in this essential cofactor and vitamin, cyanocobalamin, will result in a macrocytic anemia.

1. **Pathogenesis**

The **pathogenesis** relates to the **physiology** of vitamin B$_{12}$ in the body and the **gastrointestinal absorption** of this cofactor.

a. **Physiology.** Cyanocobalamin acts as a cofactor, in these cases as an indirect source of methyl groups, in certain biochemical reactions. There are two biochemical reactions in which it serves this function. One is the synthesis of deoxyribonucleic acid (DNA), the other is the synthesis of odd-chain fatty acids.

i. **DNA synthesis** requires the cofactor cyanocobalamin (B$_{12}$) in that the nucleotide base unique to DNA, thymidine, is a modified derivative of the nucleotide unique to ribonucleic acid, uridine. The modification entails the addition of a methyl group to uridine. The cyanocobalamin acts indirectly as a cofactor to folate in this methyl group transfer. Because the synthesis of DNA is necessary in all cell lines in which there is proliferation or cell turnover (i.e., skin, mucous membranes) and in thrombopoiesis, leukopoiesis, and erythropoiesis, any deficiency in cyanocobalamin will result in a decrease in the production of these cells.

ii. **Myelin synthesis** is disrupted by a deficiency in cyanocobalamin. A proposed mechanism is that myelin synthesis depends on the formation of odd-number carbon fatty acid chains. The synthesis of odd-chain fatty acids requires cyanocobalamin, and thus any deficiency in cyanocobalamin will result in dysfunctional myelin synthesis.

b. Gastrointestinal absorption. GI absorption of vitamin B_{12} has been well elucidated. Vitamin B_{12} occurs in high concentrations only in **meats,** especially red meat. Once ingested, it is bound in the stomach to a chemical produced by antral parietal cells and absorbed exclusively in the **terminal ileum.** If vitamin B_{12} is not bound to this chemical, called **intrinsic factor,** it cannot be absorbed.

2. **Manifestations**

The **specific manifestations** of vitamin B_{12} deficiency relate to its physiologic functions and include not only chronic anemia but also a smooth tongue (atrophic glossitis) as a result of loss of tongue papillae, and a decreased sensation to vibration and decreased position sense with an ataxic gait as a result of loss of highly myelinated axons in dorsal columns of the spinal cord. The **peripheral smear** will reveal hypersegmented polymorphonuclear cells, large platelets, and macroovalocytes (see Fig. 5-2).

3. **Underlying causes**

The **underlying causes** of cyanocobalamin deficiency reflect GI absorption of vitamin B_{12}. A deficiency can occur as a result of **nutritional deficiency,** but this is quite rare, because the storage pool of B_{12} lasts up to 2 years. Cyanocobalamin deficiency can also occur as the result of a deficiency in the binding protein, **intrinsic factor.** Intrinsic factor itself may be deficient as a result of gastric parietal cell dysfunction, gastric resection, or pernicious anemia. A final reason for vitamin B_{12} deficiency is **malabsorption of the IF–B_{12} complex** in the ileum as a result of ileal resection or inflammatory disease.

4. **Evaluation and management**

The **specific evaluation and management** include the steps listed in Box 5-1 and in Table 5-3. Serum levels of B_{12}, folate, LDH, and total bilirubin should be determined. If the serum cyanocobalamin level is less than 150 pg/mL, it is diagnostic of B_{12} deficiency. If the patient is B_{12} deficient:

a. Administer vitamin B_{12}, 1,000 μg IM, now and once a day for 4 days, then once weekly for 4 weeks, followed by 1,000 μg IM once monthly for life.

b. Perform a **Schilling test** to determine the cause of

T A B L E   5 - 4
Schilling Test

Purpose: To determine the pathophysiologic reason for the patient's
B$_{12}$ deficiency.

Part I: 1. Administer cobalt 60–labeled B$_{12}$, 500 μg PO.
         2. Collect a 24-hour urine sample for the ^{60}Co-labeled B$_{12}$.

         Results: <5% of B$_{12}$ dose is excreted in urine: abnormal
                  absorption of B$_{12}$.
                  >5% of B$_{12}$ dose is excreted in urine: normal ab-
                  sorption of B$_{12}$.
         3. Administer 1000 μg of nonradiolabeled B$_{12}$ IM exactly 2
            hours after the oral dose. This serves as a "flushing"
            dose.

Part II: To be performed only if <5% of ^{60}Co-labeled B$_{12}$ is excreted
         in urine in Part I of the test.

         1. Administer ^{60}Co-labeled B$_{12}$ and intrinsic factor 50 mg
            PO.
         2. Collect a 24-hour urine sample for the ^{60}Co-labeled B$_{12}$.

         Results: <5% of B$_{12}$ dose is excreted in urine: malabsorp-
                  tion at the terminal ileum.
                  >5% of B$_{12}$ dose is excreted in urine: lack of IF
                  due to either pernicious anemia or gastric re-
                  section.

         3. Administer 1000 μg of nonradiolabeled B$_{12}$ IM exactly 2
            hours after the oral dose. This serves as a "flushing"
            dose.

the deficiency. This test is easily performed but
is not mandatory in all cases. It is described in
Table 5-4.
   c. Monitor the **reticulocyte count** and potassium
      level, as potassium levels decrease with rapid
      erythropoiesis (increased reticulocytosis).
   d. Supplementation with **iron and folate** is indi-
      cated. Supplementation should be provided dur-
      ing the phase of reticulocytosis, i.e., approxi-
      mately over the first 4–6 months of B$_{12}$ repletion.
B. **Folate deficiency**
   A deficiency in this essential vitamin will result in a
   macrocytic anemia.
   1. **Pathogenesis**
      The **pathogenesis** relates to the **physiology** of folate
      in the body and to the **gastrointestinal absorption** of
      this cofactor.
      a. **Physiology.** Folate acts as a cofactor, in this case

as a direct source of methyl groups, in certain biochemical reactions. There are several biochemical reactions in which it serves this function, the most important one being the synthesis of deoxyribonucleic acid (DNA).

DNA synthesis requires this cofactor in that the nucleotide base unique to DNA, thymidine, is a modified derivative of the nucleotide unique to ribonucleic acid, uridine. The modification entails the addition of a methyl group to uridine, the methyl group being directly donated by a folate molecule. Because the synthesis of DNA is necessary in all cell lines in which there is proliferation or cell turnover (i.e., skin, mucous membranes) and in thrombopoiesis, leukopoiesis, and erythropoiesis, any deficiency in folate will result in a decrease in the production of these cells.

b. **Gastrointestinal absorption.** GI absorption of folate has been well elucidated. Folates are found in many foodstuffs but occur in particularly high concentrations in leafy green vegetables. Once ingested, folate is absorbed in the small intestine in general, and predominantly in the **proximal jejunum.**

2. **Manifestations**

The **specific manifestations** of folate deficiency reflect its physiology and include chronic anemia. Unlike in cyanocobalamin deficiency, there are no neurologic manifestations associated with folate deficiency. The **peripheral smear** will reveal hypersegmented polymorphonuclear cells, large platelets, and macroovalocytes (see Fig. 5-2).

3. **Underlying causes**

The **underlying causes** of folate deficiency relate to GI absorption of folate and folic acid. A deficiency can occur as a result of **nutritional deficiency,** which is not uncommon in malnourished people and chronic ethanol users. Another cause of folate deficiency is **malabsorption of folate or folic acid** in the small intestine as a result of small bowel resection or inflammatory bowel disease.

4. **Evaluation and management**

The **specific evaluation and management** of folate deficiency include the steps listed in Box 5-1 and Table 5-2. Serum levels of B_{12}, folate, LDH, and total bilirubin should be determined.

a. If the serum B_{12} is normal and the serum folate is low, replete the folate with **folate, 3–5 mg PO once daily.**

      b. Monitor the **reticulocyte count** and potassium level. Potassium levels decrease with rapid erythropoiesis (increased reticulocytosis).

VI. Normochromic normocytic anemia

Anemias in which the MCV and the MCH of the erythrocytes are within normal range are quite common. The underlying causes and specific evaluative tests for these anemias include those items listed in Table 5-2. Although the differential diagnosis is broad, only the normochromic normocytic anemia associated with **chronic renal failure** will be discussed here.

Chronic renal failure is a frequent cause of a modest to significant normochromic normocytic anemia.

A. Pathogenesis

The underlying **pathogenesis** of this anemia relates to the endocrine function of the kidneys. The kidneys produce the hormone erythropoietin. In the normal state this hormone is released when the kidneys sense a decrease in the intravascular volume. There is a direct stimulation of the normoblasts with resultant reticulocytosis. In the setting of renal failure, this function of the kidneys also becomes embarrassed. This is usually not a significant problem until there is a modest to marked overall impairment of renal function, i.e., the creatinine clearance rate is <20 mL/min.

B. Manifestations

The **specific manifestations** are minimal until the anemia is quite marked. It is not uncommon for a patient to have a hematocrit in the low to mid 20% range without any significant manifestations of such a degree of anemia. The paucity of symptoms and signs results from the slow progression and chronicity of the anemia, which allows compensatory mechanisms to take effect, and from the development of an acidosis, which further shifts the oxyhemoglobin dissociation curve to the left, increasing and optimizing the extraction of oxygen from hemoglobin by the tissues. The **peripheral smear** will reveal anemia with some spur cells (echinocytes).

C. Evaluation and management

The **specific evaluation and management** include the steps listed in Box 5-1 and in Table 5-2. In addition, the cause of the renal failure must be determined and managed (see Chapter 3, page 181). Furthermore, the initiation of **erythropoietin** is an effective modality in management. This recombinantly synthesized molecule is homologous to the natural human hormone and is quite effective. The goal is to increase the hematocrit and maintain it in the 30%–33% range.

VII. **Consultation**

Problem	*Service*	*Time*
Pancytopenia	Hematology	Urgent
Anemia of undetermined etiology	Hematology	Urgent
Hemoglobinopathies	Hematology	Elective
Chronic renal failure	Nephrology	Elective

VIII. **Indications for admission:** Any evidence of hemodynamic instability, any sickle cell anemia crisis, or an acute loss of blood, either by hemorrhage or hemolysis.

Excessive Bleeding States

Hemostasis is complex and integral to the survival of any human being. **Hemostasis** is the ability of the blood and its components to patch leaks in blood vessels. The leak is usually acquired as a result of trauma. By patching the acquired defect, hemostasis prevents the loss of fluid and blood from the intravascular tree. The **patch** so formed is a **clot** or **thrombus.**

Thrombus generation involves several sets of proteins and one formed element in the blood. The **protein sets** are grouped into the intrinsic and extrinsic coagulation cascades which, when either or both are activated, form the protein **thrombin.**

The **intrinsic coagulation cascade** consists of factors VIII, IX, and X and is activated by any breakdown of plasma membrane, such as endothelial breakdown. The **extrinsic coagulation cascade** consists of factors II, V, VII, IX, and X.

Platelets are the formed elements in the blood that are involved in thrombus formation. Concurrently with thrombin formation, platelets, via a mechanism involving the large protein, **von Willebrand factor,** will adhere to any area of endothelial breakdown. This results in the activation of and aggregation with other platelets. This platelet aggregate with the early thrombin fibrils is termed a **primary thrombus.** The primary thrombus matures by the development of covalent linkages between thrombin molecules to form the stable **secondary thrombus.**

I. **Overall manifestations**

The **overall manifestations** of excessive bleeding include the dermatologic findings of **petechiae** (red, nonblanching macules on the skin), **purpura** (nonblanching patches), and **ecchymoses.** Hematologic manifestations may include recurrent epistaxis (nosebleeds), hemarthroses, and upper or lower GI bleeding. The patient may report episodes of frank hematuria (blood in urine), and women may describe **men-**

orrhagia (heavy menstrual flow) or **menometrorrhagia** (abnormal menstrual bleeding between normal periods). The time of onset and whether the condition has been present since youth or is of recent onset are important because one can thus differentiate **congenital** from **acquired** coagulation defects. The patient must be questioned about the use of anticoagulants, especially heparin or warfarin, and the use of the antiplatelet agent aspirin.

Once the clinical diagnosis of an excessive bleeding state has been made and the evaluations listed in Box 5-3 have been performed, the coagulopathy (excessive bleeding state) can be subcategorized into one of three overall groups. These groups are discussed below.

II. **Elevated prothrombin time (PT)**
   A. **Pathogenesis**

   The underlying **pathogenesis** is a decrease in the production or effectiveness of the factors in the **extrinsic** coagulation pathway. These coagulation factors include factors II, V, VII, IX, and X. A deficiency of these coagulation factors may be acquired as a result of vitamin K deficiency or of severe hepatic dysfunction.

   1. A deficiency in **vitamin K,** a vitamin required for the production of all of the extrinsic coagulation factors except factor V, will manifest with an elevated PT and an increased bleeding tendency. The **differential diagnosis** includes entities that decrease vitamin K absorption in the ileum or its effectiveness in coagulation factor synthesis. Therefore, **malnutrition** (especially of leafy green vegetables), or any **malabsorption** syndrome, or the use of the oral anticoagulant **warfarin** will decrease vitamin K stores and increase PT.

   2. **Severe hepatic dysfunction.** All of the coagulation factors of the extrinsic pathway are produced in the liver, including factor V. Therefore, severe liver disease results in an elevated PT and an increased bleeding tendency.

   B. **Specific manifestations**

   The **specific manifestations** of excessive bleeding due to an elevated PT are similar to those listed under **I. Overall manifestations.** In addition, there is a history of Coumadin (sodium warfarin) use, poor nutrition, or ileal disease, or manifestations of severe hepatic insufficiency (see section on End-Stage Hepatic Dysfunction in Chapter 2, page 91).

   C. **Evaluation**

   Further **evaluation** includes making the clinical diagnosis and performing the tests listed in Box 5-3. One can

B O X 5 - 3

Basic Evaluation and Management of an Increased Bleeding Tendency

Evaluation

1. Determine the **platelet count**. This is central to evaluation and management, which depend on whether this value is low or normal.
2. Determine the **complete blood cell count** for baseline purposes.
3. Determine the **prothrombin time (PT)**. This is central to evaluation and management, which depend on whether this value is low or normal.
4. Determine the **activated partial thromboplastin time (aPTT)**. This is central to evaluation and management, which depend on whether this value is low or normal.
5. Determine the **bleeding time** to reproducibly quantify the coagulopathy.
6. Elicit the **family history**. If there is any family history of excessive bleeding, a family tree specific to the problem of excessive bleeding should be made.
7. Determine the patient's **nutritional status**. Estimate the quantity of leafy green vegetables that the patient ingests. Leafy green vegetables are rich in vitamin K.
8. Determine the **age at onset** of the increased bleeding tendency, which will help differentiate an acquired defect from a congenital defect.
9. Elicit the **medication history**, including the use of prescribed and over-the-counter agents.
10. To easily and rapidly differentiate an **acquired inhibitor** from a **factor deficiency**, mix the patient's plasma 1 : 1 with fresh frozen plasma (FFP). If a **factor deficiency** is present, the coagulopathy will correct; if an **acquired inhibitor** is present, no correction occurs.

Management

1. **Fresh frozen plasma** can be used on an emergency basis to control most coagulopathies (except inhibitors). It is rich in all factors required for coagula-

(continued)

B O X 5 - 3 *(continued)*

> tion; therefore, it can be used in any condition caus-
> ing an extrinsic or intrinsic coagulation deficit.
> Because it is a blood product and there is an inher-
> ent risk of transmitting HIV and hepatitis with trans-
> fusion, its use should be reserved for clear emer-
> gencies. Insofar as is possible, use specific factor
> concentrates if the deficiency type is known.
> 2. Instruct the patient not to use **aspirin** until the co-
>   agulopathy has been defined and corrected.

differentiate vitamin K deficiency from liver failure by
the following measures.

1. **Administer 10 mg of vitamin K subcutaneously.** If
   the PT elevation is due to vitamin K deficiency of
   any cause, the PT will correct, whereas in liver failure, the PT elevation will not correct.
2. The plasma level of **factor V,** which is not dependent
   on vitamin K, will be normal in vitamin K deficiency
   but low in liver disease.
3. **Liver function test results** are usually normal in vitamin K deficiency but abnormal in hepatic failure.
4. If surreptitious warfarin use is suspected, the **plasma
   warfarin level** should be determined.

D. **Management**

The **management** of excessive bleeding due to an isolated elevated PT includes determining the underlying
cause and treating that specific entity.

1. If the patient is **bleeding acutely,** administer FFP
   acutely to give coagulation factors and reverse the
   coagulopathy, unless an inhibitor is present.
2. If the condition is due to **vitamin K deficiency,** provide supplemental vitamin K and instruct the patient
   to eat leafy green vegetables. If the deficiency is due
   to malabsorption, SC or IM administration may be
   required. The usual dosage of vitamin K is 10 mg PO
   q. A.M.
3. In patients with **liver failure,** vitamin K supplementation can be attempted but is usually of little utility.
   The liver disease must be treated in order to correct
   the coagulopathy.
4. If any invasive procedures are planned, the PT must
   be decreased to less than 15 seconds. If the PT is

elevated as the result of warfarin, the clinician can use one of three methods to decrease the PT:

a. Instruct the patient not to take the warfarin for 2–3 days prior to the procedure.

b. Administer 0.5–1.0 mg vitamin K IV 4 hours before the procedure.

c. If the procedure is emergent, FFP may be administered.

If the PT is elevated as the result of hepatic dysfunction, FFP may be administered prior to the procedure.

III. **Elevation of the activated partial thromboplastin time (aPTT)**

A. **Pathogenesis**

The **underlying pathogenesis** is a decrease in the production or effectiveness of factors in the **intrinsic coagulation pathway.** These factors include VIII, IX, and X. A deficiency in these coagulation factors may be either **congenital** or **acquired.**

1. The **differential diagnosis** of congenital deficiencies in these intrinsic coagulation factors and thus an elevated aPTT includes the X-linked recessive **hemophilia A** (factor VIII deficiency), the X-linked recessive **hemophilia B** (factor IX deficiency), the **dysfibrinogenemias,** and **von Willebrand disease** (a deficiency of von Willebrand factor, a large protein that is necessary for factor VIII function and platelet adhesion).

2. The **differential diagnosis** of acquired deficiencies in these intrinsic coagulation factors and thus an elevated aPTT includes the use of **heparin** or the development of the pathogenic entity **disseminated intravascular coagulation (DIC).**

B. **Manifestations**

The **specific manifestations** of this group are similar to those listed under **I. Overall manifestations.** In addition, there is a history of hemarthroses which are quite classic for factor VIII or IX deficiency states; furthermore, a history of heparin use is helpful in defining the process.

C. **Evaluation**

The further **evaluation** of this subgroup includes making the clinical diagnosis and performing the tests listed in Box 5-3. One can differentiate congenital from acquired disorders by the **clinical history** in virtually all cases. The specific evaluation is dependent on this differentiation.

1. In a presumed **congenital deficiency** (i.e., if there is

a history of increased bleeding since childhood), evaluation for a deficiency of factor VIII or IX or von Willebrand factor is indicated.

   a. Determine **plasma levels** of **factor VIII** and **factor IX.**

   b. Perform a ristocetin aggregation test for von Willebrand factor deficiency. Normal platelets aggregate in vitro in the presence of the chemical ristocetin, but platelets from patients with von Willebrand disease do not aggregate in vitro in the presence of ristocetin. A caveat to this test is that it measures aggregation; however, in vivo, the platelet dysfunction in von Willebrand disease is one of adhesion. Adhesion is not easily measured, but aggregation can be measured reproducibly.

2. The **acquired deficiency states** include heparin use and DIC, both of which generally are clinically evident. In DIC there is an abnormal consumption of coagulation factors and platelets with a resultant elevation of the aPTT and PT, a decrease in fibrinogen, and the development of thrombocytopenia.

   a. "DIC" panel of aPTT, PT, platelets, and fibrinogen.

   b. If there is any question in differentiating heparin use from hypofibrinogenemic states (e.g., DIC), one can measure the **thrombin time (TT) *and*** perform the **reptilase test.**

      i. The **thrombin time** measures the time required to convert fibrinogen to fibrin and is **increased** in patients with low or dysfunctional fibrinogen states (e.g., DIC) and in heparin use.

      ii. The **reptilase time** is the TT measured by using reptilase, a coenzyme that is not affected by heparin; therefore, the reptilase time is elevated in low or dysfunctional fibrinogenemia states but **not elevated in heparin use.** In summary, heparin use increases TT but is accompanied by a normal reptilase time.

D. Management

The **management** of this group includes determining the underlying cause and treating that specific entity.

1. **Hemophilia A**

   a. To treat **emergently,** and if no factor VIII concentrate is available, use **FFP.**

   b. **Factor VIII concentrate** should be used therapeutically to treat any bleeding and prophylactically before any procedure. The goals of therapy include:

Minor bleeding: To attain >25% of normal plasma levels.

Major bleeding: To attain >50% of normal plasma levels.

Preoperatively: To attain a 100% level initially, then >50% for 10 days.

   c. The usual **dosage** is 60 units/kg IV initially, then 20–30 units/kg IV for 10 days.

2. Hemophilia B

   a. To treat **emergently,** and if no factor IX concentrate is available, use **FFP.**

   b. **Factor IX concentrate** should be used therapeutically to treat any bleeding and prophylactically before any procedure. The goals of therapy include:

Minor bleeding: To attain >25% of normal plasma levels.

Major bleeding: To attain >50% of normal plasma levels.

Preoperatively: To attain a 100% level initially, then >50% for 10 days.

   c. The usual **dosage** is 80 units/kg IV initially, then 30–40 units/kg IV for 10 days.

3. von Willebrand disease

   a. **DDAVP**—A synthetic vasopressin analogue that releases stored factor VIII:ag multimers from the endothelium.

Dosing regimen:

Initial: 0.3 μg/kg in 50 mL of normal saline infused **intravenously** over 30 minutes.

Maintenance: 0.3 μg/kg in 50 mL of normal saline infused **intravenously** over 30 minutes, once per day as long as the patient is at risk for bleeding.

   b. **Cryoprecipitate**—A blood product that is rich in factor VIII:ag multimers.

Dosing regimen:

Initial: 1 bag/10 kg administered as IV bolus.

Maintenance: 1 bag/10 kg administered as IV bolus once per day as long as the patient is at risk for bleeding.

Either one of these—DDAVP or cryoprecipitate—can be used acutely for bleeding or as prophylaxis prior to a surgical procedure.

4. **Heparin use.** If the patient is bleeding, discontinue heparin. Heparin anticoagulation can be rapidly reversed with protamine sulfate if the bleeding is significant.
5. **DIC.** Determine the underlying cause. Often the patient has impending or clinical septicemia, usually with gram-negative organisms. The clinician must aggressively **determine** and **treat the underlying cause.**

IV. **Increased bleeding time (BT)**
   A. **Pathogenesis**
      The **underlying pathogenesis** is a decrease in the production, life span, or effectiveness of the formed elements involved in thrombus formation, the platelets. Platelet dysfunction may result from a **quantitative** deficiency of platelets (i.e., thrombocytopenia as defined by a platelet count of <150,000/mm^3) or from a **qualitative** defect in platelets.
      1. The **differential diagnosis** of the **quantitative disorders** (i.e., thrombocytopenia) includes disorders that decrease production of platelets and disorders that increase peripheral destruction.
         a. Disorders that **decrease the production of platelets** in the bone marrow include **aplastic anemia, megaloblastic processes** (vitamin B_{12} or folate deficiency), **myelophthistic processes** (i.e., the replacement of bone marrow with tumor or granulomatous infection), or **amegakaryocytic thrombocytopenia** (i.e., the primary loss of megakaryocytes within the bone marrow).
         b. Disorders that result in **premature peripheral destruction**—that is, a decrease in the normal 9-day life span of the platelet—include the immune-mediated process of **autoimmune thrombocytopenia purpura** (ITP), SLE, **Evan's syndrome** (autoimmune hemolysis and autoimmune thrombocytopenia), and **drug-related thrombocytopenia.**
      2. The **differential diagnosis** of qualitative disorders includes anything that decreases the platelet's ability to perform its two fundamental functions—adhering to the endothelium and aggregating. These include the **acquired** entities of aspirin use and uremia and

the **congenital** entities of von Willebrand disease, Glanzmann's thrombasthenia, and Bernard–Soulier syndrome. The most common cause is aspirin use.

B. Manifestations

The **specific manifestations** of this group are similar to those listed under **I. Overall manifestations.** In addition, there is a marked number of petechiae as these skin and mucous membrane manifestations are quite specific for quantitative and qualitative platelet disorders. A history of aspirin use can be helpful in defining the process.

C. Evaluation

The further **evaluation** of this subgroup includes making the clinical diagnosis and performing the tests listed in Box 5-3. (Qualitative defects other than those due to aspirin are rare and beyond the scope of this text; therefore, the remaining discussion will be directed toward thrombocytopenia.) Specific evaluations include measuring levels of **platelet-associated antibodies,** IgM, IgG, and drug-specific antibodies; reviewing the peripheral smear; and determining serum folate and vitamin B_{12} levels. A bone marrow examination may be considered but is not mandatory.

D. Management

The **specific management** of thrombocytopenia is based on the degree of the deficit and the underlying cause.

1. If there is any **evidence of bleeding,** or if **surgery is contemplated,** or if the **platelet count is <10,000/ mm³,** platelet transfusions are indicated. The dosage of **random-donor platelets** is 1 pack/10 kg of patient's body weight. Each random-donor platelet pack should raise the peripheral count by 10,000/ mm³. Transfusion of **HLA-typed platelets** is effective but extremely expensive, requires an active and large blood bank, and is time-consuming for the donor of the platelets. Thus, HLA-matched platelets should be reserved for refractory cases.

2. If the process is thought to be **immune-mediated,** discontinue the potentially offending medications and initiate a course of **steroids.** The steroid dose is either prednisone, 60–80 mg PO once per day with a taper, or Solumedrol, 40 mg q.8h. IV with a taper. The steroid taper should be titrated to the platelet count.

   a. If the patient is not bleeding, transfusion with platelets in patients with immune-mediated processes is of **little benefit** because of the rapid peripheral destruction of normal host and donor platelets.

3. Until stabilized, platelet counts should be determined daily. After the steroid taper begins, less frequent measurement is acceptable.
4. **Aspirin is contraindicated.**

V. Consultation

Problem	Service	Time
Elevated PT unresponsive to vitamin K	Hematology	Urgent
Elevated aPTT, except for heparin use	Hematology	Urgent
Thrombocytopenia	Hematology	Urgent/emergent

VI. **Indications for admission:** Any active bleeding, any consumptive coagulopathy such as DIC, or any profound thrombocytopenia (i.e., platelet count < 20,000/mm^3).

Breast Malignancy

The **normal breast** is composed of multiple glands that, under appropriate hormonal stimulation, lactate (produce milk). The milk produced flows to the nipples through ducts. The **epithelium** lining these ducts is the source of the vast majority of malignant neoplastic lesions in the breast.

The **underlying pathogenesis** of breast malignancy is not completely known; however, certain endocrine and genetic factors are involved.

Specific **risk factors** for the development of breast malignancy include the **endocrine factors** of an early onset of menarche (before age 12 years), a late menopause (after age 50 years), the long-term use of high-dose estrogens, and a late first completed pregnancy (after age 30 years). **Genetic risk factors** include, prominently, a family history of breast cancer or in a first-degree female relative (mother, daughter, or sibling). A final risk factor is a personal history of breast carcinoma in the contralateral breast.

The **incidence** of this malignant neoplastic lesion is very high. In 1987 approximately 130,000 new cases of breast carcinoma were diagnosed in the United States and western Europe. The incidence and death rate for this malignancy are, in women, **second** only to bronchogenic carcinoma. Based on various epidemiologic calculations, a woman has a **1 in 9** risk of developing this malignancy in her lifetime.

I. Overall manifestations
The **overall manifestations** of breast carcinoma are usually minimal until relatively late in its course.

A. **Early manifestations**

   Early manifestations may include a painless lump in the breast, with or without concurrent lumps in the ipsilateral axilla. On **examination,** early signs include a painless, firm to rock-hard nodule or mass with or without palpable ipsilateral lymph nodes. A not uncommon early manifestation is an abnormal area of small calcifications on a **mammogram** in a patient with **no palpable abnormalities** on physical examination.

B. **Advanced manifestations**

   Manifestations of **advanced disease** include weight loss, bone pain, local skin pain, swelling, retraction of the overlying skin with *peau d'orange* sign, and ulceration of the skin overlying and adjacent to the breast mass. The ulceration occurs as a result of tumor invading the skin in locally advanced disease.

II. **Screening tests**

   The **screening tests** for breast carcinoma as recommended by the American Cancer Society include:

   A. **Breast self-examinations**

      Breast self-examination should be performed on a monthly basis, starting at menarche. It is best for the patient to perform the examination on the 5th day after the onset of menstrual flow.

   B. **Physician breast examination**

      Annual breast examinations should be performed by a physician, starting when the patient is 20.

   C. **Mammography**

      A baseline mammogram should be obtained at age 35, then mammography should be performed every other year until age 50, after which annual mammograms should be obtained. The baseline mammogram may be obtained at age 30 in patients who are at high risk for breast carcinoma.

III. **Evaluation and management of a lump**

   The **specific evaluation and management** of a **lump** discovered on palpation or by mammography include the following schemas. These schemes are put into effect **before** the diagnosis of breast carcinoma has been made.

   A. **Clinically suspicious lumps**

      If the **lump** is in any way **suspicious** for a neoplastic lesion, the patient should be referred expeditiously to a general surgeon with experience in breast disorders for an **excisional biopsy. Characteristics of the lump** that increase the suspicion for malignancy include painlessness, firmness (even to the point of being hard), concurrent ipsilateral axillary lymph node enlargement, and the mammographic demonstration of **minute calcifications** within its substance. **Patient characteristics** that increase the suspicion for malignancy include **any** of the risk factors for breast carcinoma development described above.

B. **Clinically benign lumps**

If the **lump** is clinically benign, it can be followed with a repeated physical examination in 2–3 months and a repeated mammogram at that time. The defining physical features of a **benign lump** include the absence of any features listed under **A** that would define a suspicious lesion and, if it is in a young patient, the lump is **intermittently tender,** especially waxing and waning in discomfort and size during the menstrual cycle, and there are **no microscopic calcifications** in the lump detected mammographically. If on repeat examination there is any **increase in suspicion** for malignancy, referral to a surgeon is indicated for excisional biopsy.

C. **Surgical options**

Once the **decision** to perform an excisional biopsy is made, the surgeon, primary care physician, and the patient should decide how to proceed if the **frozen section results** of the excisional biopsy are positive for carcinoma. It is at this time, **before the procedure** and before the diagnosis is histopathologically confirmed, that the strategy for surgical management must be determined. If the lump is histopathologically demonstrated to be carcinoma, the surgical options include:

1. A **modified radical mastectomy with axillary dissection,** in which the entire breast along with the underlying pectoralis muscle and the adjacent axillary lymph nodes are resected in one piece; *or*
2. A **lumpectomy with axillary dissection and postoperative adjuvant irradiation,** in which the breast lump is resected and, in a concurrent procedure, the axillary nodes are dissected and resected. Postoperative local adjuvant irradiation is mandatory.

IV. **Evaluation and staging of histopathologically diagnosed carcinoma**

The **evaluation and staging** of clinically and **histopathologically diagnosed (via biopsy)** breast carcinoma usually occur after a definitive surgical intervention. The evaluation and staging are based on the **natural history** of the disease. **Early metastases** of breast carcinoma are to the lymph nodes. If the primary lesion is in the outer quadrants of the breast, disease will spread to the ipsilateral axillary lymph nodes, whereas if the primary lesion is in the inner quadrants of the breast, disease will spread to the ipsilateral

B O X   5 - 4

Overall Evaluation and Staging of Breast Carcinoma

Evaluation

1. **Bilateral mammography** should already have been performed in the evaluation of a breast mass.
2. Obtain **chest radiographs** in PA and lateral views to stage the disease, looking especially for any nodules in the pulmonary fields.
3. Perform **liver function tests,** including alkaline phosphatase, LDH, SGOT, SGPT, and total bilirubin. If any of these indices are elevated, disease may have metastasized to the liver; therefore, further evaluation with CT of the abdomen is indicated.
4. Perform a radionuclide **bone scan** to look for any "hot spots," areas of increased uptake indicative of metastatic disease.
5. If there is any hepatomegaly or if any liver function test results are abnormal, perform **abdominal CT** to look for space-occupying lesions consistent with metastatic disease.
6. All **biopsy specimens** must be tested for estrogen and progesterone receptors. The presence or absence of these receptors on the tumor is an integral factor in determining further management.
7. If there is any neurologic deficit, perform **CT of the head** to look for any space-occupying lesion consistent with metastatic disease.

Staging

The overall staging is important not only in prognosis but also in determining the best modalities to use in addition to surgery in the treatment of breast carcinoma. The **TNM (tumor, node, metastases) staging system** is listed in Table 5-5.

---

mediastinal nodes. In **advanced disease** metastases occur to the supraclavicular lymph nodes, liver, lungs, brain, and/or bones. Components in the evaluation and staging of the carcinoma are listed in Box 5-4.

V. Overall management

The **overall management** of breast carcinoma entails effectively screening for breast lesions, making the diagnosis

T A B L E 5-5
TNM Staging Classification of Breast Carcinoma

Stage	Description
T1	Lesion size: <2 cm in diameter
T2	Lesion size: 2 cm to 5 cm in diameter
T3	Lesion size: >5 cm in diameter
T4	Lesion fixed to the chest wall and/or skin
N0	No nodal metastases
N1	Mobile axillary nodes
N2	Axillary nodes fixed to the skin and/or fascia
N3	Supraclavicular nodes
M0	No distant metastases
M1	Any distant metastases

early, using the described strategies, and effecting appropriate surgical intervention. **After surgery** and staging, the clinician assesses the risk for disease recurrence and thus the need for further nonsurgical therapy. Unlike many other malignant neoplasms, breast carcinoma is responsive to chemotherapy and hormonal therapy, but the more advanced the stage, the poorer is the prognosis for the patient. Postoperative management is discussed here for three categories, based on the risk for recurrence of the disease.

A. **Minimal risk**

There is no evidence of metastatic disease, including no metastatic disease in the ipsilateral axillary lymph nodes. After the surgical procedure, **no adjuvant chemotherapy** is needed.

B. **Moderate risk**

There is no evidence of metastatic disease outside of the local area, but **one to three lymph nodes are positive** for metastatic carcinoma. Although the tumor has been surgically resected, there is the risk for micrometastatic disease, and therefore, **adjuvant chemotherapy is indicated.**

C. **High risk**

There is documented metastatic disease outside the axillary lymph nodes, or more than four lymph nodes are positive for disease. Not adjuvant but therapeutic chemotherapy and/or hormonal intervention is needed.

VI. **Chemotherapy and hormonal therapy**

A. **Chemotherapy**

Adjuvant or therapeutic chemotherapy includes regimens of **CMF** (cyclophosphamide, methotrexate, and 5-FU) or regimens based on **anthracycline** (e.g., Adriamycin). Adjuvant regimens are of shorter duration but not necessarily of lower intensity than therapeutic regimens.

B. **Hormonal therapy**

Endocrine manipulation includes the use of the antiestrogen agent **tamoxifen,** which is effective in controlling metastatic disease in estrogen receptor (ER)–positive patients. Tamoxifen is most useful in postmenopausal women with ER-positive, metastatic disease. The **dosage** of tamoxifen is 10 mg/day PO. A potential **side effect** is hypercalcemia in patients with metastatic disease to the bones.

VII. **Consultation**

Problem	*Service*	*Time*
Any suspicious lesion	General surgery	Urgent
Adjuvant local irradiation	Radiation oncology	Urgent (if a lumpectomy with axillary node dissection is planned)
Adjuvant or therapeutic chemotherapy is indicated	Medical oncology	Urgent

VIII. **Indications for admission:** Scheduled admissions for the initiation of chemotherapy or for surgical intervention.

Bronchogenic Carcinoma

The **normal lung** is composed of a branching network of hollow tubes or **bronchi** that become incrementally smaller until they reach the sites of gas exchange, the **alveoli.** The bronchi, which are lined with simple ciliated columnar epithelium, are designed to **filter** inhaled atmospheric air and **move** the atmospheric air to and from the alveoli. The alveoli are unique structures where the **exchange of gases** between the erythrocytes and the atmospheric air occurs with great alacrity. These cells can be exposed to many harmful and potentially carcinogenic agents and therefore are not uncommon sites of malignant transformation and form primary or **bronchogenic carcinoma.**

The **underlying pathogenesis** of bronchogenic carcinoma is unclear, but the cells of origin of the malignant neoplastic growth are in the lung tissue and have been postulated to be from a common stem cell or from malignant transformation of mature cells in the airways, the alveoli, or the neuroectoderm—Kulchitsky's cells. Thus, there can be significant diversity in the histopathologic types of bronchogenic carcinomas.

The **risk factors** for the development of all bronchogenic carcinoma except the specific non-small cell carcinoma, adenocarcinoma, include **smoking** of any **tobacco** product, **smoking marijuana,** exposure to **asbestos fibers,** and exposure to **heavy metals** or **irradiation.** Smoking of tobacco and exposure to asbestos **synergistically** increase the risk of bronchogenic carcinoma development.

The **risk factors** for **adenocarcinomas** include any process that results in scarring or fibrosis of the lung tissue, irradiation, and exposure to asbestos. Adenocarcinoma has been referred to as "scar carcinoma."

The **incidence** of these malignant neoplastic disorders is high and increasing at an alarming rate. This entity is the most common cause of cancer **and** cancer-related deaths in the United States and probably in the western world. In 1988 more than 150,000 new cases of bronchogenic carcinoma were diagnosed in the United States alone.

I. Overall manifestations

The **overall manifestations** of bronchogenic carcinoma are usually quite minimal until late in the disease course. These manifestations can be as a **direct result** of the tumor in the lung or of **metastatic disease;** they may also occur as **paraneoplastic syndromes.**

A. Manifestations attributable to the tumor

Manifestations **directly attributable** to the tumor include a **cough** that is chronic or subacute, intermittent **hemoptysis,** unintentional **weight loss,** and a history of recurrent **pneumonias** in the same lobe. Further manifestations include **wheezing localized** to the affected areas and **chest radiographic** findings of a nodule (<4 cm in diameter), a mass (>4 cm in diameter), or a persistent radiographic infiltrate. Other manifestations that may occur as a direct result of locally advanced disease include those described below.

1. **Horner's syndrome,** which manifests with the triad of **unilateral miosis, unilateral ptosis,** and **unilateral anhydrosis,** all as a result of tumor in the **ipsilateral** upper lobe that directly invades the ipsilateral superior cervical ganglion. This ganglion supplies sympathetic innervation to the ipsilateral face and head.

2. The development of a **brachial plexopathy,** which manifests with weakness **(paresis), pain, paresthesias,** and **dysthesias,** all as a result of tumor in the ipsilateral upper lung that has invaded the brachial plexus.

B. Manifestations of metastatic disease

These manifestations include bone pain, especially in the low back, and even pathologic fractures, all as a

result of **bony metastases.** Furthermore, neurologic deficits and hepatomegaly can develop as a result of metastatic disease to the **brain** or **liver.**
C. **Manifestations of paraneoplastic syndromes**
Several of these syndromes will be discussed in the specific discussion of small cell and non-small cell carcinoma.

II. Screening
Bronchogenic carcinoma would be a perfect disorder for a screening examination. Unfortunately, there is no effective screening technique, including scheduled chest radiography, that is useful in the detection of this malignant disorder.

III. Overall evaluation and staging
The **overall evaluation and staging** of these lesions include assessing the probability that bronchogenic carcinoma is present, based on findings on chest radiographs and clinical observations, especially in patients with a moderate to high risk factor profile. In many respects, the overall evaluation is quite similar to that described for a solitary pulmonary nodule (see Chapter 4). The overall evaluation is listed in Box 5-5.

B O X 5 - 5

Overall Evaluation of Suspected Bronchogenic Carcinoma

Evaluation

1. Take a thorough **history** and perform a **physical examination,** with emphasis on the findings listed under **I. Overall manifestations.**
2. Obtain **chest radiographs** in **PA and lateral views,** a central component of the evaluation. The radiographs are useful in demonstrating the size of the lesion and the presence or absence of concurrent manifestations such as pleural effusions or hilar enlargement.
3. Obtain **sputum** for cytology, AFB smear, and Gram

(continued)

B O X 5 - 5 (continued)

stain q. A.M. for 3 days. The cytologic findings, if positive, will clinch the diagnosis, and further invasive evaluation is usually unnecessary. Negative cytologic findings, however, do not rule out a malignant neoplastic lesion.

4. If pleural fluid is accessible, perform thoracentesis for diagnostic purposes (see section on Pleural Effusions, Chapter 4, page 223). The cytologic findings on the pleural fluid, if positive for a malignant, neoplastic lesion, will clinch the diagnosis and in most cases obviate the need for other invasive evaluation.

5. Perform **CT imaging** of the lesion with and without contrast media. This imaging technique demonstrates the extent of local disease: the size of the mass, any mediastinal lymph node enlargement, and any concurrent pleural disease.

6. If the previous steps **do not produce** a histopathologic diagnosis, more invasive evaluation is indicated.
   a. If the lesion is **peripheral** in location, percutaneous needle biopsy under CT guidance should be performed by a radiologist with expertise in this procedure.
   b. If lesion is **central,** bronchoscopy for biopsy of the lesion should be performed by a pulmonologist.

7. Perform **pulmonary function tests,** including FEV_1, FVC, and arterial blood gases. PFTs are particularly important if any surgical intervention for resection of the lesion is being considered, as an **FEV_1 of** **<1.5 L** is a contraindication to pneumonectomy.

8. If a **solitary pulmonary nodule** is discovered, see the section on Solitary Pulmonary Nodule in Chapter 4.

9. Determine levels of serum calcium, phosphorus, albumin, electrolytes, and a CBC with differential for baseline purposes. These indices are important, as several of the malignant neoplastic lesions can manifest with hypercalcemia and/or profound hyponatremia as a result of a paraneoplastic syndrome.

10. Differentiate the tumor type into one of two groups: **small cell carcinoma** or **non-small cell carcinoma.** The specific evaluation and management are based on this differentiation.

IV. **Specific evaluation and management by tumor type**

The **specific evaluation, natural history, staging,** and **management** of the various primary bronchogenic carcinomas are best outlined if the lesions are divided into two broad categories, **small cell carcinoma** and **non-small cell carcinoma.**

A. **Small cell carcinoma**

Small cell carcinoma is a unique but common form of bronchogenic carcinoma, possibly derived from cells of neuroectoderm origin.

1. **Manifestations**

The **specific manifestations** of small cell carcinoma include those listed under **I. Overall manifestations.** This specific type of neoplasia will often manifest with a paraneoplastic syndrome. In fact, the paraneoplastic syndrome is frequently the initial manifestation of this lesion. These **paraneoplastic syndromes** include but are not limited to the following:

a. The **syndrome of inappropriate antidiuretic hormone secretion (SIADH),** with resultant hyponatremia. The hyponatremia may be marked and may result in delirium, lethargy, and seizures.

b. The **syndrome of ectopic ACTH,** with resultant increased skin pigmentation and findings of hypercortisolism. The secondary hypercortisolism will manifest with truncal obesity, hypertension, hyperglycemia, hypokalemia, and hypernatremia.

c. **Eaton–Lambert syndrome,** a diffuse, myasthenia-like muscle weakness that, unlike myasthenia gravis, improves with repeated motor activity.

2. **Natural history**

Small cell carcinoma grows rapidly and metastasizes early and significantly: to adjacent lung tissue, the contralateral lung, the bones, bone marrow, brain, liver, or adrenal glands.

3. **Evaluation**

The **specific evaluation** of this entity includes the steps listed in Box 5-5 and making the histopathologic diagnosis. Evaluation is based on the natural history of the tumor and is tantamount to staging. Evaluation entails a CT imaging of the head, the thorax, and abdomen. Further evaluation includes performing a bone scan and bone marrow aspiration.

4. **Staging**

The **staging** of small cell carcinoma entails categorizing the disease as **limited** or **extensive.** In the **limited stage,** tumor is restricted to one hemithorax; in the **extensive stage,** disease is demonstrated outside the affected hemithorax. The stage is a marker for prognosis and also aids in therapeutic decision-making.

5. **Management**

The **management** of small cell carcinoma is based on disease stage at the time of presentation and on the fact that it is a malignant neoplasm that responds to chemotherapy. In the limited stage, this tumor is potentially **curable.** Therefore, therapeutic intervention must be aggressive. Chemotherapy regimens include those based on **anthracycline** (e.g., daunorubicin) or **etopside (VP-16).**

Follow-up should be conducted by a medical oncologist on a regular basis.

A caveat to management is that a **solitary pulmonary nodule** that has been resected and diagnosed to be small cell carcinoma should be treated, at a minimum, as limited disease. Therefore, unlike in a solitary pulmonary nodule with non-small cell carcinoma, **adjuvant chemotherapy is indicated in small cell carcinoma.**

B. **Non-small cell carcinoma**

Non-small cell carcinomas include adenocarcinomas, squamous cell carcinomas, and large cell anaplastic carcinomas. Each of these malignant neoplasms is biologically distinct but, from a clinical point of view, all behave and respond to therapy in similar ways, and as such are discussed together.

1. **Manifestations**

The **specific manifestations** of these lesions include those listed under **I. Overall manifestations.** Non-small cell carcinomas often manifest with a paraneoplastic syndrome, which may be the initial manifestation of a lesion. The paraneoplastic syndromes include but are not limited to the following:

a. The **syndrome of ectopic secretion of a parathormone (PTH)-like substance** with resultant hypercalcemia. This will often manifest with polyuria, polydipsia, constipation, intravascular volume depletion, lethargy, and even coma.

b. The development of **hypertrophic pulmonary osteoarthropathy,** which manifests with bilateral clubbing and a diffuse, symmetric, polyarticular, small joint arthritis.

2. **Natural history**

Non-small cell carcinomas grow quite slowly and metastasize first to the local mediastinal lymph nodes, then to bone and liver.

T A B L E 5 - 6
TNM Staging Classification of Non-Small Cell Carcinomas

Stage	Descriptors
T1	mass <3 cm in diameter
T2	mass ≥3 cm in diameter and/or there is extension to the hilum
T3	T2 and the presence of atelectasis and/or pleural effusion
N0	No nodal metastases
N1	Hilar nodes present
N2	Mediastinal nodes present
M0	No extrathoracic metastases
M1	Any extrathoracic metastasis

3. **Evaluation**

   The **specific evaluation** of non-small cell carcinoma includes the steps listed in Box 5-5 and making the histopathologic diagnosis. Evaluation is based on the natural history of the tumor and is tantamount to staging. Evaluation entails CT imaging of the thorax and abdomen and, if clinically indicated, of the head. Further evaluation includes performing a bone scan to look for bony metastases.

4. **Staging**

   The **staging** of non-small cell carcinomas is best done by the TNM (tumor, node, metastases) method (see Table 5-6).

5. **Management**

   The **management** of non-small cell carcinoma is based on disease stage at the time of presentation and on the fact that these lesions are **refractory** to irradiation and chemotherapy. After disease has spread from the primary site, the condition is essentially **incurable.** Therefore, early-stage lesions, especially those that are a solitary pulmonary nodule, should be treated aggressively surgically, but for advanced disease only palliative therapy is indicated. Thus, irradiation should be saved until the patient has become symptomatic, i.e., the disease can be palliated.

V. **Prevention**

   Prevention is a major factor in the management of bronchogenic carcinoma. Instructing the patient to **discontinue smoking** tobacco and developing strategies to minimize exposure of people to **second-hand smoke** and to **carcinogenic fibers** (e.g., asbestos) are of paramount importance.

VI. **Consultation**

Problem	Service	Time
CT-directed biopsy of peripheral lesion	Radiology	Urgent
Bronchoscopy for central lesion	Pulmonology	Urgent
Small cell carcinoma	Oncology	Urgent
Non-small cell carcinoma	Oncology	Urgent
Non-small cell carcinoma	Radiation oncology	Elective
Superior vena cava syndrome	Radiation oncology	Emergent
Any solitary pulmonary nodule in a high-risk patient	Cardiothoracic surgery	Urgent

VII. **Indications for admission:** Any symptomatic paraneoplastic syndrome, any active pneumonia, any severe side effects of chemotherapy, Horner's syndrome, a superior vena cava syndrome.

Colon Carcinoma

The **colon,** although not essential for life, has several important functions. These include absorbing water from and acting as a short-term storage container for fecal material. In the normal state, the colon is lined with **simple columnar,** mucus-secreting epithelium.

The **underlying pathogenesis** of colon carcinoma is not completely clear, but it is known that colon adenocarcinoma usually develops from **adenomatous polyps in the colon.** These polyps are lesions in which there is the nonmalignant neoplastic growth of the colonic mucosa. Such polyps may be pedunculated or sessile. They grow slowly and can transform into malignant neoplastic disease, i.e., colon adenocarcinoma. The risk factors for polyp development are essentially the same as for the development of colon adenocarcinoma.

Risk factors include the presence of **adenomatous polyps** in the colon, in general, and the polyposis syndromes, many of which are hereditary, in specific. Several polyposis syndromes are described in Table 5-7. Other risk factors include a **low-fiber, high-fat diet** and the inflammatory bowel disorder, **ulcerative colitis.** Ulcerative colitis is independent of polyps in the development of colon adenocarcinoma.

T A B L E 5 - 7
Polyposis Syndromes

Syndrome	Genetics	Components
Turcot's syndrome	Autosomal recessive	Multiple adenomatous polyps Supratentorial glioblastomas Increased risk of colon adenocarcinoma
Canada–Cronkhite syndrome	Not inherited	Generalized hyperplastic polyps throughout the GI tract Generalized alopecia Hyperpigmentation of skin and nails Diarrhea with hypoalbuminemia No increase in colon adenocarcinoma
Peutz–Jegher's syndrome	Autosomal dominant	Hyperpigmented GI and/or GU and/or respiratory polyps Increased risk of intussusception No increased risk of colon adenocarcinoma
Gardner's syndrome	Autosomal dominant	Multiple adenomatous polyps Skeletal osteoma Retroperitoneal fibrosis Neurofibromas Desmoid tumors Increased risk of colon adenocarcinoma
Familial polyposis syndrome	Autosomal dominant	Multiple adenomatous polyps Increased risk of colon adenocarcinoma

The **incidence** of colon cancer is **high** in North America and western Europe. Various sources have reported an overall incidence of almost 50 cases per 100,000 population per year in the U.S. population over 30 years of age. Moreover, colon cancer is second only to bronchogenic carcinoma as a cause of **cancer-related death** in the United States today.

I. Overall manifestations

The **overall manifestations** of colon carcinoma depend on the stage of the disease and the antecedent risk factors.

A. Early manifestations

The disease process is minimally symptomatic until quite late in its course. **Adenomatous polyps,** even those with areas of carcinoma in situ, usually manifest with intermittently guaiac-positive stools and only

rarely become **symptomatic.** The exception to the paucity of early manifestations is if the antecedent disease
process is **ulcerative colitis.** In the case of ulcerative
colitis, bloody diarrhea, fevers, and abdominal pain are
usually quite evident; in fact, the patient usually already has that diagnosis.

B. **Late manifestations**

Manifestations of advanced colon adenocarcinoma include constipation, obstipation, melena, hematochezia,
weight loss, a pale color to the skin and mucous membranes due to anemia, and occasionally findings referable to large bowel obstruction, i.e., diffuse abdominal
pain, tympanic abdominal distention, and a significant
decrease in flatus.

II. **Screening tests**

Screening tests for colon carcinoma and colon polyps include stool guaiac examinations and flexible proctosigmoidoscopy. The screening test is based on the fact that adenomatous polyps and early colon adenocarcinomas bleed
intermittently.

A. **Recommended screening schedule**

The **screening schedule** as recommended by the American Cancer Society includes the following elements:

1. **Annual rectal examination,** starting at age 40 years.
2. **Annual stool guaiac test,** starting at age 50 years.
3. **Flexible proctosigmoidoscopy,** with a baseline study
   performed at age 50 years. If results are normal, the
   test is repeated every 3 years thereafter.

B. **Subsequent studies based on screening results**

1. When a **stool guaiac screen** is **positive,** further evaluation is indicated. The evaluation entails *either* flexible proctosigmoidoscopy **and** an air contrast barium
   enema examination, which can be performed by the
   primary care physician, *or* colonoscopy, which is
   performed by the gastroenterologist.
2. If **flexible proctosigmoidoscopy** or the air contrast
   barium enema examination discloses one or more
   polyps, full colonoscopy and **biopsies of all polyps**
   are indicated.
3. The **histopathology** of these lesions is of paramount
   import. If **adenocarcinoma** is demonstrated, further
   evaluation and management are indicated, whereas
   if a **nonmalignant polyp** is demonstrated, follow-up
   colonoscopy in 1 year is indicated.
4. If **ulcerative colitis** is demonstrated, yearly surveillance colonoscopy is indicated starting 10 years after
   the initial diagnosis. Multiple biopsy specimens

should be obtained, especially of any suspicious looking areas.

III. Evaluation and staging

Evaluation and staging are based on the **natural history** of the disease. The malignant neoplastic disease starts as a focus of malignant transformation, i.e., carcinoma in situ, in the polyp and, with growth, invades the colonic wall. **Early metastases** of the carcinoma are to the local lymph nodes, to the liver via the portal venous system, and later to the lungs, bone, and brain.

A. Evaluation

Once the **histopathologic diagnosis has been made** by biopsy of a polyp via flexible proctosigmoidoscopy or colonoscopy, the overall evaluation is tantamount to a staging evaluation. Components of evaluation and staging are listed in Box 5-6.

B. Staging

The **staging** of colon adenocarcinoma is described in Table 5-8. The **prognosis is related to stage:** the later the stage, the poorer the prognosis. **Preoperative staging** will only demonstrate extracolonic metastases and thus only **dichotomizes the staging** into **Dukes' D** and **non-Dukes' D lesions.** Further Dukes' staging requires the surgical specimen.

IV. Overall management

The **overall management** of colon carcinoma entails screening for the lesions, especially in patients at **high risk,** and making the diagnosis expediently via invasive endoscopy and biopsy. Once the diagnosis is made, the management schemas differ according to whether the stage of the cancer is non-Dukes' D or Dukes' D.

A. Non-Dukes' D lesions

All **non-Dukes' D lesions** demand surgical intervention. **Surgical interventions** include hemicolectomy on the side involved by the adenocarcinoma, or a total proctocolectomy in polyposis syndromes or ulcerative colitis. Surgical intervention in the early stages is essentially curative. If the **stage is B2 or C,** adjuvant chemotherapy may be of benefit.

B. Dukes' D lesions

All **Dukes' D carcinomas** are candidates for chemotherapy. Although the response rates are low (10%–15%), some significant partial and even complete remissions can occur with chemotherapy. The most commonly used regimens include **continuous infusion of 5-fluoruracil (5-FU)** and/or levamisole. Surgical interven-

B O X 5 - 6

Overall Evaluation of Known Colon Adenocarcinoma

Evaluation

1. **Colonoscopy,** if not yet performed, is necessary to look for any **metachronous lesions.** The reasoning is that if one carcinoma or polyp is discovered, there is an increased risk of **concurrent** colonic lesions.
2. A **serum carcinoembryonic antigen (CEA)** level should be determined at baseline. An elevated CEA level is a marker for disease regression or recurrence. A normal CEA level, however, **does not rule out** metastatic or recurrent disease.
3. Obtain **chest radiographs in PA and lateral views** to look for any nodules that might be consistent with metastatic colon carcinoma. The classic pattern is one of multiple nodular lesions in both pulmonary fields.
4. Determine the **complete blood cell count** for baseline purposes and to look for any evidence of an iron deficiency anemia.
5. Perform **liver function tests** to look for any abnormal elevations that might be consistent with metastatic disease to the liver. The classic pattern is one of a moderate increase in GGT and alkaline phosphatase levels and a mild increase in SGOT, SGPT, and LDH levels.
6. Perform **CT of the abdomen** if there is any clinical evidence of hepatomegaly or any LFT abnormalities. CT is used to look for any metastatic disease to the liver. The classic pattern is one of multiple space-occupying lesions in the liver.

tion in stage Dukes' D disease is indicated only for **palliation.**

V. Consultation

Problem	Service	Time
Dukes' B2 and C lesions	Oncology	Postoperatively: required
Dukes' D lesions	Oncology	At time of diagnosis: urgent
All non-Dukes' D lesions	General surgery	Urgent

T A B L E   5 - 8
Astler–Coller Modification of the Dukes' Staging Classification

Stage	Definition	Prognosis (5-Year Survival)
A	Limited to mucosa	95%
B1	Extends to the muscularis propria, lymph nodes negative	80%
B2	Extends through the entire wall; lymph nodes negative	70%
C1	Extends to the muscularis propria; lymph nodes positive	50%
C2	Extends through the entire wall; lymph nodes positive	30%
D	Distant metastases	10%

VI. **Indications for admission:** Evidence of bowel obstruction, or for scheduled surgical interventions.

Erythrocytosis

Erythrocytosis is an abnormal excess of erythrocytes in the peripheral blood. The laboratory parameters that define this entity include, in men, a hemoglobin above 18 g/dL and/or a hematocrit above 55% (in women the parameters are hemoglobin above 16 g/dL and/or a hematocrit above 50%). From the outset, it is important to differentiate erythrocytosis from polycythemia. **Erythrocytosis** is a nonspecific increase in hemoglobin or hematocrit, whereas **polycythemia** is a specific form of erythrocytosis that occurs as a result of a primary myeloproliferative neoplastic disorder.

I. **Overall pathogenesis**
The **overall pathogenesis** of erythrocytosis is an increase in hemoglobin or hematocrit that, irrespective of the underlying cause, above a given threshold results in the **sludging of blood,** an **increase in blood viscosity,** and a paradoxical **decrease in the delivery of oxygen** to the tissues. Although these events may occur in all tissues and organ systems, the ones most sensitive to changes in perfusion and oxygen delivery, the cardiovascular and cerebrovascular systems, will be the sites of the initial and potentially most devastating manifestations. The specific pathogenetic mechanisms of each etiology are discussed subsequently.

II. **Overall manifestations**
The overall manifestations are referenced to the pathogenesis, although the majority of patients are asymptomatic at

the time of presentation. The overall manifestations may be divided into two groups, cardiovascular and cerebrovascular.

A. **Cardiovascular manifestations**
   Cardiovascular manifestations include dyspnea, orthopnea, crackles, and a third heart sound, all as a result of left ventricular failure due to profound volume overload and sludging of blood in the coronary arteries. Furthermore, the patient may have angina pectoris, again as a result of sludging of blood in the coronary arteries and poor oxygen delivery to the tissues.

B. **Cerebrovascular manifestations**
   Cerebrovascular manifestations include lethargy, mental status changes (including delirium), and even cerebrovascular accidents, all as a result of the sludging of blood and poor oxygen delivery to the cerebral tissue.

   A further manifestation is an overall reddened complexion, sometimes referred to as a "ruddy" appearance of the face.

III. **Differential diagnosis**
   The underlying causes of erythrocytosis are quite diverse. A simple approach is to classify the erythrocytosis as **primary,** i.e., the neoplastic myeloproliferative disorder, polycythemia rubra vera, or **secondary,** i.e., due to another underlying process. The pathogenesis, manifestations, evaluation, and management for each of these two broad classifications are discussed below.

   A. **Primary erythrocytosis**
      Primary erythrocytosis, or **polycythemia rubra vera (PRV),** is a not uncommon malignant neoplastic process. The underlying **pathogenesis** is uncontrolled proliferation of normoblasts with a resultant increase in the number of erythrocytes in the bone marrow and the peripheral blood. The **specific manifestations** include an insidious onset of the overall findings and splenomegaly.

      1. **Evaluation**
         The **evaluation** of primary erythrocytosis includes making the clinical diagnosis. If polycythemia rubra vera is suspected, further evaluation is necessary to confirm the diagnosis. The laboratory examinations and criteria used in the diagnosis of polycythemia rubra vera are listed in Table 5-9. If and when a bone marrow biopsy is performed, a karyotypic analysis should be performed on the aspirate.

      2. **Management**
         The **management** of PRV includes making the diagnosis and involving hematologists from the outset.

T A B L E   5 - 9
Criteria for the Diagnosis of Polycythemia Rubra Vera

1. Oxygen saturation on room air: >92%
2. Splenomegaly
3. RBC mass: males, >36 mL/kg; females, >32 mL/kg
4. Altitude below 5,000 feet
5. Thrombocytosis: >450,000 platelets per mm^2
6. Elevated vitamin B_{12} binding capacity
7. Elevated leukocyte alkaline phosphatase (LAP) score
8. Leukocytosis
9. Bone marrow aspirate revealing erythrocytic hyperplasia.

All of the various therapeutic modalities may be applied with the advice of a hematology consultant. These therapeutic modalities include **phlebotomy** and, potentially, the initiation of **chemotherapy**, either chlorambucil or hydroxyurea. The goal is to decrease the **hematocrit** to the asymptomatic levels of **48%–50%**.

  a. **Phlebotomy** is a first-line therapeutic modality. It is easily performed by a primary care physician in the outpatient setting and is the cornerstone of the treatment of PRV. Phlebotomy consists of placing a large-bore intravenous catheter (18–16 gauge) into a peripheral vein and removing 500 mL of blood each time. The frequency of phlebotomy is directly related to the level of hematocrit elevation or the presence of symptoms. The initial frequency is phlebotomy every 2–5 days until the target hematocrit is reached. The frequency is then decreased to maintain the target hematocrit.

  b. **Chemotherapy** is not indicated in the acute setting, is a second-line modality, and should only be administered by a hematologist. It is beyond the scope of this text and is not discussed further here.

  In all cases CBC must be determined frequently and regularly. A hematologist is involved in follow-up, and a Pneumovax vaccine is administered.

B. **Secondary erythrocytosis**

  The **secondary causes** of erythrocytosis include a wide range of entities. Two distinct categories of secondary erythrocytosis are described here: **chronic hypoxemia,** and erythrocytosis as a result of a **paraneoplastic syndrome.**

1. **Categories of secondary erythrocytosis**
   a. **Chronic hypoxemia** is a not uncommon cause of erythrocytosis. The underlying **pathogenesis** is referenced to a natural compensatory mechanism. If there is chronic hypoxemia or a chronic low delivery of oxygen to the tissues, the kidneys increase the production and release of erythropoietin in order to effect an erythrocytosis and thus increase the total oxygen-carrying capacity of the blood. The increase in erythrocytes is effective until the erythrocytosis becomes of such magnitude as to result in symptomatic erythrocytosis. Some causes of chronic hypoxemia include living at **high altitudes** with lower atmospheric oxygen tension, states of **chronic hypoxemia** (e.g., severe COPD or cor pulmonale), any **right-to-left intracardiac shunts** (e.g., tetralogy of Fallot), and **hemoglobins with a high affinity for oxygen** (i.e., oxyhemoglobin dissociation curve shifted to the left). **Specific manifestations** of these entities include cyanosis, wheezing, bilateral clubbing, murmurs or gallops, and edema.
   b. **Paraneoplastic syndromes** also result in erythrocytosis. The underlying **pathogenesis** is excessive erythropoietin production from a tumor or disease process unrelated to hypoxemia. **Entities of interest** include primary hepatocellular carcinoma, renal cell carcinoma, and the nonneoplastic entity, polycystic kidney disease. **Specific manifestations** include hematuria, either microscopic or gross, flank mass, and hepatomegaly.

2. **Evaluation**
   The **evaluation** of secondary erythrocytosis entails making the clinical diagnosis of erythrocytosis and suspecting a secondary etiology as the underlying cause. Secondary erythrocytosis is usually easily discerned because the patient does not meet the diagnostic criteria for polycythemia rubra vera (see Table 5-9) but does have other manifestations attributable to the underlying entity. In addition to the examinations listed in Box 5-7 and Table 5-9, the erythropoietin level may be determined. Further evaluation is directed toward defining the underlying cause.

3. **Management**
   Management focuses on treating the underlying cause and alleviating manifestations attributable to the elevated hematocrit. **Phlebotomy** is useful in decreasing the hematocrit to asymptomatic levels, i.e.,

BOX 5-7

Overall Evaluation of Erythrocytosis

Evaluation

1. Perform a **physical examination,** looking for enlarged lymph nodes or splenomegaly. Lymph node enlargement and splenomegaly are more indicative of a primary myeloproliferative disorder.
2. Determine the **altitude** at which the patient **usually** lives.
3. Determine **complete blood cell count** with differential. This is central to the definition and diagnosis of erythrocytosis.
4. Review and **examine visually** the peripheral smear for any abnormal erythrocytes, leukocytes, or platelets.
5. Determine the **platelet count.** An elevated platelet count is more indicative of a primary myeloproliferative disorder.
6. Determine **arterial blood gas values while the patient is breathing room air** (i.e., Fio_2 = 21%). This is central to the evaluation: if the Pao_2 is normal, the differential diagnosis is markedly different from that of an abnormally low Pao_2.
7. Obtain **chest radiographs in PA and lateral views** for baseline purposes.
8. Perform **urinalysis with microscopic examination** to look for hematuria as an early diagnostic marker for a clear cell carcinoma of the kidney.
9. Determine levels of serum electrolytes, BUN, and creatinine for baseline purposes.

a target of 48%–50%. Further details on evaluation and management may be found in the sections on Hematuria (Chapter 3) and Chronic Obstructive Lung Disease (Chapter 4).

IV. Consultation

Problem	Service	Time
All suspected or diagnosed cases of PRV	Hematology	Urgent
Hematuria	Genitourinary	Urgent
Renal mass	Genitourinary	Urgent
COPD	Pulmonary	Urgent

V. **Indications for admission:** Any evidence of left ventricular failure, cerebrovascular insufficiency, or unstable angina pectoris.

Hodgkin's Disease

Lymphoid tissue consists of lymphocytes and cells of the reticulo-endothelial system and is normally present in various collections in every organ system of the body. Among the most common collections of such tissue are the **lymph nodes.** The functions of **normal** lymphoid tissue include acting as a line of host defense against invading pathogens and as a repository of the cells of humoral and cell-mediated immunity, B-lymphocytes and T-lymphocytes respectively. **Hodgkin's disease** is a specific form of malignant lymphoproliferative transformation of this lymphoid tissue.

The **incidence** of Hodgkin's disease is bimodal, with a sharp peak in the population in the third decade of life and a lesser peak in the sixth decade.

I. **Underlying pathogenesis**
   The **underlying pathogenesis** of this malignant lymphoproliferative disease is unknown, but one of the postulated mechanisms involves a viral infection. The virus that has been most highly correlated with the development of Hodgkin's disease is the DNA virus of **Ebstein–Barr.** The **cell type** that becomes malignant is similarly unknown but is postulated to be a stromal or a reticuloendothelial cell within the lymph node that manifests histopathologically as a **Reed–Sternberg cell.**

II. **Overall manifestations**
   The **overall clinical manifestations** of Hodgkin's disease are variable and depend on the site of lymph node tissue disease and the stage of the disease at the time of presentation. **Early in the course** of the disease the patient may be asymptomatic, presenting to the physician only with a "lump in the neck" or "enlarged glands." On examination there often is lymph node enlargement with a rubbery texture.

   In advanced disease, **B symptoms** may appear. B symptoms have staging implications and, when present, are consistent with an advanced stage and portend a poorer prognosis. **B symptoms** include an **unintentional weight loss of more than 10 pounds, drenching night sweats,** and/or **fevers,** especially fevers with a fever curve of the Pel–Ebstein pattern, i.e., clusters of multiple spikes separated by several days without fever.

B O X   5 - 8

***Overall Evaluation and Staging of Presumed
Hodgkin's Disease***

1. **Biopsy** of an accessible lymph node should be per-
    formed by a general surgeon. The biopsy can be inci-
    sional or excisional, and the specimen must be sent
    for histopathologic analysis. The pathologist should
    be informed of the clinical suspicion that the patient
    may have Hodgkin's disease.
2. Determine the **complete blood cell count with differ-
    ential** for baseline purposes and to look for any con-
    current anemia. It is quite uncommon to have a leu-
    kocytosis or left shift.
3. Perform **liver function tests** for baseline purposes.
    Elevated transaminase levels may be indicative of
    hepatic involvement by the lymphoproliferative
    disease.
4. Obtain **chest radiographs in PA and lateral views** for
    staging purposes, as the mediastinum is a common
    site of Hodgkin's-related lymphadenopathy.
5. Determine **serum uric acid levels** at baseline. Any
    lymphoproliferative disorder may, as a result of in-
    creased cell turnover, be accompanied by elevated
    levels of this catabolite of purine bases. The serum
    uric acid level may markedly increase at the time of
    treatment, and therefore a baseline value is indi-
    cated.
6. Perform a **direct Coombs test,** especially in patients
    with anemia, as Hodgkin's disease can result in
    Coombs-positive hemolytic anemia.
7. Obtain **CT scans** of the thorax, abdomen, and pelvis
    as part of the staging evaluation. The CT scans dem-
    onstrate, and grossly define, any lymphadenopathy
    in the mediastinum, the periaortic areas, or the retro-
    peritoneal areas. Furthermore, CT is excellent for
    demonstrating any concurrent hepatomegaly or sple-
    nomegaly.
8. **Bilateral bone marrow aspirates** and trephine biop-
    sies are indicated for staging. If Hodgkin's disease is
    present, it is, by definition, stage IV disease. Bone
    marrow aspirates are obtained bilaterally to increase
    the sensitivity of the testing procedure.

T A B L E 5 - 1 0
Stages of Hodgkin's Disease

Stage I: Disease in one lymph node group on one side of the dia-
           phragm
Stage II: Disease in more than one lymph node group on one side of
           the diaphragm
Stage III: Disease in more than one lymph node group on both sides
           of the diaphragm
Stage IV: Extralymphatic involvement (i.e., in the liver or bone
           marrow)

NOTE: Each stage may be further qualified by A, denoting absence of B
symptoms, or B, denoting presence of B symptoms such as unintentional weight loss, drenching night sweats, and episodic fevers (see
text).

III. **Screening**
     There are no effective screening techniques for this disease.

IV. **Overall evaluation and staging**
    A. **Evaluation**
       The **overall evaluation** is based on the **natural history**
       of the disease. This malignant lymphoproliferative dis-
       ease starts in one lymph node group and spreads contig-
       uously to other lymph node groups. Once the histopath-
       ologic diagnosis has been made via biopsy, further
       evaluation, ostensibly for staging, includes the steps de-
       scribed in Box 5-8.
    B. **Staging**
       Using the results and data gleaned from the evaluation
       described in Box 5-8 and the information regarding B
       symptoms, it is quite easy to stage the disease. In Hodg-
       kin's disease, as in many other malignant conditions,
       the stage is important in **determining prognosis** and **di-
       recting therapy**—radiation, chemotherapy, or both. The
       stages of Hodgkin's disease are listed in Table 5-10.

V. **Histopathologic classification**
   The **histopathologic classification** of Hodgkin's disease is
   listed in Table 5-11. This classification is quite useful, because the overall prognosis is somewhat **correlated** with
   the histopathologic type.

VI. **Overall management**
    The **overall management** of Hodgkin's disease entails mak-
    ing the diagnosis and staging the disease using the outline
    given in Box 5-8 and Table 5-10. **Aggressive treatment** with

T A B L E   5 - 1 1
Histopathologic Types of Hodgkin's Disease, Based on Biopsy of Lymph Nodes

Type	Age Group	Prognosis	Features
Lymphocyte predominate	Young	Good	Many lymphocytes on biopsy, rare to no Reed–Sternberg cells
Nodular sclerosing	Young	Good	Most common; many lymphocytes interspersed with sheets of birefringent stroma; rare to no Reed–Sternberg cells
Lymphocyte depleted	Old	Poor	Very few lymphocytes, many Reed–Sternberg cells
Mixed cellularity	Young or old	Fair/good	A mixture of the above three; Reed–Sternberg cells present but not prominent

early and mandatory oncology consultation is indicated. Referral to general surgery for lymph node biopsy is also indicated.

A. Management strategies

1. **Mantle irradiation** can be used for stage IA and IIA disease if the disease is above the diaphragm. The radiation field includes cervical and mediastinal lymph nodes and the spleen.

2. **Total body irradiation** is used in stage IIA disease if the disease is below the diaphragm.

3. **Chemotherapy** is indicated in most patients with B symptoms or if the disease is stage III or IV. Chemotherapy regimens include either **MOPP** (mechlorethamine, vincristine, procarbazine, and prednisone) or **ABVD** (doxorubicin, bleomycin, vinblastine, and dacarbazine).

B. Side effects

The male patient should be queried regarding the desire to produce progeny, as the treatment regimens for Hodgkin's disease can result in irreversible infertility. Therefore, if possible, a semen sample should be obtained and stored for potential future use. Patient care after the diagnosis should be orchestrated by the medical oncologist and the primary care physician.

C. Adjuvant therapy

Allopurinol, 300 mg PO q. A.M., should be initiated immediately before therapy is initiated. Allopurinol prevents renal dysfunction and gout as a result of the significant release of purines and uric acid from the tumor cell nuclei as they are destroyed.

VII. Consultation

Problem	Service	Time
Any suspicious lymph nodes	General surgery	Urgent
Hodgkin's disease	Oncology	Urgent

VIII. Indications for admission: initiation of chemotherapy under the direction of a medical oncologist.

Bibliography

Anemia

Beutler E: The common anemias. JAMA 1988;259:2433–2437.

Clementz GL, Schade SG: The spectrum of vitamin B-12 deficiency. Am Fam Pract 1990;41:150–161.

Fischer SL, Fischer SP: Mean corpuscular volume. Arch Intern Med 1983;143:282–283.

Hansen R, et al: Failure to suspect and diagnose thalassemic syndromes. Arch Intern Med 1985;145:93–94.

Konatey-Ahulu F: The sickle cell diseases: Clinical manifestations including the sickle cell crisis. Arch Intern Med 1974;133:611.

Platt OS, et al: Pain in sickle cell disease. N Engl J Med 1991;325:11–15.

Steinberg MH, Dreiling BJ: Microcytosis: Its significance and evaluation. JAMA 1983;249:85–87.

Witte DL, et al: Prediction of bone marrow iron findings from tests performed on peripheral blood. Am J Clin Pathol 1986;85:202–206.

Excessive Bleeding States

Burns TR, Saleem A: Idiopathic thrombocytopenic purpura. Am J Med 1983;75:1001–1007.

Holmberg L, Nilsson IM: Von Willebrand's disease. Clin Haematol 1985; 14:461–488.

George JN, Shattil SJ: The clinical importance of acquired abnormalities of platelet function. N Engl J Med 1991;324:27–38.

Kasper CK, et al: Hematologic management of hemophilia A for surgery. JAMA 1985;253:1279–1283.

Lind SE: Prolonged bleeding time. Am J Med 1984;77:305–311.

Breast Malignancy

AMA Council on Scientific Affairs: Mammographic screening in asymptomatic women aged 40 years and older. JAMA 1989;261:2535–2542.

Basset LW, Butler DL: Mammography and early breast cancer detection. Am Fam Pract 1991;43:547–557.

Chittoor SR, Swain SM: Adjuvant therapy in early breast cancer. Am Fam Pract 1991;44:453–462.

Eddy DM: Screening for breast cancer. Ann Intern Med 1989;111:389–399.

Fisher B, et al: Systemic therapy in patients with node-negative breast cancer. Ann Intern Med 1989;111:703–712.

Legha SS: Tamoxifen in the treatment of breast cancer. Ann Intern Med 1988;109:219–228.

Weiss RB, et al: Adjuvant chemotherapy after conservative surgery plus irradiation versus modified radical mastectomy. Am J Med 1987;83:455–462.

Bronchogenic Carcinoma

Brower M, et al: Treatment of extensive stage small cell bronchogenic carcinoma. Am J Med 1983;75:993–1000.

Bunn PA, et al: Chemotherapy alone or chemotherapy with chest radiation therapy in limited stage small cell lung cancer. Ann Intern Med 1987; 106:655–662.

Cohen MH: Signs and symptoms of bronchogenic carcinoma. Semin Oncol 1974;I:183–187.

Eddy DM: Screening for lung cancer. Ann Intern Med 1989;111:232–237.

Johnson BE, et al: Non-small cell lung cancer. Am J Med 1986;80:1103–1110.

Johnson DH, et al: Thoracic radiotherapy does not prolong survival in patients with locally advanced, unresectable non-small cell lung cancer. Ann Intern Med 1990;113:33–38.

Colon Carcinoma

Bulow S: Colorectal polyposis syndromes. Scand J Gastroenterol 1984;19: 289–293.

Dodds WJ: Clinical and roentgen features of the intestinal polyposis syndromes. Gastrointest Radiol 1976;1:127–142.

Fletcher RH: Carcinoembryonic antigen. Ann Intern Med 1986;104:66–73.

Hansen RM: Systemic therapy in metastatic colorectal cancer. Arch Intern Med 1990;150:2265–2269.

Krook JE, et al: Effective surgical adjuvant therapy for high risk rectal carcinoma. N Engl J Med 1991;324:709–715.

Provenzale D, et al: Risk for colon adenomas in patients with rectosigmoid hyperplastic polyps. Ann Intern Med 1990;113:760–763.

Ransohoff DF, Lang CA: Screening for colorectal cancer. N Engl J Med 1991;325:37–41.

Erythrocytosis

Berk PD, et al: Therapeutic recommendations in polycythemia vera study group protocols. Semin Hematol 1986;23:132–143.

Golde DW, et al: Polycythemia: Mechanisms and management. Ann Intern Med 1981;95:71.

Kaplan ME, et al: Long-term management of polycythemia vera with hydroxyurea: A progress report. Semin Hematol 1986;23:167–171.

Hodgkin's Disease

Buzaid AC, et al: Salvage therapy of advanced Hodgkin's disease. Am J Med 1987;83:523–531.

Fuller LM, Hagemeister FB: Hodgkin's disease in adults: Stages I and II, in Hodgkin's Disease and Non-Hodgkin's Lymphomas in Adults and Children, Fuller LM, Hagemeister FB, Sullivan MP, Velasquez WS (eds). New York: Raven Press, 1988;230–246.

Gibbs GE, et al: Long-term survival of patients with Hodgkin's disease. Arch Intern Med 1981;141:897–900.

Kaplan HS: Hodgkin's disease: Biology, treatment, prognosis. Blood 1981; 57:813.

—D.D.B.

Dale Berg, Ed. *Handbook of Primary Care Medicine.* Copyright © 1993 J. B. Lippincott Company.

CHAPTER 6

Infectious Diseases

Bacterial Skin Diseases

Descriptions of and treatments for bacterial skin diseases are presented in Table 6-1.

Bite Wounds

I. **Human bite wounds**
   Bite wounds inflicted by humans are a not uncommon problem.
   A. **Mechanisms**
      There are basically two mechanisms through which a human bite wound is incurred: **indirect** and **direct.**
      1. In the **indirect method,** injuries are incurred by hitting or cutting the hand, fingers, or knuckles on another person's teeth. This method is commonly associated with a fistfight.
      2. **Direct bite wounds** occur when another person directly bites the patient. Direct bite wounds commonly occur on the fingers, hands, genitals, and breasts.
   B. **Pathogenesis**
      The **underlying pathogenesis** of disease in human bite wounds involves damage resulting in **skin breakdown,** damage to adjacent soft tissue structures, and **exposure to infectious agents** from the mouth and body secretions (e.g., saliva). Infectious agents include **bacterial** and **viral agents.**
      1. The two requisite components in the development of **bacterial skin infections** are a **disruption** of the normal integrity of the skin and a **source of bacteria.**
         a. The bacteria normally present on the **skin of the patient** result in infection when the integrity of

(Text continues on page 317)

TABLE 6-1
Bacterial Skin Infections

Disease	Clinical Findings	Organism	Treatment
Impetigo	Superficial skin infection Pruritic Significant oozing and crusting can occur Highly contagious; patient may autoinfect other parts of skin by touching originally infected area Types: a) Vesiculopustular type (yellow colored) b) Bullous type c) Ecthyma: An ulcerative type of impetigo that is quite deep	*Streptococcus* or *Staphylococcus* *Staphylococcus aureus* with phage	Contact isolation Mupirocin (Bactroban) 2% applied b.i.d. to affected skin Dicloxicillin, 250–500 mg PO q.6h. for 7–10 days, *or* cephalexin (Keflex), 500 mg PO q.i.d. for 7–10 days Hydroxyzine, 25 mg PO q.i.d. PRN for pruritus
Ecthyma	A deep impetigo infection		
Erysipelas	Superficial infection that is sharply demarcated Usually has significant rubor, tumor, dolor, and calor Usually unilateral on the face No vesicles Nonpruritic	*Streptococcus*	Penicillin, 600,000–1,200,000 units IV q.4h., *or* erythromycin, 500–1,000 mg IV q.6h. Usually should admit patient Watch for rapid dissemination Contact isolation Infectious disease consultation

Condition	Features	Organism	Treatment
	Has associated systemic signs and symptoms: fever, chills, nausea Can rapidly disseminate through the skin, subcutaneous tissues, and blood Even in immunocompetent hosts may be life-threatening		
Folliculitis	Area of pus and erythema in and adjacent to hair follicle Single or multiple Patient may autoinfect during shaving	Staphylococcus aureus	Mupirocin (Bactroban) 2% b.i.d. for 5–7 days
Furuncle	Deep abscess due to folliculitis Very painful; also called "boil"	Staphylococcus aureus	Erythromycin, 500 mg PO q.i.d. for 7 days, or cephalexin, 500 mg PO q.i.d. for 7 days, or dicloxicillin, 250–500 mg PO q.i.d. for 7 days Avoid "squeezing" lesion Incise and drain when "mature"
Carbuncle	Multiple interconnecting abscesses Usually on neck and back Often recurrent Diabetes mellitus is a predisposing factor for this sequela of folliculitis	Staphylococcus aureus	As for furuncle, and screen for and aggressively manage diabetes mellitus
Hidradenitis suppurativa	Chronic infection of apocrine glands of axillae or inguinal areas Multiple abscesses and nodules develop in axillae and inguinal areas Develops in postpubertal period	Staphylococcus spp.	As for furuncle: usually requires surgical drainage and debridement

(continued)

T A B L E 6 - 1 *(continued)*

Disease	Clinical Findings	Organism	Treatment
Cellulitis	Deeper skin infection Nonpitting edema with other signs of in-flammation Usually less well demarcated Predisposition includes: a) Lacerations or any skin break b) Bites, human or animal (see Bite Wounds, page 313) c) Lower extremity edema d) Tinea infections (cracks in skin) e) Diabetes mellitus f) Intravenous drug use	*Streptococcus* *Staphylococcus aureus* Anaerobes Specific pathogens in bites	If **severe:** Admit Blood cultures Leading edge aspirate and Gram stain of little value Incise and drain any abscess Minimize handling of area (keep elevated) If bite, see Bite Wounds, page 313 Treat underlying tinea infection, if present Antibiotics: Ampicillin–sulbactam (Unasyn), 1.5–3.0 q.6h. IV, *or* Clindamycin, 900 mg q.8h. IV and an aminoglycoside If **not severe:** Elevation Cephalexin (Keflex), 500 mg PO q.i.d. for 10 days, and/or clindamycin, 600 mg PO t.i.d. for 10 days For **both:** Tetanus toxoid, if indicated Debride any necrotic tissue Control blood glucose

the skin is disrupted. These include the aerobic **gram-positive coccal** organisms of the genera *Streptococcus* and *Staphylococcus.*

   b. The bacteria present in the assailant's mouth may cause infection in the bite victim. **Anaerobic bacteria** are common if the assailant has gingival disease, as massive quantities of anaerobes would be present. Another bacterium, unique to the human mouth, that can cause bite-related wound infections is the gram-negative rod *Eikenella corrodens.* The gram-positive rod *Clostridium tetani,* the bacterial organism that results in tetanus, can also be transmitted.

 2. The two requisite components for the transmission of viral agents from the assailant to the victim are a **disruption** of the normal integrity of the skin and a **source of virus.** The source of any virus is the bodily secretions of the assailant. These viruses include, but are not limited to, hepatitis B and the human immunodeficiency virus (HIV).

C. **Evaluation and management**

The **specific evaluation and management** of human bites include the steps listed in Box 6-1.

II. Domestic animal bite wounds

Bite wounds inflicted by domestic animals are more common than bite wounds inflicted by humans.

A. **Mechanism**

There is basically one mechanism of incurring a bite wound from an animal: by a **direct bite.** The most common domestic animals in the United States, and therefore the most common sources of animal bites, are dogs and cats. Common sites of animal bite wounds are the fingers, hands, face, and feet.

B. **Pathogenesis**

The **underlying pathogenesis** of disease in animal bite wounds involves damage resulting in **skin breakdown,** damage to adjacent soft tissue structures, and **exposure to infectious agents** from the mouth and body secretions (e.g., saliva) of the animal. Infectious agents include **bacterial** and **viral agents.**

 1. The two requisite components in the development of **bacterial skin infections** are a **disruption** of the normal integrity of the skin and a **source of bacteria.** **Dog bites** usually are avulsive wounds associated with significant areas of adjacent crush injury. **Cat bites,** invariably puncture-type wounds, may penetrate deep into the soft tissue.

BOX 6-1

Overall Evaluation and Management of Bite Wounds, Human or Animal

Evaluation

1. **Examine** the patient's bite wound for adjacent soft tissue or structural damage (e.g., tendon damage if the bite is in the finger or wrist). Clean the wound vigorously and debride all necrotic tissue in and adjacent to the wound. Determine who or what bit the patient and when the bite wound occurred.
2. If the wound is clean and if the patient presents within 24 hours of the bite, one can safely **primarily close** the wound with **sutures.**
3. If there is any evidence of infection or if the wound is more than 24 hours old, healing should be by **secondary intent.**
4. If **cosmesis** is a concern or if there is a large defect or any significant concurrent damage, referral to plastic surgery is indicated.
5. In all cases of human bite wounds a serum HIV and hepatitis panel should be obtained from the assailant and the victim.
   a. If at risk, **hepatitis gammaglobulin** or, if available, **hepatitis B immune globulin** and **hepatitis B vaccine** should be administered to the patient (see section on Hepatitis in Chapter 2).
   b. If the assailant is HIV positive, manage the bite as for a **needle stick** (see section on HIV Infection, page 328).

Management

1. Administer, as necessary, **tetanus toxoid** (see Table 6-2).
2. **Antibiotics** are indicated in all cases. Regimens can include one of the following:
   a. Ampicillin–clavulinic acid (Augmentin), 250 mg PO t.i.d. for 7 days, *or*
   b. A second-generation cephalosporin (e.g., Ceftin, 500 mg PO q.i.d.) for 7 days, *or*
   c. Ciprofloxacin, 500 mg PO b.i.d., and clindamycin, 600 mg PO t.i.d. for 7 days. (Ciprofloxacin has minimal antibacterial activity against anaerobes.)

(continued)

B O X   6 - 1 *(continued)*

> 3. Follow-up should be quite close, and sutures, if placed, should be removed in 3–5 days. Any signs of infection should result in immediate opening of the wound and removal of the sutures.
> 4. **In all cases of animal bites,** the risk of rabies in the animal should be assessed. If at risk, the animal should be observed and, as necessary, destroyed for diagnostic purposes. The definitive method of diagnosing rabies in these animals is by demonstrating via microscopy the presence of Negri bodies in the hippocampus. If there is **any suspicion** that the animal is rabid, rabies vaccine should be administered to the patient. Table 6-3 provides specifics in the administration of and indications for the rabies vaccine.

    a. The bacteria normally present on the **skin of the patient** may result in infection when the integrity of the skin is disrupted. These include the aerobic **gram-positive coccal** organisms of the genera *Streptococcus* and *Staphylococcus.*

    b. The bacteria present in the animal's mouth may cause infection in the bite victim. Bacteria include the gram-negative rod *Pasteurella multocida,* the gram-negative rod **DF-2 (***Capnocytophaga spp.***),** and some **anaerobes.** Anaerobes are less of a problem in animal bites relative to hu-

T A B L E   6 - 2
Tetanus Immunizations

1. If patient was **never immunized** and has a dirty wound:
   a. Administer TIG (tetanus immune globulin), 250 IU IM, *and*
   b. DT (diphtheria + tetanus toxoid) IM.
2. If patient was **immunized in the past** and has a dirty wound:
   a. Administer a DT booster IM, if the last booster was given more than 5 years before presentation.
3. Every adult should have DT booster every 10 years.

(Modified from: CDC. Recommendations of the Immunization Practice Advisory Committee: Diphtheria, Tetanus, and Pertussis: Guidelines for vaccine prophylaxis and other preventive measures. MMWR 1985; 34:405–414, 419–426.)

T A B L E 6 - 3
Rabies Vaccination

Domestic Animal Bites:

1. If the animal is healthy and has received a rabies vaccine, observe the animal for 10 days. If the animal remains asymptomatic, no vaccination for the patient is needed.
2. If the animal is rabid, or if it has escaped capture and cannot be observed, administer rabies vaccine to the patient. See dosing schedule below.

Non-Domestic Animal Bites:

1. Bites from skunks, bats, fox, coyotes, and racoons require the initiation of rabies vaccine.
2. Rabbits, rodents, squirrels, and livestock rarely have rabies; however, one must check with the local **Public Health Service** for further information on these animals in the community. Rabies vaccine need not be administered.

Schedule of Administration for Rabies Vaccine:

1. **Rabies immune globulin (RIG),** 20 mg/kg; one-half of the dose at the wound site, one-half of the dose **IM.**
2. **HDCV** (human diploid cell vaccine) **IM,** on the following days (after bite):

   Day 0
   Day 3
   Day 7
   Day 14
   Day 28

Report the bite to the Public Health Service.
Destroy the rabid animal.

(Modified from: CDC. Recommendations of the Immunization Practices Advisory Committee of the U.S. Public Health Services. Rabies Prevention, United States, 1984. MMWR 1984;33:393–402, 407–408.)

man bites. *Clostridium tetani,* the bacterial organism that results in tetanus, can be transmitted by animal bites.
2. The **viral agent** that can be transmitted by animal bites is **rabies virus.**
C. Evaluation and management
The **specific evaluation and management** of animal bites include the steps listed in Box 6-1.

III. **Consultation**

Problem	Service	Time
Infection refractory to antibiotics	Infectious diseases	Urgent

Problem	Service	Time
HIV risk high	Infectious diseases	Required
Bite to face	Plastic surgery	Urgent
Large wound	Plastic surgery	Urgent
Concurrent tendon or nerve damage	Plastic surgery	Urgent
Suspected rabies	Public Health Service	Urgent

IV. **Indications for admission:** Few. If plastic surgery is needed, admission is usually required.

Bacterial Endocarditis

Prophylactic measures for the prevention of bacterial endocarditis are presented in Table 6-4.

HIV Infection

I. **Epidemiology**
Over the past decade both the **incidence of infection** with human immunodeficiency virus **(HIV)** and the **incidence of the disease process** resulting from this infection, acquired immunodeficiency syndrome **(AIDS),** have significantly increased in the United States and around the world. Recent estimates by the Centers for Disease Control (CDC) revealed that between 1 and 1.5 million people in the United States were HIV infected in 1992. Furthermore, almost 160,000 people in the United States have AIDS, and 20,000 people died of AIDS in 1990 alone. Finally, the infection is involving a **more diverse group of people.** No longer is AIDS restricted to homosexual men or intravenous drug users in urban centers. In fact, in Africa, heterosexual transmission far outweighs any other route of transmission. These data alone clearly portend a dire problem in the fields of public health and professional health care.

II. **Pathophysiology**
The human immunodeficiency virus is an RNA virus of the lentivirus family. HIV uses the enzyme **reverse transcriptase** and the **host cell's mechanisms** to produce, by the process of **reverse transcription,** DNA specific to the virus. Once the DNA specific to the virus is produced, it can be stored in the nucleus of the host cell, or the host cell's mechanisms can be used to produce, via **transcription,** either new RNA viral particles or messenger RNA. This

T A B L E   6 - 4
Endocarditis Prophylaxis

Cardiac lesions in which prophylaxis is indicated:

Prosthetic cardiac valves, metallic or bioprosthetic	High-risk lesion
Surgically constructed systemic–pulmonary shunts	High-risk lesion
Congenital heart malformations **except ASD**	High-risk lesion
Rheumatic heart disease	High- or low-risk lesion
Idiopathic hypertrophic subaortic stenosis (IHSS)	Low-risk lesion
Past history of bacterial endocarditis	High-risk lesion
Mitral valve prolapse **with** mitral regurgitation	Low-risk lesion

Procedures in which prophylaxis is indicated, if the patient has one or more of the above lesions:

Dental procedures inducing gingival bleeding
   Professional cleaning
   Dental extractions
   Endodontic procedures
Tonsillectomy
Bronchoscopy, especially if rigid, and/or if biopsies are to be performed
Incision and drainage of any abscess in the oral cavity
Cystoscopy
Any prostatic surgery
Vaginal hysterectomy
Any colonic surgery
Any urinary tract surgery
Sclerotherapy for esophageal varices
Esophagogastroduodenoscopy (EGD) with biopsy
Flexible/rigid proctosigmoidoscopy with biopsies
Colonoscopy

Antibiotic regimens (1990):

Dental and respiratory procedures:
  Low-risk lesions
    Amoxicillin, 3 g PO 1 hour before and 1.5 g PO 6 hours after the procedure,
       or
    Erythromycin, 1 g PO 1 hour before and 500 mg 6 hours after,
       or
    Clindamycin, 600 mg PO 1 hour before and 300 mg PO 6 hours after
  High-risk lesion
    Ampicillin, 2 g IV, and gentamicin, 1–1.5 mg/kg, 1 hour before and 8 hours after the procedure,
       or
    Vancomycin, 1 g IV, 1 hour before, over the hour before the procedure
Genitourinary and/or gastrointestinal procedures, all lesions:
    Ampicillin, 2 g IV, and gentamicin, 1–1.5 mg/kg 1 hour before and 8 hours after the procedure,

T A B L E   6 - 4 *(continued)*

or

Vancomycin, 1 g IV over 1 hour, and gentamicin, 1–1.5 mg/kg, both 1 hour before the procedure and 12 hours after the procedure

The above regimens are also recommended in the prevention of peri-procedure prosthetic joint infections.

(Modified from: Prevention of bacterial endocarditis: Recommendations of the American Heart Association. JAMA 1990;264:2919–2922.)

mRNA may then, again through host cell mechanisms, be **translated** to produce specific proteins. One or more of these specific proteins result in the death of the host cell itself.

A. **Disease mechanisms**

HIV enters the body via blood or body secretions. Once in the body the virus may enter any cell, but it has a propensity to **infect cells of the immune system** (i.e., monocytes and lymphocytes) in general and T-cell lymphocytes in specific.

1. HIV has a particular affinity for **lymphocytes** bearing the **CD4 receptor** on their surface, as this receptor aids viral entry into the cell. The cells with CD4 receptors on their surface are known as **T-helper lymphocytes.** By infecting and eventually destroying these cells, which are of central importance to cell-mediated immunity, they will become depleted. **T-helper cell depletion** results in increased susceptibility of the patient to infections by opportunistic organisms. These include a diverse set of viral, fungal, bacterial, and parasitic organisms that would not cause infection in an immunocompetent patient.

2. HIV also has a propensity to infect monocytes and macrophages, thus forming an effective **reservoir** for the virus.

3. HIV can produce damage and manifestations through mechanisms independent of cell-mediated immunity. This is particularly evident in the **central nervous system,** where HIV causes **direct neuronal infection** and eventual cell death, with resultant dementia.

B. **Transmission**

Transmission of the virus, and therefore of the disease, occurs by direct contact of a patient's blood or body secretions with the blood or body secretions of a person infected with HIV. Any human can become infected with HIV and develop AIDS, but certain activities are associated with a higher risk of infection. These include, but are not limited, to the following:

1. Unprotected anal, oral, or vaginal sex with multiple partners, heterosexual or homosexual.
2. Unprotected sexual intercourse with an HIV-positive person.
3. Intravenous drug abuse.
4. Blood transfusions outside the United States or during the years 1977–1985 inside the United States. The risk of HIV transmission from a transfusion of blood in the United States today is extremely low, i.e., 1:45,000.
5. Unprotected sexual intercourse with a person who has a recent or past history of sexually transmitted disease, such as purulent urethritis, purulent cervicitis, or genital herpes.

III. Natural history and overall manifestations of HIV infection

A. Acute period
In the **acute setting** there is usually an acute viremia that, in a minority of cases, results in a flu-like syndrome of myalgias, arthralgias, and fevers, but is self-limited and resolves in days to weeks. The HIV antibody test is nonreactive.

B. Quiescent period
In the **quiescent period** the patient is asymptomatic. The virus has infected and remains in the cells designed to destroy it, the cells of the immune system. The largest reservoir of virus is the cells of the monocyte–macrophage lineage. During the quiescent period the patient is HIV antibody reactive and infectious. The quiescent period is variable in duration, but theoretically may last for years to decades.

C. Symptomatic period
In the **symptomatic period** the virus has destroyed a significant quantity of T-helper lymphocytes. This decrease in T-helper cells results in cell-mediated immunosuppression, and the patient develops opportunistic infections. The HIV antibody test is reactive and the patient is infectious. Symptomatic HIV infection effectively defines AIDS (see subsequent discussion).

IV. Evaluation of an asymptomatic patient
The **evaluation of an asymptomatic patient at risk for HIV infection** includes obtaining a history for the specific risk factors. The history and physical examination should also look for any early infectious manifestations that are harbingers of early immunocompromise, such as recurrent **herpes**

zoster in a young patient or the development of **oral thrush.** Another important evaluative tool is the **serum HIV antibody titer.**

A. **Indications for determining the serum HIV antibody titer**
1. The patient has any of the known risk factors for the transmission of infection.
2. The patient has sustained a needle stick injury (see Box 6-3).
3. A young patient has had the onset of recurrent herpes zoster or oral thrush.
4. To confirm HIV infection in a patient with an opportunistic infection and thus, by definition, has AIDS.

B. **Rationale**
The **reasoning** behind determining the serum HIV antibody titer in such patients is not only to confirm the diagnosis, but also to put into effect preventive and therapeutic interventions.
1. **Preventive interventions,** which should be taught to all humans, not only those who are HIV antibody reactive, include the following:
   a. The institution of **safe sexual practices,** including the use of **condoms.** The clinician should reinforce that **abstinence** or monogamy with complete fidelity are the only true forms of safe sex.
   b. **No sharing of needles** by people who abuse drugs intravenously. The clinician should reinforce that the best way to prevent this form of transmission is to **discontinue IV drug abuse.**
2. **Therapeutic interventions.** Some recent and compelling evidence from the National Institutes of Health indicates that **early intervention** with **azidothymidine** (AZT) in selected asymptomatic HIV-infected patients does slow the progression of HIV infection to AIDS.

C. **Protocol**
The serum **HIV antibody test** consists of two separate tests, both of which are highly sensitive and specific. The two tests should be performed in a specific sequence.
1. The first test uses the **ELISA** method to detect the presence of antibody in the patient's serum. This is a fairly inexpensive test and is quite useful as a first-line screening test. If this test is negative, it should be repeated twice at 6-month intervals and patient measures to prevent viral transmission should be reinforced. Because the test's specificity, although high, is not 100%, any positive result must be confirmed by a second test, the Western blot technique.

B O X   6 - 2

Overall Evaluation and Management of Newly Diagnosed HIV Infection

Evaluation

1. Take a thorough history and perform a physical examination, focusing on sexual practices and partners.
2. Determine the complete blood cell count with differential analysis for baseline purposes.
3. Determine the platelet count for baseline purposes.
4. Determine levels of alkaline phosphatase, LDH, total bilirubin, SGOT, SGPT, and GGT to document the overall functioning of the liver at baseline.
5. Determine electrolyte, BUN, creatinine, and glucose levels for baseline purposes.
6. Determine albumin, calcium, PO_4, and magnesium levels for baseline purposes.
7. Perform the serum **VDRL** test to rule out concurrent infection with syphilis.
8. Obtain hepatitis A, B, and C panels to rule out concurrent infection with or past exposure to viral hepatitis.
9. Determine serum titers of **cytomegalovirus** and **Toxoplasma** at baseline. If in the future an acute infection with one of these agents is suspected, a baseline titer will be of great clinical utility.
10. Obtain chest radiographs in PA and lateral views for baseline purposes and to rule out any concurrent infiltrates.
11. Perform urinalysis for baseline purposes.
12. Perform a **PPD skin test with controls** to determine if the patient has been exposed to mycobacterial disease and if the patient is anergic. If the patient does not react to any of the applied skin tests, he or she is, by definition, anergic. Anergy is a significant manifestation of cell-mediated immunocompromise.
13. Determine **T-cell subsets** (i.e., CD4 and CD8 counts). This is a pivotal test in that there is a clear correlation between the number of CD4 T-cells and rate of progression to AIDS: the lower the CD4 count, the faster the progression to AIDS. This is

(continued)

BOX 6-2 *(continued)*

the most reproducible method of measuring cell-mediated immunity. Furthermore, the absolute number of T-helper cells—the CD4 count—can be used as a marker for the initiation of therapy.

a. If the **CD4 count is above 500 cells,** follow the counts every 4–6 months. No intervention is required.

b. If the **CD4 count is below 500 cells,** initiate AZT, 100 mg PO 5 times per day. Follow the CBC and renal function on a biweekly basis, then on a bimonthly basis. Follow the CD4 counts every 4–6 months. AZT, once initiated, should be continued indefinitely.

c. If the **CD4 count is below 200 cells,** initiate *Pneumocystis carinii* prophylaxis with trimethoprim-sulfamethoxazole (Bactrim DS, one tablet PO q.d.) or inhaled pentamidine every 2 weeks, and initiate herpes simplex prophylaxis with acyclovir, 200 mg PO b.i.d. Both regimens, once initiated, should be continued indefinitely.

14. Other serologic tests that act as markers for progression to AIDS include:

a. **β_2-microglobulin.** This small molecular weight protein, when **elevated,** is a harbinger of the development of AIDS (i.e., of a poor prognosis).

b. **P-24 antigen.** This antigen is a component of the HIV organism and, when **elevated,** is indicative of rapid progression to AIDS.

Management

1. **Immunizations**
   a. Pneumovax, polyvalent.
   b. Influenza B.
   c. Hepatitis B (see section on Hepatitis in Chapter 2).
2. **Education**
   a. "Safe sex" techniques (e.g., condoms).
   b. No sharing of needles.
   c. No sharing of toothbrushes or razors.
3. **Stage** the disease using the scheme in Table 6-5. Staging is useful in prognosis and in treating the patient.
4. Obtain an infectious diseases consult.

B O X   6 - 3

Management of Needle Sticks

Management

1. Minimize the risk of needle sticks. Place used needles in a "sharps" box, do not recap them, and
   never leave needles lying around. Wear latex gloves
   when examining any patient.
2. If a needle stick occurs:
   i. Immediately cleanse the wound with copious
      amounts of soap and water.
   ii. Assess the risk of the patient for HIV.
   iii. If the HIV status of the patient is unknown: Ob-
      tain HIV and hepatitis A and B panels.
   iv. If the HIV status of the patient is positive
      (known at outset), obtain hepatitis panel from
      patient.
   v. Obtain HIV, hepatitis panel, baseline CBC, elec-
      trolytes, and LFTs on caregiver.
   vi. Perform a pregnancy test to the caregiver, if ap-
      propriate.
   vii. Administer tetanus toxoid, if indicated, to the
      caregiver.
   viii. Administer hepatitis B gamma globulin IM to
      the caregiver if the patient's hepatitis B positive
      and the caregiver has no hepatitis B antibody.
   ix. If the patient is known to be HIV positive, initi-
      ate AZT, 100 mg PO 5 times per day, for 4–6
      weeks. This recommendation is based on anec-
      dotal and theoretical evidence; there is no ran-
      domized controlled study to support any effi-
      cacy of this prophylactic regimen.
   x. Determine CBC, electrolytes, and renal function
      at 6 weeks, 12 weeks, 6 months, and 12 months.
   xi. Determine HIV antibody titer at 3, 6, and 12
      months.
   xii. Use contraception for at least the first 3 months
      after exposure.

2. The **Western blot** examination, when positive, has a
   specificity of virtually 100%, thereby minimizing the
   false positive rate. If this test is positive, the patient
   should undergo the overall evaluation and management described in Box 6-2.

T A B L E 6 - 5
Staging Scheme for HIV-Positive Patients

Stage I: **Recent Infection with HIV**

Usually the acute infection is subclinical, but it may manifest myalgias, arthralgias, and a "flu-like" syndrome

The patient is HIV antibody positive, although a window of several months may exist during which the patient is HIV antibody negative

CD4 count normal (>500)

Stage II: **Asymptomatic, Healthy**

HIV positive
CD4 count > 500

Stage III: **Asymptomatic, Poor Prognosis**

HIV positive
CD4 count < 500

Stage IV: **Symptomatic, Mild**

HIV positive
CD4 count < 500, usually < 200
Presence of thrush, hairy tongue (hairy leukoplakia), and/or herpes zoster
In the past, the stage was referred to as AIDS-related complex (ARC).

Stage V: **AIDS**

Any opportunistic infection
CD4 counts are invariably very low

(Modified from: CDC. Classification for human T-lymphotropic virus Type III/lymphadenopathy-associated virus infections. MMWR 1986;35:1334–1339.)

   a. If the Western blot is **negative,** it should be repeated along with the ELISA assay in 1 month.
   3. If there are any questions as to the interpretation of these tests, an infectious diseases consult to aid in interpretation should be sought.

V. Early management

In the early stages of HIV infection, the primary care physician will be managing these patients. A subspecialist should be consulted early in the course of the disease, but the overall management until late in the disease will be orchestrated by the primary care physician.

VI. Manifestations of HIV infection

The **specific manifestations,** along with their evaluation and the management of AIDS, are very diverse but can be classified into the following scheme.

A. Pulmonary manifestations

Pulmonary manifestations virtually all occur as a result of opportunistic infections caused by HIV-induced immunocompromise. The three most common opportunistic infections involving the lungs are *Pneumocystis carinii* infection, mycobacterial infections, and cytomegalovirus infections. The immunocompromised patient is at risk for infection by a diverse set of pathologic agents, including the common community-acquired pathogens. Thus, in addition to the following discussion, the reader is referred to the section on Community-Acquired Pneumonitis in Chapter 4 for further information and a discussion of pneumonia.

1. ***Pneumocystis carinii.*** This is a protozoan organism that may be present in the lungs of a normal patient but does not cause disease. In the cell-mediated immunosuppressed patient, especially a patient with HIV-induced immunocompromise, these organisms proliferate and result in life-threatening opportunistic infection. This infection is extremely common in AIDS patients.

   a. The **specific manifestations** of *P. carinii* infection include dyspnea, decreased exercise tolerance, and a nonproductive cough. Often the patient will have crackles in the lungs and fevers, but there may be surprisingly few signs on physical examination.

   b. The **specific evaluation** of this disorder entails having an appropriate clinical suspicion in a patient who presents with the specific manifestations of *P. carinii* infection and is, or is suspected to be, HIV positive. Chest radiographs and arterial blood gas determinations are mandatory in all cases. The **chest radiograph** usually shows a diffuse interstitial infiltrate, and the **arterial blood gas values** usually reveal hyperventilation with a respiratory alkalosis, and hypoxemia with an increased A–aO$_2$ gradient. An additional specific examination is **bronchoscopy with bronchoalveolar lavage (BAL)** for *P. carinii* organisms or other potential concurrent processes or causes of interstitial pneumonitis, including CMV viral titers and mycobacterial smears and cultures.

   c. The **specific management** includes admitting the patient to the hospital, providing supplemental oxygen to keep PaO$_2$ above 65 mm Hg, and initiating empirical treatment. Effective **therapeutic regimens** include TMP/sulfa, or pentamidine, or Dapsone (see Table 6-6 for dosages). The antibiot-
(*Text continues on page 334*)

Agent	Indications	Dosing	Mechanism	Side Effects
Acyclovir	Prophylaxis for HSV Treatment of HSV pneumonitis encephalitis	100 mg PO b.i.d. 5–10 mg/kg IV in 8-hour dosing	Thymidine synthetase inhibitor	Tremors Mild renal dysfunction
Amphotericin B	Treatment of disseminated fungal infections	0.5–1.0 mg/kg/day IV to 2 g, then 0.5 mg/kg/day IV 2 times/wk		Wheezing Chills Hypocationemia (K, Mg) Renal failure Type I renal tubular acidosis To prevent wheezing and chills, the patient should be pretreated with: a) Diphenhydramine (Benadryl), 25–50 mg PO/IV, *and* b) Acetaminophen, 1 g PO, *and* c) Hydrocortisone, 25–50 mg IV, all before infusion *(continued)*

Agent	Indications	Dosing	Mechanism	Side Effects
Azidothymidine (AZT) (Zidovudine)	HIV positive, asymptomatic, CD4 < 500 HIV positive, symptomatic AIDS	100 mg PO 5 times/day 200 mg PO q.4h. for 4 wk, then 100 mg PO 5 times/day Same	Anti-reverse transcriptase; inhibits HIV replication	Nausea Vomiting Headache Pancytopenia
Clindamycin–primaquine	Treatment of *Pneumocystis carinii*	Clindamycin, 900 mg IV/PO q.8h. Primaquine, 30 mg PO of the base q. A.M.		Diarrhea Hemolysis in patients with G-6-PD deficiency
Clotrimazole (Mycelex troches)	Prophylaxis and treatment of thrush	10 mg 5 times/day		Minimal
Dapsone	Prophylaxis of *Pneumocystis carinii*	25 mg PO b.i.d. to q.i.d.		Anemia Rash Increased methemoglobinemia
Fluconazole	Treatment of cryptococcal meningitis Treatment of candidal esophagitis	200 mg PO/IV q.d. Same		Very few
Foscarnet	CMV retinitis	Induction: 60 mg/kg IV q.8h. for 3 wk; then Maintenance: 90 mg/kg IV q.d. indefinitely	Viral DNA polymerase inhibitor	Seizures Hypomagnesemia Hypocalcemia Renal dysfunction
Flucytosine	Treatment of *Cryptococcus* (adjuvant)	75–100 mg/kg/day in q.6h. doses		Pancytopenia

Drug	Indication	Dosage	Mechanism	Side Effects
Gancyclovir (DHPG)	Treatment of CMV retinitis and pneumonitis	5 mg/kg/day IV	Guanine nucleoside analogue	Granulocytopenia Thrombocytopenia AZT relatively contraindicated
Nystatin	Treatment of thrush	200,000–600,000 units q.i.d. by swish and swallow		Minimal
Pentamidine	Prophylaxis for *P. carinii*	300 mg by hand-held nebulizer every 2–4 wk		Hypoglycemia
	Treatment of *P. carinii*	4 mg/kg IV q.d.		
Pyrimethamine–sulfadoxine (Fansidar)	Prophylaxis for *P. carinii*	One tablet (Fansidar) PO q.d.	Antimetabolite	Rash Stevens–Johnson syndrome Cytopenias To minimize side effects, place on folinic acid, 5 mg/kg/day PO
	Prophylaxis for *T. gondii*	One tablet (Fansidar) PO q.d., or pyrimethamine, 25 mg PO, and sulfadoxine, 1 g PO q.d.		
	Treatment of *T. gondii*	Pyrimethamine, 100 mg PO q.d. for 2 days, then 50 mg PO q.d. and sulfadoxine, 1 g PO q.d., for 4–6 wk		
Trimethoprim–sulfamethoxazole	Prophylaxis for *P. carinii*	Bactrim DS, one tablet PO q.d.	Inhibits DNA synthesis	Anaphylaxis Stevens–Johnson syndrome Pancytopenia
	Treatment of *P. carinii*	15–20 mg/kg/day IV in 6-hour dosing, using the trimethoprim component for dosing		

ics should be initiated even before confirmatory bronchoscopy is performed.

   Steroid administration. Administration of steroids to patients with severe *P. carinii* pneumonitis offers a clear advantage in acute survival and in quality of life, as measured by an increased exercise tolerance. The indications for steroid use early in the course of the disease include severe disease as manifested by an increased A–aO_2 gradient, decreased PaO_2, and decreased O_2 saturation. Specific regimens include methylprednisolone, 40–60 mg IV q.8h. for 5 days, or prednisone, 60 mg PO q. A.M. for 5 days, either followed by a tapering dose of prednisone.

   d. Prophylaxis. Once treated, all of these patients require long-term prophylaxis with trimethoprim–sulfamethoxazole, inhaled pentamidine, or Dapsone (see Table 6-6 for dosages and potential side effects).

2. **Mycobacteria.** The acid-fast-staining mycobacteria, transmitted in respiratory secretions, cause infection and disease in both immunocompetent and immunosuppressed hosts. In fact, diseases due to both **typical** (i.e., *M. tuberculosis*) and **atypical** (i.e., *M. avium-intracellulare* and *M. kansasii*) mycobacteria are rapidly increasing in prevalence in HIV-positive patients.

   a. The **natural history** of mycobacterial disease is markedly different between immunocompetent and immunosuppressed hosts (see section on Mycobacterial Diseases in Chapter 4). Relative to the immunocompetent patient, the natural history of mycobacterial disease in HIV-positive patients includes the following features.

      i. A marked increase in risk for atypical mycobacterial disease in HIV patients.

      ii. A rapidly progressive course of either typical or atypical mycobacterial disease in HIV patients.

      iii. The propensity of either primary or reactivation disease to manifest as the diffuse and severe variant, **miliary mycobacterial disease,** in HIV patients.

   b. The **specific manifestations** include those described in the section on Mycobacterial Diseases in Chapter 4 and include fever, unintentional weight loss, cough productive of sputum, and occasionally a nodular skin rash.

c. The **specific evaluation** entails having an appropriate clinical suspicion in a patient with specific manifestations of mycobacterial infection and is, or is suspected to be, HIV positive. Chest radiographs, arterial blood gas determinations, sputum for acid-fast bacilli smear and culture, and a PPD test (unless reactive in the past) with controls are mandatory in all cases.

   i. The **chest radiographic** appearance may be variable, ranging from the typical manifestations of Ghon or Simon foci in reactivation disease manifesting with cavitary lesions to a miliary pattern in either primary or reactivation mycobacterial disease.

   ii. The **arterial blood gas values** are variable but may reveal hyperventilation with a respiratory alkalosis and hypoxemia with an increased $A-aO_2$ gradient.

   iii. The **PPD test** may be reactive, and if it is reactive, it is of use. However, in the immunocompromised host, lack of reactivity may occur as a result of the depressed cell-mediated response and not of nonexposure. Therefore, controls must be used to differentiate a nonreactive test due to no exposure from a nonreactive test due to cell-mediated immunocompromise.

   iv. If there is any evidence of **active disease,** especially if the AFB smear is positive or any cavitary lesions are seen on the chest radiograph, the patient must be placed in **respiratory isolation.**

   v. If the patient is febrile or has systemic or miliary manifestations, **blood** should be obtained for **mycobacterial culture.**

   vi. A further specific examination, if using the above procedures no diagnosis has been made, is **bronchoscopy with BAL** to detect AFB organisms. BAL will also assist in evaluating for other potential concurrent processes or causes of interstitial pneumonitis, including fungi, CMV, and *P. carinii.* The timing of bronchoscopy depends on the severity of the disease. A **miliary** (interstitial) pattern requires immediate bronchoscopy with BAL, whereas a stable patient may undergo bronchoscopy as an elective procedure.

d. The **specific management** includes admission to

the hospital, providing supplemental oxygen to keep $PaO_2 > 65$ mm Hg, and initiating empirical treatment.

    i. *M. tuberculosis* is best treated with three drugs: 9 months of isoniazid, 300 mg PO q.d., and rifampin, 600 mg PO q.d., with a third drug, either ethambutol, 25 mg/kg/day PO, or pyrazinamide, 25 mg/kg/day PO, for the first 2 months. Response rates are usually quite good.

    ii. In **atypical mycobacterial disease** the response rates are poor, even with very aggressive regimens. Aggressive regimens include the administration of five drugs, including INH, rifampin, ethambutol, pyrazidamide (all in same doses as above), and streptomycin, 1 g IM q.d. for the first 60 days of therapy. Treatment is usually long term and complex. Side effects will eventually limit the duration of therapy. The care of patients with atypical mycobacterial disease should be coordinated by an infectious disease or pulmonary disease expert.

3. Cytomegalovirus. This is a DNA virus that is transmitted by blood and body secretions. CMV infection is quite common but underrecognized because it is often subclinical. This is a systemic infection to which the patient was exposed in the past and now, as a result of HIV-induced immunocompromise, has become reactivated.

    a. The **specific manifestations** include shortness of breath, a quite nonproductive cough, and subjective fevers, chills, and night sweats. Examination usually discloses tachypnea, tachycardia, and a low-grade fever. Auscultation of the lungs reveals diffuse crackles. Otherwise there is a paucity of cardiac or pulmonary signs.

    b. The **specific evaluation** of CMV infection entails having an appropriate clinical suspicion in a patient with specific manifestations and who is, or is suspected to be, HIV positive. Chest radiographs and arterial blood gas determinations are mandatory in all cases. The **chest radiograph** usually shows a diffuse interstitial infiltrate. **Arterial blood gas values** reveal hyperventilation with a respiratory alkalosis, and hypoxemia with an increased $A-aO_2$ gradient. A further specific examination is **bronchoscopy with BAL** to determine CMV titers and to look for other concurrent processes or causes of interstitial pneumonitis, including *P. carinii* and mycobacterial smears and cultures.

c. The **specific management** includes admission to the hospital, providing supplemental oxygen to keep $PaO_2 > 65$ mm Hg, and initiating empirical treatment. Effective **therapy** includes, once CMV titers are positive, the immediate initiation of **DHPG (ganciclovir),** 5 mg/kg given IV over 1 hour per day. Once therapy is initiated it is **long term,** and therefore a catheter must be placed for permanent IV access, such as a Hickman catheter. Because the concomitant use of AZT with DHPG is relatively contraindicated, the **diagnosis of CMV must be confidently made** before committing the patient to long-term DHPG.

   CMV retinitis. CMV retinitis is a significant problem that may be concurrent with or antedate the pneumonitis. Therefore, an ophthalmology consult should be obtained to look for and diagnose early CMV retinitis. DHPG is also used to treat this entity and should be limited when CMV retinitis is diagnosed (see Table 6-6 for dosages). The therapy is, again, long term. An alternative agent for the treatment of CMV infections is **foscarnet.** This agent has been demonstrated to be effective in the therapy of CMV and has several advantages over DHPG: it can be used concurrently with AZT, and early data suggest that it may have an inherent anti-HIV effect and prolong overall patient survival.

B. **Neurological manifestations**

   Neurological manifestations of HIV infection can result from the **direct effects** of the virus on the nervous system or from immunocompromise, with a resultant increased risk for and incidence of opportunistic infections in the CNS. As such, a brief discussion of both the direct and indirect manifestations of HIV involving the CNS will be presented.

1. **Direct HIV infection**

   a. The **underlying pathogenesis** of direct damage to the nervous system by HIV is as follows. The virus crosses the blood–brain barrier, usually via cells of the monocyte–macrophage lineage. Once in the central or peripheral nervous system the virus directly infects the neurons themselves. Infected cells die, resulting in the loss of irreplaceable neurons.

   b. The **natural history** involves a slowly and irreversibly progressive course. Because virtually all patients with AIDS have a direct neuronal infection with the virus, the prevalence of this process is very high among patients with AIDS.

c. The **specific manifestations** of these entities thus include those related to the actual loss of neuronal tissue in the central or peripheral nervous systems. These manifestations can be quite variable and depend on the relative damage to various parts of the central and peripheral nervous systems. The manifestations vary from a **dementing process** as the result of cortical neuronal loss to a **peripheral neuropathy** as the result of loss of peripheral neurons.

   i. A **dementing process** manifests with a slowly progressive loss of memory, both short term and long term; a decrease in cognitive ability; and disorientation. The patient can develop seizures, tremor, or parkinson-like manifestations if the neuronal destruction affects the basal ganglia.

d. The **specific evaluation** entails making the clinical diagnosis and excluding all potentially treatable causes or exacerbating processes. This includes excluding any concurrent opportunistic infection (see below), obtaining a serum VDRL, and, if reactive, performing a lumbar puncture and VDRL on the CSF to rule out neurosyphilis; performing thyroid function tests; and obtaining a serum B_{12} level.

e. The **specific management** includes treating the HIV infection, diagnosing and treating any reversible opportunistic intracranial infections, and treating any reversible causes of a dementing process. If the process is due to HIV, supportive care and structuring of the patient's environment are of therapeutic assistance.

2. **Toxoplasmosis.** This is a disease process due to a eukaryotic opportunistic parasite, *Toxoplasma gondii.*

   a. **Transmission and natural history.** Like other opportunistic organisms, *T. gondii* results in disease only in patients with antecedent immunosuppression. The portal of entry or exposure is thought to be the **respiratory mucosa.** Once exposed, the immunosuppressed patient may develop an intracerebral or retinal infection, or both. Cats are vectors, and disease may be acquired as a result of exposure to infected cat feces.

b. The **specific manifestations** of toxoplasmosis include recurrent generalized headaches which over days to weeks progressively worsen in intensity, frequency, or duration. Concurrent with the headaches are, quite invariably, fevers, chills, and occasional night sweats. The patient may present with delirium or seizures. The seizures, if present, not uncommonly have a focal component and may be followed by postictal localized paresis or plegia—Todd's paralysis.

c. The **specific evaluation** of toxoplasmosis includes having the appropriate clinical suspicion in a patient with known or suspected HIV infection. The evaluation includes:

   i. Perform a thorough history and physical examination looking for any focal sensory or motor deficits.

   ii. The patient should undergo head imaging.

      (a) The first imaging technique should be a **CT scan with and without contrast.** CT of the head in a patient with toxoplasmosis lesions will demonstrate multiple, relatively small (1–2 cm in diameter) lesions with peripheral ring contrast enhancement.

      (b) If the **CT scan is normal** and the suspicion for a space-occupying lesion remains, **MRI of the head** should be obtained. MRI of the head is the most sensitive imaging technique for toxoplasmosis lesions, because MRI is the most specific and sensitive technique for imaging of processes that affect the white matter.

   iii. An ophthalmologic consultation for a retinal examination to look for concurrent toxoplasmosis retinitis should be obtained.

   iv. A **lumbar puncture** can be considered, unless an intracranial mass makes the risk of herniation high. The CSF obtained should be submitted for routine tests (see section on Meningitis in Chapter 14) and a *Toxoplasma gondii* antibody titer.

   v. Admission to the hospital as well as consultation with infectious diseases and neurosurgery should be performed in an expedient fashion.

      vi. **Biopsy** of the lesions, performed by neuro-surgeons, should be considered if there is no response to initial treatment or if CSF titers are negative for toxoplasmosis. Biopsy is the only definitive method of establishing the diagnosis and thus of ruling out any other cause, such as lymphoproliferative disease, mycobacterial disease, or abscesses.

    d. Management

      i. **Antibiotic regimens** that are effective against toxoplasmosis in the acute setting should be initiated empirically. These regimens include **pyrimethamine,** 100 mg PO q.d. for 2 days, then pyrimethamine, 25–50 mg PO q.d. *and* **sulfadiazine,** 1 g PO q.6h., *and,* to minimize pancytopenia, **folinic acid,** 5–10 mg/kg/day PO (not folic acid, as this inhibits pyrimethamine activity). This regimen should be continued for a duration of 6 weeks (see Table 6-6).

      ii. **Prophylaxis.** Once the diagnosis is secured, either by a high clinical suspicion or by increased toxoplasmosis titers or by direct biopsy of a lesion, lifelong **prophylactic therapy** is required. This regimen includes **pyrimethamine,** 25 mg PO q.d., *and* **sulfadiazine,** 1 g PO q.d. *or* **clindamycin,** 600 mg PO q.d., along with folinic acid, 5 mg/kg/day PO (see Table 6-6).

3. Cryptococcosis is a disease process that is due to the eukaryotic opportunistic fungal organism, *Cryptococcus neoformans.*

    a. Transmission and natural history. Like all opportunistic organisms, *C. neoformans* results in disease only in patients with antecedent immunosuppression. The portal of entry or exposure is thought to be the **respiratory mucosa.** Once exposed, the patient can develop a localized pneumonitis or a solitary intracranial mass infection. In either case, the end result is spread to the leptomeninges, which invariably results in severe **leptomeningitis.**

    b. The **specific manifestations** of cryptococcosis include the subacute onset of recurrent generalized headaches, fevers, and chills. The symptoms then progress to delirium and/or generalized tonic–clonic seizures. On examination, there are often the meningeal signs of nuchal rigidity, Brudzinski's sign and/or Kernig's sign. In a small minority of cases the process manifests with focal neurologic findings.

c. The **specific evaluation and management** of this entity include having the appropriate clinical suspicion in a documented or suspected HIV-positive patient. After a history and physical examination looking for any focal sensory or motor deficits, the patient should undergo head imaging.

  i. The first imaging study should be a **CT scan, with and without contrast.** CT of the head in a patient with cryptococcal lesions will demonstrate multiple, relatively small (1–2 cm in diameter) lesions with peripheral ring enhancement.

  ii. A **lumbar puncture** should be considered, unless an intracranial mass makes the risk of herniation high. The CSF obtained should be submitted for routine tests, a *Toxoplasma gondii* antibody titer, an **India ink stain** for cryptococcal organisms (the organism, but not the peripheral capsule, will stain), and, by latex agglutination, a **cryptococcal antigen titer.**

  iii. Admission to the hospital should be performed as well as consultation with infectious diseases and neurosurgery in an expedient fashion.

  iv. A **chest radiograph** to look for a nodule or infiltrate consistent with a cryptococcal infection should be obtained.

  v. Serum cryptococcal antigen and blood cultures should be obtained.

  vi. **Antibiotic regimens** that are effective against this opportunistic infection include **amphotericin B,** 0.5–1.0 mg/kg/day IV on a daily basis to a total dose of 2 g, **and,** concurrently, **flucytosine,** 75–100 mg/kg/day, **or fluconazole,** 200–400 mg PO q.d., until the dose of amphotericin has reached 2 g. While the patient is taking amphotericin B, the clinician must closely **monitor renal function** and cations, as hypokalemia and a decreased serum magnesium level often develop, and must monitor CBC frequently (i.e., 1–2 times per week).

d. **Prophylaxis.** Once the diagnosis is secured, lifelong prophylactic therapy is required. This prophylactic regimen includes **amphotericin B,** 40 mg IV 2–3 times per week, or **fluconazole,** 100–200 mg PO q.d. to q.o.d., lifelong. The amphotericin B regimen requires the placement of a Hickman catheter and close monitoring of the cation, renal, and fluid status of the patient.

C. **Gastrointestinal manifestations**

The gastrointestinal manifestations of HIV and AIDS are very diverse. The virus itself can directly damage the GI tract, and much more commonly, can indirectly increase the risk of opportunistic infections involving any area of the GI tract. The two manifestations of HIV-related GI disease are **diarrhea** and **dysphagia/odynophagia.** The reader is referred to these specific sections in Chapter 2.

VII. **Consultation**

Problem	*Service*	*Time*
HIV positive	Infectious diseases	Required
Any opportunistic infection	Infectious diseases	Urgent/emergent
Any intracranial lesion not diagnosed by "routine" tests	Neurosurgery	Emergent/urgent
Interstitial pneumonitis	Pulmonology	Urgent/emergent bronchoscopy
Intractable diarrhea	Gastroenterology	Required, for flexible proctosigmoidoscopy
Odynophagia not responsive to antifungal agents	Gastroenterology	Urgent for EGD

VIII. Indications for admission: New interstitial pneumonitis in an HIV-positive patient, severe vomiting with intravascular volume contraction, any neurologic manifestations of HIV, or any evidence of profound diarrhea.

Sexually Transmitted Diseases

Sexually transmitted diseases (STDs) are extremely common in the United States today. As a group, these diseases have several disconcerting and malignant features. First, the **incidence** of disease, in the United States and the world, is quite high and in some cases increasing. Second, there is a **significant morbidity** and even mortality in patients who are undiagnosed and thus untreated.

Third, STDs are disease processes that can be overlooked by physicians who are not attuned to the manifestations of sexually transmitted diseases. Finally, HIV is spread through the same mechanisms as are other STDs, and HIV has a disconcertingly **high prevalence** in patients with other STDs.

I. Sexual history
The **sexual history** is an integral component of the overall history but may be quite challenging to obtain, even when the patient's presenting complaint may be due to an STD.

A. Historical information
The **history** consists of the physician querying the patient regarding very personal, intimate, and potentially embarrassing activities. These include:

1. The patient's selection of partners, including sexual orientation, i.e., if the partners are of the same sex (homosexual), the opposite sex (heterosexual), or of either sex (bisexual).
2. The number of sexual partners over a given period of time.
3. Specific sexual practices, including vaginal intercourse, anal intercourse, receptive anal intercourse, oral sex (including fellatio and/or cunnilingus, and the use of erotic devices).
4. The patient's knowledge of and use of barrier methods and/or "safer sex" techniques, in general, and condoms, in specific.
5. If the patient has had sexual contact with anyone who is HIV positive or at high risk for being HIV positive. High-risk groups include people who abuse IV drugs or who are promiscuous, whether homosexual, bisexual, or heterosexual.

B. Tips for history taking
Helpful tips in obtaining a sexual history include the following:

1. Explain to the patient the importance of an accurate history.
2. Reassure the patient that the questions are not meant to embarrass.
3. The queries should be asked in a matter-of-fact manner.
4. The physician must be comfortable asking the patient these questions.
5. The questions, as in all history taking, should begin with general queries and move on to specifics.
6. The physician should become cognizant of and use, when appropriate, the slang terms for various anatomic structures or activities. A penis may be referred to as "my nature," masturbation as "mashing"

or "beating off," fellatio as "a blow job" or "giving head." The use of these terms may make the patient understand your queries and even make her or him more comfortable.

7. Have the patient describe in his or her own words the activities and symptoms.

II. Bacterial diseases

Bacteria that can cause STDs include *Neisseria gonorrhoeae*, *Chlamydia trachomatis*, and *Treponema pallidum*. These organisms are the causative agents in the vast majority of symptomatic STDs. Each is discussed below.

A. *Neisseria gonorrhoeae*

This gram-negative intracellular diplococcus results in a significant percentage of symptomatic STDs in the United States and the world. It is transmitted by the exchange of infected body fluids and can be transmitted during any sexual activity. It infects and affects the mucosal surfaces of any part of the body. The vast majority of symptomatic cases involve the male urethra or female cervix, but the pharynx and rectum can also be affected. The manifestations, complications, evaluation and management of specific syndromes caused by this pathogenic bacterium include the following:

1. **Urethritis in males**

   a. The **specific manifestations** of this entity include a fairly acute onset of moderate to severe dysuria with associated hesitancy, urgency, and pyuria. There are usually no associated fevers or hematuria. Patients often complain that a yellow discharge is present in the underpants or on bedlinen in the morning. A history of unprotected intercourse in the proximate past can usually be obtained from the patient. **Complications** of this infection include transmission to others and the development of systemic disease, which may manifest with a monoarticular arthritis.

   b. The **specific evaluation and management** of this entity entail making the clinical diagnosis by performing the examinations and management steps outlined in Box 6-4. Cultures should be plated out onto agar medium at the time of specimen procurement. *Chlamydia* infections should, in most cases, be concurrently treated.

2. **Cervicitis or urethritis in females**

   a. The **specific manifestations** of this entity include a fairly acute onset of a moderate amount of yellow vaginal discharge with concurrent pruritus, a burning sensation, or pain in the vaginal area.

B O X   6 - 4

***Overall Evaluation and Management of
a Suspected STD***

Evaluation

1. Obtain a **sexual history,** central to the evaluation and management (see text).
2. **Assess the patient's risk** for HIV (see section on HIV Infection, page 321).
3. Perform a physical examination, looking for any rashes or any evidence of purulent pharyngitis in the oropharynx, and of the genitourinary system. In all **males,** a GU and rectal examination is mandatory: in all **females** a pelvic and rectal examination is mandatory.
4. Perform **chlamydial cultures** of the **cervix** in females and of the **urethral orifice** in males.
5. Perform a **gonococcal (GC) smear and culture** of the **cervix** in females and of the **urethral orifice** in males. If pharyngitis of proctitis is clinically suspected, perform GC cultures from those sources. The culture should be swabbed onto the Thayer–Martin or New York City agar at the time of specimen procurement.
6. Obtain a serum **VDRL** in all patients. If reactive, confirm with **FTA-abs** and treat as described in the text.
7. Determine the **serum HIV antibody titer** in all patients at risk.
8. Obtain a **hepatitis B panel** in all patients at risk.
9. Obtain a **Tzank smear** of any painful vesicular lesions to look for multinucleated giant cells, a finding indicative of herpes simplex infection.
10. Perform a **darkfield examination** on scrapings from any painless, raised lesions present. Such a lesion is consistent with a chancre. The darkfield analysis is a microscopic assessment used to diagnose primary syphilis.
11. Perform a **urine pregnancy test** in all women who have not previously undergone a hysterectomy or bilateral oophorectomy. This test is **mandatory.**

(continued)

B O X 6 - 4 *(continued)*

Management

1. Antibiotic regimens
   a. Treatment for *Neisseria gonorrhoeae*
      Ceftriaxone, 250 mg IM in one dose, *or*
      *Amoxicillin, 3 g, and probenicid, 1 g PO in one
      dose, *or*
      Spectinomycin, 2 g IM in one dose (the agent
      of choice for GC proctitis).
      *NOTE: **Ceftriaxone** is the **drug of choice** in com-
      munities in which the resistance of *N. gonor-
      rhoeae* to penicillin and penicillin analogues is
      above 1%.
                    AND
   b. Treat *Chlamydia* infections. Because GC and non-
      GC urethritides co-occur in 50%–60% of cases,
      both must be treated concurrently. Therefore, in
      addition to the GC treatment, a regimen for *Chla-
      mydia* should be instituted. These regimens in-
      clude:
      Tetracycline, 500 mg PO q.i.d. for 7 days, *or*
      Doxycycline, 100 mg PO b.i.d. for 7 days, *or*
      Erythromycin, 500 mg PO q.i.d. for 7 days.
      Azithromycin, 1,000 mg PO for one dose (take
      on an empty stomach).
2. Treat genital herpes simplex with acyclovir, 200 mg
   PO 5 times per day for 7 days.
3. Foster prevention. Educate patient in safe sexual
   practices (monogamy, barrier methods) or abstinence.
4. Report all cases to the Public Health Service.

There often are associated dyspareunia (pain during coitus) and a mild to moderate dysuria with
associated hesitancy, urgency, and pyuria. There
usually are no associated fevers or hematuria. A
history of unprotected intercourse in the proximate past can usually be obtained from the patient.
   b. The **complications** of this infection include:
      i. **Transmission to others.**
      ii. The development of **systemic disease,** which
          manifests with a monoarticular arthritis.
      iii. The development of **pelvic inflammatory**

disease (PID). PID is the infection and resultant purulent inflammation of the fallopian tubes by the underlying bacterial pathogen. The pathogen may be either *N. gonorrhoeae* or *C. trachomatis.* The **natural history** of this specific complication is the development of an acute tubal abscess, septicemia, and spread of infection to the upper peritoneum with resultant peritonitis. This peritonitis, also known as perihepatitis or the Fitz–Hugh–Curtis syndrome, can lead to intra-abdominal abscess formation and death.

   iv. A **long-term complication** of PID is **scarring** of the fallopian tubes with a resultant increased risk of **infertility** or **tubal pregnancy.**

c. The **specific evaluation and management** of this entity entail making the clinical diagnosis by performing the examinations and management steps outlined in Box 6-4. Cultures should be plated out onto agar medium at the time of specimen procurement. *Chlamydia* infections should, in most cases, be concurrently treated.

   i. If the patient has any evidence of **adnexal fullness** on pelvic examination or any evidence of systemic dissemination (e.g., fevers), further specific evaluation and management include:

   (a) A complete blood cell count to look for anemia or leukocytosis.

   (b) **Ultrasound of the pelvis** to look for an abscess in the fallopian tubes.

   (c) Consultation with and probably admission to the **gynecologic service** is indicated.

   ii. Once PID is suspected or diagnosed, the initiation of parenteral antibiotics, e.g., ceftriaxone, a **third-generation cephalosporin,** 2 g IV q.24h., and **clindamycin,** 900 mg IV q.8h., to cover anaerobic bacteria, is indicated.

3. **Pharyngitis**

a. The **specific manifestations** of this entity include the fairly acute onset of a moderate to severe sore throat. Often the patient has concurrent urethral or cervical manifestations, as described above. A history of unprotected intercourse and fellatio in the proximate past is generally present. Examination discloses purulent pharyngitis with marked cervical lymphadenopathy. **Complications** of this infection include transmission to others and the development of systemic disease, which may manifest with a monoarticular arthritis.

    b. The **specific evaluation and management** of this entity entail making the clinical diagnosis by performing the examinations and management steps outlined in Box 6-4. Cultures should be plated out onto agar medium at the time of specimen procurement. *Chlamydia* infections should, in most cases, be concurrently treated. Once GC pharyngitis is suspected or diagnosed, the initiation of parenteral antibiotics, e.g., ceftriaxone, a **third generation cephalosporin,** is indicated. If indeed it is GC pharyngitis, it usually responds rapidly to the ceftriaxone.

  4. **Proctitis**

    a. The **specific manifestations** of this entity include the fairly acute onset of moderate to severe perianal and/or rectal discomfort that is exacerbated by defecation. It is not uncommon in heterosexual or homosexual patients who practice anal intercourse, especially **receptive anal intercourse.** It is not uncommon for the patient to have concurrent urethritis or cervicitis, depending on sexual practices. A history of unprotected intercourse in the proximate past is generally present. Examination discloses marked tenderness in the rectal vault. **Complications** of this infection include transmission to others and the development of systemic disease, which manifests with a monoarticular arthritis.

    b. The **specific evaluation and management** of this entity entail making the clinical diagnosis by performing the examinations and management scheme outlined in Box 6-4. Cultures should be plated out onto agar medium at the time of specimen procurement. *Chlamydia* should, in most cases, be concurrently treated. Once GC proctitis is diagnosed or suspected, treatment is with regimen described in Box 6-4. The strain of *N. gonorrhoeae* that is associated with this entity is markedly resistant to beta-lactams, and thus the drug of choice is **spectinomycin, 2 g IM** for one dose.

  B. *Chlamydia trachomatis*

    This is an atypical bacterium that results in a significant percentage of symptomatic STDs in the United States and the world; in fact, it is one of the most common causes of STDs in the world today. The organism is transmitted by the exchange of infected body fluids and can be transmitted during any sexual activity. It can infect and affect the mucosal surfaces of any part of the body. The vast majority of asymptomatic and symptomatic cases involve the male urethra or female cervix. The manifestations, complications, evaluation and management of specific syndromes caused by this pathogenic bacterium are described below.

1. **Urethritis in males**
   a. The **specific manifestations** of this entity cover a wide spectrum, ranging from the fairly acute onset of moderate to severe dysuria with associated hesitancy, urgency, and pyuria, quite similar to gonococcal urethritis, to virtually no symptoms even when the disease is acute. There usually are no associated fevers or hematuria. Unlike in GC urethritis, patients rarely report that a yellow discharge is present on underpants or on bedlinen in the morning. A history of unprotected intercourse in the proximate past can usually be obtained from the patient. **Complications** of this infection include transmission to others and the development of epididymitis with abscess formation in the future.
   b. The **specific evaluation and management** of this entity entail making the clinical diagnosis by performing the examinations and management steps outlined in Box 6-4. Urethral culture for *Chlamydia trachomatis* and urethral smear and culture for *N. gonorrhoeae* are indicated. Cultures should be plated out at the time of specimen procurement. If there is any suspicion of concurrent GC, it should be concurrently treated. Once the condition is diagnosed or suspected, treatment should be with the regimen given in Box 6-4.

2. **Cervicitis or urethritis in females**
   a. The **specific manifestations** of this entity range from the fairly acute onset of a moderate amount of yellow vaginal discharge with pruritus in the vaginal area with a modest amount of associated dyspareunia and a mild to moderate dysuria with associated hesitancy, urgency, and pyuria, all quite similar to gonococcal urethritis, to virtually no symptoms even when the disease is acute. Women most often present with **minimal to no symptoms.** There usually are no associated fevers or hematuria. A history of unprotected intercourse in the proximate past can usually be obtained from the patient.
   b. The **complications** of this infection include:
      i. **Transmission to others.**

    ii. The development of **systemic disease,** which may manifest with a monoarticular arthritis.

    iii. The development of **pelvic inflammatory disease (PID).** PID is the infection and resultant purulent inflammation of the fallopian tubes with the underlying bacterial pathogen. The pathogen can be either *N. gonorrhoeae* or *C. trachomatis.* The **natural history** of this specific complication is the development of an acute tubal abscess, septicemia, and spread of the infection to the upper peritoneum with resultant peritonitis. This peritonitis, also known as perihepatitis or Fitz–Hugh–Curtis syndrome, can lead to intra-abdominal abscess formation and death.

    iv. A **chronic complication** of PID is **scarring** of the fallopian tubes with a resultant increased risk of **infertility** or **tubal pregnancy.**

    v. The complication of **neonatal chlamydial pneumonitis or conjunctivitis** can occur in neonates born of mothers who deliver vaginally when the disease is active.

  c. The **specific evaluation and management** of this entity entail making the clinical diagnosis by performing the examinations and management steps outlined in Box 6-4. Urethral culture for *C. trachomatis* and urethral smear and culture for *Neisseria gonorrhoeae* are indicated. Cultures should be plated out at the time of specimen procurement. If there is any suspicion of concurrent GC, it should be concurrently treated. Once the condition is diagnosed or suspected, treatment should be with the regimen listed in Box 6-4.

    i. If the patient has any evidence of **adnexal fullness** on pelvic examination or any evidence of systemic dissemination (e.g., fevers), further specific evaluation and management include the following steps.

      (a) A complete blood cell count to look for anemia or leukocytosis.

      (b) **Ultrasound of the pelvis** to look for an abscess in the fallopian tubes.

      (c) Consultation with and probably admission to the **gynecology service** are indicated.

    ii. Once PID is suspected or diagnosed, the initiation of erythromycin or tetracycline for 10 days and, to empirically cover for GC, parenteral antibiotics (e.g., ceftriaxone, a third-generation cephalosporin) is indicated.

iii. All pregnant woman who have evidence of or are at risk for *Chlamydia* infection should undergo the examinations listed in Box 6-4. Specific therapy for *Chlamydia* infection is more difficult, and management should be undertaken by the patient's obstetrician.

C. *Treponema pallidum*

This non-gram-staining spirochetal organism causes the local and systemic disease called **syphilis** or **lues venereum.** This STD, although still uncommon, has been increasing in incidence in the United States. The organism is **transmitted** by the exchange of infected body fluids and can be transmitted during any sexual activity. It can infect and affect the mucosal surfaces of any part of the body. The vast majority of asymptomatic and symptomatic cases initially involve the male urethra or female cervix. The manifestations, complications, evaluation, and management are best described by categorizing the disease into one of the well-described **discrete stages,** based on the **natural history** of this infectious disease process.

1. **Primary lues**

a. The **specific manifestations** of this temporal stage of treponemal infection are the result of the initial exposure and infection. These manifestations occur **1–2 weeks after exposure.** They are limited to the development of a **chancre,** a **raised, indurated, painless lesion** with raised borders and a central depression (Fig. 6-1). The chancre develops in an area of sexual contact, usually the vulva, penis, scrotum, or oral mucosa. The lesion is self-limited, resolving spontaneously, without sequelae, in 7–10 days. It is, however, a lesion in which transmission of the spirochete is highly likely if intimate contact is made with another person; i.e., it is highly infectious.

b. The **specific evaluation and management** of this entity entail making the clinical diagnosis by performing the examinations and management steps outlined in Box 6-4. A **serum VDRL** and a scraping of the lesion's base for **darkfield assessment** should be performed for diagnostic purposes. Once the diagnosis is made, therapy should be initiated. The therapy for primary lues is penicillin G benzathine, 2.4 million units IM once, or erythromycin, 500 mg PO q.i.d. for 15 days, or ceftriaxone, 250 mg IM once (see Table

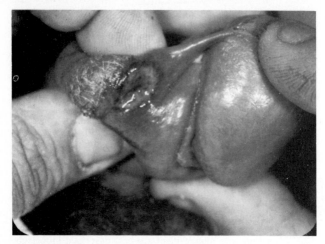

F I G U R E   6 - 1
The chancre of primary lues venereum.

6-7). The regimen of ceftriaxone, 250 mg IM, that
is used for GC is also curative for primary lues.
Therefore, if GC needs to be treated, ceftriaxone
will cure the GC and the lues venereum.

2. Secondary lues

   a. The **specific manifestations** of this temporal stage
   of treponemal infection result from systemic dissemination of the spirochetes after the initial infection in a host who has not been effectively
   treated. These manifestations occur **8–10 weeks
   after exposure,** and thus approximately 8 weeks
   after chancre resolution. They include low-grade
   fever, fatigue, night sweats, and one or more of
   the following dermatologic manifestations:

   i. A **generalized, painless, erythematous macular rash** which involves the soles and
   palms.

   ii. A self-limited, **painless, generalized papular
   rash,** called **condyloma latum.** This phase of
   lues venereum is self-limited and lasts up to
   several weeks. Many times this phase is only
   modestly symptomatic. The specific lesions
   of condylomata lata also have treponemes
   present and are infectious in nature.

   b. The **specific evaluation and management** of this

T A B L E   6 - 7
Regimens for the Treatment of Syphilis (Lues Venereum)

Syndrome	Drug of Choice	Alternate Regimens
Primary lues Secondary lues Early latent lues	Penicillin G benzathine, 2.4 million units IM *or* Ceftriaxone, 250 mg IM once	Erythromycin 500 mg PO q.i.d. for 15 days
Late latent lues	Penicillin G benzathine, 2.4 million units IM once a week for 3 wk	Erythromycin, 500 mg PO q.i.d. for 30 days
Neurosyphilis Cardiovascular lues	Penicillin G, 2–4 mil- lion units IV q.4h. for 10 days	Erythromycin, 500 mg PO q.i.d. for 30 days

(Based on: CDC treatment guidelines for sexually transmitted disease.
MMWR 1989;38[Suppl]:5.)

entity entails making the clinical diagnosis by
performing the examinations and management
steps outlined in Box 6-4. A **serum VDRL** as well
as a scraping of the lesional base of a papule
in condyloma latum for **darkfield assessment**
should be performed for diagnostic purposes.
Once the diagnosis is made, therapy should be
initiated. The therapy for secondary lues is penicillin G benzathine, 2.4 million units IM once, or
erythromycin, 500 mg PO q.i.d. for 15 days, or
ceftriaxone, 250 mg IM once (see Table 6-7). The
regimen of ceftriaxone, 250 mg IM, that is used
for GC is also curative for secondary lues. Therefore, if GC needs to be treated, ceftriaxone will
cure the GC and the lues venereum.

3. **Latent lues**
   a. The **specific manifestations** of this temporal stage
      of treponemal infection are as the result of the
      host controlling and in some cases effectively
      eradicating the body of the spirochetes, in a host
      who has not been effectively treated. This **stage,**
      by definition, **begins at the termination of the
      manifestations of the secondary lues** phase and
      may continue for life. As this is defined to be a
      "latent" period, there are no clinical manifesta-
      tions of disease. The patient may, in the sexual
      history, relate a past history of a chancre that was
      not treated. The **latent stage** can be further di-
      vided into two subgroups, **early** and **late.**

        i. **Early latent**—The **first year** after the exposure to the disease.

        ii. **Late latent—more than 1 year** after exposure to the disease.

b. The **specific evaluation and management** of this entity entail making the clinical diagnosis by performing the examinations and management steps outlined in Box 6-4. A **serum VDRL** and a **serum FTA-abs** are indicated. It is not uncommon for the **VDRL to become nonreactive** in the latent stage; however, the **FTA-abs remains reactive permanently.** If the patient has latent lues, a lumbar puncture to obtain CSF for a VDRL test needs to be performed to rule out asymptomatic neurosyphilis (see discussion below). Once the diagnosis is made, therapy should be initiated.

        i. The therapy for **early latent lues** is penicillin G benzathine, 2.4 million units IM once, or erythromycin, 500 mg PO q.i.d. for 15 days, or ceftriaxone, 250 mg IM once. The regimen of ceftriaxone, 250 mg IM, that is used for GC is also curative for early latent lues. Therefore, if GC needs to be treated, ceftriaxone will cure the GC and the lues venereum (see Table 6-7).

        ii. The therapy for **late latent lues** requires a more intensive course of antibiotics, i.e., penicillin G benzathine, 2.4 million units IM once weekly for 3 consecutive weeks, or erythromycin, 500 mg PO q.i.d. for 30 days (see Table 6-7).

4. Tertiary lues. This temporal stage of treponemal infection is as the result of the infection becoming clinical again after a variable period of subclinical latency. The manifestations of tertiary lues can begin years to decades after the primary infection. The manifestations of this stage of the disease are effectively and clinically divided into several subtypes relating to the location of manifestations. The patient with tertiary lues venereum may have one or more of the following manifestations, including more than one type of neurosyphilis.

    a. Late benign gummatous lues

        i. The **specific manifestations** of this form of tertiary lues are the result of the development of **gummata,** or chronic inflammatory areas due to lues. Gummata can develop anywhere in the body tissues. The manifestations thus depend on where the gummata develop. For example, if they develop in the heart, AV nodal block can occur, whereas if they develop in the skin, a nodule can be palpated.

ii. The **specific evaluation** of this entity entails making the clinical diagnosis by performing the examinations listed in Box 6-4. A **serum VDRL** and **serum FTA-abs** are indicated. It is not uncommon for the **VDRL to become and remain nonreactive** in the latent stage; however, the **FTA-abs remains reactive permanently.** Any suspicious nodules in the skin can be biopsied. The presence of a gumma is diagnostic of tertiary lues. If the patient has tertiary lues, a **lumbar puncture** to obtain CSF for a VDRL test needs to be performed to rule out asymptomatic neurosyphilis (see discussion below). Once the diagnosis is made, therapy should be initiated.

iii. The **specific management of gummatous lues** requires an intensive course of antibiotics, i.e., penicillin G, 2–4 million units IV q.4h. for 10 days, or erythromycin, 500 mg PO q.i.d. for 30 days (see Table 6-7).

b. **Cardiovascular lues**

i. The **specific manifestations** of this form of tertiary lues are the result of spirochetes infecting and invading the large arteries of the cardiovascular system. This results in the development of aortic insufficiency or a thoracic aortic aneurysm, with their attendant manifestations, i.e., a diastolic murmur best heard at the base with an increased pulse pressure and bounding peripheral pulses.

ii. The **specific evaluation** of this entity entails making the clinical diagnosis by performing the examinations listed in Box 6-4. A serum VDRL and serum FTA-abs are clearly indicated. Any evidence of a diastolic murmur should be aggressively evaluated with a thorough cardiovascular examination, chest radiography in PA and lateral views to look for mediastinal widening, and echocardiography to look at the aortic valve. If the patient has cardiovascular lues, a lumbar puncture to obtain CSF for a VDRL test needs to be performed to rule out asymptomatic neurosyphilis (see discussion below). Once the diagnosis is made, therapy should be initiated.

iii. The **specific management** for **cardiovascular**

lues requires an intensive course of antibiotics, i.e., penicillin G, 2–4 million units IV q.4h. for 10 days, or erythromycin, 500 mg PO q.i.d. for 30 days (see Table 6-7). Furthermore, a referral to cardiology and/or a cardiothoracic surgeon for management of the aortic insufficiency and/or thoracic aneurysm is clearly indicated in an expedient manner. Virtually all of these patients require acute, inpatient surgical intervention.

   c. **Neurosyphilis**
      See Table 6-8 for **manifestations, evaluation,** and **management.**

III. **Viral diseases**
   Viral organisms that cause STDs include **herpes simplex II, hepatitis A virus, hepatitis B virus,** the **human immunodeficiency virus (HIV),** and **human papillomavirus (HPV).**
   A. **Herpes simplex II**
      This DNA virus causes a significant percentage of symptomatic STDs in the United States and the world. It is transmitted by the exchange of infected blood and body fluids and can be **transmitted** during any sexual activity. It can infect and affect the mucosal surfaces of any part of the body. The vast majority of symptomatic cases involve the male urethra or female cervix, but the pharynx and rectum can also be infected or affected.
      1. The **specific manifestations** include the acute onset of multiple **vesicular lesions** that are **very painful** (Fig. 6-2). The vesicular lesions remain present for 7–10 days and then spontaneously resolve. The virus is present in very high concentrations within these vesicles; therefore, the vesicular lesions are very infectious.
      2. **Natural history.** The virus remains in the ganglia of the cutaneous nerves supplying the infected area. At various times after the initial infection there can be a recurrence, which manifests very similarly to the initial infection with multiple vesicular lesions. Whenever the disease is active—that is, whenever vesicular lesions are present—the disease is transmissible.
      3. The **specific evaluation and management** entail making the clinical diagnosis by examination and performing the tests described in Box 6-4. It is usually not necessary to perform a Tzanck smear on all cases as the clinical diagnosis is often quite straightforward. The **specific management** includes that de-

T A B L E 6 - 8
Syndromes of Neurosyphilis

Syndrome	Manifestations	Cerebrospinal Fluid Findings	Management
Asymptomatic	No specific manifestations Past history of untreated STD or chancre	VDRL reactive Mild increase in protein Cell count normal	See Table 6-7
Tabes dorsalis	Sensory neuropathy to fine touch, position, and vibration in a "stocking-glove" distribution Diffusely decreased deep tendon reflexes Argyl–Robertson pupil: constricts normally to accommodation, but not to direct or consensual light	VDRL reactive Mild increase in protein Cell count normal	See Table 6-7 Refer to occupational therapy
Meningovascular	Generalized headaches Low-grade fevers Cranial nerve defects, unilateral or bilateral, including peripheral cranial nerve VII and XII deficits Mild to modest neck stiffness; rarely any acute meningeal signs	VDRL reactive Mild increase in protein Marked increase in number of cells with a predominance of lymphocytes	See Table 6-7
General paresis	Insidious, progressive onset of dementia	VDRL reactive Mild increase in protein Mild increase in number of cells, mainly lymphocytes	See Table 6-7

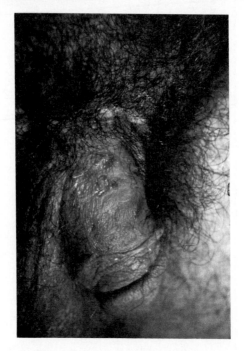

FIGURE 6-2
The vesicular, painful rash of herpes simplex genitalis.

scribed in Box 6-4. **Acyclovir,** 200 mg PO 5 times a day for 7 days, decreases the duration and intensity of symptoms, decreases the duration of the vesicles, and thus decreases the duration of infectivity. It is not a curative regimen and is most effective only in the first episode of herpes simplex infection. Acyclovir ointment on a twice daily basis will also decrease symptoms and duration of vesicles; however, there is no benefit to the concurrent use of topical and oral acyclovir.

B. **Other viruses**

The reader is referred to the section on Hepatitis in Chapter 2 for a discussion of **viral hepatitis,** to the section on HIV Infection, page 321, for details on that disease process, and to the section on Viral Skin Infections in Chapter 8 for a discussion of **HPV infection.**

IV. Consultation

Problem	Service	Time
Latent or tertiary lues	Infectious diseases	Urgent
HIV positive	Infectious diseases	Required
Condyloma latum	Dermatology	Elective
Cardiovascular lues	Cardiology	Urgent
Adnexal mass	Gynecology	Urgent
Evidence of systemic spread of GC	Gynecology	Emergent
Pregnancy concurrent with STD	Ob/Gyn	Urgent
Painful scrotal mass	Urology	Emergent
Any STD	Public Health	Required

V. **Indications for admission:** Neurosyphilis, any evidence of cardiovascular lues venereum, any adnexal mass on pelvic examination, any evidence of ectopic pregnancy, and any evidence of systemic spread of *Neisseria gonorrhoeae*.

Bibliography

Bacterial Skin Infections
Hook E, et al: Microbiologic evaluation of cutaneous cellulitis in adults. Arch Intern Med 1986;146:295–298.

Reagan D, et al: Elimination of coincident *Staphylococcus aureus* nasal and hand carriage with intranasal application of mupirocin calcium ointment. Ann Intern Med 1991;114:101–106.

Suss SJ, Middleton DB: Cellulitis and related skin infections. Am Fam Pract 1987;36:126–136.

Wheat LJ, et al: Diabetic foot infections. Arch Intern Med 1986;146:1935–1940.

Bite Wounds
Goldstein E, Richwald G: Human and animal bite wounds. Am Fam Pract 1987;36:101–109.

Klein M: Nondomestic mammalian bites. Am Fam Pract 1985;32:137–141.

Marcy SM: Infections due to dog and cat bites. Pediatr Infect Dis 1982;1:351–356.

Suwanagool S, et al: Pathogenicity of *Eikenella corrodens* in humans. Arch Intern Med 1983;143:2265–2268.

Bacterial Endocarditis
American Heart Association: Prevention of bacterial endocarditis. JAMA 1990;264:2919–2922.

Baltch AL, et al: Bacteremia in patients undergoing oral procedures. Arch Intern Med 1988;148:1084–1088.

HIV Infection

Barnes PF, et al: Tuberculosis in patients with human immunodeficiency virus infection. N Engl J Med 1991;324:1644–1650.

Bloom J, Palestine A: The diagnosis of cytomegalovirus retinitis. Ann Intern Med 1988;109:963–969.

Broder S, et al: Antiretroviral therapy in AIDS. Ann Intern Med 1990; 113:604–608.

Gabuzda D, Hirsch M: Neurologic manifestations of infection with human immunodeficiency virus. Ann Intern Med 1987;107:383–391.

Gemson DH, et al: Acquired immunodeficiency syndrome prevention. Arch Intern Med 1991;151:1102–1108.

Laskin OL, et al: Ganciclovir for the treatment and suppression of serious infections caused by cytomegalovirus. Amer J Med 1987;83:201–207.

Makadon HJ: Assessing HIV infection in primary care practice. J Gen Intern Med 1991;6(Suppl):S2–S7.

Miles SA: Diagnosing and staging of HIV infection. Am Fam Pract 1988; 38:248–256.

Montaner J, et al: Corticosteroids prevent early deterioration in patients with moderately severe *Pneumocystis carinii* pneumonia and the acquired immunodeficiency syndrome (AIDS). Ann Intern Med 1990;113:14–20.

Palestine AG, et al: A randomized, controlled trial of foscarnet in the treatment of cytomegalovirus retinitis in patients with AIDS. Ann Intern Med 1991;115:665–673.

Powderly WG, et al: A controlled trial of flucohazole or amphotericin B to prevent relapse of cryptococcal meningitis in patients with the acquired immunodeficiency syndrome. N Engl J Med 1992;326:793–798.

Small PM, et al: Treatment of tuberculosis in patients with advanced human immunodeficiency virus infection. N Engl J Med 1991;324:289–294.

Vinson RP, Epperly TD: Counseling patients on proper use of condoms. Am Fam Pract 1991;43:2081–2085.

Sexually Transmitted Diseases

Boslego JW, et al: Effect of spectinomycin use on the prevalence of spectinomycin-resistance and of penicillinase-producing *Neisseria gonorrheae*. N Engl J Med 1987;317:272–278.

Guinan M: Oral acyclovir for treatment and suppression of genital herpes simplex virus infection. JAMA 1986;255:1747–1757.

Hart G: Syphilis tests in diagnostic and therapeutic decision making. Ann Intern Med 1986;104:368–376.

Hutchinson C, et al: Characteristics of patients with syphilis attending Baltimore STD clinics. Arch Intern Med 1991;151:511–516.

Kirchner J: Syphilis—An STD on the increase. Am Fam Pract 1991;44: 843–854.

Morgan R: Clinical aspects of pelvic inflammatory disease. Am Fam Pract 1991;43:1725–1732.

Pruessner HT, et al: Diagnosis and treatment of chlamydial infections. Am Fam Pract 1986;34:81–92.

Romanowski B, et al: Serologic response to treatment of infectious syphilis. Ann Intern Med 1991;114:1005–1009.

Schwarcz SK, et al: National surveillance of antimicrobial resistance in *Neisseria gonorrhoeae*. JAMA 1990;264:1413–1421.

Stone K, et al: Primary prevention of sexually transmitted diseases. JAMA 1986;255:1763–1767.

Stott GA: New macrolide antibiotics: clarithromycin and azithromycin. Am Fam Pract 1992;46:863–869.

—D.D.B.

Dale Berg, Ed. *Handbook of Primary Care Medicine.* Copyright © 1993 J. B. Lippincott Company.

C H A P T E R   7

Musculoskeletal Disorders

Nonsteroidal Anti-Inflammatory Agents

Nonsteroidal anti-inflammatory agents are listed in Table 7-1.

Elbow (Box 7-1)

The **elbow** is the articulation of the distal humerus and the proximal radius and ulna. The **normal movements** of this joint and the normal range of motion for each movement are as follows:

Extension: 0°
Flexion: 160°
Pronation: 90°
Supination: 90°

I. Specific clinical syndromes
   A. Medial epicondylitis (golf elbow)
      1. **Manifestations**
         The **manifestations** of this entity include the acute onset of pain and tenderness over the **medial epicondyle.** There usually is associated limitation of forearm flexion due to pain, but rarely is there associated swelling or redness. The patient usually relates a past history of similar manifestations, usually after performing certain activities, including many common household activities, isometric exercises that use these muscles, or the **golf foreswing.**
      2. **Pathogenesis**
         The **underlying pathogenesis** is noninfectious inflammation at the common origin of the forearm flexor muscles, immediately adjacent to the medial epicondyle.
      3. **Evaluation**
         The **evaluation** of medial epicondylitis includes making the clinical diagnosis. **Radiographs** of the elbow

B O X   7 - 1

***Overall Evaluation and Management of
Elbow Discomfort***

Evaluation

1. Take a history and perform a physical examination,
   evaluating range of motion and looking for any joint
   effusion. If effusion is present, treat as described in
   the section on Monoarticular Arthritis (page 423).
2. Obtain radiographs of the elbow if fractures are suspected.

Management

The specific management of musculoskeletal disorders
affecting the elbow is discussed in the text.

are invariably normal; therefore, unless there is an
antecedent history of trauma or other manifestations
are present, radiographs are unnecessary.
4. **Management**
   a. For **acute management,** i.e., in the first hour after
      symptoms commence, ice is applied to the elbow
      for 30–45 minutes.
   b. **After the acute period,** treatment modalities in-
      clude nonsteroidal anti-inflammatory drugs PRN
      (see Table 7-1), and temporary avoidance of the
      exacerbating activity. Physical therapy for range of
      motion and strengthening activities may be indi-
      cated.
   c. If the manifestations are **severe** and **refractory** to
      initial treatment, a radiograph of the elbow should
      be obtained. Triamcinolone, 10–20 mg, may be in-
      jected **over the medial epicondyle.** If the manifes-
      tations are severe enough to warrant radiography
      and triamcinolone injection, referral to orthope-
      dics should be considered.
5. **Consultation**

Service	Time
Physical therapy	Elective
Orthopedics	Elective

TABLE 7-1
Nonsteroidal Anti-Inflammatory Agents

Agent	Mechanism of Action	Dose	Side Effects
Acetylsalicylic acid (aspirin)	Cyclooxygenase inhibition Decreases prostaglandin levels systemically	600 mg PO t.i.d. (therapeutic range 100–200 mg/dL) in serum	Tinnitus Metabolic acidosis Gastropathy
Ibuprofen (Motrin)	Same	400–800 mg PO t.i.d.	Nephropathy Gastropathy
Piroxicam (Feldene)	Same	20 mg PO q.d.	Nephropathy Gastropathy
Sulindac (Clinoril)	Same	150–200 mg PO b.i.d.	Nephropathy Gastropathy
Naproxen (Naprosyn)	Same	275 mg PO q.d.	Nephropathy Gastropathy
Magnesium choline salicylate (Disalcid)	Same	Two 750-mg tablets b.i.d.	Decreased risk of gastropathy relative to other agents

B. **Elbow tunnel syndrome**
1. **Manifestations**
   The **manifestations** of elbow tunnel syndrome include progressively worsening pain and tingling on
   the medial (ulnar) side of the forearm, hand, and digits 4 and 5. These findings are present on **both the
   palmar and dorsal aspects.** The patient often reports
   having had similar episodes in the past that resolved
   spontaneously. There is rarely a history of antecedent
   trauma or any significant weakness of the upper extremity. **Examination** may disclose no signs of weakness of finger abduction/adduction or any atrophy of
   the hypothenar musculature until late in the course
   of the disease process. A particularly useful sign is
   the reproduction of symptoms when the clinician palpates the ulnar groove.
2. **Pathogenesis**
   The **underlying pathogenesis** is entrapment of the ulnar nerve as it passes through the ulnar groove, a
   groove between the medial epicondyle and the olecranon on the dorsal aspect of the elbow. Entrapment
   can occur as a result of **nonspecific inflammation** or
   recurrent mild trauma to that area.
3. **Evaluation**
   The **evaluation** of this disorder includes making the
   clinical diagnosis. **Radiographs** of the elbow are invariably normal; therefore, unless there is an antecedent history of trauma or other manifestations are present, radiographs are unnecessary. The diagnosis can
   be confirmed by performing nerve conduction studies
   and electromyography on the upper extremities.
4. **Management**
   Specific management includes rest of the involved
   extremity and the initiation of NSAID (see Table 7-1).
   If the findings are **severe** or **refractory** to first-line
   therapy, referral to orthopedics for **surgical release** of
   the nerve entrapment is indicated.

C. **Olecranon bursitis**
1. **Manifestations**
   The **manifestations** of this entity include the onset of
   pain and swelling over the dorsal aspect of the elbow,
   immediately dorsal and adjacent to the **olecranon** of
   the ulna. On **examination** the area is tender, fluctuant,
   and often transilluminable. The area of swelling may
   become rather large. Patients often report similar episodes in the past, each of which was transient and
   self-limited. If the condition is due to an infectious
   cause, there invariably are concurrent fevers, signs of

inflammation in the adjacent skin (i.e., cellulitis), and marked tenderness.

2. **Pathogenesis**

   The **underlying pathogenesis** is inflammation of the olecranon bursa as a result of trauma, especially recurrent, mild trauma (e.g., leaning on the elbow, occupational activities with recurrent bumping of the elbow); **inflammatory arthritides,** crystal-related processes including tophaceous gout; and, rarely, **infectious** processes. The **organisms** that cause infectious bursitis are most commonly the gram-positive organisms *Streptococcus* and *Staphylococcus.*

3. **Evaluation**

   The **evaluation** entails making the clinical diagnosis and assessing the likelihood that the underlying process is infectious. **Radiographs** of the elbow are invariably normal; therefore, unless there is an antecedent history of trauma or other manifestations are present, radiographs are unnecessary.

4. **Management**

   a. If there is a **moderate to high level** of suspicion that it is **septic or infectious,** a diagnostic and therapeutic **needle drainage procedure** should be performed. If the procedure is performed, all fluid should be removed. The fluid is grossly examined visually and sent for Gram stain, culture, and crystal analysis. If the Gram stain reveals PMNs and gram-positive organisms, the specific management includes placing the patient on **systemic antibiotics** for 7–10 days (e.g., Keflex, 500 mg PO q.i.d.) and instructing the patient to rest the elbow for several days. **Follow-up** should be in 1–3 days and drainage repeated at that time if fluid has reaccumulated. The elbow joint itself must be examined each time to detect early evidence of concurrent arthritis. Consultation with orthopedics or rheumatology can be made on an elective basis.

   b. If the clinical suspicion for an infectious process is **low** or if the Gram stain shows no organisms, the **specific management** is conservative with resting of the joint, an NSAID (see Table 7-1), and follow-up in 3–5 days. If at that time the bursitis has not resolved, needle drainage for diagnosis and therapy can be performed. Again, unless there is evidence of concurrent monoarticular septic arthritis or of a systemic inflammatory arthritis, consultations are necessary only on an elective basis.

5. Consultation

Service	Time
Physical therapy	Elective
Orthopedics	Elective

D. Lateral epicondylitis (tennis elbow)
  1. **Manifestations**
     The **manifestations** of this quite common entity include the fairly acute onset of pain and tenderness over the lateral aspect of the elbow, immediately over and adjacent to the lateral epicondyle, and painful **limitation to extension** of the elbow. The patient relates a history of similar complaints in the past, especially after certain activities, such as knitting, repeated handshaking and practicing the backhand swing in tennis.
  2. **Pathogenesis**
     The **underlying pathogenesis** is noninfectious inflammation of the origin of the extensor muscles adjacent to the **lateral epicondyle** of the distal humerus.
  3. **Evaluation**
     The **evaluation** of lateral epicondylitis includes making the clinical diagnosis. **Radiographs** of the elbow are invariably normal; therefore, unless there is an antecedent history of trauma or other manifestations are present, radiographs are unnecessary.
  4. **Management**
     a. **For acute management,** i.e., the first hour after symptoms commence, ice is applied to the elbow for 30–45 minutes.
     b. **After the acute period** the modalities that can be used include NSAIDs PRN (see Table 7-1) and temporary avoidance of the exacerbating activity. Physical therapy for range of motion and strengthening activities is indicated.
     c. If the manifestations are **severe** and **refractory** to initial treatment, a radiograph of the elbow should be obtained. Triamcinolone, 10–20 mg, can be injected **over the lateral epicondyle.** If the manifestations are severe enough to warrant radiography and triamcinolone injection, referral to orthopedics should be considered.
  5. Consultation

Service	Time
Physical therapy	Elective

II. **Indications for admission:** Admission is rarely necessary.

B O X 7 - 2

> ### Overall Evaluation and Management of Foot and Ankle Pain
>
> *Evaluation*
>
> 1. Take a history and perform a physical examination, including evaluating range of motion.
> 2. Obtain radiographs of the ankle if trauma, including sprains, is a possibility.
>
> *Management*
>
> The specific management for different disorders is given in the text.

Foot and Ankle (Box 7-2)

The **anatomy** of the foot and ankle is complex and beyond the scope of this discussion. Several structures, however, deserve special mention. The two largest bones of the foot are the **calcaneus bone,** which forms the heel and is the bone into which the Achilles tendon inserts, and the **talus bone,** which is immediately superior to the calcaneus and forms an integral part of the tibiotalar joint.

The ligaments in this region may be divided into those on the medial side of the foot and ankle and those on the lateral side.

1. The ligament on the medial ankle is the **deltoid ligament,** which is large and thick and attaches the medial malleolus (the distal tibia) to the talus.

2. The ligaments on the lateral aspect of the ankle include the **calcaneofibular ligament** and the anterior and posterior **talofibular ligaments.** These ligaments attach the lateral malleolus (the distal fibula) to the calcaneus and the talus.

The **normal movements** of the joints of the toes, feet, and ankles are complex and quite diverse. A selected list of basic movements and the normal range of motion for each are as follows:

Dorsiflexion of the ankle:	20°
Plantar flexion of the ankle:	45°
Inversion of the foot (great toe side tilted up):	30°
Eversion of the foot (great toe side tilted down):	20°

I. Ankle sprains

A **sprain** is a tear in the fibers of a ligament. A ligament is a band of connective tissue that binds two adjacent bony structures, usually at a joint. Ligaments commonly injured in the ankle include the deltoid, which is medial, and the calcaneofibular and anterior and posterior calcaneofibular ligaments, which are lateral.

A. Medial sprains

1. Manifestations

The **manifestations** of this relatively uncommon entity include the acute onset of medial ankle pain, medial ankle tenderness, decreased range of motion of the ankle joint due to pain, and significant swelling, usually on both the medial and the lateral aspects of the ankle. Medial sprains of the ankle are invariably due to trauma.

2. Pathogenesis

The **underlying pathogenesis** is trauma with damage to the deltoid ligament. The trauma is due to forced **eversion,** i.e., trauma to the joint with the great toe tilted down. Medial sprains are relatively uncommon because the deltoid ligament is thick and not easily injured unless there is significant trauma.

3. Evaluation

The **evaluation** of a medial ankle sprain includes making the clinical diagnosis and obtaining radiographs of the injured area. Radiographs are necessary because there may be a concurrent avulsive fracture of the distal tibia or proximal talus.

4. Management

The **specific management** is based on the time that has elapsed since the injury occurred.

a. In the **acute setting,** i.e., immediately after the injury, apply an ice pack for 20–30 minutes and wrap the ankle with a tight elastic bandage for several hours. These interventions decrease local edema and decrease the potential for secondary damage.

b. **After the acute intervention,** management includes resting and immobilizing the joint. A large elastic wrap may provide the necessary support for mild sprains, but splinting may be necessary for a moderate to severe sprain. Further management includes the initiation of NSAIDs (see Table 7-1) and the use of crutches for 10–14 days to minimize weight-bearing. Physical therapy is usually indicated. If the sprain is severe, defined as the need for splinting or the presence of a concurrent avulsive fracture or a hypermobile joint, expedient referral to orthopedics is required. A rule of thumb is to apply **ice packs early** and **heat later,** i.e., >24–48 hours after the injury.

5. Consultation

Problem	*Service*	*Time*
Fracture	Orthopedics	Required
Hypermobile joint	Orthopedics	Elective
	Physical therapy	Elective

B. Lateral sprains
1. Manifestations
The **manifestations** of these common sprains include the acute onset of marked pain and tenderness on the lateral aspect of the foot with concurrent, usually significant, swelling and ecchymosis on the lateral aspect of the ankle. There is invariably an antecedent history of trauma. Further examination of severe sprains may disclose an **anterior drawer sign,** i.e., an anterior shift of the calcaneus under the tibia of more than 4 mm. This sign is elicited by the examiner grasping the distal tibia in one hand and the calcaneus in the other and applying anterior pressure on the distal tibia.

2. Pathogenesis
The underlying **pathogenesis** is a forced **inversion injury,** i.e., trauma occurring with the great toe tilted up. The sprain is a tear of the **calcaneofibular** or **anterior or posterior talofibular ligaments.** The most common site of a sprain is the **calcaneofibular ligament.**

There are three degrees of severity to this sprain: **first degree**—ligament stretching; **second degree**—a partial tear; and **third degree**—a complete tear, usually associated with the anterior drawer sign or avulsive fractures.

3. Evaluation
The **evaluation** of lateral ankle sprains includes making the clinical diagnosis and obtaining radiographs of the ankle. Radiographs are necessary because there may be a concurrent avulsive fracture of the distal fibula or the proximal calcaneus.

4. Management
The **specific management** of this entity is based on the time that has elapsed since injury.

a. In the **acute setting,** i.e., immediately after injury, apply ice packs for 20–30 minutes and wrap the ankle with a tight elastic wrap for several hours. These interventions decrease local edema and decrease the potential for secondary damage.

b. After the acute intervention, management includes resting and immobilizing the joint. A large elastic bandage may provide the necessary support for mild sprains, but splinting is often necessary for a moderate to severe sprain. Further management includes the initiation of NSAIDs (see Table 7-1) and the use of crutches for 10–14 days to minimize weight-bearing. Physical therapy is usually indicated. If the sprain is severe, defined as one that needs splinting or is associated with a concurrent avulsive fracture or a hypermobile joint, expedient referral to orthopedics is indicated. A rule of thumb is to apply **ice packs early** and **heat later,** i.e., >24–48 hours after the injury.

5. **Consultation**

Problem	Service	Time
Fracture	Orthopedics	Required
Hypermobile joint	Orthopedics	Elective
	Physical therapy	Elective

II. Foot and ankle fractures

Although trauma can result in fracture of any of the bony structures of the foot, one fracture is unique and common enough to merit special discussion. This fracture is a **Jones' fracture.**

A. Jones' fracture

1. **Manifestations**

The **manifestations** of a Jones' fracture include the acute onset of pain and swelling of the lateral foot and ankle with associated decreased range of motion of the ankle joint and ecchymosis. There is also a history of antecedent trauma to the foot.

2. **Pathogenesis**

The **underlying pathogenesis** is trauma to the foot with forced **inversion,** i.e., trauma occurring with the great toe tilted up. The damage is a simple fracture of the **base of the fifth metatarsal,** often as a result of or concurrent with a severe lateral sprain.

3. **Evaluation**

The **evaluation** of a Jones' fracture includes making the clinical diagnosis and obtaining radiographs of the ankle. Radiographs are needed to demonstrate the fracture and because there is a potential for a concurrent avulsive fracture of the distal tibia or the proximal talus.

4. **Management**

The **specific management** of this entity is based on the time that has elapsed since injury.

a. In the **acute setting,** i.e., immediately after the injury, apply ice packs for 20–30 minutes and wrap the area with a tight elastic wrap for several hours.

These interventions decrease local edema and decrease the potential for secondary damage.

b. **After the acute intervention,** management includes resting and immobilizing the joint. In virtually all cases splinting is required. Further management includes the initiation of NSAIDs (see Table 7-1) and the use of crutches for 21–28 days to minimize weight-bearing. Physical therapy is usually indicated. Expedient orthopedics intervention is required.

5. **Consultation**

Problem	Service	Time
Fracture	Orthopedics	Required
	Physical therapy	Elective

III. Neuromuscular dysfunction

A set of peripheral nerves supplies the foot. Each nerve supplies an area of sensation and a set of muscles, which in turn perform various specific aspects of foot motor activity.

A. Tarsal tunnel syndrome

1. **Manifestations**

The **manifestations** of this uncommon entity include the development of paresthesias and numbness on the sole of the affected foot and paresis of the intrinsic foot musculature that is manifested as a decrease in the ability to adduct and abduct the toes. Palpation over the posterior aspect of the medial malleolus precipitates or exacerbates the paresthesias.

2. **Pathogenesis**

The **underlying pathogenesis** is a peripheral neuropathy due to damage to or constriction of the **tarsal tunnel.** The tarsal tunnel is located immediately **infero-posterior to the medial malleolus.** It is the structure through which the posterior tibial nerve passes to supply sensation to the sole of the foot and direction to the intrinsic foot musculature. The syndrome can be exacerbated by or associated with the systemic disorders of diabetes mellitus, acromegaly, hypothyroidism, or rheumatoid arthritis; **or** it can occur as a result of local trauma or inflammation.

3. **Evaluation**

The **evaluation** of tarsal tunnel syndrome entails making the clinical diagnosis and looking for any underlying disorder. The diagnosis is confirmed by electromyography and nerve conduction studies of the affected lower extremity.

4. **Management**

The **specific management** is based on the acuity of the syndrome.

a. **Acute management** includes aggressive treatment and reversal of any underlying or associated systemic disorder *and* local treatment. Local treatment includes rest of the foot with, if severely symptomatic, splinting of the ankle and the initiation of an NSAID (see Table 7-1). If the condition is severe or recurrent, referral to orthopedics or podiatry for a surgical procedure to **release** the tarsal tunnel is indicated.

b. In the **chronic setting,** if there are any deficits that do not respond to therapy, including surgical intervention, the patient will have minimal recovery of nerve function. This underscores the need for **early diagnosis** and intervention. Once present, chronic hypesthesia of the foot may place the patient **at higher risk for foot infections.** Thus, the patient must be educated in the need for meticulous foot care.

5. **Consultation**

Service	Time
Orthopedics/podiatry	Elective

B. **Foot drop syndrome**

1. **Manifestations**

The **manifestations** of this not uncommon entity include inability to **dorsiflex** the affected foot and ankle. A steppage or "foot drop" gait develops and is especially prominent during stair climbing. Further examination often discloses atrophy of the anterior compartment leg musculature.

2. **Pathogenesis**

The **underlying pathogenesis** is an acquired or congenital dysfunction of the **common peroneal nerve,** which supplies direction to the musculature of the anterior compartment of the leg. Conditions that can result in such dysfunction of the common peroneal nerve include **trauma** (e.g., proximal fibular fracture), an **infiltrative process** (e.g., diabetes mellitus), and **Charcot–Marie–Tooth disease,** a congenital, autosomal dominant disorder that involves the common peroneal nerves bilaterally.

3. **Evaluation**

The **evaluation** of foot drop syndrome entails making the clinical diagnosis and looking for any underlying disorder. Radiographs of the leg are indicated to look for and document any old fracture of the proximal fibula. The diagnosis is confirmed with electromyography and nerve conduction studies of the affected lower extremity.

4. **Management**

The **specific management** includes the aggressive treatment and reversal of any underlying or associated systemic disorder and physical therapy to strengthen the anterior compartment musculature. The patient should be referred to podiatry for special shoes, which will assist the patient in ambulation.

5. **Consultation**

Service	Time
Physical therapy	Elective
Podiatry	Elective

IV. Toes and foot
A. Hammer toe

1. **Manifestations**

The **manifestations** of this relatively common acquired entity include the development of pain in the toe(s), with a deformity in which the **distal interphalangeal (DIP) joint** is normal, the **proximal interphalangeal (PIP) joint** has a flexion contracture, and the **metatarsophalangeal (MTP) joint** has a contracture of hyperextension. There is invariably an associated corn—an abnormal thickening of normally thin stratum corneum of the skin—on the affected toe.

2. **Pathogenesis**

The **underlying cause** is ill-fitting shoes.

3. **Evaluation**

The **evaluation** of hammer toe includes making the clinical diagnosis. Unless there are concurrent atypical findings or a history of antecedent trauma, it is rarely necessary to obtain radiographs of the foot and ankle.

4. **Management**

The **specific management** includes rest of the affected foot, the initiation of NSAIDs PRN, and referral to a podiatrist for fitting of special shoes to aid in reversing the process. Podiatric surgery may be necessary in severe or chronic cases.

5. **Consultation**

Service	Time
Podiatry	Elective

B. Hallux valgus

1. **Manifestations**

The **manifestations** of this quite common disorder include chronic, recurrent pain and tenderness over the dorsomedial aspect of the first metatarsophalangeal head. Concurrently, the great toe is invariably **laterally displaced.**

2. **Pathogenesis**

The **underlying pathogenesis** is inflammation followed by deviation of the first MTP joint, all as a result of ill-fitting shoes or of an inflammatory arthritis involving the anterior foot (rheumatoid arthritis). There is often a **corn** or a **callus**—an abnormal excessive thickening of the normally slightly thick stratum corneum—adjacent to the hallux valgus.

3. **Evaluation**

The **evaluation** of this disorder includes making the clinical diagnosis and obtaining radiographs of the affected great toe. Radiographs show an increased angle between the first and second metatarsals. The angle normally is <**10 degrees.** A common complication is the development of a bunion adjacent to the hallux valgus.

4. **Management**

The **specific management** includes rest of the affected foot, the initiation of NSAIDs PRN, and referral to a podiatrist for the fitting of special shoes to aid in reversing the process. Podiatric surgery may be necessary in severe or chronic cases.

5. **Consultation**

Service	*Time*
Podiatry	Elective

C. **Bunion**

1. **Manifestations**

The **manifestations** of this quite common entity include the acute onset of pain and tenderness over the MTP joints on any or all of the toes. It can be and often is associated with decreased range of motion of the affected joints and may be recurrent in nature.

2. **Pathogenesis**

The **underlying pathogenesis** is a noninfectious inflammation of one or more bursae on the toes. A bunion is commonly associated with hallux valgus and, like hammer toe with hallux valgus, is often the result of ill-fitting shoes.

3. **Evaluation**

The **evaluation** of this disorder includes making the clinical diagnosis. Radiographs are of little benefit unless hallux valgus is concurrently present or atypical features are present.

4. **Management**

The **specific management** includes rest of the affected foot, initiation of NSAIDs PRN, and referral to a podiatrist for the fitting of special shoes to aid in reversing the process. Podiatric surgery may be necessary in severe or chronic cases.

5. **Consultation**

Service	Time
Podiatry	Elective

D. Metatarsalgia

1. **Manifestations**

The **manifestations** of this common, often recurrent process include the acute development of pain and tenderness in the plantar aspect of the forefoot directly over the heads of the metatarsal bones. The pain is worse on weight-bearing. The condition is associated with callus development over the affected metatarsal heads.

2. **Pathogenesis**

The **underlying pathogenesis** is nonspecific inflammation of the affected metatarsal heads, usually as a result of ill-fitting shoes or an inflammatory arthritis (e.g., rheumatoid arthritis) involving the anterior foot.

3. **Evaluation**

The **evaluation** includes making the clinical diagnosis. Radiographs of the foot and ankle are rarely necessary unless there are concurrent findings or a history of antecedent trauma.

4. **Management**

The **specific management** includes rest of the affected foot, the initiation of NSAIDs PRN, and referral to a podiatrist for the fitting of special shoes. The specific modification is placement of a "metatarsal bar" in the sole of the shoe to support the foot and aid in reversing the process. Podiatric surgical intervention may be necessary in severe or chronic cases.

5. **Consultation**

Service	Time
Podiatry	Elective

E. Morton's neuroma

1. **Manifestations**

Morton's neuroma is uncommon but quite dramatic when present. **Manifestations** include the acute or subacute onset of a burning pain on the plantar surfaces of the proximal aspect of the 3rd and 4th toes about the MTP joints. The patient often reports that tight shoes precipitate or exacerbate the symptoms and gentle foot massage and warmth relieve the symptoms. Examination discloses **Mulder's sign,** or pain and a click sensation when the clinician places palpable pressure over the distal 3rd MTP joint.

2. **Pathogenesis**

The **underlying pathogenesis** is compression of the 3rd MTP space by excessive fibro-osseous material, usually as a result of chronic or recurrent mild trauma to the area.

3. **Evaluation**

The **evaluation** of Morton's neuroma includes making the clinical diagnosis. Radiographs of the foot and ankle are rarely necessary unless there are concurrent findings or a history of antecedent trauma.

4. **Management**

The **specific management** includes rest of the affected foot, the initiation of NSAIDs PRN, and referral to a podiatrist for the development of special shoes. The specific modification is widening the shoe to aid in reversing the process. In severe cases refractory to rest, shoe widening, and NSAIDs, injection of glucocorticoids (triamcinolone, 10–15 mg) into the plantar aspect of the fibro-osseous ring may be quite effective. Podiatric surgery may be necessary in severe or chronic cases.

5. **Consultation**

Service	*Time*
Podiatry	Elective

F. **Sesamoid bone disorders**
   1. **Manifestations**

   The **manifestations** of these not uncommon disorders include the acute or recurrent onset of pain, tenderness, and swelling on the plantar side of the MTP joint of the affected digits. The most common toe involved is the great toe. The patient often relates that the symptoms are exacerbated by bearing weight on the joint.

   2. **Pathogenesis**

   The **underlying pathogenesis** is an inflammation of one or all of the sesamoid bones at the base of the first MTP. The first MTP joint usually has a lateral and a medial sesamoid bone. These sesamoid bones normally assist in MTP joint mobility and, with stress or trauma, can become inflamed or even fracture. As such, sesamoid bone disorders are not uncommon in patients who are avid **joggers** or **dancers.**

   3. **Evaluation**

   The **evaluation** of sesamoid bone disorders includes making the clinical diagnosis and obtaining radiographs of the affected foot in AP, lateral, and sesamoid axial views. The **axial sesamoid views** increase the sensitivity of the examination in demonstrating fractures of the sesamoid bones.

4. **Management**

The **specific management** includes rest of the affected foot, the initiation of NSAIDs PRN, and referral to a podiatrist for special shoes. The specific modifications are stiffening the sole of the shoe and decreasing the size of the heel to aid in reversing the process. Podiatric surgery may be necessary in severe or chronic cases, but is rarely necessary even when sesamoid fractures are demonstrated.

5. **Consultation**

Service	Time
Podiatry	Elective

G. Plantar fasciitis

1. **Manifestations**

The **manifestations** of this quite common entity include the acute onset of pain and tenderness over the medial and plantar aspects of the foot immediately anterior (distal) to the heel. The pain, which is often recurrent, is worse in the morning and improves through the day. A classic phenomenon is the "first step" symptom, in which the pain is maximal upon bearing weight the first time in the morning.

2. **Pathogenesis**

The **underlying pathogenesis** is a noninfectious inflammation of the **plantar fascia** as a result of excessive use of the feet. This is a common disorder after marathon runs, in which small tears occur in the origin of the plantar fascia with secondary inflammation.

3. **Evaluation**

The **evaluation** of plantar fasciitis includes making the clinical diagnosis. Radiographs of the feet and ankles are invariably unremarkable, and thus, if there is no history of antecedent trauma or any atypical features, radiographs are not indicated.

4. **Management**

The **specific management** includes rest of the involved foot, i.e., the proscription of running for 5–7 days, the initiation of NSAIDs PRN (see Table 7-1), and, if the condition is severe or recurrent, referral to a podiatrist for potential surgical intervention. This intervention can take the form of release of the plantar fascia.

5. **Consultation**

Service	Time
Podiatry	Elective

H. **Infracalcaneal bursitis**
   1. **Manifestations**
      The **manifestations** of this relatively common entity include the development of acute or recurrent pain in the ball of the heel with concurrent tenderness over the calcaneal tuberosity of the affected foot.
   2. **Pathogenesis**
      The **underlying pathogenesis** is noninfectious inflammation of the infracalcaneal bursa, usually as a result of jogging or weight-bearing activities.
   3. **Evaluation**
      The **evaluation** of this disorder includes making the clinical diagnosis. Radiographs of the feet and ankles are invariably unremarkable, and thus, if there is no history of antecedent trauma or any atypical features, radiographs are not indicated.
   4. **Management**
      The **specific management** includes rest of the involved feet, limiting running for a short period of time, the initiation of NSAIDs PRN (see Table 7-1), and, if the condition is severe or recurrent, referral to a podiatrist for shoe modification to prevent recurrences.
   5. **Consultation**

Service	*Time*
Podiatry	Elective

I. **Posterior calcaneal bursitis**
   1. **Manifestations**
      The **manifestations** of this common disorder include the acute or recurrent development of pain and tenderness in and about the **Achilles tendon,** especially at its **insertion on the calcaneus bone.**
   2. **Pathogenesis**
      The **underlying pathogenesis** is noninfectious inflammation of the bursa adjacent to the insertion of the Achille's tendon on the calcaneus, often as a result of wearing high-heeled shoes or an excessively firm heel base in the shoes.
   3. **Evaluation**
      The **evaluation** of this disorder includes making the clinical diagnosis. Radiographs of the feet and ankles are invariably unremarkable, and thus, if there is no history of antecedent trauma or any atypical features, radiographs are not indicated.
   4. **Management**
      The **specific management** includes rest of the involved feet, the limitation of running for a short period of time, the initiation of NSAIDs PRN (see Table

7-1), and, if the condition is severe or recurrent, referral to podiatry for shoe modification to prevent recurrences. Wearing of high-heeled shoes is temporarily **proscribed.**

5. **Consultation**

Service	Time
Podiatry	Elective

J. Achilles tendinitis

1. **Manifestations**

   The **manifestations** of this common problem include recurrent or chronic pain in the Achilles tendon with concurrent tenderness and even palpable swelling within the tendon itself, specifically in the area immediately superior to the calcaneus, adjacent to the tendon insertion. Patients often relate that the symptoms and signs are exacerbated after exercise and relieved with rest.

2. **Pathogenesis**

   The **underlying pathogenesis** is noninfectious inflammation of the Achilles tendon (the tendon of the gastrocnemius muscle), usually as a result of mild trauma.

3. **Evaluation**

   The **evaluation** of this disorder includes making the clinical diagnosis. Radiographs of the feet and ankles are invariably unremarkable, and thus, if there is no history of antecedent trauma or any atypical features, radiographs are not indicated.

4. **Management**

   The **specific management** includes rest of the involved feet, the limitation of running for a short period of time, the initiation of NSAIDs PRN (see Table 7-1), and, if the condition is severe or recurrent, referral to a podiatrist for shoe modification to prevent recurrences. A further useful referral is to **physical therapy.** The physical therapist can often instruct the patient as to the proper techniques of pre-exercise gastrocnemius muscle stretching, as proper pre-exercise stretching will help prevent this entity.

5. **Consultation**

Service	Time
Podiatry	Elective
Physical therapy	Elective

V. Indications for admission: Admission is virtually never required.

B O X 7 - 3

*Overall Evaluation and Management
of Hand Dysfunction*

Evaluation

1. Take a history and perform a physical examination, including range of motion of the various articulations, sensory examination, and motor examination of the digits, hand, and wrist; see normal ROM measurements, above.
2. Determine the patency of the ulnar artery by performing the Allen test: the examiner compresses the radial and ulnar arteries for 30 seconds, then releases the ulnar side. If ulnar arterial disease is present, there will be a retarded flush of blood into the hand.
3. Obtain radiographs of the digits, hand, and wrist as clinically indicated.
4. Refer to an occupational therapist as needed.
5. Immobilize the joint(s) if a fracture is suspected.

Management

The management of specific hand dysfunctions is discussed in the text.

Hand (Box 7-3)

The normal movements and **range of motion** of various joints in the hands and fingers are listed below. These movements and their normal values are important in the physical examination and evaluation of hand injuries.

Metacarpophalangeal (MCP) joint movements
    Flexion: 90°
    Extension: 30°
Proximal interphalangeal (PIP) joint movements
    Flexion: 120°
    Extension: 0°
Distal interphalangeal (DIP) joint movements
    Flexion: 80°
    Extension: 0°

I. **Fingers**
 A. **Felon**
  1. **Manifestations**

   The **manifestations** of a felon, or "collar button abscess," include the acute onset of severe pain, swelling, modest erythema, and exquisite tenderness in the **palmar aspect** of the **distal digit.** There often is an antecedent history of a puncture wound to that area, e.g., a rose thorn wound or a cat bite. The history often is that the wound was initially tender, the tenderness decreased or even resolved, and then after several days of quiescence markedly increased in intensity and severity.

  2. **Pathogenesis**

   The **underlying pathogenesis** is an abscess in the terminal pulp cavity in the distal phalange. This is a **closed compartment** infection that is adjacent to the periosteum. As such, there is an increased risk of local edema, fingertip necrosis, osteomyelitis, and systemic infection. The infecting organisms most often are *Streptococcus* spp. or *Staphylococcus* spp. Unique to the puncture wound, *Sporotrichosis* can be associated with rose thorn wounds.

  3. **Evaluation**

   The **evaluation** of felon includes making the clinical diagnosis and determining if there are any concurrent sequelae as described above.

  4. **Management**

   The management of felon is based on the underlying pathogenesis and the potential for severe sequelae. Expedient, definitive intervention is mandatory. **Specific management** includes early and complete incision and drainage of the abscess, requiring deep drainage and placement of a small drain. Usually this procedure requires the expertise of a general surgeon and thus consultation with a surgical colleague is indicated on an urgent basis. The use of **concurrent antibiotics** is mandated, regimens include a 7–10 day course of Keflex, 500 mg PO t.i.d., or erythromycin, 250–500 mg PO q.i.d. **Immunization for tetanus** must be performed when indicated (see Table 6-2). If a bite, see section on Bite Wounds in Chapter 6.

  5. **Consultation**

Service	*Time*
Surgery (general or plastic)	Urgent

B. Heberden's and Bouchard's nodes

1. Manifestations

The **manifestations** of this quite common entity include the presence of nontender nodules on the distal interphalangeal (DIP) or proximal interphalangeal (PIP) joints of the digits. They usually occur on the digits of hands or feet in middle-aged or older patients. Often they are quite asymptomatic and go unnoticed by the patient until brought to their attention by the examining physician.

2. Pathogenesis

The **underlying pathogenesis** is the development of small synovium-lined cysts in the bone adjacent to these joints. These cysts are prevalent in degenerative joint disease. Specifically, **Heberden's nodes** affect the DIP joint and **Bouchard's nodes** affect the DIP joint. There is a significant amount of overlap between the two nodular types, and both are consistent with underlying degenerative joint disease.

3. Evaluation and management

The **evaluation and management** of these nodes entail making the clinical diagnosis and managing the underlying arthritis when it is symptomatic. No evaluation or management specific to these lesions is required, nor is any referral to any specific subspecialist required.

4. Consultation

No consultations are indicated.

C. Clubbing

See section on Clubbing in Chapter 4.

D. Sclerodactyly

1. Manifestations

The **manifestations** of sclerodactyly include a diffuse and painless decreased range of motion of the digits, particularly evident in the DIP joints. There often is thickening of the skin and underlying connective tissue about the digits. The patient may have Raynaud's phenomenon concurrently. This is the presence of pain, with white to red discoloration of the digits, upon exposure of the digits to the cold. Finally, symptoms and signs related to the underlying condition are also present, including synovitis, morning stiffness, and weight loss. A history of painful episodes precipitated by the smoking of cigarettes is quite suggestive of Buerger's disease.

2. Pathogenesis

The **underlying pathogenesis** is not completely known but probably has a strong autoimmune component. The differential diagnosis includes the autoimmune and rheumatologic disorders of mixed connective tissue disease, CREST syndrome, rheumatoid arthritis, scleroderma, and Buerger's disease. The end result is a thickening and fibrosis of the overlying skin.

3. **Evaluation**

The **evaluation** of this disorder entails making the clinical diagnosis and aggressively determining the underlying cause. Evaluation includes a thorough examination, especially of the joints, and determining the erythrocyte sedimentation rate (ESR), rheumatoid factor (RF) titer, antinuclear antibody (ANA) titer, complete blood cell count with differential, and performing urinalysis. Complications include flexion contractures of the digits with a significant decrease in hand function.

4. **Management**

The **specific management** is directed toward the underlying cause and toward preventing digital contractures. Consultations with rheumatology and occupational therapy are strongly indicated. The OT consult is to maintain ROM and prevent contractures.

5. **Consultation**

Service	Time
Rheumatology	Elective
Occupational therapy	Elective

E. **Swan neck/boutonnière deformity**
  1. **Manifestations**

The **manifestations** of these entities include the acquired development of contractures of the DIP and PIP joints of the digits. These contractures are painless but lead to a significant decrease in function of the fingers and hands and thus functional morbidity for the patient. These can involve any and all of the digits and, to be present, must involve the DIP and PIP of the same digit. **Swan neck deformity** is hyperextension contracture of the PIP and flexion contracture of the DIP joint **Boutonnière deformity** is the converse: the PIP joint has a significant flexion contracture and the DIP joint has a contracture of hyperextension.

  2. **Pathogenesis**

The **underlying pathogenesis** is not completely defined but in general involves one of the inflammatory arthritides. The classic underlying inflammatory arthritis which manifests in this way is **rheumatoid arthritis**.

3. **Evaluation and management**

The **evaluation and management** include making the clinical diagnosis and that described in the section on Polyarticular Arthritis (see page 432).

F. **Mallet finger**

1. **Manifestations**

The **manifestations** of this uncommon yet readily recognizable entity include an attitude of flexion of the DIP joint of the involved digit and loss of active digital extension, although passive extension of the digit remains intact. There is invariably a past history of hand trauma at which time the dysfunction of the finger began.

2. **Pathogenesis**

The **underlying pathogenesis** is traumatic avulsion of the finger extensor tendon with a resultant defect.

3. **Evaluation**

The **evaluation** includes making the clinical diagnosis, especially in a patient with the above findings and a recent history of trauma to the hand and/or finger. **Radiographs** of the affected hands and digits should be obtained to assess for any concurrent fractures.

4. **Management**

To effectively manage and prevent any permanent dysfunctional sequelae, early consultation with orthopedics is indicated, as is early and effective splinting of the digit. Furthermore, it is important to consult OT for short- and long-term management of the problem from the outset.

5. **Consultation**

Service	Time
Orthopedics	Urgent
OT/PT	Required

G. **Subungual hematoma**

See section on Nails in Chapter 8, page 470.

II. **Fractures**

Although there are a great number of potential fractures involving the hands and digits, any and all of which require clinical diagnosis, radiography, splinting, and early consultation with orthopedics and occupational therapy, one fracture is quite common and is described in further detail. This fracture is the "**boxer's fracture.**"

A. **Boxer's fracture**

1. **Manifestations**

The **manifestations** of this entity include the acute onset of pain and swelling over the medial aspect (ulnar side) of the hand due to trauma incurred when the patient forcibly hit an object with a closed fist. The fracture is a simple fracture of the diaphysis of the 5th metacarpal bone.

2. Evaluation and management

The **evaluation and management** include making the clinical diagnosis and performing radiography of the hand (see Fig. 7-1). Once diagnosed, the hand should be splinted and referral to orthopedics made in an expedient fashion. Again, as with many, if not all, hand dysfunctional states, consultation with OT/PT for short- and long-term therapy needs to be made.

3. Consultation

Service	*Time*
Orthopedics	Required
OT/PT	Elective

III. Tendons and bursae
A. Tenosynovitis
1. Manifestations

The **manifestations** of this fairly uncommon disease process include the acute or subacute (over hours to days) development of edema over the dorsum of the affected hand with associated **minimal active movement** of fingers in the affected hand and severe pain on passive extension of the affected fingers. The fingers are invariably held in an attitude of mild flexion. If the cause is infectious, the patient can present with concurrent systemic symptoms and signs of infection, including fever and other toxic findings.

2. Pathogenesis

The **underlying pathogenesis** is active inflammation (due to an infectious or noninfectious cause) of the tendons or their adjacent sheaths. Thus the patient often has a recent history of inflammatory arthritis (e.g., rheumatoid arthritis) or a recent wound (e.g., bite) on the affected hand.

3. Evaluation

The **evaluation** of this disorder is to make the diagnosis and to ascertain the extent of the inflammation and the underlying cause of the tenosynovitis. Often the underlying cause is readily evident from history and is a bite, laceration, or an inflammatory arthritis.

4. Management

The **management** is to treat the underlying condition and thus prevent any complications of this potentially severe and morbid condition. **Complications** can include the permanent loss of flexion/extension

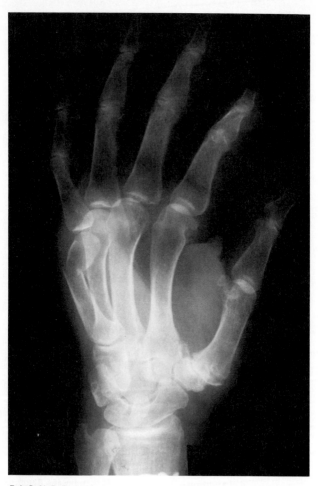

F I G U R E   7 - 1
Boxer's fracture, i.e., a simple, slightly displaced fracture of the
diaphysis of the 5th metacarpal.

mobility of the affected finger(s) and sepsis, if the underlying cause is infectious.

  a. If the underlying cause is **polyarticular inflammatory arthritis,** consultation with rheumatology and orthopedics is indicated, along with treatment of the underlying arthritis and splinting of the joint to rest it. Refer to the section on Polyarticular Arthritis, page 432.

  b. If the underlying cause is **infectious,** consultation with orthopedics for aggressive intervention and potential drainage and debridement is indicated on an emergency basis. In virtually all cases, admission to the hospital with aggressive parenteral antibiotics and surgical intervention is indicated. If the infection occurred as the result of a bite, refer to the section on Bite Wounds in Chapter 6.

5. Consultation

Service	Time
Orthopedics/Hand (infectious or noninfectious)	Emergent
Rheumatology (noninfectious)	Urgent

B. Radial bursitis

1. Manifestations

The **manifestations** of this entity include significant pain and tenderness over the flexor pollicis longus tendon. This is over the distal radial aspect of the forearm. Passive and active extension of that pollux (thumb) will increase the pain and, concurrently, the distal pollux phalanx is passively flexed. The onset of the manifestations can be acute to subacute (days to weeks).

2. Pathogenesis

The **underlying pathogenesis** is inflammation, invariably noninfectious, of the radial bursa.

3. Evaluation

The **evaluation** of this uncommon entity includes making the clinical diagnosis. Unless there are atypical findings or concurrent trauma, radiographs of the hand are rarely indicated.

4. Management

The **specific management** includes rest of the hand, splinting the involved wrist joint, and the initiation of an NSAID (see Table 7-1). Consultations are rarely indicated, although referral to OT for short- and long-term management can be of benefit.

5. **Consultation**

Service	Time
OT	Elective

C. Trigger finger

1. **Manifestations**

   The **manifestations** of this common entity include triggering or locking of the affected fingers. **Triggering** is a snapping sensation of the digit on flexion or extension. **Locking** is the reversible inability to extend the affected finger, usually at the PIP joint. There is rarely any antecedent trauma and virtually never any concurrent pain or tenderness of the hand or digits.

2. **Pathogenesis**

   The **underlying pathogenesis** is inflammation at the site where the long flexor tendons pass through the metacarpophalangeal (MCP) joint pulley. The inflammation is noninfectious and increases in incidence with age.

3. **Evaluation**

   The **evaluation** of trigger finger includes making the clinical diagnosis. Unless there is an antecedent history of trauma or any atypical features, radiographs of the involved digits and hand are rarely indicated. Trigger finger is troubling to the patient but has a benign natural history.

4. **Management**

   The **basic management** includes resting the affected fingers, splinting those fingers, initiating NSAIDs (see Table 7-1), and, if the condition is refractory and recurrently problematic, injection of 10 mg of triamcinolone into the tendon sheath (**not the tendon**) at the level of the MCP joint. Consultations with orthopedics and OT are often of benefit, especially in refractory or recurrent cases.

5. **Consultation**

Service	Time
Orthopedics/Hand	Elective

D. Ganglion

1. **Manifestations**

   The **manifestations** of this very common entity include the development of soft, fluid-filled, nontender lesions on the palmar or dorsal side of the hand or wrist. Often the patient is concerned that the lesion is growing and is malignant; or the patient may present for cosmetic reasons. These lesions, which are often multiple, have a natural history of symptomatic waxing and waning, with the lesions enlarging to various sizes then resolving for a period of time, only to recur and repeat the cycle. These lesions are usually fixed to deep tissues or tendon sheaths of the hands or wrists. They are well-defined cystic structures derived from and lined with **synovium.** The term *ganglion* or *ganglion cyst* can be misleading, because the structures have nothing to do with the nervous system.

  2. **Evaluation**

The **evaluation** of these lesions includes making the clinical diagnosis and reassuring the patient as to the benign nature of the lesions and that they often will resolve without any treatment. If the lesion is atypical, aspirate the ganglion with a 20-gauge needle. The aspirate normally reveals a viscous translucent material.

  3. **Management**

The lesions require treatment only if they are troublesome to the patient. **Specific management modalities** include aspiration with or without concurrent injection of 10–15 mg of triamcinolone into the ganglion, or surgical resection. The patient must be informed that in all cases, irrespective of the treatment modality used, the recurrence rate is quite high. Consultation with orthopedics is indicated only if the patient desires surgical intervention.

  4. **Consultation**

Service	*Time*
Orthopedics	Elective

E. **Saluting hand**

  1. **Manifestations**

The **manifestations** of this quite uncommon problem include the acquired development of a flexion contracture of the thumb with concurrent loss of all active extension of that thumb. Often the findings are acute in onset and follow an episode of trauma to the hand. There rarely is any associated pain or tenderness.

  2. **Pathogenesis**

The **underlying pathogenesis** is rupture of the extensor pollicis longus, usually due to a late complication of a Colles' fracture.

  3. **Evaluation**

The **evaluation** of this entity includes making the clinical diagnosis, and obtaining radiographs of the wrist and forearm of the affected upper extremity to look for evidence of a Colles' or Smith fracture.

4. **Management**
   The **specific management** includes referral to orthopedics and to OT for specific management.
5. **Consultation**

Service	Time
Orthopedics/Hand	Urgent
OT/PT	Elective

F. **Dupuytren's disease**
   1. **Manifestations**
      The **manifestations** of this entity, which is quite common, especially in the elderly, include permanent flexion contracture of the affected digits (i.e., the affected digits cannot be actively or passively extended). The most common and the initial digit affected is the 5th digit. The disease then progresses to involve the adjacent digits laterally.
   2. **Pathogenesis**
      The **underlying pathogenesis** is progressive contracture of the connective tissue within the flexor retinaculum of the hand, often associated with other fibrosing disorders, including **Ledderhose's disease** (flexion contractures of the toes) and **Peyronie's disease** (penile contractures and fibrosis).
   3. **Evaluation and management**
      The **evaluation and management** of this disorder include making the clinical diagnosis and referral to orthopedics or a general surgeon for surgical intervention on an elective basis. Intervention involves release of the flexor retinaculum.
   4. **Consultation**

Service	Time
Orthopedics/Hand	Elective

G. **Typewriter finger**
   1. **Manifestations**
      The **manifestations** of this quite uncommon entity include an acquired permanent flexion contracture of the PIP joint with no active extension possible in that digit. Rarely is there any concurrent pain or tenderness. A click sensation may be present during active or passive flexion of the DIP joint.
   2. **Pathogenesis**
      The **underlying pathogenesis** is rupture of the extensor tendon where it inserts into the middle phalanx. Rupture can occur as the result of inflammatory arthritides, including active rheumatoid arthritis; infectious processes; or trauma to the affected digit.

3. **Evaluation**

The **evaluation** of this entity involves making the clinical diagnosis and determining the cause. Radiographs of the affected hand are indicated only if there is a history of trauma. If the cause is an inflammatory arthritis, refer to the section on Polyarticular Arthritis (page 432) for further details.

4. **Management**

The **specific management** is to refer to orthopedics and OT in an expedient fashion for specific therapy.

5. **Consultation**

Service	*Time*
Orthopedics/Hand	Urgent
OT	Elective

H. de Quervain's disease

1. **Manifestations**

The **manifestations** of this relatively uncommon disorder include tenderness over the tendons of the anatomic "snuffbox." These tendons include those of the abductor pollicis longus muscle, the extensor pollicis longus muscle, and the extensor pollicis brevis muscle. The symptoms and signs are usually precipitated or exacerbated by activities like peeling vegetables or knitting. Examination usually discloses the Finkelstein's sign, i.e., pain is reproduced when the patient attempts to grasp the thumb with adjacent digits and ulnarly and palmarly flex the wrist.

2. **Pathogenesis**

The **underlying pathogenesis** is nonspecific, noninfectious inflammation of the tendons in the anatomical snuffbox. The inflammation can occur as a result of an inflammatory arthritis, occupational activity, or pregnancy.

3. **Evaluation and management**

The **evaluation and management** of this entity include making the clinical diagnosis, resting the hand and wrist, discontinuing the precipitating or exacerbating activity, splinting the wrist in mild dorsiflexion and with radial deviation of the thumb, and initiation of NSAIDs (see Table 7-1). If symptoms are refractory to therapy, the use of steroids (10 mg of triamcinolone injected **above** the abductor pollicis longus tendon) can be attempted, along with referral to orthopedics colleagues.

4. **Consultation**

Service	*Time*
PT	Urgent
Orthopedics	Elective

IV. **Muscles and nerves**
   A. **Volkmann's disease**
      1. **Manifestations**
         The **manifestations** of this severe but uncommon process include the insidious onset and progressive worsening of swelling, pain, and diffuse weakness of the affected hand. The fingers of the involved hand are held in an attitude of flexion. A modest amount of passive extension of the fingers is permitted. The classic description is of the **5 P's:** pain, pallor, pulselessness, puffiness, and paralysis. There invariably is a history of antecedent trauma, usually in the distant past.
      2. **Pathogenesis**
         The **underlying pathogenesis** is a forearm or arm fracture or direct trauma to the arteries themselves. This trauma results in chronic ischemia of the hand and the above described findings.
      3. **Evaluation**
         The **evaluation** of this process includes making the clinical diagnosis and obtaining radiographs of the affected forearm and arm to locate old fractures.
      4. **Management**
         This problem requires the early intervention of an orthopedist, in particular a **hand specialist,** and OT consultation for assistance in management.
      5. **Consultation**

Service	Time
Orthopedics/Hand	Urgent/emergent
OT	Elective

   B. **Claw hand**
      1. **Manifestations**
         The **manifestations** of this uncommon process include hyperextension of one or several MCP joints with concurrent flexion of PIP and DIP joints of the affected digits. Any digit may be affected. There is invariably a recent or distant history of trauma to the upper extremity.
      2. **Pathogenesis**
         The **underlying pathogenesis** is intrinsic muscle weakness in the affected digits due to peripheral nerve damage, usually as a result of trauma to the nerves. If findings involve fingers 4 and 5, it is invariably due to **ulnar nerve damage,** whereas if findings involve all of the digits on one hand, both the **ulnar and median nerves** are damaged.
      3. **Evaluation**
         The **evaluation** of this entity includes making the

clinical diagnosis, documenting motor and sensory deficits, and obtaining radiographs of the wrist, forearm, and arm to look for old or recent fractures.

4. **Management**
Referral to orthopedics or a hand specialist is clearly indicated, as is referral to OT for assistance in management of this condition, which has a great potential for morbidity.

5. **Consultation**

Service	*Time*
Orthopedics/Hand	Urgent
OT	Elective

C. Benediction hand
1. **Manifestations**
The **manifestations** of this entity include acquired inability to actively extend the 2nd and 5th fingers. When the patient is instructed to actively extend all fingers, the 2nd and 5th fingers remain flexed, whereas the 3rd and 4th fingers extend fully. Although the active deficit in extension is marked, the 2nd and 5th fingers may be passively extended. The hand appears to be raised in blessing. There is often a history of trauma, especially to the medial aspects of the arm, forearm, or wrist.

2. **Pathogenesis**
The **underlying pathogenesis** is trauma that has resulted in significant damage to the **ulnar nerve.**

3. **Evaluation**
The **evaluation** of this entity includes making the clinical diagnosis, documenting motor and sensory deficits, and obtaining radiographs of the wrist, forearm, and arm to look for old or recent fractures.

4. **Management**
Referral to orthopedics or a hand specialist is indicated, as is referral to OT for assistance in management of this condition, which has a great potential for morbidity.

5. **Consultation**

Service	*Time*
Orthopedics/Hand	Urgent
OT	Elective

D. Obstetrician's hand (accoucher's hand)
1. **Manifestations**
The **manifestations** of this uncommon entity include the acute onset of involuntary tetanic flexion of the thumb, all of the MCP joints, and the wrist. Concurrent with these flexion findings is involuntary exten-

sion of the PIP and DIP joints. This may affect one or
both of the hands.

2. **Pathogenesis**

   The **underlying pathogenesis** is hypocalcemia or hy-
   pomagnesemia, or both. There will often be other
   manifestations, including seizures, cramps involving
   other musculature, and **Chvostek's sign,** or spasm of
   the facial musculature elicited by tapping over cranial
   nerve VII. Another potential but rare cause is tetanus,
   the toxic disease due to the bacterium *Clostridium
   tetani.*

3. **Evaluation**

   The **evaluation** includes making the clinical diagnosis, attempting to elicit Chvostek's sign, and determining the serum calcium, magnesium, and albumin
   levels. If all of the above are normal, one must include
   tetanus in the differential diagnosis.

4. **Management**

   The **specific management** is to determine the underlying cause and treat it, i.e., replete the cations if low.
   Evaluation of such cation deficiencies must be aggressively performed with the assistance of endocrinology
   consultants. Virtually all cases require placement of
   an intravenous catheter and admission to the inpatient service.

5. **Consultation**

Problem	*Service*	*Time*
Hypocalcemia	Endocrinology	Emergent
Hypomagnesium	Endocrinology	Emergent
Tetanus is sus- pected	Infectious dis- eases	Emergent

E. **Wrist drop hand**

   1. **Manifestations**

      The **manifestations** of this not uncommon condition
      include the development of significant weakness in
      hand extension at the wrist joint. The patient has a
      limp wrist that can be passively but not actively ex-
      tended.

   2. **Pathogenesis**

      The **underlying pathogenesis** is damage to the radial
      nerve, usually a result of trauma to the arm, forearm,
      or wrist. The two most common causes are a Colles'
      fracture of the radius and a spiral fracture of the hu-
      meral shaft.

   3. **Evaluation**

      The **evaluation** of this entity includes making the
      clinical diagnosis, documenting motor and sensory

deficits, and obtaining radiographs of the wrist, forearm, and arm to look for old or recent fractures.
4. **Management**
    Referral to orthopedics or a hand specialist is indicated, as is referral to OT for assistance in management of this condition, which has a great potential for morbidity.
5. **Consultation**

Service	Time
Orthopedics/Hand	Urgent
OT	Elective

F. **Carpal tunnel syndrome**
    1. **Manifestations**
        The **manifestations** of this very common entity include the development of paresthesias and numbness on the volar (palmar) side of digits 1, 2, and 3. Further manifestations include thenar (thumb) muscular atrophy, Tinel's sign (paresthesias are reproduced by tapping over the median nerve), and Phalen's sign (paresthesias are reproduced by flexing the wrist for more than 1 minute). This syndrome usually occurs in middle-aged women, is often exacerbated by typing, and is often relieved by "shaking" the hand.
    2. **Pathogenesis**
        The **underlying pathogenesis** is acquired impingement of the median nerve as it enters the hand through the carpel tunnel of the wrist. Conditions leading to the development of impingement of the median nerve include **occupational disorders** (e.g., excessive typing) and the **systemic disorders** of diabetes mellitus, acromegaly, hypothyroidism, and rheumatoid arthritis.
    3. **Evaluation**
        The **evaluation** of this entity includes making the clinical diagnosis, documenting any deficits, and determining the underlying cause. Unless there is an antecedent history of trauma, radiographs of the wrist and forearm are invariably normal and therefore are not indicated. A fasting blood glucose level, TSH determination, and an occupational history are of evaluative usefulness. In order to confirm and document the degree of median nerve impairment, electromyography and nerve conduction studies of the affected extremity should be performed.
    4. **Management**
        The **specific management** includes splinting the wrist, keeping the wrist in a slightly dorsiflexed atti-

tude with the splint applied on a daily basis at
night. Further management includes the initiation of
NSAIDs (see Table 7-1), and modifying activities to
limit or discontinue those activities that exacerbate
or precipitate the attacks. If symptoms are refractory,
recurrent, or severe, referral to orthopedics for release
of the connective tissue about the tunnel is indicated.
If the patient opposes surgery, a one-time injection of
glucocorticoids (triamcinolone, 10–15 mg) above the
flexor reticulum can be administered. Consultation
with OT is indicated in the acute and long-term management of this disorder.
5. **Consultation**

Service	Time
Orthopedics	Elective (after 3 months of symptoms resistant to treatment)
OT	Elective

Hip, Thigh, and Bony Pelvis (Box 7-4)

Range of motion evaluation of the hips can be done with the knee
straight or flexed, or, **preferably, both.**

Knee straight
   Flexion: 90°
   Extension: 15°
   Abduction: 45°–60°
   Adduction: 30°
Knee flexed
   Flexion: 120°
   Extension: 0°
   Abduction: 40°
   Adduction: 40°

I. **Femoral neck fracture**
  A. **Manifestations**
    The **manifestations** of this not uncommon entity include
    an antecedent history of trauma, usually as a result of a
    fall to the floor or a fall down a flight of stairs. On **exami-
    nation** the hip is painful and tender with a significant
    decrease in range of motion; furthermore, there is sig-
    nificant tenderness over the proximal femur. The lower
    extremity is invariably **shortened** and **externally rotated
    to 90 degrees.** This is the most common fracture of the
    lower extremities in the geriatric population; it is partic-
    ularly common in patients who have osteoporosis.

B O X 7 - 4

***Overall Evaluation and Management of Hip
and Pelvic Pain***

Evaluation

1. Take a history and perform a physical examination,
   including evaluation of range of motion.
2. Obtain radiographs of the hip, especially if there is a
   history of trauma or falls, looking for a fracture of
   the femur or pelvis.
3. Involve physical therapy.
4. Rule out intrapelvic lesions by genitourinary examination, a pelvic examination in women, and examination of the testes and rectum in men.
5. Immobilize the joint if a fracture is suspected.
6. Determine the complete blood cell count if any
   trauma occurred.

Management

The management of specific problems involving the hip
and pelvis is discussed in the text.

B. **Pathogenesis**

   The **underlying pathogenesis** is a traumatic fracture.

C. **Evaluation**

   The **evaluation** of this entity includes making the clinical diagnosis and assessing the patient for concurrent
   trauma. Furthermore, it is important to determine why
   the fall occurred, so as to prevent future falls. **Radiographs** of the hip, pelvis, and femur are mandatory.

D. **Management**

   The **specific management** is based on the fact that there
   can be a significant amount of internal blood loss. Therefore, even with a simple fracture, the patient's hemodynamic status must be monitored carefully. In all cases,
   intravenous access and laboratory examinations including a CBC count and typing and cross-matching of blood
   for packed RBCs for potential transfusion are indicated.
   Emergency consultation with orthopedics is necessary,
   as the patient will invariably require surgical intervention with **internal reduction** of the fracture.

   Once the diagnosis is made and consultations are completed, an effective modality to prevent deep venous thrombosis should be recommended to the surgeon. A particularly useful modality is the application of **intermittent compression devices** to the lower extremities. From the outset, physical therapy should be consulted for rehabilitation purposes.

E. **Consultation**

Service	Time
Orthopedics	Emergent/urgent
Physical therapy	Elective

II. Bursitis or tendinitis

These are very common but sometimes overlooked causes of pain in the lower back and upper thigh. These inflammatory conditions must be included in the differential diagnosis of lower back pain and hip pain and should be clinically sought in all patients who present with such complaints.

A. **Ischiogluteal bursitis**

1. **Manifestations**

   The **manifestations** of this entity include the acute onset of or recurrent pain in the buttock that is exacerbated by sitting or performing a Valsalva maneuver. The pain is usually worse at night. It may often radiate into the hip and thus **simulate sciatica.** On examination the back has a normal range of motion, there is a negative straight leg raising test bilaterally, and there is discrete tenderness over the ischial tuberosity on the affected side.

2. **Pathogenesis**

   The **underlying pathogenesis** is noninfectious inflammation of the ischiogluteal bursa, located between the gluteal muscles and the ischium of the pelvis.

3. **Evaluation**

   The **evaluation** of this entity includes making the clinical diagnosis. **Radiographs** are invariably normal and thus, unless atypical findings are present or there is a recent history of trauma, radiographs are not indicated.

4. **Management**

   The **specific management** includes instructing the patient to sit in a position that does not result in pain. This can be facilitated by the use of a pillow or other supportive object. Further intervention includes the use of heating pads locally and the initiation of NSAIDs PRN (see Table 7-1). Referral to physical therapy may be made for short- and long-term adjunctive therapy.

5. **Consultation**

Service	Time
Physical therapy	Elective

B. **Psoas bursitis**
   1. **Manifestations**

      The **manifestations** of this quite uncommon entity include the acute onset of significant unilateral groin pain without antecedent trauma. The patient invariably relates a history of recurrent but milder "joint" pain in the ipsilateral hip over the preceding several years. On **examination** there is a negative straight leg raising test. The back examination is unremarkable, but there is a painful, **fluctuant mass** palpable immediately beneath the inguinal ligament on the affected side. Palpation of the mass reproduces the discomfort.

   2. **Pathogenesis**

      The **underlying pathogenesis** of this entity is noninfectious inflammation of the bursa adjacent to the psoas muscle; this is almost always associated with antecedent chronic osteoarthritis involving the ipsilateral hip joint.

   3. **Evaluation**

      The **evaluation** of this entity includes making the clinical diagnosis. **Radiographs** are invariably normal and thus, unless atypical findings or a recent history of trauma are present, are not indicated. If there is any evidence of **abdominal discomfort** or the potential for an abscess, a complete blood cell count with differential, an abdominal series looking for free air in the abdomen, and referral to general surgery are indicated. If there is no abdominal discomfort, these examinations are not necessary.

   4. **Management**

      The **specific management** includes the use of local heating pads and the initiation of NSAIDs PRN (see Table 7-1). Referral to physical therapy can be made for short- and long-term adjunctive therapy.

   5. **Consultation**

Service	Time
Physical therapy	Elective
Orthopedics	Elective, if refractory to first-line therapy

C. **Greater trochanteric bursitis**
   1. **Manifestations**

      The **manifestations** of this, the most common of the bursitides involving the hip, include acute or recurrent pain over the **lateral hip and thigh.** On examina-

tion the back is unremarkable and has a normal range
of motion and the straight leg raising test is normal bilaterally; however, there is significant tenderness over
the lateral aspect of hip immediately **posterior to the
greater trochanter.** The pain is exacerbated by direct
pressure or internal rotation of the hip with hip flexion.

2. **Pathogenesis**

The **underlying pathogenesis** is noninfectious inflammation of the bursa immediately over and adjacent
to the greater trochanter.

3. **Evaluation**

The **evaluation** of this entity includes making the clinical diagnosis. Radiographs are invariably normal and
thus, unless atypical findings or a recent history of
trauma are present, are not indicated.

4. **Management**

The **specific management** includes resting the involved lower extremity and the use of heating pads
over the area of discomfort. The initiation of NSAIDs
PRN (see Table 7-1) can be quite effective. Referral to
physical therapy can be made for short- and long-term
adjunctive therapy. If the condition is severe or refractory to first-line therapy, triamcinolone, 15–20 mg, can
be injected into the affected bursa.

5. **Consultation**

Service	Time
Physical therapy	Elective

III. **Osteoarthritis**

1. **Manifestations**

The **manifestations** of this very common entity, one
that increases in prevalence with increasing age, include chronic dull pain in the affected hip. The pain is
exacerbated by bearing weight and by activity involving or using the joint. The pain is typically worse in the
afternoon than in the morning, and often radiates into
the ipsilateral inguinal area. Over time there is a significant decrease in range of motion of the joint. On **examination** the patient will keep the thigh and leg in an
attitude of **adduction, flexion,** and **external rotation** to
minimize the pain. There is a decreased range of motion of the joint and occasionally mild crepitus. Finally, **Trendelenburg's sign** may be elicited: when the
patient is instructed to place weight on the opposite
leg, the affected buttock abnormally falls, which is indicative of abductor muscle weakness in the affected
hip.

2. **Pathogenesis**

The **underlying pathogenesis** is unknown, but specific risk factors for its development and progression include **trauma,** Legg–Calvé–Perthes disease, and **obesity.**

3. **Evaluation**

   The **evaluation** of this disorder includes making the clinical diagnosis. **Radiographs** of the hips should be obtained to look for the degenerative changes of osteophytes and a decrease in the joint space of the hip.

4. **Management**

   The **specific management** includes referral to **physical therapy** for range of motion and strengthening exercises. The patient should be **prescribed a cane** and instructed in its proper use. Adjunctive therapy may include the use of heat compresses on the diseased hip, weight loss if the patient is obese, and the initiation of NSAIDs (see Table 7-1). If the disease is severe or refractory to therapy or is affecting the quality of the patient's life, referral to orthopedics for total hip replacement is indicated.

5. **Consultation**

Service	*Time*
Physical therapy	Elective
Orthopedics	Elective

IV. **Indications for admission:** Any fracture. Admission is usually to the orthopedics service.

Knee (Box 7-5)

The **anatomy** of the knee is relatively simple. The **ligaments** of the knee include:

1. The **anterior cruciate ligament.** This is the largest ligament in the knee and directly connects the **anterior tibia** to the **lateral femoral epicondyle.**
2. **Posterior cruciate ligament.** This ligament directly connects the **posterior tibia** to the **medial femoral epicondyle.**
3. **Medial collateral ligament.** This ligament directly connects the **medial tibial condyle** to the **medial femoral epicondyle.**
4. **Lateral collateral ligament.** This ligament directly connects the **lateral tibial condyle** to the **lateral femoral epicondyle.**

The **normal movements** of the knee joint and the normal range of motion for each movement are described below.

Flexion:	130°
Extension:	5°
Adduction and abduction:	Minimal
Internal and external rotation:	Minimal

B O X 7 - 5

Overall Evaluation and Management of Knee Pain

Evaluation

1. Take a history and perform a physical examination, including evaluation of range of motion.
2. Obtain radiographs of the knee, especially if there is any history of trauma or falls.
3. Involve physical therapy.

Management

1. Immobilize the joint if fracture is suspected.
2. The specific management of knee disorders is discussed in the text.

I. Bursitis
The knee has a number of bursae, any one of which may become inflamed and cause significant discomfort. Five different bursitides or bursitis-related syndromes are discussed here.

A. Prepatellar bursitis
1. Manifestations
The **manifestations** of this entity include the acute onset of painless swelling and fluctuance over the lower half of the patella and the upper portion of the patellar ligament. Although it may occur in any active occupation, it is classically and colloquially known as **"housemaid's knee."**

2. Pathogenesis
The **underlying pathogenesis** is noninfectious inflammation of the prepatellar bursa, a bursa located immediately anterior (superficial) and inferior to the patella.

3. Evaluation
The **evaluation** of this entity includes making the clinical diagnosis. **Radiographs** are of little diagnostic benefit and, unless there are atypical features present or the patient has a recent history of trauma, are not indicated.

4. Management
The **specific management** includes rest of the joint and refraining from the specific activity that precipitated or exacerbates the process. If the process is quite

severe, one may attempt NSAIDs PRN (see Table 7-1), and/or perform needle aspiration of the bursa to remove the fluid. There usually is no need for subspecialty consultations.

5. Consultation

None indicated.

B. Infrapatellar bursitis

1. Manifestations

The **manifestations** of this entity include the acute onset of a painful, tender swelling on one or both sides of the inferior aspect of the patellar ligament. The most marked manifestations are located immediately **deep and inferior** to the **patella.** Because kneeling is a common exacerbating or precipitating event, the condition is often referred to as **"clergyman's knee."**

2. Pathogenesis

The **underlying pathogenesis** is a noninfectious inflammation of the infrapatellar bursa, a bursa located immediately deep and inferior to the patella itself. It is the result of mild, recurrent trauma to the tibial tuberosity and thus this specific bursa.

3. Evaluation

The **evaluation** of this entity includes making the clinical diagnosis. **Radiographs** are of little diagnostic benefit and, unless there are atypical features present or the patient has a recent history of trauma, are not indicated.

4. Management

The **specific management** includes rest of the joint and refraining from the specific activity that precipitated or exacerbates the process. If the process is severe, one may attempt NSAIDs PRN (see Table 7-1) and/or perform needle aspiration of the bursa to remove the fluid. There usually is no need for subspecialty consultations.

5. Consultation

None indicated.

C. Semimembranous bursitis

1. Manifestations

The **manifestations** of this form of bursitis include a painful, tender mass in the **superior medial aspect** of the **popliteal fossa.** Maneuvers on physical examination to further define and diagnose this entity include palpation of the popliteal fossa in extension and flexion of the leg at the knee. The bursa tenses **upon extension** and becomes **palpable and tender,** whereas the bursa relaxes upon **knee flexion** and becomes **nonpalpable and less tender.**

2. **Pathogenesis**

The **underlying pathogenesis** is noninfectious inflammation of the semimembranous bursa, a bursa located deep in the superior medial popliteal fossa and immediately adjacent to the **head of the gastrocnemius** and the **insertion of the semimembranous muscle.**

3. **Evaluation**

The **evaluation** of this entity includes making the clinical diagnosis. **Radiographs** are of little diagnostic benefit and, unless there are atypical features present or the patient has a recent history of trauma, are not indicated.

4. **Management**

The **specific management** includes rest of the joint and refraining from the specific activity that precipitated or exacerbates the process. If the process is severe, one can attempt NSAIDs PRN (see Table 7-1) and/or perform needle aspiration of the bursa to remove the fluid. There usually is no need for subspecialty consultations.

5. **Consultation**

None indicated.

D. **Anserine bursitis**

1. **Manifestations**

The **manifestations** of this entity include a painful, tender, fluctuant mass over the extreme **medial aspect** of the knee, immediately inferior to the medial femoral condyle.

2. **Pathogenesis**

The **underlying pathogenesis** is noninfectious inflammation of the **pes anserine** (goose's foot) bursa. This bursa is adjacent to the insertions of the tendons of the sartorius, gracilis, and semitendinous muscles.

3. **Evaluation**

The **evaluation** of this entity includes making the clinical diagnosis. **Radiographs** are of little diagnostic benefit and, unless there are atypical features present or the patient has a recent history of trauma, are not indicated.

4. **Management**

The **specific management** includes rest of the joint and refraining from the specific activity that precipitated or exacerbates the process. If the process is severe, one can attempt NSAIDs PRN (see Table 7-1) and/or perform needle aspiration of the bursa to remove the fluid. There usually is no need for subspecialty consultations.

5. **Consultation**
   None indicated.

II. Ligamentous and meniscal damage
A. Anterior cruciate tear
1. **Manifestations**
   The **manifestations** of this specific ligamentous tear include the acute onset of severe pain, the immediate development of a significant effusion, and severe instability of the joint, especially when ambulation is attempted. Further examination discloses the **anterior drawer sign,** i.e., the tibia slides anteriorly over the femur when the knee is flexed to 90°, and **Lachman's sign,** i.e., the tibia slides anteriorly over the femur when the knee is flexed to 30°. These two signs can be difficult to demonstrate if the injury is acute, owing to pain and swelling.
2. **Pathogenesis**
   The **underlying pathogenesis** is a partial or complete tear of the anterior cruciate ligament, usually as a result of a **force** applied to the **tibia anteriorly.** (This ligament connects the anterior tibia with the femur.)
3. **Evaluation**
   The **evaluation** of this entity includes making the clinical diagnosis and assessing for any concurrent effusion in the injured knee. **Effusion,** which invariably is present, is virtually always a **hemarthrosis;** therefore, **arthrocentesis** for diagnostic and therapeutic benefit is indicated. Because an anterior cruciate tear usually occurs as a result of significant trauma, **radiographs** of the knee and leg are indicated to rule out concurrent bony abnormalities.
4. **Management**
   The **specific management** includes immobilization of the knee and the initiation of effective analgesia, including NSAIDs PRN (see Table 7-1) or narcotic agents. Referral to orthopedic colleagues on an emergency basis is indicated. **Physical therapy** should be involved early for assistance in management.
5. **Consultation**

Service	*Time*
Orthopedics	Urgent/emergent
Physical therapy	Elective

B. Posterior cruciate tear
1. **Manifestations**
   The **manifestations** of this entity include the acute onset of significant instability of the affected knee

with associated pain and, often, concurrent joint effusion. On further examination, there is a **posterior drawer sign,** i.e., the tibia slides posteriorly over the femur with the knee flexed to 30°.

2. **Pathogenesis**

The **underlying pathogenesis** is a partial or complete tear of the posterior cruciate ligament. (The posterior cruciate ligament attaches the posterior tibia with the femur.) The tear usually occurs as a result of a direct blow to the head of the tibia when the knee is flexed.

3. **Evaluation**

The **evaluation** of this entity includes making the clinical diagnosis and assessing for the potentially present effusion. Effusion, if present, is virtually always a hemarthrosis, and thus arthrocentesis for diagnosis and therapy is indicated. Because this entity usually occurs as a result of significant trauma, other lesions, especially fractures of adjacent bony structures, need to be looked for with radiographs of the knee.

4. **Management**

The knee should be immobilized. Effective analgesia with NSAIDs or narcotic agents is indicated, and referral to orthopedic colleagues on an emergency basis is indicated. Physical therapy should be involved early for intermediate and long-term assistance in management.

5. **Consultation**

Service	*Time*
Orthopedics	Urgent/emergent
Physical therapy	Elective

C. **Medial meniscus tear**

1. **Manifestations**

The **manifestations** of this entity, whether acute or chronic, include pain and tenderness over the medial collateral ligament which are exacerbated by knee flexion, and a history of recurrent knee locking, i.e., the knee temporarily cannot be flexed. Usually no significant joint instability or effusion is present. Upon further examination, there is a positive **McMurray test,** i.e., a click during forced adduction or abduction of the knee with the patient prone and the knee flexed to 90°. Furthermore, there often is a positive **Apley's test:** with the patient prone and the symptomatic knee flexed to 90°, the examiner pushes upon the heel with valgus and varis angulation; if pain is present medially it is indicative of medial meniscus damage, whereas if pain is present laterally it is indicative of lateral meniscus damage. A final test is the **Childress test,** or "**duck waddle test**": the patient is unable to fully flex the affected knee when instructed to move in a duck waddle, which is indicative of a selective rupture of the **posterior horn** of the **medial meniscus.**

2. **Pathogenesis**

   The **underlying pathogenesis** is damage to the cartilage (meniscus) in the medial compartment of the knee. The damage occurs when the knee is twisted medially and flexed with concurrent weight-bearing.

3. **Evaluation**

   The **evaluation** of this entity includes making the clinical diagnosis and assessing for any concurrent effusion in the injured knee. **Effusion,** which is rarely present, virtually always is a **hemarthrosis;** therefore, **arthrocentesis** for diagnosis and therapy is indicated. Because a medial meniscus tear usually occurs as a result of significant trauma, **radiographs** of the knee and leg are indicated to rule out concurrent bony abnormalities.

4. **Management**

   The **specific management** includes immobilization of the knee and the initiation of effective analgesia with NSAIDs (see Table 7-1) or narcotic agents. Referral to orthopedics on an emergency basis is indicated. **Physical therapy** should be involved early for assistance in management.

5. **Consultation**

Service	Time
Orthopedics	Urgent
Physical therapy	Elective

D. **Lateral meniscus tear**
   1. **Manifestations**

      The **manifestations** of this entity, whether acute or chronic, include pain and tenderness over the lateral collateral ligament which are exacerbated by knee flexion. The knee rarely locks and rarely is unstable. On further examination there is a positive **McMurray test,** i.e., a click during forced adduction or abduction of the knee with the patient prone and the knee flexed to 90°. Furthermore there often is a positive **Apley's test:** with the patient prone and the symptomatic knee flexed to 90°, the examiner pushes upon the heel with valgus and varis angulation; if pain is present medially it is indicative of medial meniscus damage, whereas if the pain is present laterally it is indicative of lateral meniscus damage. A final test is the **Childress test,** or "**duck waddle test**": the patient is unable to fully flex the affected knee when instructed to move in the duck waddle, which is indicative of a selective rupture of the **posterior horn** of the lateral meniscus.

2. **Pathogenesis**

The **underlying pathogenesis** is damage to the cartilage (meniscus) in the medial compartment of the knee. The damage occurs when the knee is twisted laterally and flexed, with concurrent weight-bearing.

3. **Evaluation**

The **evaluation** of a lateral meniscus tear includes making the clinical diagnosis and assessing for any concurrent effusion in the injured knee. **Effusion,** which is rarely present, it virtually always is a **hemarthrosis;** therefore, **arthrocentesis** for diagnosis and therapy is indicated. Because this usually occurs as a result of significant trauma, radiographs of the knee and leg are indicated to rule out concurrent bony abnormalities.

4. **Management**

The **specific management** includes immobilization of the knee and the initiation of effective analgesia with NSAIDs (see Table 7-1) or narcotic agents. Referral to orthopedics on an emergency basis is indicated. **Physical therapy** should be involved early for assistance in management.

5. **Consultation**

Service	Time
Orthopedics	Urgent
Physical therapy	Elective

E. **Medial collateral ligament tear**
   1. **Manifestations**

   The **manifestations** of this quite uncommon entity include the acute onset of pain or even chronic pain and tenderness over the medial aspect of the knee. On examination the affected knee often has **slight medial mobility** that is even more prominent if there has been concurrent damage to the **anterior cruciate ligament.** Unless there is concurrent damage to the menisci, **McMurray's** and **Apley's signs** are not present.

   2. **Pathogenesis**

   The **underlying pathogenesis** is a partial or complete tear of the **medial collateral ligament,** usually as a result of excessive **valgus bending** of the knee during activity.

   3. **Evaluation**

   The **evaluation** of this entity includes making the

clinical diagnosis and assessing for any effusion in the injured knee. **Effusion,** which is rarely present, virtually always is a **hemarthrosis;** therefore, **arthrocentesis** for diagnosis and therapy is indicated. Because this usually occurs as a result of significant trauma, **radiographs** of the knee and leg are indicated to rule out concurrent bony abnormalities. Furthermore, because it is often concurrent with an anterior cruciate tear, an examination for this lesion must also be made.

4. **Management**

The **specific management** includes immobilization of the knee and the initiation of effective analgesia with NSAIDs (see Table 7-1) or narcotic agents. Referral to orthopedics on an emergency basis is indicated. **Physical therapy** should be involved early for assistance in management.

5. **Consultation**

Service	Time
Orthopedics	Urgent
Physical therapy	Elective

F. **Lateral collateral ligament tear**

1. **Manifestations**

The **manifestations** of this quite uncommon entity include the acute onset of pain or even the presence of chronic pain and tenderness over the lateral aspect of the knee. Upon examination the affected knee often will have **slight lateral mobility** which is even more prominent if there has been concurrent damage to the **anterior cruciate ligament.** Unless there is concurrent damage to the menisci, **McMurray's** and **Apley's signs** are not present.

2. **Pathogenesis**

The **underlying pathogenesis** is a partial or complete tear of the **lateral collateral ligament,** usually as a result of excessive **varus bending** of the knee during activity.

3. **Evaluation**

The **evaluation** of this entity includes making the clinical diagnosis and assessing for any concurrent effusion in the injured knee. **Effusion,** which is rarely present, is virtually always a hemarthrosis; therefore, **arthrocentesis** for diagnosis and therapy is indicated. Because this is usually as the result of significant trauma, **radiographs** of the knee and leg are indicated to rule out any concurrent bony abnormalities. Furthermore, given the fact that this is often concurrent

to an anterior cruciate tear an examination for this
lesion must also be made.

4. **Management**

The **specific management** includes immobilization of
the knee and the initiation of effective analgesia with
NSAIDs (see Table 7-1) or narcotic agents. Referral
to orthopedics on an emergency basis is indicated.
Physical therapy should be involved early for assistance in management.

5. **Consultation**

Service	Time
Orthopedics	Urgent
Physical therapy	Elective

III. Patellar dysfunction

A. Patellar ligament rupture

1. **Manifestations**

The manifestations of this entity include pain and
tenderness over the tibial tuberosity and the patella
abnormally present in the area **medial or lateral** to
the knee. On further examination there often are concurrent swelling about the tibial tuberosity and gross
hypermobility of the patella.

2. **Pathogenesis**

The **underlying pathogenesis** of a rupture of the patellar (also called the tendon of the quadriceps femoris)
ligament is most commonly trauma-related but may
occur spontaneously. This rupture manifests with patellar hypermobility because the patella is located
completely within the substance of the ligament, i.e.,
it is a sesamoid bone.

3. **Evaluation**

The **evaluation** of this condition includes making the
clinical diagnosis. Radiographs of the knee are usually unremarkable and thus not indicated.

4. **Management**

The **specific management** includes rest and immobilization of the knee in the acute setting, analgesia with
an NSAID (see Table 7-1), and an orthopedics referral
on an urgent basis. Physical therapy is appropriate
after the acute symptoms have resolved in order to
strengthen the **quadriceps femoris musculature.** This
intervention may **decrease** the risk of recurrence in
the future.

5. **Consultation**

Service	Time
Orthopedics	Urgent
Physical therapy	Elective

B. Chondromalacia patellae

1. Manifestations

The **manifestations** of this not uncommon entity include pain in the anterior aspect of the knee that is exacerbated by kneeling. It is the most common form of chronic and recurrent knee pain in **joggers** and **runners.** Upon examination, there is tenderness upon pressing the **patella against the tibial condyles,** but no significant decrease in the range of motion of the joint. Furthermore, there rarely is any effusion present in the knee. **Crepitus,** a nonspecific finding, is invariably present in this condition.

2. Pathogenesis

The **underlying pathogenesis** is degeneration of the articular surface of the patella that may be idiopathic or related to recurrent mild trauma.

3. Evaluation

The **evaluation** includes making the clinical diagnosis. **Radiographs** of the knees are invariably normal but may be obtained if there are any atypical features or a recent history of significant trauma.

4. Management

The **specific management** of this entity includes rest of the joint; however, immobilization of the joint is rarely necessary. The patient should continue exercising but should change to a different activity for a short period of time, such as swimming.

5. Consultation

Service	Time
Orthopedics	Urgent
Physical therapy	Elective

C. Recurrent patellar dislocation

1. Manifestations

The **manifestations** of this entity include the knee "giving out" acutely, associated with moderate to severe pain in the affected knee. On examination the patella is **hypermobile** and **displaced laterally.** There often are extended asymptomatic periods between acute events. There often is no history of antecedent trauma.

2. Pathogenesis

The **underlying pathogenesis** is trauma-related or congenital weakness of the quadriceps femoris tendon.

3. Evaluation

The **evaluation** of this condition includes making the clinical diagnosis. **Radiographs** of the knee are usually unremarkable and thus not indicated.

4. Management

The **specific management** includes rest and immobilization of the knee in the acute setting, analgesia with NSAIDs, and an orthopedics referral on an urgent basis. **Physical therapy** is appropriate after the acute symptoms have resolved in order to **strengthen** the **quadriceps femoris musculature.** This intervention may **decrease** the risk of recurrence in the future and prevent the most common **complication,** atrophy of the quadriceps femoris musculature.

5. Consultation

Service	*Time*
Orthopedics	Urgent
Physical therapy	Elective

IV. Degenerative joint disease

1. Manifestations

The **manifestations** of this common, chronic problem include **pain** in one or both knees. The pain is usually worse in the afternoon, after activities, and better in the morning. On **examination, crepitus** in the affected knee is present, as well as a decreased range of motion. A small amount of effusion may be present in the involved knee. The **natural history** is a slow, steady worsening of the process.

2. Pathogenesis

The **underlying pathogenesis** is degenerative arthritic changes, i.e., a loss of articular cartilage in the affected knee joint, through an unknown mechanism. Factors associated with its development include **obesity** and **recurrent trauma.**

3. Evaluation

The **evaluation** of this entity includes making the clinical diagnosis and ruling out any concurrent processes. **Radiographs** of the knee, in AP and lateral views, reveal narrowing of one, two, or all three **articular compartments.**

4. Management

The **specific management** includes rest PRN, NSAIDs PRN, weight loss if the patient is obese, and physical therapy. If the disease is severe and disabling, an intra-articular injection of triamcinolone, 35–50 mg, may be performed. Markedly symptomatic patients should be referred to orthopedics for consideration of total knee replacement.

Lower Back (Box 7-6)

The anatomy of the back in general and of the lumbosacral area in specific is relatively complex and beyond the scope of this discussion.

The range of motion and normal values are referred to the level of the lower back, with the pelvis stabilized by the examiner.

Extension:	30°
Flexion:	75°–90°
Lateral bending:	30°, left and right
Rotation:	30°, left and right

I. **Overall manifestations**

The **overall manifestations** include discomfort in the lower back, referred to colloquially as the small of the back. The discomfort can be pain of any type and intensity. The pain may be limited to the back or may radiate to various locations in the lower extremities.

II. **Examination**

On **examination,** the paraspinous musculature and spinous processes must be palpated for **tenderness** or muscle spasm. The **range of motion** must be assessed, as it is often limited. Furthermore, the clinician must test for a **radicular** (radicle = nerve root) component to the process. This is best assessed by testing lower extremity motor strength and performing a straight leg raising test on the patient.

A. The lower extremity muscles are innervated by the first sacral nerve root (**S1**), the fifth lumbar nerve root (**L5**), and the fourth lumbar nerve root (**L4**). These are the roots most commonly affected by processes resulting in low back pain. **S1** involvement is best assessed by having the patient perform the **tiptoe walk, L5** involvement is best assessed by the **heel walk,** and **L4** involvement is best assessed by **leg extension at the knee** against resistance.

B. The **straight leg raising examination** is performed by placing the patient supine and passively flexing each leg at the hip. If pain occurs in the leg as the leg is flexed at the hip, and especially if the pain radiates into the posterolateral thigh and leg, it is consistent with a radicular origin.

C. Examine the patient for **sensory deficits** in the lower extremities.

III. **Differential diagnosis**

The **differential diagnosis** of low back pain is quite diverse (Table 7-2). The vast majority of patients have low back pain

TABLE 7-2
Low Back Pain Syndromes

Diagnosis	History	Signs	Pathophysiology
Musculoskeletal/ligamentous	Symptoms begin acutely after specific lifting episode; can have a "tearing" sensation in the back; pain often radiates into the thigh but no further	Spasm Tenderness No radicular findings	Actual tearing of muscle and ligamentous fibers
Sciatica	Recurrent episodes of mild to moderate low back pain; over time increases in frequency, intensity; pain radiates into distal leg and is accompanied by weakness	a) L4–L5: L5 root—great toe extensors weak, dorsal foot pain b) L5–S1: S1 root—calf atrophy, decreased ankle reflex, lateral foot pain	Disk annulus herniates posteriorly
Facet disease (spondylolisthesis)	Chronic low back pain Rarely has radicular component	Minimal Radiographs showing 20% subluxation	Anterior subluxation of a vertebral body due to DJD of the facets
Compression fracture	Sudden onset of sharp pain at the level of the fracture	Tender over affected vertebra	Traumatic, or spontaneous, especially in the thoracic vertebra
Epidural disease	History of IV drug abuse, fevers, neoplasia, infections Slow, steady progression of pain, usually worse at night	Incontinence Fever Level of weakness or sensory deficit	Abscesses or tumor can form space-occupying compressive lesions
Ankylosing spondylitis	Morning stiffness Young males Systemically ill	Stiff	Rheumatoid variant

B O X 7 - 6

Overall Evaluation and Management of Low Back Pain

Evaluation

1. Take a history and perform a physical examination, including evaluating the range of motion and radicular findings (see text).
2. Obtain radiographs of the lumbosacral spine (see Table 7-3 for indications).
3. Perform urinalysis if any urinary symptoms are present to rule out urinary tract infection, pyuria, nephrolithiasis, or hematuria.
4. If the patient has sustained recent trauma, place on backboard until fracture is ruled out radiographically.

---

as a result of acute or chronic musculoskeletal or degenerative arthritic processes. Some of the most common causes are described below.

A. **Acute musculoskeletal or ligamentous sprain or strain**

　1. **Manifestations**

　　The **specific manifestations** of this cause include the acute onset of low back pain, usually unilateral but occasionally bilateral, precipitated by lifting heavy objects with improper technique. Often the patient relates a tearing sensation while lifting a heavy object and the acute onset of pain, or will present with discomfort within hours of the activity. The patient often describes short periods of similar pain in the past. When asked to describe or demonstrate the technique used to lift objects, the patient may describe lifting an object without flexing and extending the knees. **Examination** discloses spasm and tenderness of the involved back musculature but no radicular findings, including no neurologic deficits.

　2. **Pathogenesis**

　　The **underlying pathogenesis** is stretching or tearing of muscles and ligaments with resulting pain and inflammation.

　3. **Evaluation**

　　The **evaluation** of this common entity includes making the clinical diagnosis. **Radiographs** of the lumbosacral spine are of little to no benefit unless there are

T A B L E 7 - 3
Indications for Lumbosacral Radiography

Neoplastic process suspected
Compression fracture suspected
Ankylosing spondylitis suspected
Recent trauma
Recurrent pain
Fever with low back pain

atypical features to the pain syndrome or other data
make them indicated (see Table 7-3 for specific indications).

4. **Management**
   Specific management includes the following acute
   and long-term modalities.
   a. In the **acute** setting, **bed rest** for 7–14 days is nec-
      essary. Bed rest is central to management. The pa-
      tient must remain in bed, getting up only to use
      the bathroom, to minimize further trauma to the
      muscles and allow them to heal. Furthermore, an-
      algesia with an NSAID (see Table 7-1) or narcotic
      agents should be initiated. A **benzodiazepine** may
      be useful as an aid for **sleeping** only. There is no
      clear benefit to scheduled benzodiazepines for use
      as "muscle relaxants."
   b. **Long-term modalities** include educating the pa-
      tient in how to **sleep.** The patient should minimize
      sleeping on the back and instead sleep on the side
      with the knees flexed and a pillow between the
      knees. Furthermore, one can, with the guidance of
      a physical therapist, teach the patient to perform
      exercises including Williams' type exercises. The
      patient should be instructed on how to lift objects
      using the muscles of the legs and thighs, and not
      the back. Obese patients should be instructed to
      lose weight.

5. **Consultation**

Service	*Time*
Physical therapy	Elective

B. **Sciatica/herniated disk**
   1. **Manifestations**
      The **specific manifestations** of a herniated disk in-
      clude the acute or recurrent onset of mild to moderate
      low back pain radiating into one or, rarely, both distal
      lower extremities. Over time, the pain increases in
      intensity and frequency and may be associated with

weakness of the involved lower extremity. Upon **examination** there is weakness of the muscles innervated by the **L5** and **S1** nerve roots as manifested by great toe weakness and inability to perform a tiptoe walk for **S1** and a decreased ankle jerk with inability to perform a heel walk for **L5**. There invariably are concurrent posterolateral thigh and leg pain, paresthesias, and sensory deficits.

2. **Pathogenesis**

   The **underlying pathogenesis** is an acquired posterior herniation of an intervertebral disk, which may result in impingement or entrapment of the adjacent nerve root unilaterally.

3. **Evaluation**

   The **evaluation** of this common entity includes making the clinical diagnosis. **Radiographs** of the lumbosacral spine are of little to no benefit unless there are atypical features to the pain syndrome or unless other data make them indicated (see Table 7-3 for specific indications). **Nerve conduction studies** and EMG testing of the lower extremity to document the radiculopathy are indicated, as **slowing of conduction** will be present.

4. **Management**

   Specific management includes the following acute and long-term modalities.

   a. In the **acute setting, bed rest** for 7–14 days is necessary. Bed rest is central to management. The patient must remain in bed, getting up only to use the bathroom, to minimize further trauma to the muscles and allow them to heal. Furthermore, analgesia with an NSAID (see Table 7-1) or narcotic agents should be initiated. A **benzodiazepine** may be prescribed as an aid for **sleeping** only. There is no clear benefit to scheduled benzodiazepines for use as "muscle relaxants." If there is any evidence of muscle weakness or if the acute symptoms are refractory to basic management, **CT** and **myelography** or **MRI** of the lumbosacral spine are indicated, as these imaging studies will define the location and size of the herniation.

   b. **Long-term modalities** include educating the patient in how to **sleep.** The patient should minimize sleeping on the back and instead sleep on the side with the knees flexed and a pillow between the knees. Furthermore, one can, with the guidance of a physical therapist, teach the patient to perform exercises, including Williams' type exercises. Also, the patient should be instructed on how to

lift objects **using the legs and thighs,** and not the
back. Obese patients should be instructed to lose
weight.
5. **Consultation**

Service	Time
Physical therapy	Elective
Orthopedics	Elective

C. **Vertebral compression fracture**
   1. **Manifestations**
   The **specific manifestations** of this disorder include
   the acute onset of severe, sharp pain at the level of
   the fracture. An antecedent history of trauma is not
   necessary, as these fractures may occur spontaneously. The trauma that most commonly causes a compression fracture is a jump or fall onto the feet. The
   pain may radiate unilaterally or bilaterally in a band-
   like distribution. On **examination** there is significant
   tenderness over the affected vertebra. The pain is localized and can be severe. Concurrent findings are
   usually due to the underlying process. "Dowager's
   hump" is an accentuated thoracic kyphosis in patients with past compression fractures, especially in
   osteoporosis.
   2. **Pathogenesis**
   The **underlying pathogenesis** is loss of height (i.e.,
   compression) of a vertebral body. The compression
   may occur as a result of trauma or of loss of bone
   substance, which weakens the individual vertebral
   body. These disorders include **osteoporosis, neoplastic diseases,** and **infectious diseases.** The fractures
   can occur in any vertebral body, but some processes
   have a predilection for certain vertebral areas. In **osteoporosis,** usually the **thoracic vertebrae** are affected, whereas if the compression fracture is due to
   a **neoplastic process** (e.g., multiple myeloma) or an
   infectious process (e.g., osteomyelitis), it usually affects the **lumbar vertebrae.**
   3. **Evaluation**
   The **evaluation** of this entity includes making the
   clinical diagnosis. **Radiographs** of the affected areas
   will demonstrate the compression fracture. If there is
   any suspicion that this is a neoplastic or infectious
   process the ESR will be elevated, and serum protein
   electrophoresis should be performed, looking for a
   monoclonal gammopathy. If such a process is suspected, a bone scan, CT, and myelography or MRI are
   indicated to look for an epidural mass and concurrent

lesions. If an infectious or neoplastic process is suspected, CT-directed or direct (by orthopedics) biopsy is indicated for a specific diagnosis.

4. **Management**

   Specific management includes the following acute and long-term modalities.

   a. In the **acute setting, bed rest** for 7–14 days is necessary. Bed rest is central to management. The patient must remain in bed, getting up only to use the bathroom, to minimize further trauma to the muscles and allow them to heal. Analgesia with an NSAID or narcotic agents should be initiated. **Narcotic agents** may be necessary to treat the pain. A **benzodiazepine** may be prescribed as an aid for **sleeping.** There is no clear benefit to scheduled benzodiazepines for use as "muscle relaxants."

      i. If the fracture occurred as a result of **infection,** a bone biopsy, initiation of antibiotics, referral to infectious diseases and orthopedics, and admission are indicated.

      ii. If the fracture occurred as a result of a **neoplastic process,** referral to orthopedics and oncology is indicated.

   b. **Long-term modalities** include educating the patient on how to **sleep.** The patient should minimize sleeping on one's back and instead sleep on one's side with the knees flexed and a pillow between the knees. Furthermore, one can, with the guidance of a physical therapist, teach the patient to perform exercises including Williams' type exercises. Also, the patient should be instructed on how to appropriately lift objects **using the legs and thighs** and not the back. Finally, if the patient is obese he should be instructed to lose weight. If there is any evidence of muscle weakness, or if the acute symptoms are refractory to basic management, a **CT scan and myelogram,** or a **MRI** of the lumbosacral spine are indicated of the affected area, as these will define the location and size of the herniation.

5. **Consultation**

Problem	Service	Time
Neoplasia is suspected	Orthopedics	Urgent
Infection is suspected	Orthopedics	Urgent
Any weakness	Orthopedics	Emergent
	Physical therapy	Elective

D. **Facet disease (spondylolisthesis)**
1. **Manifestations**

   The **manifestations** of this disease include **chronic—** with acute exacerbations—or **recurrent** unilateral or bilateral low back pain. There is rarely any radicular component. On **examination** there is usually a **paucity** of specific findings, even when the patient presents with an **acute exacerbation** of the pain syndrome.

2. **Pathogenesis**

   The **underlying pathogenesis** is acquired anterior subluxation of a vertebral body upon an adjacent vertebral body, or spondylolisthesis. This condition occurs as a result of **degenerative joint disease (DJD)** of the facet joints.

3. **Evaluation**

   The **evaluation** of this common entity includes making the clinical diagnosis. **Radiographs** of the lumbosacral spine are of little to no benefit unless there are atypical features to the pain syndrome or unless other data make them indicated (see Table 7-3). **Nerve conduction studies** and EMG testing of the lower extremity to document the radiculopathy are indicated, as **slowing of conduction** will be present.

4. **Management**

   Specific management includes the following acute and long-term modalities.

   a. In the **acute setting, bed rest** for 7–14 days is necessary. Bed rest is central to management. The patient must remain in bed, getting up only to use the bathroom, to minimize further trauma to the muscles and allow them to heal. Analgesia with an NSAID (see Table 7-1) or narcotic agents should be initiated. A **benzodiazepine** may be prescribed as an aid for **sleeping.** There is no clear benefit to scheduled benzodiazepines for use as "muscle relaxants." If there is any evidence of muscle weakness or if the acute symptoms are refractory to basic management, **CT and myelography** or **MRI** of the lumbosacral spine are indicated, as these imaging studies will define the location and size of the herniation.

   b. **Long-term modalities** include educating the patient in how to **sleep.** The patient should minimize sleeping on the back and instead sleep on the side with the knees flexed and a pillow between the knees. Furthermore, one can, with the guidance of a physical therapist, teach the patient to perform exercises including Williams' type exercises. Also, the patient should be instructed on how to appropriately lift objects **using the legs and thighs** and not the back. Obese patients should be instructed to lose weight. In refractory cases, referral to orthopedics for potential surgical intervention is indicated.

5. **Consultation**

Service	Time
Physical therapy	Elective
Orthopedics	Elective

E. Ankylosing spondylitis

1. Manifestations

The **specific manifestations** include low back pain with a significant component of **morning stiffness.** The condition usually affects younger males and is associated with malaise, fatigue, and other systemic constitutional findings. On **examination** there is a marked abnormal **straightening** of the back, manifested specifically in loss of the normal thoracic kyphosis and lumbar lordosis. There is palpable tenderness over the sacroiliac joints, and a significant decrease in the normal range of motion of the back.

2. Pathogenesis

The **underlying pathogenesis** is a seronegative inflammatory arthritis that affects the central (**axial**) skeleton more than the peripheral (**appendicular**) skeleton. The specific inflammatory sites usually are in the **sacroiliac joints** bilaterally.

3. Evaluation

The **evaluation** of this disorder includes making the clinical diagnosis. **Radiographs** of the thoracic spine, the lumbosacral spine, and the pelvis reveal straightening of the spine and dense areas in and about the sacroiliac joints bilaterally. **Laboratory test** results are usually **normal**, including rheumatoid factor, although in active disease the erythrocyte sedimentation rate (ESR) is often elevated.

4. Management

The **specific management** includes **rest** and initiation of **scheduled NSAIDs** (see Table 7-1). The patient should be referred to physical therapy for exercises to increase the range of motion of the back and axial skeleton. Finally, expedient referral to rheumatology is indicated.

5. Consultation

Service	Time
Rheumatology	Urgent
Physical therapy	Elective

F. **Epidural disease**
   1. **Manifestations**
      The **manifestations** of this uncommon but serious form of low back pain include the subacute onset of a dull, boring pain that is constant and usually is worse at night. The pain can result in insomnia for the patient. There may be associated weakness of the lower extremities and the development of rectal and urinary bladder incontinence and retention of urine within the urinary bladder. An antecedent history of fevers, chills, and IV drug abuse should raise suspicion of an **infectious process** (i.e., an epidural abscess), whereas a past history of a **malignant neoplasm,** especially breast carcinoma, prostate carcinoma, or lymphoma, should raise suspicion of a metastatic epidural tumor. On **examination** there may be fever and, quite often, pain over the affected vertebra. There can be weakness of the musculature innervated by **L4, L5,** and the **sacral nerves.** This weakness is manifested by great toe weakness, weakness of foot dorsiflexion and foot plantar flexion, and inability to walk on the toes or heels. The **anal sphincter** may be weakened. Percussion may disclose an **enlarged fluid-filled urinary bladder.**
   2. **Pathogenesis**
      The **underlying pathogenesis** is disease from an **infectious source,** either endocarditis or an adjacent osteomyelitis, or from a malignant **neoplastic source.** The primary disease spreads either hematogenously (i.e., it metastasizes) or by contiguous spread from an adjacent site. The disease enters the epidural space and, with growth or an increase in size, results in **compression** of the spinal cord and thus damage to it. The most common pathogenic bacteria include *Streptococcus* and *Staphylococcus* spp. The most common malignant processes are the primary lesions of breast carcinoma, prostate carcinoma, and lymphoma.
   3. **Evaluation**
      The **evaluation** of this disorder includes making the clinical diagnosis and having an appropriately high clinical suspicion. **Radiographs** of the affected vertebral areas are indicated. Relevant **laboratory studies** include a complete blood cell count, blood cultures, ESR, bone scan, gallium scan, and emergency CT with myelography or, better, MRI. All of these studies are done on an emergency basis. The **CBC** will demonstrate a leukocytosis in an infectious process but will usually be normal in neoplastic disease. **Blood cultures,** if the process is infectious, will be positive for

the organism. **Bone scans** in neoplastic disease and infectious disease, including osteomyelitis, will show increased uptake in the area of bone adjacent to the epidural disease. A **gallium scan** will show greater uptake in infectious diseases relative to neoplastic disease. **MRI** will demonstrate and define the extent and size of the epidural mass.

4. **Management**

    Specific management includes emergent admission and consultation with the neurosurgery service for biopsy or drainage of the lesion. If the disease is neoplastic, the radiation oncology service should be consulted on an emergency basis. If the disease is infectious, drainage of the abscess, intravenous antibiotics, and consultation with infectious diseases are indicated.

5. **Consultation**

Service	*Time*
Neurosurgery	Emergent, in all cases
Infectious diseases	Urgent
Radiation oncology	Emergent, if neoplastic

G. **Indications for admission:** New neurologic deficits, intractable pain, any fevers (especially if osteomyelitis or endocarditis is possible), traumatic fracture, or any epidural mass demonstrated on MRI or myelography.

Monoarticular Arthritis

All mobile joints in the body are lined with the simple squamous epithelium, **synovium.** The synovium in the normal healthy state produces a small amount of fluid that functions as a lubricant for the joint. An inflammation of this lining or its adjacent structures within the joint is entitled **synovitis,** or, more colloquially, **arthritis.** If the arthritis involves only one joint, it is called **monoarticular arthritis.**

By definition, **acute arthritis** is the onset of specific findings within 2 weeks of presentation, whereas **chronic arthritis** consists of findings present for more than 2 weeks at the time of presentation.

I. **Crystal-induced arthropathies**

    These are not uncommon processes in which crystals of various chemical composition are deposited in the synovium of one or more joints with resultant acute arthritis.

    A. **Gout**

    1. **Manifestations**

        The **specific manifestations,** in addition to those described in Box 7-7, include the fact that gout has a

B O X 7 - 7

Overall Evaluation of Monoarticular Arthritis

Evaluation

1. Take a **history** and perform a **physical examination.**
   The classic findings of inflammation involving the affected joint are quite easily demonstrated. These
   findings include *tumor* (swelling), *dolor* (pain), *rubor*
   (redness), *calor* (warmth), and **decreased range of
   motion** of the involved joint. The patient may have a
   history of antecedent trauma or of similar manifestations in the same or different joint in the past. An
   effusion may be present in the affected joint.
2. Obtain **radiographs** in two views of the affected joint
   to look for fractures and soft tissue swelling (see Fig.
   7-2).
3. **Arthrocentesis** of the affected joint is mandatory.
   The following laboratory tests should be performed
   on the fluid in all cases:
   a. Gross assessment: bloody vs. clear vs. purulent.
   b. Crystal analysis using a polarizing microscope
      (see text).
   c. Gram stain of fluid, looking for polymorphonu-
      clear (PMN) cells and bacteria.
   d. Culture and sensitivity testing of fluid.
4. **Immobilize** the joint acutely if there is any evidence
   of trauma.
5. **Categorize** the process as crystal-induced, traumatic,
   or infectious.

---

predilection for certain joints. These joints include
the first metatarsophalangeal (MTP) joint (**podagra**),
the knee joint (**gonogra**), and the wrist (**chiragra**). The
patient rarely has any associated systemic manifestations and is virtually always afebrile.

2. **Pathogenesis**
   The **underlying pathogenesis** is an elevated total body
   uric acid level that sometimes manifests with an elevated serum uric acid level. Uric acid is a catabolite
   of the purine nucleosides. The rapid shift in serum
   uric acid levels, either an increase or a decrease, can
   precipitate deposition of **sodium monourate** crystals
   in a synovial space. The crystals induce inflammation

via several mechanisms, including prostaglandins and leukotrienes. The most clearly understood mechanism is the release of **crystal chemotactic factor (CCF)** from PMNs. The elevated total body uric acid levels may result from one or more of the following processes:

a. Excessive consumption of foods rich in purines and uric acid.

b. A partial or total congenital deficiency of the enzyme hypoxanthine-guanine phosphoribosyl transferase, an enzyme necessary for the catabolism of purines.

c. Saturnine gout, in which the ingestion of moonshine with lead (plumbism) will lead to renal failure and gout.

d. Lymphoproliferative disorder with increased nuclear catabolism and thus purine release and uric acid elevation.

3. Evaluation

The **specific evaluation** of this entity includes making the diagnosis by performing crystal analysis on the synovial fluid. The crystal chemical type is **sodium monourate.** These crystals have the physical property of **negative birefringence** as demonstrated on polarizing microscopy. Their polarizing properties are as follows:

a. Crystals parallel to the light: **yellow** crystals.

b. Crystals perpendicular to the light: **blue** crystals.

4. Management

The **specific management of gout** includes making the clinical diagnosis and initiating intervention in the acute setting (see Box 7-8), then preventing recurrence of the disease process. **Chronic therapy** for gout is based on the facts that there are several modalities to prevent future attacks and that once a patient has an episode of acute gout, he will desire never to experience another. **Preventive modalities** include the **abortion of an acute attack** with colchicine or an NSAID, an overall **adjustment in risk factor profile,** and initiation of **allopurinol.**

a. **Abortion of acute attacks.** This preventive method is effective, easy, and obviates long-term, potentially lifelong, daily medication. The abortion of an acute attack can be done with an NSAID, but the best agent to use is **colchicine.** The patient is instructed to take a dose of colchicine by mouth **as soon as** the attack starts, and to use the regimen described in Box 7-8.

b. **Decrease weight if obese** and decrease ethanol use,

B O X   7 - 8

Management of Acute Gout

Management

1. **Colchicine**
   a. The **mechanism of action** of this highly effective
      modality in the treatment of acute gout is that it
      inhibits the release of crystal chemotactic factor
      (CCF) from PMNs, thus specifically inhibiting in-
      flammation in gout. This agent is only mildly ef-
      fective in the treatment of pseudogout.
   b. **Dosage**
      i. **Oral:** The vast majority of patients can receive
         colchicine in the oral form. The dosage is 0.6
         mg PO now, repeated hourly until one of three
         things occurs: relief of symptoms, a total of six
         doses has been given, or diarrhea occurs. If
         relief occurs, continue dose of 0.6 mg PO b.i.d.
         If there is no response, rethink the diagnosis
         and attempt an NSAID (see Table 7-1).
      ii. **Intravenous:** 2 g of colchicine in normal saline
         over 15 minutes; give in house as a one-time
         dose and only if the patient clearly has gout
         and is unable to take PO.
   c. **Side effects** include diarrhea, which can be severe
      and dose limiting.
   d. The **duration** of therapy is 4–6 weeks and/or 2
      weeks after the initiation of chronic therapy, i.e.,
      allopurinol (if chronic therapy is indicated).
   e. A **caveat to therapy** is that colchicine is specific
      for gout; therefore, if relief occurs, it is **tanta-
      mount** to a diagnosis of gout.
2. **NSAIDs** (see Table 7-1)
   a. The **mechanism of action, dosages,** and **side ef-
      fects** are described in Table 7-1.
   b. The **duration** of therapy is 4–6 weeks and/or 2
      weeks after the initiation of chronic therapy, i.e.,
      allopurinol (if chronic therapy is indicated).
   c. A **caveat to therapy** with one of these agents is
      that these agents are nonspecific in their anti-
      inflammatory effects. Therefore, one must have
      evidence, based on arthrocentesis, to rule out any
      infectious etiology before initiating this treat-

(continued)

B O X   7 - 8 *(continued)*

> ment, which could easily mask but not treat an
> infection.
> 3. *Intra-articular steroids*
>   This modality is clearly effective. It should be re-
>   served for patients with arthrocentesis-proven mono-
>   articular gout who cannot take anything by mouth or
>   who have relative or absolute contraindications to
>   colchicine and an NSAID. Dose depends on the size
>   of the joint. In small joints (e.g., the metatarsopha-
>   langeal joint): 15–20 mg triamcinolone; in large
>   joints (e.g., the knee): 35–50 mg triamcinolone
>   should be intra-articularly administered.

both of which will decrease the risk of gout attacks.

   c. Allopurinol
      i. **Mechanism of action:** Agent is a xanthine oxi-
         dase inhibitor, i.e., it decreases the production
         of uric acid in the catabolism of purines.
     ii. **Dose:** 300 mg PO q.d. In patients with renal
         insufficiency the dosage must be adjusted
         downward to 100 mg PO q.d.
    iii. **Indications:** Limited, because aborting attacks
         is the prophylactic treatment of choice. In a
         minority of cases, however, allopurinol needs
         to be initiated and continued. These include
         patients with **recurrent gouty attacks,** pa-
         tients with **HGPRT deficiency,** patients who
         have concurrent **uric acid nephrolithiasis,** pa-
         tients with **tophaceous gout,** and patients who
         have or are being treated for **lymphoprolifera-
         tive disorders.**
     iv. **Side effect profile:** Limited. Side effects in-
         clude the rare cases of hepatic dysfunction,
         usually mild in nature.
      v. **Goals of use:** Not only the prevention of gouty
         attacks and uric acid nephrolithiasis, but also
         maintenance of the serum uric acid level in
         the 6–8 mg/dL range.
     vi. **Caveat:** During the first 2–3 weeks of therapy,
         the serum and body uric acid levels may para-
         doxically increase, with resultant increased
         risk of gouty attacks; thus, colchicine or an

NSAID must be administered for the first 2 weeks of therapy with allopurinol.

B. Pseudogout

1. Manifestations

The **specific manifestations** are similar to those listed in Box 7-7. The patient rarely has significant systemic manifestations and rarely, if ever, has a fever.

2. Pathogenesis

The **underlying pathogenesis** is the acute precipitation of **calcium pyrophosphate crystals** in the synovial space. The crystals induce inflammation by several mechanisms, including the release of prostaglandins and leukotrienes from PMNs. The underlying reason for the precipitation of such crystals is not completely known, but certain disease processes have been associated with it. These include primary hyperparathyroidism, secondary hyperparathyroidism, and chronic mild hypercalcemia of any cause.

3. Evaluation

The **specific evaluation** of this entity includes making the diagnosis by performing crystal analysis on the synovial fluid. The crystal chemical type is **calcium pyrophosphate.** These crystals have the physical property of **positive birefringence** on polarizing microscopy. Their polarizing properties are as follows:

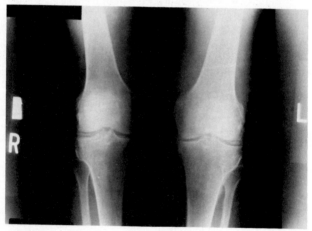

FIGURE 7-2
Radiograph of the knees, AP. The presence of calcium within the lateral compartments of the knees is consistent with the chondrocalcinosis of pseudogout.

a. Crystals parallel to the light: **blue** crystals.

b. Crystals perpendicular to the light: **yellow** crystals.

Furthermore, the evaluation should include determining the serum calcium, phosphorus, and albumin levels. If the calcium level is elevated, especially with a mild to modestly decreased serum phosphorus, an **intact PTH** (parathormone) level should be determined to rule out hyperparathyroidism.

4. **Management**

The **specific management of pseudogout** includes making the clinical diagnosis and initiating intervention in the acute setting (see Box 7-8), then preventing recurrence of the disease process. In the **acute setting** the drug of choice is an NSAID, as the efficacy of colchicine in pseudogout is significantly less than in gout. The **chronic therapy of pseudogout** is based on the facts that several modalities are helpful in preventing future attacks and that once a patient has had an episode of acute pseudogout, he will desire never to experience another. **Preventive modalities** include **aborting an acute attack with an NSAID,** and effective diagnosis and treatment of any of the associated or secondary causes (see Chapter 9).

C. **Consultation**

Service	*Time*
Rheumatology	Elective

II. **Inflammatory, nonseptic arthritis**

Polyarticular inflammatory arthritides of a chronic or acute nature (e.g., rheumatoid arthritis) can and do present with one joint affected before progressing (see section on Polyarticular Arthritis, page 432).

III. **Septic arthritis**

A. **Manifestations**

The **specific manifestations** of this entity, which is also known as infectious arthritis, include, in addition to those described in Box 7-7, the systemic features of fevers, chills, night sweats, and, quite often, an antecedent history of dysuria and pyuria. This etiology can result in severe sequelae, including loss of joint function and even death. Therefore, the diagnosis must be effectively ruled out in all patients presenting with monoarticular arthritis.

B. **Pathogenesis**

The **underlying pathogenesis** is bacterial infection of the synovial lining of the affected joint. The route of infection can entail **hematogenous spread, contiguous spread** from an adjacent cellulitis, bursitis, or osteomyelitis, or **traumatic** or **iatrogenic invasion** of the joint space by a compound fracture involving the joint or by arthrocentesis. The most common organisms that cause septic arthritis are *Neisseria gonorrhoeae, Hemophilus influenzae, Streptococcus* spp., and *Staphylococcus* spp.

1. *Neisseria gonorrhoeae*

   This **gram-negative diplococcus** is the most common organism to cause infectious arthritis in adults. The **natural history** is one in which there is, via sexual contact and transmission, an antecedent untreated gonococcal urethritis, proctitis, cervicitis, or pharyngitis with a concomitant bacteremia. The organism spreads **hematogenously** to the joint space, where inflammation/infection occurs.

2. *Hemophilus influenzae*

   This **gram-negative coccobacillus** is uncommon in adults but one of the most common causes of infectious arthritis in children. The **natural history** is one of **contiguous** spread of *H. influenzae* to the joint from an adjacent area of epiphyseal osteomyelitis, or by hematogenous spread from another source.

3. *Streptococcus* and *Staphylococcus*

   These **gram-positive cocci** in chains and clusters, respectively, are not uncommon causes of septic arthritis. The **natural history** is development by **contiguous spread,** either from an adjacent cellulitis or infectious bursitis or by introduction of organisms via arthrocentesis (rare) or, more commonly, via trauma (e.g., a compound fracture).

C. **Evaluation**

The specific **evaluation** includes the steps described in Box 7-7 and making the diagnosis by Gram stain and culture of the synovial fluid. In virtually all cases the diagnosis can be made from the Gram stain. If the organism is thought or diagnosed to be *N. gonorrhoeae*, examination and gonococcal cultures using Thayer–Martin plate media of the urethra, cervix, pharynx, and rectum are indicated.

D. **Management**

The specific **management** of infectious arthritis includes making the diagnosis using the evaluative tools listed above and intensive therapy, including the following measures:

1. **Complete drainage** of the fluid from the joint. If the fluid reaccumulates, as it often will, repeat needle drainage is necessary. Placement of a surgical drain

may be needed to completely and effectively drain the joint.

2. **Immobilize** the affected joint with appropriate splintage.
3. **Consultation** with orthopedics and infectious diseases experts is mandatory.
4. Initiation of **parenteral antibiotics,** including
    a. If *Neisseria gonorrhoeae* is suspected or diagnosed: Ceftriaxone, 1–2 g IV q.8h. for 10 days (see section on Sexually Transmitted Diseases in Chapter 6 for other mandatory concurrent antibiotic treatment).
    b. If **gram-positive cocci:** Nafcillin, 2 g IV q.8h., or cefazolin, 2 g IV q.8h., **and** an aminoglycoside for 10 days. An alternative is vancomycin, 1 g IV q.12h., for 10 days.
    c. If *Hemophilus influenzae:* Ampicillin, 2 g IV q.8h., or cefuroxime, 1.5 g IV q.8h., for 10 days.

E. **Consultation**

Problem	*Service*	*Time*
All	Orthopedics	Urgent
All	Infectious diseases	Urgent
Any STD	Public Health Service	Required

IV. Hemarthrosis

A. **Manifestations**

The **specific manifestations** of this entity include, in addition to those described in Box 7-7, an antecedent history of recent trauma to the joint. There are rarely any systemic manifestations and the patient is invariably afebrile.

B. **Pathogenesis**

The **underlying pathogenesis** is, in the vast majority of cases, traumatic damage to the intrinsic structures of the joint. The classic example is hemarthrosis associated with an acute tear of the anterior cruciate ligament of the knee. **Spontaneous** (non-trauma-related) hemarthrosis can occur as a result of **hemophilia A** or **hemophilia B,** in which bleeding into the joint can occur at any time and without any antecedent trauma.

C. **Evaluation**

The **evaluation** includes that described in Box 7-7. It is necessary to obtain **radiographs** of bones around the joint. Usually there is little doubt as to the diagnosis as the synovial fluid is grossly bloody; however, the fluid should be sent for all of the routine studies listed in Box 7-7, especially joint fluid culture to rule out concurrent or early infectious arthritis. Further assessment includes a detailed orthopedics examination of the affected joint and determining the platelet count, PT, and aPTT to rule out concurrent coagulopathy.

D. Management

The **specific management** of a hemarthrosis includes making the diagnosis and initiating intensive therapy, including the following steps:

1. **Complete drainage** of the joint of all fluid. Repeat arthrocentesis as necessary to keep the joint free of excess fluid.
2. **Immobilize** the affected joint with appropriate splintage.
3. Consult **orthopedics** on an urgent/emergent basis.
4. Initiate effective **analgesia,** including narcotics as necessary.
5. If the underlying cause is **hemophilia,** see section on Excessive Bleeding States in Chapter 5 for further evaluation and management.

E. Consultation

Service	Time
Orthopedics	Urgent
Physical therapy	Elective

V. Indications for admission: Septic arthritis, uncontrolled coagulopathy, or concurrent fracture of the bone involved in the articulation.

Polyarticular Arthritis, Acute or Chronic

The **synovium,** the simple squamous epithelial lining of the joint, may become inflamed as a result of a systemic inflammatory process or damaged by chronic trauma. As with monoarticular arthritis, the difference between **acute** and **chronic polyarticular arthritis** is based on the duration of symptoms—less than or more than 2 weeks—at the time of presentation.

I. Overall manifestations

The **overall manifestations** of polyarticular arthritis include those resulting from joint inflammation and those resulting from systemic inflammatory or from noninflammatory disease itself.

A. Joint manifestations

The **manifestations of joint inflammation** include the classic findings of *tumor* (swelling), *dolor* (pain), *rubor* (redness), *calor* (warmth), and loss of function. The pattern of joint involvement can be stratified using certain qualifying features. These features, which can be used to aid in the diagnosis of the underlying systemic disease, include:

1. The **number of joints** involved. Involvement of two to four joints is pauciarticular arthritis, whereas involvement of more than four joints is termed polyarticular arthritis.

2. The **degree of symmetry** of joint involvement. Various disease processes have varying degrees of symmetry, i.e., the concurrent involvement of same joints on contralateral sides.

3. The **size of the joints involved.** Some disease processes predominantly involve small joints (e.g., hands) or large joints (e.g., axial skeleton).

B. Systemic manifestations

The **systemic manifestations** can include those specific to the underlying disease itself, which will be discussed below, and the presence of the constitutional findings of fevers, easy fatigability, malaise, and stiffness of the joints, especially **morning stiffness.** As a rule of thumb, **inflammatory arthritides** (e.g., rheumatoid arthritis, Lyme, etc.) often have the systemic findings of malaise, fevers, and significant morning stiffness, whereas **noninflammatory processes** (e.g., osteoarthritis) manifest with pain but without any systemic findings.

II. Rheumatoid arthritis

A. Manifestations

The **specific manifestations** of this disorder can be divided into those occurring **early** in the course of the disease and those occurring **later.**

1. **Early manifestations** include an insidious onset of fatigue, morning stiffness, and arthralgias with an associated **symmetric** arthritis, usually initially involving the **small joints.** The first joints involved are in the digits of the hands and feet, i.e., the PIP and DIP joints. Furthermore, there can often be the acute development of **nontender rheumatoid nodules** over the extensor surfaces in 20%–40% of patients.

2. The **late manifestations** include sequelae of the inflammatory processes and include, but are far from limited to, **ulnar deviation** of the digits, joint **contractures,** and the development of "swan neck" deformities in the digits of the hands and feet, i.e., the PIP joint is hyperextended, the DIP has a flexion contracture or boutonnière deformities (the PIP has a flexion contracture, the DIP is hyperextended). Concurrent manifestations often include **carpal tunnel syndrome, tarsal tunnel syndrome,** and fevers.

B. **Pathogenesis**

The **underlying pathogenesis** is an immunologically mediated systemic disease that produces chronic inflammatory and destructive arthritis. The immune-mediated process can be demonstrated with a reactive rheumatoid factor (RF) test. Some variant syndromes will have different immune-mediated mechanisms and will be RF negative (see Table 7-5).

C. **Evaluation**

The **evaluation** of this disorder includes making the clinical diagnosis with the tools described in Box 7-9.

D. **Management**

The **specific management** includes **rest,** both **overall** and of the **affected joints.** One modality to rest the specific joints is to splint those which have active disease. In all cases, the patient should be referred to physical therapy for initiation of ROM exercises. NSAIDs (see Table 7-1) should be initiated. In all cases, especially when there is evidence of **active, erosive disease,** refer the patient to a **rheumatologist** for the initiation of treatment with **remission-inducing agents.** These include the first-line agent, **gold,** followed by one or more of the following:

Glucocorticoids systemically
Hydroxychloroquine
Penicillamine
Cyclophosphamide

B O X   7 - 9

Overall Evaluation of Polyarticular Arthritis

Evaluation

1. Take a **thorough history** and perform a **physical examination,** with particular emphasis on the **history** of any recent skin rashes, sore throat, exposure to ticks, exposure to hepatitis B, or past manifestations of inflammatory bowel disease. On **physical examination,** look for the presence of any rashes or erythema, conjunctivitis, pharyngitis, nodules over tendons, or tender hepatomegaly. Furthermore, a

(continued)

B O X 7 - 9 *(continued)*

thorough examination of all joints is mandatory, looking for decreased ROM, inflammatory findings, and contractures.
2. Based on the above findings, stratify the arthritis into inflammatory and noninflammatory types. The inflammatory arthritides produce systemic manifestations and all of the signs of inflammation, whereas the noninflammatory arthritides cause only pain and loss of function. The schemas for evaluation are based on this and include:
   a. **Noninflammatory and inflammatory**
      i. Arthrocentesis of any joint with an effusion to rule out any crystal-induced or septic arthritis.
      ii. Serum uric acid, calcium, phosphorus, albumin.
      iii. Radiographs of affected joints, especially if there is any loss of function, looking for any concurrent fractures and narrowing of the joint space size.
      iv. Chest radiographs in PA and lateral views, looking for any mass which may represent a non-small carcinoma causing the paraneoplastic syndrome, hypertrophic pulmonary osteoarthropathy.
      v. Lyme titer, serum; an ELISA assay for antibodies to *Borrelia burgdorferi*. If IgM elevated, indicative of recent infection.
      vi. Hepatitis B serology and LFTs to rule out any recent hepatitis B infection which can, in its prodrome, manifest with such an arthritis.
   b. **Inflammatory only**
      i. ESR. This nonspecific test for inflammation should be elevated if inflammatory.
      ii. Rheumatoid factor to aid in evaluation for rheumatoid arthritis. If negative, can still be a "rheumatoid variant."
      iii. Complete blood cell count with differential to look for concurrent autoimmune cytopenia.
      iv. ANA (see Table 7-4 for types and interpretation).
      v. BUN and serum creatinine to look for concurrent renal dysfunction.
      vi. Urinalysis with microscopic to look for concurrent renal dysfunction.

T A B L E 7 - 4
Types of Antinuclear Antibodies

Specific Antigen	Antigen Description	Associated Disease States and Sensitivity
ds DNA	Native, double-stranded DNA	Systemic lupus erythematosus Sensitivity: 70%
Histone	Protein associated with native, double-stranded DNA	Drug-induced DNA Sensitivity: 95% SLE Sensitivity: 70%
SS-A	Also known as Ro Non-histone protein associated with RNA	Sjögren's syndrome Sensitivity: 80%–85% SLE Sensitivity: 15%–20%
SS-B	Also known as La Non-histone protein associated with RNA	Sjögren's syndrome Sensitivity: 80%–85% SLE Sensitivity: 20%–25%
Sm	Smith antigen Non-histone protein associated with RNA	SLE Sensitivity: 35%–40% Specificity: 95%–100%
Nucleolar	Intranuclear processor of ribosomal RNA	Progressive systemic sclerosis (scleroderma) Sensitivity: 45%–50%
Centromere	Protein to which the chromatids attach during meiosis and mitosis	Progressive systemic sclerosis (scleroderma) Sensitivity: 50%–60% CREST syndrome Sensitivity: 80%–90%

    E. **Consultation**

Service	Time
Rheumatology	Urgent
Physical therapy	Required

III. **Osteoarthritis**
    A. **Manifestations**
        The **specific manifestations** of this very common disorder, one which has a prevalence of 20%–30% in the geriatric population, include chronic and/or recurrent dull pain in any or all joints. The most commonly involved joints are **large joints** and include the knees, hips, and hands. The distribution can be symmetric or asymmetric in nature. The manifestations usually improve with activity or after a hot bath. There is no associated stiffness

T A B L E 7 - 5
Rheumatoid Variant Syndromes

Syndrome	HLA-B27	Rheumatoid Factor	Appendicular Joints	Axial Skeleton	Associated Manifestations
Reiter's syndrome	Positive	Negative	Lower extremity more involved than upper extremity joints	Mild disease Asymmetric	Uveitis Conjunctivitis Urethritis Aortic insufficiency
Ankylosing spondylitis	Positive	Negative	Lower extremity more involved than upper extremity joints	Marked disease Symmetric Sacroiliitis	Aortic insufficiency
Psoriatic arthropathy	Negative	Negative	Upper extremity more involved than lower extremity joints	Mild disease Asymmetric	Psoriasis
Inflammatory bowel disease	Negative	Negative	Lower extremity more involved than upper extremity joints	Mild disease Symmetric	Crohn's disease Ulcerative colitis Sclerosing cholangitis Uveitis Aortic insufficiency

or swelling of the affected joints, nor are there any systemic manifestations. On **examination,** there often is the nonspecific finding of **crepitus** in the affected joints, especially at the base of the thumb. There usually are **Bouchard's nodes** (nontender nodules at the PIP joints) and/or **Heberden's nodes** (nontender nodules at the DIP joints of the digits of the hands and/or feet).

B. **Pathogenesis**

The **underlying pathogenesis** of this disorder is an idiopathic degenerative noninflammatory arthritis that is nonsystemic. Predisposing factors include **trauma** to the joints, Legg–Calvé–Perthes disease of the hips, and **obesity.**

C. **Evaluation**

The **evaluation** of this entity includes making the clinical diagnosis with the tools described in Box 7-9. Laboratory findings in this type of arthritis are invariably normal, and thus routine laboratory evaluative tests for the clinical diagnosis of osteoarthritis are not indicated.

D. **Management**

The **specific management** of this disorder includes **rest** of the affected joint(s), including the use of a **cane** if the joint affected is the hip or knee. Obese patients should lose weight. Referral to **physical therapy** for ROM exercises and muscle strengthening exercises is indicated. For pain relief, especially to encourage activity, NSAIDs can be prescribed.

1. If the patient is refractory to the above therapy, especially if one joint is significantly more symptomatic than the rest, injection of the affected joint with triamcinolone, 15–20 mg for a **small joint,** 35–50 mg for a **large joint,** is an effective modality that usually affords 3–6 months of relief. Before intra-articular glucocorticoids are administered, however, the patient must be informed that this treatment modality may accelerate the osteoarthritic process.

2. If refractory manifestations develop, referral to **orthopedics for surgical intervention** involving replacement of the affected joint, especially if the joint is a hip or knee, is indicated.

E. **Consultation**

Service	Time
Orthopedics	Elective
Physical therapy	Elective

IV. **Systemic lupus erythematosus**

A. **Manifestations**

The **specific manifestations** of this not uncommon disorder include an insidious onset of fatigue; diffuse, symmetric **arthralgias;** fevers; and frothy urine as a result of proteinuria. Further manifestations can include recurrent Raynaud's phenomenon and recurrent aphthous ulcers in the mouth. The patient also often has **pleuritic and pericardial chest pain** as a result of inflammation of these mesothelial linings. On examination there may be a malar **erythematous rash** of the face, mild inflammation of some joints, especially the small joints of the hands and feet, and **pitting edema,** which can approach anasarca if the patient has developed nephrotic syndrome.

B. **Pathogenesis**

The **underlying pathogenesis** is an autoimmune systemic disease that manifests with **inflammation** of many of the organ systems of the body, including the CNS, kidneys, hematologic system, and joints. The specific pathogenesis remains unclear, although there is a component of an **abnormal immune surveillance system** and a probable **decrease** in the overall number of **T-suppressor cells** relative to helper cells.

C. **Evaluation**

The **evaluation** of this entity includes making the clinical diagnosis with the tools described in Box 7-9. The American Rheumatologic Association (ARA) criteria for the diagnosis of systemic lupus erythematosus are given in Table 7-6.

T A B L E   7 - 6
Criteria for Systemic Lupus Erythematosus

Cytopenias
    Anemia, may be Coombs positive
    Granulocytopenia
    Immune-mediated thrombocytopenia
Malar rash, erythematous
Serositis
    Peritonitis
    Pericarditis
    Pleuritis
Alopecia
Proteinuria, may be nephrotic range
Photosensitivity
RBC casts on urinalysis
Cerebritis, may manifest as psychosis or seizure disorder
Raynaud's phenomenon
Discoid lupus
False-positive VDRL
Recurrent aphthous-type ulcers
Positive serology, including ANA (see Table 7-4)

(From Tan EM et al: The 1982 revised criteria for the classification of systemic lupus erythematosus (SLE). Arthritis Rheum 1982;25:1271.)

D. Management

The **specific management** is directed toward symptomatic relief and the treatment of the systemic disorder, which will help resolve the symptoms. As with other inflammatory processes, cornerstones of therapy include **rest,** initiation of **NSAIDs,** and referral to **rheumatology** and **physical therapy** in an expedient fashion. If there is evidence of an active glomerulonephritis (i.e., renal failure and red cell casts on urinalysis), consultation with **nephrology** is indicated for assistance and for the potential of performing a diagnostic renal biopsy. Furthermore, in active disease, the initiation of **high-dose glucocorticoids,** e.g., prednisone, 60–80 mg PO q.d., is clearly indicated.

1. Specific indications for **initiation of glucocorticoids** include:
    a. Severe serositis.
    b. Hemolysis (Coombs positive).
    c. Immune-mediated thrombocytopenia.
    d. Psychosis as a result of lupus cerebritis.
    e. Glomerulonephritis, especially membranous type.
2. Other **immunosuppressive agents** which can be initiated under the direction of a rheumatologist in patients with severe symptomatic SLE include cyclophosphamide (Cytoxan) and hydroxychloroquine. Hydroxychloroquine in a dose of 200 mg PO b.i.d. is especially effective if there is a significant component of **discoid lupus,** i.e., significant skin and mucosal involvement.

E. Consultation

Service	Time
Rheumatology	Urgent
Physical therapy	Elective

V. Rheumatic fever

A. Manifestations

The **specific manifestations** of this rare yet important entity include an antecedent exudative pharyngitis which was not treated with antibiotics but has recently clinically resolved. The patient now presents with a several-day history of fevers, constitutional signs and symptoms, the development of heart valve dysfunction as manifested by murmurs, and polyarticular arthritis. Other manifestations include those described as **Jones' criteria: polyarticular arthritis, pancarditis** (i.e., pericarditis, myocarditis with heart failure, and valvulitis with new heart murmurs), **erythema marginatum, subcutaneous nodules,** and **choreiform movements.**

B. **Pathogenesis**

The **underlying pathogenesis** is a systemic immune-mediated illness occurring as a result of recent infection with Group A β-hemolytic streptococci.

C. **Evaluation**

The **specific evaluation** includes that described in Box 7-9 and obtaining a **pharyngeal culture** on the chance that β-hemolytic streptococci are present. Also, in order to document a recent streptococcal infection, a serum **antistreptolysin antibody (ASO) titer** should be obtained. Echocardiography to document valvular, myocardial, and pericardial function is indicated.

D. **Management**

The **specific management** includes initiation of NSAIDs and an antistreptococcal antibiotic, either penicillin or erythromycin, for 10 days. Once the diagnosis is made or highly suspected, the patient will need **long-term prophylaxis** with penicillin. An effective regimen is benzathine penicillin (Bicillin) IM every 2 weeks or erythromycin, 250 mg PO b.i.d. Finally, the patient will need one of the **"high-risk" prophylactic antibiotic regimens** for any invasive or dental procedures (see section on Bacterial Endocarditis in Chapter 6).

E. **Consultation**

Service	*Time*
Infectious diseases	Urgent
Cardiology	If any heart failure; urgent

VI. **Other causes of polyarticular arthritis**

A. **Hepatitis B prodrome**

In the prodromal stage of acute hepatitis B, before there is any evidence of hepatic inflammation, there may be a period of weeks to months of pauciarticular to polyarticular arthralgias and even frank arthritis (see section on Hepatitis in Chapter 2).

B. **Lyme disease**

This infectious disease can, in its late, untreated stages, manifest with chronic polyarticular arthritis. The patient often vacationed at or lives in a geographic area where this infection, due to the spirochete *Borrelia burgdorferi*, is endemic. These geographic areas include the northeastern and the upper midwestern areas of the United States. A history of a tick bite, the rash of **erythema chronicum migrans,** and an IgM Lyme titer elevation are helpful in making the diagnosis. The **specific management,** after making the diagnosis or suspecting it, includes the initiation of antibiotics, either **doxycycline,**

100 mg PO b.i.d., and/or a **third-generation cephalosporin** IV for a duration of **4–6 weeks.** Consultations with infectious diseases and rheumatology are clearly indicated.

VII. **Indications for admission:** Recurrent fevers of undetermined origin, acute renal failure, intensely active acute inflammatory disease, the acute onset of lupus cerebritis, or evidence of valvular failure in acute rheumatic fever.

Shoulder (Box 7-10)

The **normal movements** of the shoulder joint and the normal range of motion for each are described below. These motions and ranges are relative to the neutral position, i.e., the anatomic position with the arm hanging down at the side.

External rotation:	90°
Internal rotation:	90°
Extension:	50°
Flexion:	180°
Abduction:	180°
Adduction:	50°

B O X 7 - 1 0

Overall Evaluation and Management of Shoulder Pain

Evaluation

1. Take a history and perform a physical examination, including range of motion and assessment of the function of the arteries and nerves of the upper extremity, as deficits may occur as a result of shoulder damage.
2. Obtain radiographs of the shoulder, especially if there is a history of trauma or falls, looking for fractures, dislocations, or separation.

Management

1. Immobilize the joint if fracture is suspected.
2. Refer to physical therapy.

I. Dislocation of the glenohumeral joint

There are two types, anterior and posterior glenohumeral shoulder dislocations.

A. Anterior glenohumeral dislocation

1. **Manifestations**

   The **manifestations** include an acute onset of unilateral shoulder pain and markedly decreased range of motion of the joint. Often the patient has had similar episodes in the past. On examination, the acromion is inappropriately prominent and the head of the humerus is anteriorly and medially displaced to a position beneath the coracoid process. Furthermore, there is a "Napoleon Bonaparte" presentation: the patient holds the arm close to the body with the elbow flexed. There is complete loss of passive or active adduction of the arm at the shoulder.

2. **Pathogenesis**

   The **underlying pathogenesis** is **anterior and medial** displacement of the head of the humerus from the glenohumeral joint (Fig. 7-3). This usually occurs during an activity which requires **hyperextension of the arm,** such as pitching a baseball or an overhand tennis serve. Overall, 95% of all shoulder dislocations are of this type.

3. **Evaluation**

   The **evaluation** of this disorder is to make the clinical diagnosis and to carefully assess and document the function of the axillary nerve and artery, as these structures can be damaged during the dislocation. **Radiographs** of the shoulder and humerus are required to document the dislocation and determine if a concurrent humeral head fracture is present.

4. **Management**

   The **specific management** is one of analgesia and reduction of the dislocation. If the primary care physician has not been trained in reducing an anteriorly dislocated shoulder or if there is any evidence of neurovascular compromise or if there is a concurrent fracture, emergency consultation with orthopedics should be obtained.

   After reduction, the patient must keep the shoulder immobilized in a shoulder sling for **4–6 weeks.** Physical therapy should be consulted for long-term assistance in management of this entity.

5. **Consultation**

Service	*Time*
Orthopedics	Urgent/emergent
PT	Elective

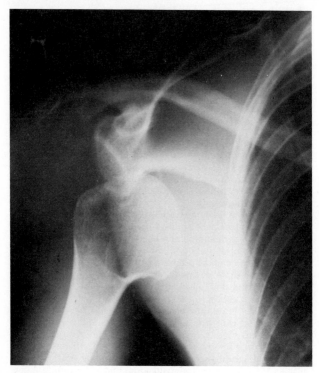

F I G U R E 7 - 3
Radiograph of shoulder, AP: Anterior dislocation of the humerus from
the glenohumeral joint. Note the position of the humeral head
inferior and even slightly medial to the coracoid process.

B. **Posterior glenohumeral dislocation**
   1. **Manifestations**
      The **manifestations** of this rare type of dislocation
      include the sudden inability to use the shoulder for
      any movement with the development of pain and dis-
      comfort in that joint. There may be no history of ante-
      cedent trauma that the patient recalls. This entity can
      be a sequela of a generalized tonic–clonic seizure.
      Upon examination, the arm is usually hanging in a
      neutral position and upon examination, it is difficult,
      if not impossible, to assess where indeed the humeral
      head is located.

2. **Pathogenesis**

   The **underlying pathogenesis** is **posterior** and **inferior displacement** of the head of the humerus from the glenohumeral joint. The humerus is located immediately posterior to the acromion. Displacement usually occurs as a result of weakening of the joint due to old trauma. Overall, less than 5% of shoulder dislocations are of this type.

3. **Evaluation**

   The **evaluation** of this disorder is the make the clinical diagnosis and to assess and document the function of the axillary nerve and artery as these structures can often be damaged during the dislocation. **Radiographs** of the shoulder and humerus are required to document the dislocation and determine if a concurrent humeral head fracture is present.

4. **Management**

   The **specific management** is one of analgesia and reduction of the dislocated humeral head. In all cases emergency consultation with orthopedics to reduce the dislocation should be obtained.

   After reduction, the patient must keep the shoulder immobilized in a shoulder sling for **4–6 weeks.** Physical therapy should be consulted for long-term assistance in management.

5. **Consultation**

Service	*Time*
Orthopedics	Emergent
PT	Elective

II. **Shoulder separation syndromes**

   There are two basic types of shoulder separation, **acromioclavicular** and **sternoclavicular.**

   A. **Acromioclavicular separation**

   1. **Manifestations**

      The **manifestations** of this entity include an acute onset of severe pain and swelling over the acromion, usually precipitated by an episode of trauma involving the symptomatic shoulder. On **examination,** the distal clavicle is superiorly displaced from the acromion. The patient is unable to actively abduct or flex the ipsilateral arm. In most cases the separation of the clavicle from the acromion is palpable and thus the diagnosis is quite evident on examination.

   2. **Pathogenesis**

      The **underlying pathogenesis** is trauma involving force exerted against the shoulder with an inferoposterior thrust, e.g., running into a door with the shoulder or being tackled by a football linebacker.

3. **Evaluation**

The **evaluation** is to make the clinical diagnosis and to immobilize the shoulder. Shoulder **radiographs** will confirm the clinical diagnosis and may demonstrate concurrent fractures or lesions.

4. **Management**

After immediate immobilization and initiation of analgesia, an orthopedic surgeon must be consulted on an emergency or urgent basis. Physical therapy should be consulted for long-term assistance in management.

5. **Consultation**

Service	*Time*
Orthopedics	Urgent/emergent
PT	Elective

B. **Sternoclavicular separation**

1. **Manifestations**

The **manifestations** include the acute onset of severe pain and some swelling about the sternoclavicular joint. The examining physician will hear or the patient will report a clicking sensation or sound with any movement of the affected upper extremity. This quite uncommon entity is the result of significant trauma to the superior chest wall. On examination the patient is usually in great discomfort and the clavicle on the affected side is displaced anteriorly from the sternum, thus making the diagnosis quite evident on inspection and palpation of the structures involved.

2. **Pathogenesis**

The **underlying pathogenesis** is significant trauma to the chest and chest wall, such as blunt trauma sustained during a motor vehicle accident during which the patient sustained a rapid deceleration impact against the steering wheel.

3. **Evaluation**

The **evaluation** of this entity is to make the clinical diagnosis and to immobilize the shoulder. **Radiographs** of the shoulder, sternum, chest, and clavicle should be obtained to confirm the clinical diagnosis and to look for any concurrent fractures or sequelae, such as pneumothorax as a result of the blunt trauma.

4. **Management**

The **specific management** includes, after immediate immobilization and initiation of analgesia, emergent consultation with an orthopedic surgeon for surgical intervention. Physical therapy should be consulted for acute and chronic assistance in management.

5. Consultation

Service	Time
Orthopedics	Emergent
PT	Elective

III. **Fractures**

The two most common fractures of bony structures involving the shoulder are fractures of the **humeral head** and the **clavicle.**

A. **Humeral head fracture**

1. **Manifestations**

The **manifestations** of this entity include an acute onset of severe pain in the proximal arm and shoulder with severe limitation of shoulder and arm movement. It is not uncommon for the patient to have a concurrent **anterior glenohumeral dislocation.** There invariably is a recent history of significant trauma to the affected shoulder, at which time the manifestations began.

2. **Pathogenesis**

The **underlying pathogenesis** is trauma to the shoulder with associated hyperextension of the humerus. Many of the same traumatic experiences that result in anterior glenohumeral dislocations also can result in humeral head fractures. The fracture itself is either a simple or a compound fracture of the **proximal humerus.**

3. **Evaluation**

The **evaluation** is to make the clinical diagnosis and to immobilize the shoulder and arm in an expedient manner. One must assess the patient for a concurrent anterior glenhumeral dislocation. Furthermore, the function of the axillary artery and nerve must be assessed and documented from the outset, as these structures can be damaged. **Radiographs** of the shoulder and humerus are indicated and confirm the diagnosis.

4. **Management**

Emergent consultation with orthopedics is clearly indicated. Physical therapy should be consulted for assistance in the acute and chronic management of this entity.

5. **Consultation**

Service	Time
Orthopedics	Emergent
PT	Elective

B. Clavicular fracture

1. **Manifestations**

   The **manifestations** of this not uncommon entity include an acute onset of pain and swelling over the collarbone (clavicle). Upon examination, the patient is unable to abduct or elevate the entire upper extremity and, upon inspection and palpation, the fracture is quite evident.

2. **Pathogenesis**

   The **underlying pathogenesis** is direct trauma to the shoulder or anterior superior chest wall, usually as the result of a fall.

3. **Evaluation**

   The **evaluation** of this fracture includes making the clinical diagnosis and immediately immobilizing the upper extremity in a sling. **Radiographs** of the shoulder and clavicle are indicated to confirm the diagnosis and look for any other bony abnormalities.

4. **Management**

   Referral to orthopedics on an urgent/emergent basis is clearly indicated. Physical therapy should be consulted for assistance in acute and chronic management.

5. **Consultation**

Service	*Time*
Orthopedics	Emergent
PT	Elective

IV. Tendinitis/bursitis

A. Bicipital tendinitis

1. **Manifestations**

   The **manifestations** of this quite common entity include pain in the anterior shoulder and tenderness over the **bicipital groove,** the anatomic groove through which the long head of the biceps muscle passes on the proximal humerus, between the greater and lesser tubercles. On **examination** there is tenderness in the bicipital groove and a positive **Yergason's sign,** i.e., the reproduction of pain on flexion of the elbow and supination of the forearm.

2. **Pathogenesis**

   The **underlying pathogenesis** is noninfectious inflammation of the long head of the biceps in the bicipital groove. It usually occurs after the initiation of a new activity involving the shoulder or overuse of the shoulder in a throwing activity, classically the **overhand pitch** in baseball.

3. **Evaluation**

The **evaluation** of this disorder includes making the clinical diagnosis and **preventing** any potential **complications,** including subacromial bursitis and the disuse atrophy syndrome of adhesive capsulitis (see below). Unless other atypical manifestations are present or there is a history of recent significant trauma, **radiographs** of the shoulder and humerus are usually of little benefit.

4. **Management**

The **specific management** is time sensitive, i.e., dependent on when the patient presents with the injury.

   a. **Acute management.** If the patient is seen immediately after onset of symptoms, i.e., within 30 minutes, apply ice to the shoulder for 20–30 minutes. In all cases this is followed by a 3–4-day period of shoulder rest with **proscription** of any overhead arm activity. This can be accomplished by placing the involved arm **in a sling** to keep the arm close to the body, the elbow flexed, and shoulder movement minimized. Furthermore, the initiation of an NSAID is usually of clinical benefit.

   b. **Subacute and chronic management.** After initial therapy the patient should be referred to physical therapy and begin **Codman exercises,** pendular exercises in which the arm is dangled in front and slowly moved side to side, front to back, and in slowly increasing circles. This along with an NSAID should continue for the next 14 days. If at the end of the above therapy, i.e., approximately 3 weeks, there is no improvement, referral to an orthopedic surgeon or injection of the bicipital groove is indicated. The injection is with 15–20 mg triamcinolone around, **not into,** the biceps tendon.

5. **Consultation**

Service	Time
Orthopedics	Elective
PT	Elective

B. **Subacromial bursitis**

1. **Manifestations**

The **manifestations** include pain in the anterior aspect of the shoulder associated with painful movements of the shoulder itself. It quite often is concurrent with **bicipital tendinitis.** On examination there are significant tenderness over the anterior and inferior aspects of the acromion and the development of

signs of impingement, including a positive impingement test, i.e., pain over the anterior acromion when
the patient's arm is maximally passively flexed and
the examiner presses upon the shoulder girdle, and,
quite often, the findings of bicipital tendinitis.

2. **Pathogenesis**

    The **underlying pathogenesis** is noninfectious in-
    flammation of the subacromial bursa. This is a large
    bursa located **inferior and anterior** to the acromion.
    This entity is associated with, and can be precipitated
    or exacerbated by, the same activities as bicipital ten-
    dinitis.

3. **Evaluation**

    The **evaluation** of this disorder includes making the
    clinical diagnosis and **preventing** any potential **com-
    plications,** including the disuse atrophy syndrome of
    adhesive capsulitis (see below). Unless other atypical
    manifestations are present or there is a history of re-
    cent significant trauma, **radiographs** of the shoulder
    and humerus are usually of little benefit.

4. **Management**

    The **specific management** is time sensitive, i.e., de-
    pendent on when the patient presents with the injury.

    a. **Acute management.** If the patient is seen immedi-
       ately after onset of symptoms, i.e., within 30 min-
       utes, apply ice to the shoulder for 20–30 minutes.
       In all cases this is followed by a 3–4-day period
       of shoulder rest with **proscription** of any overhead
       arm activity. This can be accomplished by placing
       the involved arm **in a sling** to keep the arm close
       to the body, the elbow flexed, and the shoulder
       movement minimized. Initiation of an NSAID is
       usually of clinical benefit.

    b. **Subacute and chronic management.** After initial
       therapy, the patient should be referred to physical
       therapy and begin **Codman exercises,** pendular ex-
       ercises in which the arm is dangled in front and
       slowly moved side to side, front to back, and in
       slowly increasing circles. This along with an
       NSAID should continue for the next 14 days. If at
       the end of the above therapy, i.e., approximately
       3 weeks, there is no improvement, either referral
       to an orthopedic surgeon or injection of the sub-
       acromial bursa is indicated. The injection is with
       15–20 mg triamcinolone.

Service	Time
Orthopedics	Elective
PT	Elective

C. Supraspinatus tendinitis

1. Manifestations

The **manifestations** of this entity include pain in the anterior and lateral aspects of the shoulder which can be, by history, acute or recurrent or chronic with acute exacerbations. On examination there is significant tenderness over and adjacent to the greater tuberosity of the humerus and the acromion process.

2. Pathogenesis

The **underlying pathogenesis** of this entity, also known as **calcific tendinitis,** is noninfectious inflammation of the rotator cuff tendons in general and of the supraspinatus tendon in specific. This is often exacerbated or precipitated by activities that require arm and shoulder abduction or elevation. A classic example is the **side arm pitch.**

3. Evaluation

The **evaluation** of this disorder includes making the clinical diagnosis and **preventing** any potential **complications** including the disuse atrophy syndrome of adhesive capsulitis (see below). **Radiographs** of the shoulder and humerus are of benefit in the evaluation of this entity given the fact that calcium is usually present in the supraspinatus tendon.

4. Management

The **specific management** is time sensitive, i.e., dependent on when the patient presents with the injury.

   a. Acute management. If the patient is seen immediately after onset of symptoms, i.e., within 30 minutes, apply ice to the shoulder for 20–30 minutes. In all cases this is followed by a 3–4-day period of shoulder rest with **proscription** of any overhead arm activity. This can be accomplished by placing the involved arm **in a sling** to keep the arm close to the body, the elbow flexed, and the shoulder movement minimized. Initiation of an NSAID is usually of clinical benefit.

   b. Subacute and chronic management. After initial therapy, the patient should be referred to physical therapy and begin **Codman exercises,** pendular exercises in which the arm is dangled in front and slowly moved side to side, front to back, and in slowly increasing circles. This along with an NSAID should continue for the next 14 days. If at the end of the above therapy, i.e., approximately 3 weeks, there is no improvement, either referral to an orthopedic surgeon or injection of the shoulder itself is indicated. The injection is with 15–20 mg triamcinolone.

5. **Consultation**

Service	Time
Orthopedics	Elective
PT	Elective

D. **Rotator cuff tears**
   1. **Manifestations**

      The **manifestations** of this entity include pain over the deltoid muscle which is exacerbated by any overhead arm movement. Concurrently range of motion of the affected shoulder is decreased. There is a wide spectrum in the intensity of pain associated with the tear. It may be quite painful in young patients but only minimally painful in the elderly. On examination there are tenderness over the greater tuberosity of the humerus and weakness of the motions of **abduction and external rotation** of the arm at the shoulder. The **passive** range of motion of the arm is normal, but **active** motion, especially abduction, is significantly limited.

   2. **Pathogenesis**

      The **underlying pathogenesis** is a tear of one or more of the tendons or muscles which compose the rotator cuff, i.e., the supraspinatus, the infraspinatus, and/or the teres minor. The quantity of force required to cause a rotator cuff tear is largely dependent on the age and health of the patient. Significant trauma or force is required in young athletes, but in the elderly a tear can occur with minimal force.

   3. **Evaluation**

      The **evaluation** of this disorder includes making the clinical diagnosis and **preventing** any potential **complications,** including subacromial bursitis and the disuse atrophy syndrome of adhesive capsulitis (see below). Unless other atypical manifestations are present or there is a history of recent significant trauma, **radiographs** of the shoulder and humerus are usually of little benefit.

   4. **Management**

      The **specific management** is time sensitive, i.e., dependent on when the patient presents with the injury.

      a. **Acute management.** If the patient is seen immediately after initiation of symptoms, i.e., within 30 minutes, apply ice to the shoulder for 20–30 minutes. In all cases this is followed by a 3–4-day period of shoulder rest with **proscription** of any overhead arm activity. This can be accomplished by placing the involved arm **in a sling** to keep the arm close to the body, the elbow flexed, and the shoulder movement minimized. Initiation of an NSAID is usually of clinical benefit.

b. Subacute and chronic management. After initial therapy, the patient should be referred to physical therapy and begin **Codman exercises,** pendular exercises in which the arm is dangled in front and slowly moved side to side, front to back, and in slowly increasing circles. This along with the above initiated NSAID should continue for the next 14 days. Virtually all cases, especially those in young patients or if there are severe symptoms, require an orthopedics consultation.

5. Consultation

Service	Time
Orthopedics	Urgent
PT	Elective

E. Biceps tendon rupture

1. Manifestations

The **manifestations** of this entity include an acute or subacute onset of weakness in **flexion and supination** of the forearm. If acute and traumatic, there usually is associated pain in the area of the proximal biceps muscle and biceps tendon. On examination there are a significant weakness of the flexion and supination of the forearm and a **single hump** of noncontracting muscle in the area of the biceps muscle.

2. Pathogenesis

The **underlying pathogenesis** is rupture of the biceps tendon as a result of **trauma** or of **injection of steroids** into the bicipital groove.

3. Evaluation and management

The **evaluation and management** of this disorder involve making the clinical diagnosis. Radiographs are not indicated unless there is an atypical history or recent trauma. Analgesia and referral to orthopedics and physical therapy are indicated.

4. Consultation

Service	Time
Orthopedics	Urgent
PT	Elective

F. "Frozen shoulder"

1. Manifestations

The **manifestations** of this entity include chronic, diffuse pain and tenderness about the glenohumeral joint anteriorly and posteriorly. On examination there are a significant decrease in ROM both to active and passive motion, often associated significant pain, and crepitus with any movement.

2. **Pathogenesis**

The **underlying pathogenesis** of this entity, which is also known as **adhesive capsulitis,** is the end result of many of the chronic shoulder problems, especially if the shoulder is not appropriately immobilized in the acute setting, causing further damage, or is immobilized for an excessive duration of time. It is the nonspecific end result of recurrent trauma or inflammation of the shoulder joint.

3. **Evaluation and management**

The **evaluation and management** of this disorder involve making the clinical diagnosis and, most important, **prevention. Radiographs** of the shoulder may be of some utility in determining if there are any concurrent lesions, including fractures and dislocations, and thus are indicated. The **prevention** is via encouraging patients to present to a physician when they develop pain in their shoulder and aggressively manage as appropriate for each entity. Once present, NSAIDs PRN and consultation with physical therapy for activities to increase the range of motion of the shoulder are indicated on a long-term basis.

4. **Consultation**

Service	*Time*
Orthopedics	Required
PT	Required

G. **Indications for admission:** Any open fracture, the concurrent presence of a humeral head fracture with a dislocation of the humerus from the glenohumeral joint, or any evidence of neurovascular compromise in the affected upper extremity.

Bibliography

Elbow

Bernhang AM: The many causes of tennis elbow. NY State J Med 1979;79:1363.

Foot and Ankle

Cailliet R: Foot and Ankle Pain. Philadelphia, FA Davis, 1974.

Kavanaugh JH, et al: The Jone's fracture revisited. J Bone Joint Surg [Am] 1978;60:776–782.

Keene JS, Lange RH: Diagnostic dilemmas in foot and ankle injuries. JAMA 1986;256:247–251.

Mahowald ML: Examination of the foot in rheumatic disease. Postgrad Med 1986;79:258–261.

Swain RA, Holt WS: Ankle injuries. Postgrad Med 1993;93:91–100.

Hand

American Society for Surgery of the Hand: The Hand. Examination and Diagnosis, 2nd ed. New York, Churchill Livingstone, 1985.

Hoffman DF, Schaffer TC: Management of common finger injuries. Am Fam Pract 1991;43:1594–1607.

Jones JG: Ulnar tunnel syndrome. Am Fam Pract 1991;44:497–502.

Loder RT, Mayhew HE: Common fractures from a fall on an outstretched hand. Am Fam Pract 1988;37:327–338.

Hip, Thigh, and Bony Pelvis

Solomon L: Patterns of osteoarthritis of the hip. J Bone Joint Surg 1976;58B.

Knee

Baugher WH, White GM: Primary evaluation and management of knee injuries. Orthop Clin North Am 1985;16(2):315–327.

Berg E, et al: Office diagnosis of knee pain. Patient Care 1990;24:48–78.

Hawkins RJ, et al: Acute patellar dislocations: The natural history. Am J Sports Med 1986;14:117–120.

Larsson LG, Baum J: The syndromes of bursitis. Bull Rheum Dis 1986; 36:1–8.

Laskin RS (ed): Symposium on disorders of the knee joint. Orthop Clin North Am 1979;10(1):1.

Rothenberg MH, Graf BK: Evaluation of acute knee injuries. Postgrad Med 1993;93:75–86.

Lower Back

Byrne TN: Spinal cord compression from epidural metastases. N Engl J Med 1992;327:614–619.

Deyo RA: Early diagnostic evaluation of low back pain. J Gen Intern Med 1986;1:328–338.

Deyo RA, et al: Herniated lumbar intervertebral disk. Ann Intern Med 1990;112:598–603.

Frymoyer JW: Back pain and sciatica. N Engl J Med 1988;318:291–300.

Monoarticular Arthritis

Freed JF, et al: Acute monoarticular arthritis: A diagnostic approach. JAMA 1980;243:2314.

Goldenberg DL, Reed JI: Bacterial arthritis. N Engl J Med 1985;312:764.

Roberts WN, et al: Colchicine in acute gout. JAMA 1987;257:1920–1922.

Wolfe F: Gout and hyperuricemia. Am Fam Pract 1991;43:2141–2150.

Polyarticular Arthritis

Calin A: Degenerative joint disease. Am Fam Pract 1986;33:167–172.

Kelley WN, et al (eds): Textbook of Rheumatology. Philadelphia, WB Saunders, 1978.

Pinals RS: Rheumatoid arthritis: A pharmacologic overview. Am Fam Pract 1988;37:145–152.

Rahn DW, Malawista SE: Lyme disease: Recommendations for diagnosis and treatment. Ann Intern Med 1991;114:472–481.

Smith CA, Arnett FC: Diagnosing rheumatoid arthritis: Current criteria. Am Fam Pract 1991;44:863–870.

Tan EM: Antinuclear antibodies in diagnosis and management. Hosp Pract 1983;January:79–84.

Weiner SR: Emergencies in rheumatoid arthritis. Am Fam Pract 1984;29: 127–131.

Shoulder

Smith DL, Campbell SM: Painful shoulder syndromes: Diagnosis and management. J Gen Intern Med 1992;7:328–339.

Zuckerman JD, et al: The painful shoulder: Part I. Extrinsic disorder. Am Fam Pract 1991;43:119–128.

Zuckerman JD, et al: The painful shoulder: Part II. Intrinsic disorders and impingement syndrome. Am Fam Pract 1991;43:497–512.

—D.D.B.

Dale Berg, Ed. *Handbook
of Primary Care Medicine.*
Copyright © 1993 J. B.
Lippincott Company.

C H A P T E R   8

Dermatology

Acne Vulgaris

Acne vulgaris is a disorder of skin structures normally present in
the skin, the **pilosebaceous glands.** These glands, located mainly
in the skin of the **face, upper back,** and **trunk,** produce **sebum,** a
lipoproteinaceous material that aids in skin moisturization. In
acne, the pilosebaceous glands **abnormally increase** the **production** of and **content of fatty acids** in sebum. The abnormal increase in sebum production is multifactorial in nature. Underlying factors that influence its development include **heredity** and
an increase in **serum androgens** during puberty in males. Furthermore, androgen use for illicit or therapeutic purposes will also
increase sebum production.

   In certain patients the increase in sebum sets off a cascade of
events. These events include (1) **obstruction of the ducts** of the
pilosebaceous glands by keratin and the excess sebum, with resultant dilation of the gland, and (2) infection and inflammation of
the obstructed gland and adjacent tissue by **anaerobic bacteria,**
especially the species *Proprionibacterium acnes.* Acne lesions
will drain spontaneously but, if the inflammatory component was
great, will **heal with scarring.**

   I. **Overall manifestations**
      The **overall manifestations** include multiple lesions over
      the areas where pilosebaceous glands are located, i.e., the
      face, neck, upper back, and upper trunk. There are three
      discrete types of lesions—closed comedones, open come-
      dones, and cystic lesions. Patients may have some of each,
      but one type usually predominates.
      A. **Closed comedo**
         This is a mildly tender papule with a whitish yellow
         center and mild erythema peripherally. It is commonly
         referred to as a **whitehead.** It occurs as a result of ob-
         struction of the gland's duct with the accumulation of
         keratin and sebum.

B O X   8 - 1

Overall Evaluation and Management of Acne Vulgaris

Evaluation

1. The diagnosis is made clinically after a thorough history and physical examination. No special tests are required for diagnosis, **nor is biopsy required.**
2. **No specific dietary changes are necessary,** as there has been no documented association of acne with any foodstuff, including chocolate.
3. Limit face washing to twice per day. Excessive washing and picking at the face can exacerbate the acne.
4. Direct the patient not to squeeze the comedones.
5. If cosmetics are necessary, **water-based ones** should be used and should be washed off each evening before the patient retires.

Management of Comedo-Predominant Acne

1. **Benzoyl peroxide** 10% lotion or cream may be applied to the affected skin b.i.d. This agent can be used as monotherapy and will control comedo-predominant acne in the majority of cases.
   a. This agent acts as a **comedolytic agent,** decreasing the fatty acid content of the sebum and decreasing the quantity of anaerobic bacteria in the affected gland.
   b. **Side effects** include drying of the skin, which can be dose-limiting.
   c. **Benzoyl peroxide is available as an over-the-counter agent.**
2. **Tretinoin** (topical retinoic acid), 0.01%–0.025% gel, 0.05% liquid, or 0.05%–0.1% cream, may be applied to affected skin every other evening upon retiring. Because the cream is the least irritating form, it is the form most commonly used for the treatment of **comedo-predominant acne.** It should be used for at least 6–12 weeks before any improvement can be expected. The patient should be instructed that there may well be an exacerbation of the acne early in the course of therapy. There is **synergy** in efficacy when tretinoin is used with benzoyl peroxide.
   a. This agent acts as a **comedolytic.**
   b. **Side effects** include significant skin drying, which can be dose- and agent-limiting.

(continued)

B O X   8 - 1 *(continued)*

Management of Cystic/Nodular-Predominant Acne

1. **Benzoyl peroxide** 10% lotion or cream may be applied to the affected skin b.i.d. This agent can be used as monotherapy and will control cystic/nodular-predominant acne in a minority of cases.
   a. This agent acts as a **comedolytic agent,** decreasing the fatty acid content of the sebum and decreasing the quantity of anaerobic bacteria in the affected gland.
   b. **Side effects** include drying of the skin, which can be dose-limiting.
   c. **Benzoyl peroxide is available as an over-the-counter agent.**
2. **Topical antibiotics** are effective in the treatment of **inflammatory nodular acne. Specific antibiotic agents** include **erythromycin 3% cream, clindamycin 1% cream,** and **tetracycline 0.22% cream.** Any of these agents is effective when applied to the affected areas b.i.d. as long as there is an inflammatory component to the acne.
   a. These agents are very effective when used with **benzoyl peroxide.** A product that combines a topical antibiotic with benzoyl peroxide is Benzamycin 3%, which combines erythromycin 3% and benzoyl peroxide 5%. This agent is applied to the skin b.i.d.
   b. Topical antibiotics to treat the anaerobic infection and therefore decrease the inflammation.
   c. **Side effects** include irritation and drying of the skin.
3. **Systemic antibiotics** are effective and therefore indicated if the inflammatory component is marked or refractory to topical antibiotic therapy. **Specific regimens** include, in the acute setting, **tetracycline,** 500 mg PO q.i.d. for 14 days, or **erythromycin,** 250 mg PO t.i.d. to q.i.d. for 14 days, followed by **long-term tetracycline,** 250 mg PO once daily, or erythromycin, 250 mg PO once daily.
   a. Systemic antibiotics treat the bacterial infection and therefore decrease the inflammation.
   b. **Side effects** include the fact that **tetracycline is contraindicated in pregnant women.**

(continued)

B O X 8 - 1 *(continued)*

4. **Isotretinoin** (Accutane), a vitamin A derivative, can be used in the treatment of severe cystic/nodular acne refractory to other therapeutic modalities.
   a. The **dosage** is 0.5–1.0 mg/kg/day PO in a b.i.d. dosing for 16–18 weeks. The response rate is dramatic, as up to **90%** of patients will respond after 4 months of therapy.
   b. The **mechanism of action** of this agent includes decreasing sebum production and local anti-inflammatory effects.
   c. **Side effects** are significant and include severe **drying** of the skin, which can be dose- and even agent-limiting. The agent can cause an increase in serum triglycerides and has been associated with the development of hepatic dysfunction. Finally, isoretinoin is teratogenic, and therefore its use is **contraindicated in pregnant women**. In fact, it should not be used by any woman of childbearing age. Because of its side effect profile it should be reserved for the most severe cases of acne vulgaris.

B. **Open comedo**
   This is a nontender papule with a central black area, commonly called a **blackhead.** It occurs as a result of the duct or "pore" opening and allowing some of the contents of the gland to drain externally.

C. **Cystic/nodular**
   These lesions are **nodular** and are frequently accompanied by inflammation in and adjacent to them. The nodules may be quite tender and large, reaching 1–2 cm in size. They may exude purulent material, especially early in their time course. These lesions usually represent a progression from comedones and are the lesions that cause the most scarring.

II. **Consultation**

Problem	Service	Time
Refractory acne	Dermatology	Elective

III. **Indications for admission:** None.

(Text continues on page 470)

Blistering Diseases

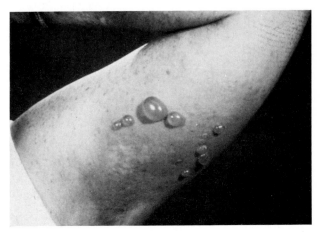

F I G U R E 8 - 1
Bullous pemphigoid on extensor surface of right upper extremity.

T A B L E 8 - 1
Blistering Diseases*†

Disease	Affected Areas	Forms	Site of Cleavage	Histopathology	Associated Laboratory	Treatment
Pemphigus	Skin Mucous membranes	Pemphigus vulgaris Pemphigus foliaceus	Intraepidermal	Acantholysis IgG to desmosomes	Antidesmosomal antibody assay positive HLA-A10	High-dose prednisone (60–80 mg/day); as the disease comes under control, add azathioprine, 100 mg/day PO, then wean from both Dermatology consultation Erythromycin, 250 mg PO q.i.d. (during active blistering)

Disease	Distribution	Variant	Histology	Immunofluorescence	Serology	Treatment
Bullous pemphigoid (see Fig. 8-1)	Skin; Mucous membranes		Subepidermal	IgG and C3 to basement membrane	Anti-basement membrane antibody present in serum	Prednisone, 60–80 mg PO q.d.; may need to add azathioprine; Erythromycin, 250 mg PO q.i.d. (during active blistering); Dermatology consultation
Cicatrical pemphigoid	Skin and mucous membranes of head and neck	Brunstag–Perry variant: skin involved only	Subepidermal	IgG and C3 to basement membrane	None	Same as for bullous pemphigoid
Dermatitis herpetiformis	Skin, especially scalp, elbows, and knees	Granular; Linear	Subepidermal; Subepidermal	Antibodies to basement membrane; IgA, linear deposits along basement membrane	HLA-B8/Dw3; Gluten-sensitive enteropathy; 70% have IgA antiendomysial antibodies present in serum	Gluten-free diet; Dapsone, 50 mg PO q.d.; Dermatology consultation

*In any and all cases it is imperative to replete any intravascular volume fluid deficit, support the patient, and if significant bullous disease is present, to manage as a burn patient. Lactated Ringer's solution is the most appropriate for IV fluid repletion.

†Indications for admission include active disease, intravascular volume depletion, and any sign of bacterial superinfection.

Dermatitis

TABLE 8-2
Dermatitis

Disease	History and Physical Examination Findings	Treatment
Contact	Erythematous Can develop secondary bacterial infections Weeping and crusting of affected areas Located on areas exposed to inciting agent (e.g., chemical, allergen, detergent) Asymmetric pattern of distribution (e.g., poison ivy) Vesicle formation	a) Remove inciting agent b) Triamcinolone, 0.1% b.i.d. to affected areas c) Calamine lotion b.i.d. to affected areas d) If lichenified, use ointment (greasy) e) If severe: prednisone, 40–60 mg PO q.d. for 3–5 days f) Hydroxyzine (Atarax), 25 mg PO q.6h. PRN for itching
Atopic (eczema) (see Fig. 8-2)	Pruritic Symmetric distribution Distribution on face, neck, trunk; also on flexor surfaces of elbows and knees Can have lichenification of lesions Strong correlation with other atopic diseases Eosinophilia is common Special type: eczema herpeticum—herpes simplex viral infection superimposed on atopic dermatitis	a) Hydroxyzine (Atarax), 25–50 mg PO q.6h. PRN for itching b) Triamcinolone 0.1% b.i.d. to affected areas c) Calamine lotion b.i.d. to affected areas d) Rarely severe enough to require oral steroids e) If eczema herpeticum, add parenteral acyclovir to above regimen (dose: 10 mg/kg/24 hr in q.8h. dosing by IV for 7–10 days) f) Dermatology consult

Drug-induced	Bright, erythematous rash Pruritic Begins on trunk and spreads to periphery Time course is different for each use of the agent (amnestic response): a) First use: onset 8–10 days after start b) Subsequent use: onset 1–3 days after start	a) Hydroxyzine (Atarax), 25–50 mg PO q.6h. PRN b) Discontinue offending agent c) Triamcinolone 0.1% topical q.6h. d) Observe patient for other anaphylactic signs (bronchospasm, hypotension); if present, epinephrine SC is indicated (see Table 4-1, page 200) e) Systemic steroids rarely necessary in treatment f) Label patient "allergic" to that specific agent
Photodermatitis (sunburn)	Development of diffuse, confluent, nonraised, warm, erythematous rash on areas exposed to sunlight or other UV light sources Nausea and diarrhea Risk factors: a) Fair-skinned b) SLE c) Porphyria cutanea tarda	Prevention: a) Limit exposure to UV light b) Use sunscreens with SPF (sunprotective factor) >15 if in sun Treatment of acute burn: a) Topical steroids (e.g., triamcinolone 0.1% cream) b) Aspirin, 325 mg PO q.4–6h. c) If severe, prednisone, 40–60 mg PO q.d. for 5 days d) If porphyria cutanea tarda is a factor, chloroquine, 125 mg PO 2× per week, and/or phlebotomy once monthly, are effective in treatment
Seborrheic	Chronic and recurrent Papulosquamous lesions Pruritic Many exacerbating and/or precipitating factors: a) Hormone changes b) Emotional stress c) Infections	Low-dose topical steroids, e.g., hydrocortisone 0.1% q.i.d. Selenium sulfide–containing shampoos (e.g., Selsun Blue, and others)

465

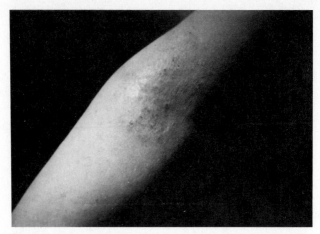

F I G U R E 8 - 2
Atopic dermatitis (eczema) on the flexor surface of an upper extremity.

Erythemas

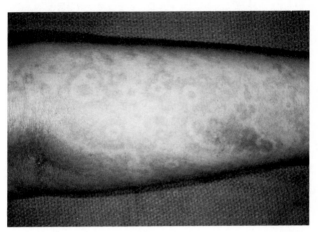

F I G U R E 8 - 3
Erythema multiforme on the flexor surface of an upper extremity.

TABLE 8-3
Erythemas

Disease	Symptoms and Signs	Precipitating Factors	Biopsy and Laboratory Findings	Treatment
Erythema nodosum	Tender, erythematous, nodular lesions 1–10 mm in size Extensor surfaces of the distal lower extremities	Streptococcal infections Coccidioidomycosis Mycobacterial infections Hepatitis B Lues venereum Sarcoidosis Ulcerative colitis Leukemia	Septal panniculitis	a) Diagnose and treat underlying cause b) KI (potassium iodide), in saturated solution, 5–15 drops to nodules t.i.d.
Erythema multiforme (see Fig. 8-3)	Multiple wheals and papules Symmetric in distribution Can progress to toxic epidermolytic syndrome and involve mucous membranes (Stevens–Johnson syndrome) Occurs on palms and soles Classically, "target" shaped	*Mycoplasma* infections Herpes simplex (HSV) infections (as a late sequela) Drug-related: Phenytoin TMP/sulfa	Nonspecific Increased cold agglutinins in serum	a) Diagnose and treat the underlying cause b) If severe, treat as a burn: Admit to burn unit Aggressively monitor for and replete fluid and electrolyte losses c) Acyclovir, 200 mg PO 5× per day, if HSV suspected d) Erythromycin, 500 mg PO/IV q.6h., if *Mycoplasma* suspected e) Consider steroids PO or IV acutely, especially if severe f) Dermatology consult

Erythema marginatum	Erythematous Rapidly spreading Flat, pale centers Raised red margins	Rheumatic fever (streptococcal infections)	Increased ASO titer in serum	Treat underlying infection (streptococcal) with appropriate antibiotics (usually penicillin based)
Erythema infectiosum	Erythematous, papular rash Trunk, back, face Central clearing present Fevers to 103 °F Can have rhinorrhea, sore throat, other URI symptoms concurrently Slapped face appearance common Pediatric age group Also known as "fifth disease"	Parvovirus B-19	Nonspecific	Symptomatic and supportive Pregnancy precautions: pregnant women should be isolated from patients with this infection
Erythema chronicum migrans	Flat with central clearing Asymmetric Nonpruritic Trunk, back, thighs Can resolve, then recur in another area Concurrent arthralgias, neuropathy, and/or cardiac manifestations not uncommon	Lyme disease (*Borrelia burgdorferi*)	Elevated Lyme titer	See section on Polyarticular Arthritis in Chapter 7, page 432

Nails

I. Problems

Specific problems that can affect the **fingernails** or **toenails** are described below.

A. Paronychia

1. Manifestations

The **specific manifestations** of this entity include the acute onset of pain and swelling about the distal finger in general, and about the **lateral nail fold** unilaterally in specific. The patient usually has a past history of trauma to the involved nail or of onychocryptosis ("in-grown nail") in the affected digit. **Examination** discloses redness, warmth, tenderness, swelling, and often an area of purulent material in and adjacent to the involved lateral nail fold.

2. Pathogenesis

The **underlying pathogenesis** is growth of the nail plate into the lateral nail fold or otherwise irritating the lateral nail fold. Irritation can occur as a result of trauma, poor nail care, or a fungal infection involving the nail plate (onychomycosis). Causative **organisms** include the gram-positive cocci (e.g., *Streptococcus* spp. and *Staphylococcus* spp.).

3. Evaluation

The **specific evaluation** of this problem includes making the clinical diagnosis and examining the patient for any concurrent processes, such as septic arthritis or cellulitis. **Radiographs** of the affected hand, foot, or digits are indicated only if there are any **atypical features,** a history of **antecedent trauma,** evidence of a concurrent **septic arthritis** as manifested by a decreased range of motion of the DIP or PIP joints of the affected digit, or if the patient has **diabetes mellitus.**

4. Management

The **specific management** includes **warm soaks** of the involved digit, **antibiotics,** and simple local surgery.

a. Specific **antibiotic regimens** include either a 7-day course of cephalexin (Keflex), 500 mg PO q.i.d., or erythromycin, 250–500 mg PO q.i.d.

b. If there is any evidence of fluctuance or if the lesion is severe, the area must be **incised and drained.** This is easily performed by the primary care physician and entails either a local drainage procedure using a No. 11 blade to incise the lesion laterally and drain it, or surgical removal of the involved half of the nail plate itself.

     c. If the primary care physician has not been trained in incising and draining such lesions, urgent referral to a general surgeon is indicated.

B. Onychorrhexis

1. Manifestations

The **specific manifestations** of this entity include the insidious development of irregular, easily broken edges on the distal surfaces of the nail plates, usually involving most or all of the nails. It is rarely symptomatic unless the patient breaks one or more of the nail plates or "catches" them while putting on socks or gloves, resulting in irritation.

2. Pathogenesis

The **underlying pathogenesis** is a weak and dysfunctional nail plate as a nonspecific manifestation of chronic disease, especially any process that leads to cachexia or malnutrition, especially protein malnutrition.

3. Evaluation and management

The **specific evaluation and management** of this problem include making the clinical diagnosis and determining the nutritional status of the patient. If the patient is cachetic or malnourished, determine the underlying reason and treat that disorder. Consultation with a dietician, as appropriate, is recommended on an urgent basis.

C. Subungual hematoma

1. Manifestations

The **specific manifestations** of this entity include the acute onset of pain in the distal digit beginning immediately after crushing or pinching trauma to that digit. **Examination** discloses a reddish blue collection of blood beneath the nail plate **in the nail bed itself** and **exquisite tenderness** on minimal palpation of the affected nail plate.

2. Pathogenesis

The **underlying pathogenesis** is trauma resulting in the collection of blood beneath the nail plate, with resultant increased pressure in the distal digit.

3. Evaluation

The **specific evaluation** of this problem includes making the clinical diagnosis. **Radiographs** of the hand, foot, or digit are indicated only if there is evidence of trauma-related concurrent damage.

4. Management

The central goal is to relieve the pressure and pain by **incising the hematoma.** Various methods may be used to achieve this goal. One of the easiest and most effective methods is to use a paper clip. The tip of the paper clip is bent perpendicularly, then heated in a flame until the **tip is red hot.** This sterilizes the tip and allows easy passage of the tip through the nail plate. The clinician firmly and rapidly presses the red-hot tip through the nail plate into the hematoma. Once drained, the symptoms rapidly resolve.

After the procedure, the nail plate will have a defect that will resolve in several weeks as the nail plate grows distally. The patient need only keep the wound clean. Antibiotics are not indicated unless a concurrent process is present.

D. Glomus tumor

1. Manifestations

The **specific manifestations** of this rare entity include pain and tenderness in the distal digit. The pain may be severe and associated with exquisite tenderness. There is no antecedent history of trauma. **Examination** discloses tenderness localized to the nail bed and a red lesion in the nail bed that is several millimeters in diameter.

2. Pathogenesis

The **underlying pathogenesis** is a benign but significantly symptomatic tumor of vascular origin localized to the nail bed. Although this lesion is nonmalignant, it causes significant pain for which the patient desires expedient intervention.

3. Evaluation and management

The **specific evaluation and management** of this problem include making the clinical diagnosis. Goals include affording **analgesia** by protecting the finger with a plastic fingerguard and analgesics, including narcotics (e.g., acetaminophen with codeine [Tylenol #3]), and, most important, referral to a **general surgeon** for surgical resection of the lesion.

E. Onychauxis

1. Manifestations

The **specific manifestations** of this rather common process include thickening and discoloration of the nail plate itself. The plate becomes brittle and will easily fracture. The nail thickness can reach 4–5 mm. The process may be limited to one nail or may involve multiple nail plates. The risk of development of onychocryptosis or a paronychium is increased in this process.

2. Pathogenesis

The **underlying pathogenesis** is a chronic infection with the fungal elements of a dermatophyte in the involved nail plate (i.e., onychomycosis).

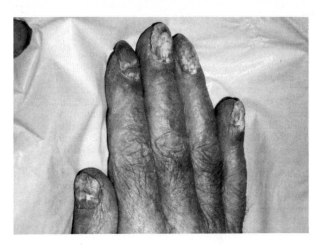

F I G U R E 8 - 4
Onychomycosis of the nail plates on all digits. Note loss of
translucency, thickening, brownish discoloration, and distal
breaking of the nail plates themselves.

3. **Evaluation and management**
The **specific evaluation and management** entail
making the clinical diagnosis and looking for complications or concurrent processes, such as tinea
pedis, tinea manus, or onychocryptosis. Treatment
involves treating the underlying cause.
F. **Onychomycosis**
1. **Manifestations**
The **specific manifestations** of this not uncommon
problem include onychauxis (i.e., thickened nail
plates), brittle nail plates, and easy fracturing of the
affected plate (see Fig. 8-4). The process may be limited to one nail or may involve multiple nails. **Examination** frequently discloses erythema of the adjacent
skin, cracking of the adjacent skin with concurrent
flaking, or even vesicle formation, all as a result of a
concurrent tineal infection. The risk of development
of onychocryptosis and of a paronychium is increased in this process.
2. **Pathogenesis**
The **underlying pathogenesis** is a chronic infection
with the fungal elements of a dermatophyte or *Can-*

dida infection. There invariably is a long history of antecedent tineal skin infections.

3. **Evaluation**

The **specific evaluation** of this problem includes making the clinical diagnosis by inspection of the affected nails. For diagnostic confirmation, one can perform a fungal culture using Sabouraud's medium on a piece or fragment of the infected/affected nail.

4. **Management**

The **specific management** includes the following measures.

  a. **Application of clotrimazole** (Lotrimin, Mycelex) 1% cream b.i.d. to affected areas. This topical antifungal agent **will not cure the onychomycosis** but will treat the underlying tineal skin infections and thus prevent spread to other nails. The feet should be kept dry.

  b. The actual nail infection is quite difficult to treat and usually **requires surgical intervention.** The surgical intervention is easily performed by a primary care physician or by a general surgeon or podiatrist. The procedure consists of **nail removal and ablation** and is **reserved for toenail infections.** The patient needs to be informed that this will permanently ablate the nail, which may not be acceptable to some individuals.

  c. If the patient desires a trial of aggressive **medical management, griseofulvin,** 500 mg t.i.d. to q.i.d. PO for 3–6 months, will effectively treat fingernail but not toenail onychomycosis. While taking griseofulvin, the patient must abstain from ethanol use and must undergo liver function tests on a scheduled basis, as griseofulvin can cause hepatic dysfunction as a side effect. Another exciting but not yet approved modality is the use of **fluconazole,** 100 mg PO once daily for several weeks. This agent may be effective for fingernail and toenail onychomycosis.

G. **Onychocryptosis**

1. **Manifestations**

The **specific manifestations** of this relatively common process include pain and tenderness in the tissue in and adjacent to the lateral nail fold, with the lateral aspect of the nail plate embedded in the lateral nail fold.

2. **Pathogenesis**

The **underlying pathogenesis** is inappropriate growth of the nail plate into the lateral nail fold. **Risk**

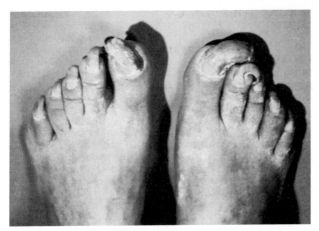

F I G U R E 8 - 5
Onychogryphosis of the nails of the feet.

factors for the development of this process include trauma, onychomycosis, onychorrhexis, and onychauxis. It can in itself be a risk factor for the development of a paronychium.

3. **Evaluation and management**
The **specific evaluation and management** of this entity entail making the clinical diagnosis and, if the condition is significant, surgically removing the involved half of the nail plate.

H. **Onychogryphosis**
1. **Manifestations**
The **specific manifestations** of this entity include a grossly elongated nail that may develop a hooked configuration (Fig. 8-5). This is invariably due to lack of manicure or pedicure, quite often in a patient with poor hygiene.

2. **Evaluation and management**
The **specific evaluation and management** of this problem include making the clinical diagnosis and performing a manicure or pedicure of the affected nails. Pedicure of large toenails may be done by **podiatrist** with a special technique.

I. **Clubbing**
This condition is also referred to as **hippocratic nails.** See section on Clubbing in Chapter 4.

II. **Consultation**

Service	*Time*
General surgery	Elective

III. **Indications for admission:** No specific indications.

Neoplasia, Benign and Malignant

I. **Basal cell carcinoma (BCCA)**
   A. **Incidence**

   BCCA is one of the most common forms of cancer in the United States today. More than 500,000 new cases are diagnosed per year. Furthermore, it is a malignant neoplasm that is **increasing in incidence. Risk factors** for its development include fair skin, increasing age, exposure to UV (A and B) light, and a past history of irradiation exposure.

   B. **Manifestations**

   The **specific manifestations** include lesions appearing on skin areas that are **frequently exposed to the sun,** i.e., the face, head, and back of the neck. There are several variations of this neoplasm, each with moderately different presenting features. These are as follows:

   1. **Nodular BCCA.** The vast majority of basal cell carcinomas are of this type. These lesions are **papular,** with a translucent quality. Invariably they have surface telangiectasias, and occasionally they ulcerate. They have been described as having a "pearly" margin (see Fig. 8-6).
   2. **Sclerosing BCCA.** This variant is easily overlooked. It is a palpable, indurated, flat lesion that can be hypopigmented and is easily overlooked as an old scar. This variant is quite uncommon.
   3. **Pigmented BCCA.** A pigmented version of the nodular BCCA, this variant can be difficult to distinguish clinically from a malignant melanoma. It is uncommon.

   C. **Natural history**

   This malignant neoplasm, although it is very invasive and quite destructive via contiguous growth, rarely metastasizes. Therefore, whereas it is locally malignant and causes significant morbidity, it rarely causes death.

   D. **Evaluation and management**

   The **specific evaluation and management** include making the clinical and histopathologic diagnosis by performing the evaluative tests described in Box 8-2. Any lesion potentially a basal cell carcinoma, especially one that is pigmented and thus slightly suspicious for melanoma, must be excisionally biopsied.

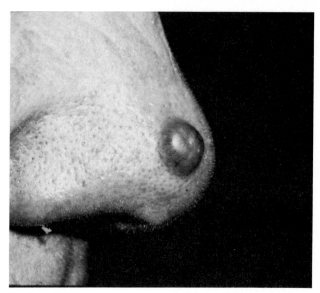

F I G U R E   8 - 6
Basal cell carcinoma of nose. Classic features include a smooth, pearly, translucent nodule with some telangiectasias within the lesion.

1. A **specific type** of surgical biopsy has been developed for BCCA. In **Mohs' surgical technique** the surgeon shaves off layers of the tumor and sends each layer for frozen section analysis to determine if the margins of the excision are free of the tumor. This allows the surgeon to resect all of the tumor, while minimizing adjacent normal tissue removal.
2. If there is a **contraindication** to surgical intervention or if the size of the tumor precludes surgical intervention, a punch biopsy for confirmation of the diagnosis followed by local irradiation should be performed. Local irradiation is an effective modality in the treatment and cosmetic effect, even with large BCCAs.

E. **Consultation**

Problem	*Service*	*Time*
Surgical excision	Dermatology	Urgent
If surgery is contra-indicated or re-fused by the patient	Radiation therapy	Elective/required

B O X 8 - 2

*Overall Evaluation and Management of
Neoplastic Skin Disorders*

Evaluation

1. **Examine** the lesion, including inspection and palpation. In the vast majority of cases, a presumptive diagnosis can be made from the examination results.
2. If there is any suspicion that a lesion is malignant or premalignant, refer the patient to dermatology or general surgery for an excisional biopsy. **Excisional biopsy** usually allows complete resection of the lesion and therefore is diagnostic and therapeutic.
3. After the **histopathology** of the lesion is known, stage the lesion. See discussion in the text for the natural history and staging of each type of malignant neoplastic lesion.

Treatment

1. Starting at age 40, each person should have a thorough skin inspection and examination to screen for early lesions.
2. The major focus is on **prevention.** Many of the malignant and premalignant skin neoplasms can be prevented by **limiting exposure to UV light.** Tanning salons and sun exposure should be minimized. If sun exposure cannot be directly limited, the use of lotions with a sun protection factor (SPF) of >**15** is strongly advised.

II. Squamous Cell Carcinoma (SCCA)
A. Incidence

This not uncommon malignant skin neoplasm is increasing in incidence in the United States. **Risk factors** for its development include exposure to UV light, exposure to ionizing radiation, recurrent trauma to the skin, and the viral-related lesions of condyloma acuminatum and periungual warts. The specific virus is the DNA **human papillomavirus (HPV). Chimney sweeps** are at occupational risk for the development of squamous cell carcinoma in the scrotum. A historical risk factor for squamous cell carcinoma is chronic exposure to or ingestion of **arsenic.**

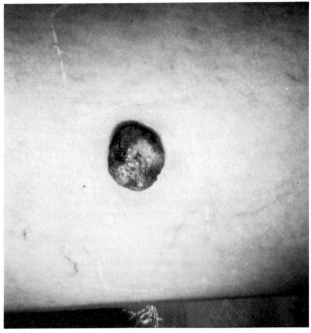

F I G U R E 8 - 7
Squamous cell carcinoma on the upper extremity. Note the features of
an ulcerated, nontender nodule.

B. Manifestations

The **specific manifestations** include lesions developing
on the face, ears, or dorsum of the hands. The patient
presents with a nontender, solitary **nodular lesion** in
the skin. The nodule invariably has a central necrotic-
appearing ulcer and some peripheral erythema (Fig.
8-7). The lesion increases rapidly in size over weeks to
months. Multiple lesions usually occur in patients with
more than one risk factor.

C. Natural history

These lesions may invade adjacent tissues and structures, and also metastasize. Thus, unlike BCCA, this
type of skin cancer can, if not treated early in its course,
cause the death of the patient. These tumors metastasize
to **local lymph nodes** early in the course of disease.
Sites of later metastases include the bone, brain, liver,
and lungs.

D. **Evaluation and management**

The **specific evaluation and management** include making the clinical and histopathological diagnosis by performing the evaluative tests described in Box 8-2. Any lesion that is potentially SCCA must be biopsied. **Excisional biopsy** is the procedure of choice. If performed early, it can be diagnostic and curative.

1. Once the diagnosis has been **histopathologically confirmed,** one must **stage** the disease. This consists of palpating any adjacent **lymph nodes,** performing **liver function studies** (LDH, alkaline phosphatase, total bilirubin, SGOT, SGPT, and GGT), and obtaining a **chest radiograph.** If there are any suspicious (i.e., indurated) lymph nodes, they should be **biopsied.** If there are any suspicious areas on the chest radiograph or LFT abnormalities, further imaging with **CT** of the suspicious areas should be performed.

2. If there is **any evidence** of metastatic disease, expedient referral to an **oncologist** is indicated. The management of metastatic squamous cell carcinoma is beyond the scope of this text.

E. **Consultation**

Problem	Service	Time
Excisional biopsy	Dermatology	Urgent
Metastatic disease	Hematology/ oncology	Urgent

III. **Dysplastic nevus syndrome**

A. **Epidemiology**

This syndrome, first described approximately 15 years ago by Clark et al., has an estimated prevalence of 2%–5% in the United States today. **Risk factors** for development are familial. The **familial form** is transmitted as an **autosomal dominant trait.** A **sporadic form** has been described that appears spontaneously.

B. **Manifestations**

The **specific manifestations** of **dysplastic nevi** are best described by comparing and contrasting them with **benign nevi.**

1. **Benign nevi,** present on every human being, usually are small (<**5 mm** in diameter); have sharp, **well-defined boundaries** with adjacent skin; are **uniformly pigmented;** are usually **macular;** and rarely have any **pink hue** to the pigment. Three different types of benign nevi and their histopathology are as follows:

a. **Junctional nevus.** A benign, classic clinical presentation as described above. Histopathologically, the melanocytes are normal-appearing and are localized into a cluster in the epidermis. These lesions either **resolve** or **evolve** into a compound nevus. There is no malignant potential associated with this lesion.

b. **Compound nevus.** Same as a junctional nevus, except that histopathologically, the melanocytes are in both the epidermis and dermis. The lesion may either **resolve** or **evolve** into an intradermal nevus. There is no malignant potential associated with this lesion.

c. **Intradermal nevus.** Same as junctional and compound types of nevi, except that the epidermal component of the melanocytes has disappeared. The lesion may either **remain** or spontaneously **resolve.** Again, there is no malignant potential.

There can be an **evolution in a benign nevus** from junctional to compound to intradermal.

2. **Dysplastic nevi** are usually **large** (>5 mm in diameter); have irregular, **ill-defined boundaries** with adjacent skin; have a **disorganized pigment;** are usually **papular,** and quite often have **pink hues** in the pigment (see Fig. 8-8). On histopathologic analysis, there are irregular, atypical-appearing melanocytes

F I G U R E 8 - 8
Dysplastic nevus. Note the irregular borders, asymmetric distribution of pigment, and different pigment colors within the nevus.

within the dermis. The lesion has a premalignant
potential.
C. **Natural history**
This syndrome results in multiple recurrent dysplastic
nevi with a great potential for malignant transformation.
There is a significant risk of the development of **malignant melanoma,** especially in patients with **familial
dysplastic nevus syndrome** where the **relative risk** can
be **50 times** that of the general population. The complications include those related to the development of **malignant melanoma.**
D. **Evaluation and management**
The **specific evaluation and management** include making the clinical and histopathologic diagnosis by performing the evaluative tests described in Box 8-2. After
the clinical diagnosis has been made, a thorough **family
history** and even examination of family members for
such lesions is required. **Photographs** of the patient's
skin should be obtained at **baseline** and again every 4–6
months for comparison. Any suspicious lesion mandates an excisional biopsy, **never a punch biopsy,** as
the lesion may be a malignant melanoma. The patient
should be instructed to perform a monthly skin self-
examination and to report any changes in the nevi.
E. **Consultation**

Service	*Time*
Dermatology	Required

IV. **Malignant melanoma**
A. **Incidence**
This malignant neoplasm of the skin is **increasing** in
incidence. Specific **risk factors** for its development include fair skin; intense sunburns, especially as a child;
a family history of melanoma; the presence of dysplastic
nevus syndrome; and exposure to UV light.
B. **Manifestations**
The **specific manifestations** of this entity include a nevus with **irregular borders,** an **irregular distribution of
pigment** within the nevus, or one that has **increased in
diameter.** Although any of these changes in a nevus
suggest a malignant melanoma, suspicion is even higher
if the patient has a history of dysplastic nevus syndrome. There are several clinical variations of malignant melanoma, which are described in Table 8-4.
C. **Natural history**
Early in its course, the malignant lesion remains quite
superficial, with little to no invasion or metastatic potential. As the tumor grows, it invades deeper into the
skin and increases the incidence of metastatic spread.

T A B L E 8 - 4
Clinical Variants of Malignant Melanoma

Lentigo-maligna

Location: Any skin areas that are recurrently exposed to UV light.
Gross manifestations: Flat, with irregular borders, various shades of brown and black pigment within the nevus.
Histologic description: Normal and malignant melanocytes within the basal area of the epidermis.
Mean age of patient at presentation: 70 years.

Superficial spreading (see Fig. 8-9)

Location: Any and all body surfaces.
Gross manifestations: Palpable lesion with irregular borders; asymmetric configuration of the lesion with multiple colors within the nevus itself: black, brown, and pink pigments.
Histologic description: Multiple malignant-appearing melanocytes within the epidermis.
Mean age of patient at presentation: 50 years.

Nodular

Location: Any and all body surfaces.
Gross manifestations: Palpable lesion; smooth borders; uniform black pigmentation with a surrounding area of decreased pigmentation.
Histologic description: Large numbers of malignant melanocytes with multiple areas of dermal invasion.
Mean age of patient at presentation: 45 years.

There is a **direct relationship** between depth of invasion and distant metastases and an **inverse relationship** between depth of invasion and survival. Thus, the lesion is staged by depth of penetration.

1. The two systems used in **staging** malignant melanoma are the Clark and Breslow staging schemas. The **Clark system** describes the depth relative to skin layer; the **Breslow system** uses depth measured in millimeters. A brief overview of these important staging systems is given in Table 8-5.
2. **Distant metastases** are to the regional lymph nodes, liver, lungs, and the brain. It can and frequently does metastasize to unique organs, including the myocardium and/or the wall of the small or large intestine.

D. **Evaluation and management**
The **specific evaluation and management** include making the clinical and histopathologic diagnosis by performing the evaluative tests described in Box 8-2. After a thorough history and physical examination, **excisional biopsy** of any suspicious lesion is **mandated.**

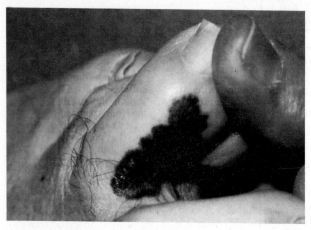

F I G U R E   8 - 9
Superficial spreading malignant melanoma of the left foot. Any
pigmented lesion on the palms of the hands or soles of the feet is a
malignant melanoma until proven otherwise.

1. The gold standard for **staging** malignant melanoma
   is the Clark/Breslow levels; therefore, extensive imaging of other organ systems is not indicated unless
   symptoms are referable to that area.
2. The **specific management** of metastatic malignant
   melanoma is beyond the scope of this text; however,
   some points can be made.
   a. There are no data to indicate that radical dissec-
      tion of regional lymph nodes is of any benefit to
      patient in the short or long term. Therefore, this
      procedure is not indicated.
   b. There is a want of effective modalities, including
      radiation and chemotherapy, in the treatment of
      advanced malignant melanoma. As such, the ma-
      jor thrust in management is on **prevention** and
      early detection.
E. Consultation

Problem	*Service*	*Time*
Any suspicious nevus	Dermatology	Urgent

V. **Actinic keratoses**
   A. **Incidence**
      As with many other neoplastic dermatologic lesions, the
      incidence of this benign neoplastic disorder is increas-

T A B L E   8 - 5
Clark Staging Systems for Malignant Melanoma

Clark Level I

Confined to the epidermis
Breslow level = <0.75 mm
0% metastases
100% cure rate

Clark Level II

Penetrates the epidermal basement membrane into the
  papillary dermis
Breslow level = <0.75 mm
5% metastases
95% cure rate

Clark Level III

Penetrates the epidermal basement membrane to a level at the junction of the papillary and reticular dermis
Breslow level = 0.75–1.5 mm
15%–25% metastases
70% cure rate

Clark Level IV

Penetrates into the deep reticular dermis
Breslow level = 1.5–3.0 mm
40% metastases
40%–50% cure rate

Clark Level V

Penetrates the entire thickness of both the epidermis and the dermis
  into the subdermal fat
Breslow level = >3.0 mm
70% metastases
20% cure rate

ing. **Risk factors** for their development include UV light
exposure, especially in individuals with fair skin, increasing age, and (of historical importance) the chronic
ingestion of or exposure to arsenic.
B. **Manifestations**
The **specific manifestations** of these lesions include occurrence on the face, neck, dorsal aspects of hands, and
forearms. There are four discrete variants, each with
different clinical features.
  1. **Atrophic variant.** The lesion is dry, scaly, and rough
     in texture. Lesions may be single or multiple, and
     are usually <5 mm in diameter.
  2. **Hypertrophic variant.** These pink papules are well
     demarcated from the adjacent skin tissue. They may

form cutaneous "horns" of keratin, a finding that, when present, is quite dramatic.

3. **Bowenoid variant** (not Bowen's disease). The scaly, red plaques can be quite large, >1 cm. They are well demarcated from the adjacent skin.

4. **Spreading variant.** These papules and plaques spread centrifugally from a central origin.

C. **Natural history**

Although the lesion is itself benign, it is **premalignant** for squamous cell carcinomas.

D. **Evaluation and management**

The **specific evaluation and management** include making the clinical and histopathologic diagnosis by performing the evaluative tests. described in Box 8-2. If there is any suspicion for a basal cell carcinoma or squamous cell carcinoma, **excisional biopsy** of the suspicious lesion is **mandated.** If there is **no clinical suspicion** for malignancy within the lesion, one of the following therapeutic modalities may be utilized.

1. **Cryosurgery.** Liquid nitrogen is applied to the lesion using a cotton swab. This procedure effects excellent results, especially for smaller lesions.

2. **Shave biopsy.** After local anesthesia, the lesion is shaved off. This modality is excellent for diagnosis and treatment, especially of smaller lesions.

3. **5-fluorouracil** cream (Efudex) applied b.i.d. for 4–6 weeks is good for the treatment of a large spreading actinic keratosis.

E. **Consultation**

Service	Time
Dermatology	Required

VI. **Seborrheic keratoses**

A. **Incidence**

These benign dermatologic lesions are **extremely common.** The prevalence approaches 100% in the elderly. **Risk factors** for development include familial factors. If familial, it is transmitted as an autosomal dominant trait. Other risk factors are Leser–Trelat syndrome, which is a marked increase in seborrheic keratoses in association with an internal adenocarcinoma, and increasing age.

B. **Manifestations**

The **specific manifestations** of these lesions include occurrence with a symmetric distribution on the trunk and proximal extremities. The lesions are often 1–1.5 cm in size, slowly increase in size over time, and are light brown to dark brown in color. They have a "stuck-on" appearance. They are nonpainful and nonpruritic.

C. **Natural history**

The lesions may remain constant or may slightly deepen in color or increase in size with time. These lesions are of the epidermis only and have **no malignant potential.**

D. **Evaluation and management**

The **specific evaluation and management** include making the clinical diagnosis by performing the evaluative tests described in Box 8-2. Usually biopsy is not required, but if there is any question as to the diagnosis clinically, excisional biopsy should be performed. The specific modalities used to remove these lesions for cosmetic purposes include cryosurgery or electrodissection.

VII. **Hemangiomas**

This is a diverse group of benign lesions. Almost every human will, over the course of life, develop one or more of these lesions. A select group of the most common types of hemangiomas is discussed here.

A. **Spider hemangiomas**

1. **Manifestations**

These not uncommon lesions are asymptomatic. The lesion consists of a pinhead-sized central vessel, usually an arteriole, with small vessels radiating centripetally from the center. It can be compared to a spider in appearance. Each lesion will blanch with the application of mild pressure. The lesions, which can be single or multiple, invariably occur on the skin of the shoulders and upper chest and back.

2. **Underlying causes**

Underlying causes include severe hepatic dysfunction, pregnancy, and the Osler–Weber–Rendu syndrome.

3. **Evaluation**

The **specific evaluation** includes a urine pregnancy test in the appropriate patient. Abdominal examination and liver function tests to look for signs of hepatic dysfunction are indicated in clinically appropriate patients. However, in most cases no acute evaluation is indicated.

4. **Management**

No specific treatment is necessary unless removal for cosmetic reasons is required. This is easily performed by electrosurgery. The electrosurgical probe on low current is placed **into** the **central** vessel.

B. **Capillary hemangiomas**

1. **Manifestations**

These not uncommon lesions are asymptomatic. The lesion is a 3–5-mm red papule that may occur singly

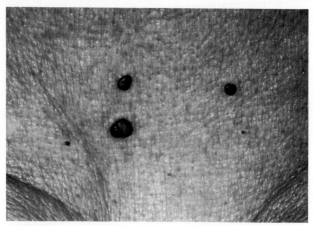

FIGURE 8-10
Several capillary hemangiomas on the right neck. These red
papules represent a benign condition.

or in multiples on any skin surface, increasing in
frequency with increasing age (see Fig. 8-10).
2. **Evaluation and management**
No specific evaluation or intervention is required
unless indicated for cosmetic purposes, in which
case surgical excision or electrosurgical removal is
effective.

C. **Port wine spots**
1. **Manifestations**
These relatively uncommon lesions are large,
asymptomatic **flat patches** that may occur anywhere
on the body. When they occur on the face, they are
associated with the **Sturge–Weber syndrome,** i.e., a
port wine nevus with concurrent **cerebellar** and **retinal hemangiomas.** They are congenital and **do not
enlarge** with increasing age.
2. **Evaluation**
No specific evaluation is indicated unless Sturge–
Weber syndrome is suspected, in which case a retinal examination looking for retinal hemangiomas
and CT of the head looking for cerebellar hemangi-
oma are indicated.
3. **Management**
The **specific management** of the local lesion is cosmetic; however, few modalities have proved effective in providing cosmesis for large lesions. Referral

to a plastic surgeon should be considered if the patient so desires.
D. Consultation

Service	Time
Dermatology	Elective

VIII. **Indications for admission:** Few. Virtually all patients with malignant or nonmalignant neoplastic dermatologic disorders can be managed as outpatients.

Parasitic Infestations

I. Scabies
A. Manifestations
The **specific manifestations** include severe pruritus affecting the trunk, back, and arms. The pruritus is especially severe at night. Because the organism that causes this entity is easily transmitted between individuals and therefore is highly contagious, epidemics can occur. Lesions from the infestation occur on the skin of the entire body except for the head. On **examination,** the lesions are classically 1–3 mm in size and usually occur in straight lines, or "runs." An excellent place to look for these lesions is on sides of the digits. These lesions usually have adjacent areas of excoriation and may become pustular as a result of secondary bacterial infection.
B. Pathogenesis
The **organism** that causes this infestation is *Sarcoptes scabiei.* The organism burrows in the skin and causes the above-described lesions.
C. Evaluation
The **specific evaluation** of this entity involves making the clinical diagnosis. If there is any question as to the diagnosis, a shave biopsy of one of the "runs" can be performed. On microscopic evaluation, the organism can often be demonstrated. A **urine pregnancy test** should be performed on all women of childbearing age.
D. Management
The **specific management** includes the following:
1. In all patients, one must **treat any secondary bacterial infection** with topical antibiotics (e.g., Polysporin) and, if **severe,** with systemic antibiotics such as cephalexin (Keflex), 500 mg PO q.i.d., or dicloxacillin, 250 mg PO q.i.d. for 5 days.
2. All **clothes and linen** must be washed in **hot water,** > 140 °F, for 1–2 hours and then dried in a hot dryer for >20 minutes.
3. All family members must be treated **concurrently.**

4. In **nonpregnant adults:**
   a. **Lindane (Kwell) 1% cream** is applied once to the entire body below the head and left on overnight. Lindane comes in 1% cream, lotion, or shampoo. It is **contraindicated in pediatric or pregnant patients.** Usually it is 100% effective.
   b. Alternatively, **Permethrin (Elimethin) 5% cream** is applied once to the entire body except for the face and left on overnight. It is **contraindicated in pregnant patients** or those **less than 2 months of age.** The advantages over lindane include the facts that it can be used in the hair and in younger patients. It is usually 95%–100% effective.
5. In **children and pregnant women, crotamiton 10% (Eurax)** cream or lotion is used. The patient first bathes, then applies the agent to all areas from the neck down. The process is repeated in 24 hours. It is more than 90% effective in eradicating the infestation.

II. Pediculosis (lice infestation)

A. Manifestations

The **manifestations** are specific to the site affected and include the acute onset of pruritus in the affected hair-containing areas. **Examination** discloses some erythema and excoriations about the affected hair-containing area and nits, or egg capsules, which appear as whitish structures on the hair filaments. Infestation occurs in or adjacent to areas of skin with hair. This organism is relatively easy to transmit and can result in epidemics.

B. Pathogenesis

The **organisms** that cause this infestation include *Pediculus humanus capitis,* the head louse; *Pediculus humanus corporis,* the body louse; and *Phthirus pubis,* the genital hair louse, commonly called "crabs." The underlying pathogenesis is that the organism infests an area of hair-containing skin. The organism is transmitted by close body contact, i.e., it can be a sexually transmitted disease, or it can be transmitted by sharing combs or bed linen.

C. Evaluation

The **specific evaluation** of this entity involves making the clinical diagnosis by physical examination.

D. Management

The **specific management** includes the following:
1. In all patients, **treat any secondary bacterial infection** with topical antibiotics (e.g., Polysporin) or, if **severe,** with systemic antibiotics such as cephalexin (Keflex), 500 mg PO q.i.d., or dicloxacillin, 250 mg PO q.i.d. for 5 days.

2. All **clothes and linen** must be washed in **hot water** (>140 °F) for 1–2 hours, then dried in a hot dryer for more than 20 minutes.
3. All family members must be treated concurrently.
4. In **nonpregnant adults, Lindane** (Kwell) 1% cream, lotion or shampoo, is applied to the affected hair and left on for 15–30 minutes. The nits should be combed out at 12 hours. This agent is contraindicated in pregnant women and children. The patient should be instructed to avoid mucous membranes with this substance.
5. In **pregnant women and children, pyrethrin 0.3% or piperonyl butoxide 3%** (Nix, Rid, others), as a gel, shampoo, or solution, is applied to affected hair and adjacent skin, then after 10–15 minutes washed out, with any nits concurrently combed out.

III. Fleas
A. Manifestations
The **specific manifestations** include the onset of generalized pruritus in a patient with a dog and/or cat at home. On **examination** there may be multiple, tiny (1–2 mm) punctate lesions on the skin. The lesions are asymmetric in distribution and may occur anywhere on the skin surface. There may be, but not necessarily are, excoriations adjacent to the lesions. Often the patient relates that the pet has been excessively or incessantly scratching itself.

B. Pathogenesis
The **organisms** that cause this infestation include *Ctenocephalides felis,* in which the cat is the preferred host, and *Ctenocephalides canis,* in which the dog is the preferred host. The organism infests an area of hair-containing skin. The organism can be transmitted by sharing combs with an infested pet or by close contact with an infested pet. Humans are not the preferred host for these blood-sucking organisms.

C. Evaluation and management
The **specific evaluation and management** of this entity involve making the clinical diagnosis and **treating the pet** with an **appropriate topical agent.** This agent may be obtained over the counter or from a veterinarian.
1. The patient should steam clean all carpets and wash all linen in **hot water and dry in a hot dryer for more than 20 minutes** to kill any adult fleas and eggs.
2. Once the preferred host—the cat or dog—is treated, the infestation resolves. **No other specific topical treatment is required for the patient.**

(*Text continues on page 499*)

Scaling Diseases

T A B L E 8 - 6
Scaling Diseases

Disease	History and Physical Examination Findings	Precipitating Factors or Events	Histopathology	Treatment
Lichen planus (Fig. 8-11)	Pruritic papules Symmetric distribution Mucous membranes and skin involved Violaceous appearing Wickham's striae present, i.e., white streaks on papular surface Koebner's sign present, i.e., lesions occur along linear scratch sites	Ulcerative colitis Vitiligo Graft-versus-host disease Medications Gold Quinine Tetracycline Streptomycin Arsenicals Others	IgG and C3 at basement membrane, and infiltration of T-cells into dermis	Anxiolytics Topical corticosteroids Discontinue and treat precipitating factor Dapsone, 50 mg PO q.d. Psoralens and PUVA (long-wave UV light) Dermatology consultation

| Psoriasis (Fig. 8-12) | Reddish plaques with scales
Mild pruritus
Nail pitting
Asymmetric arthritis
Koebner's sign present
Scalp, elbows, and knees commonly affected, usually symmetric distribution
Recurrent, chronic
Scales silvery
Auspitz's sign—minute bleeding sites when a scale is removed | Genetic predisposition
HIV related | Multiple dermal microabscesses | *Acute:* calamine with 10% coal tar q.d.; betamethasone applied b.i.d. (both to affected areas for 2 weeks)
Dermatology consultation
Goekerman regimen/PUVA |
| Pityriasis rosea | Spring and fall are periods of highest incidence
Oval, scaly lesions
Herald patch on trunk, followed by development of multiple patches on trunk, back, and chest | None | Nonspecific inflammation; biopsy rarely needed | Diphenhydramine, 25–50 mg PO q.6h.
Reassurance |

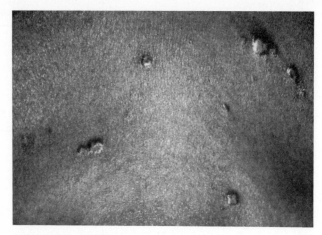

F I G U R E 8 - 1 1
Pruritic papules of lichen planus on the upper trunk.

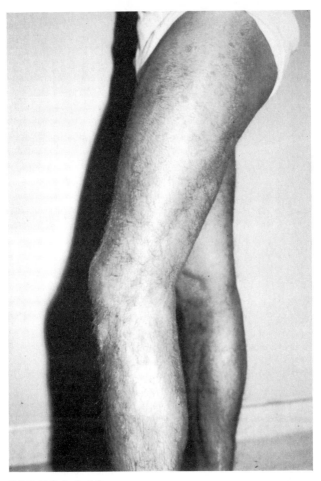

F I G U R E 8 - 1 2
Scaly, mildly pruritic plaquelike lesions of psoriasis on the extensor
surface of the extremities.

Fungal Skin Infections

T A B L E 8 - 7
Fungal Skin Infections

Disease	History and Physical Examination	Diagnosis	Treatment
Tinea capitis	Scalp Multiple scaly areas with alopecia Mildly pruritic Kerion development: nodular pustule in the scalp	Microscopic analysis of hair pretreated with KOH, and/or fungal culture of hair	Griseofulvin, 500–1,000 mg/day for 8 wk or fluconazole, 100 mg PO q.d. for 6–8 wks Clotrimazole 1% to area b.i.d. If kerion present, use above and: KI, 5–10 drops PO q.d. for 10 days Prednisone, 40 mg PO q.d. for 10 days Dermatology consult
Tinea corporis (Fig. 8-13)	Pruritic Scaly, centally clearing lesions with reddish margins Usually on trunk, back, thighs Asymmetric distribution Also known as ringworm	Scrape margins of lesion with a scalpel; add KOH to scrapings and look for hyphae	Clotrimazole 1% b.i.d. to affected areas If severe, griseofulvin, 500–1,000 mg PO q.d. for 1 wk, or fluconazole, 100 mg PO q.d. for 1 wk
Tinea cruris	Pruritic Intertriginous zones Sharply demarcated areas Moist; some superficial skin breakdown can occur Usually occur in hot, humid weather	KOH preparation of scrapings Clinical diagnosis	Loose-fitting underwear Absorbing powder (talc, Zeasorb, others) to affected areas Clotrimazole 1% b.i.d. If severe, griseofulvin, 500–1,000 mg/day PO q.d. for 14 days, or fluconazole, 200 mg PO q.d. for 14 days, and wet compresses applied once daily, saturated with 1:10,000 KMnO₂

Tinea pedis or manuum (Fig. 8-14)	Erythema, pruritus Acutely can have small vesicles and weeping fissures develop in toe and finger webs Can develop onychomycosis	KOH preparation, look for hyphae	Absorbing powder (talc, Zeasorb, others) to affected areas Change hose daily Dry between toes Clotrimazole 1% b.i.d. Aluminum subacetate solution; soak feet for 20 minutes 3 times daily
Tinea unguium	Toenails and/or fingernails friable, discolored, and brittle Also known as onychomycosis	Scrapings of nail with KOH, hyphae seen	Clotrimazole 1% b.i.d., griseofulvin 1,000 mg PO q.d., or fluconazole, 100 mg PO q.d. Difficult to eradicate
Tinea versicolor	Macules, hypopigmented Trunk Mildly pruritic Organism: *Pityrosporon orbiculare* (also known as *Malassezia furfur*)	Clinically Scrapings of affected areas with KOH, hyphae demonstrated	Lotion containing selenium sulfides* (e.g., Selsun Blue, others) q.d. for 1–2 wk Clotrimazole 1% b.i.d.
ID, "dermatophytid"	Acute onset of small, pruritic lesions on flexor surfaces of digits and on palms Quite pruritic "Allergy" to a chronic fungal skin infection in another area of body Must differentiate from tinea manuum	No hyphae seen on KOH preparations of affected skin scrapings	Treat tineal infection at other sites Hydrocortisone 0.1% b.i.d. to ID areas

*The appropriate use of selenium sulfide–containing lotion (1%–2.5%) is as follows. The patient should bathe and dry completely, then apply the lotion to all skin areas from the neck to the pubis and allow the lotion to dry. The lotion is washed off 24 hours later. This process is repeated on a weekly basis for 4 weeks.

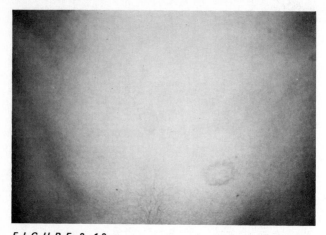

FIGURE 8-13
Tinea corporis on lower abdomen. Note peripheral erythema with central clearing. Lesions are mildly pruritic.

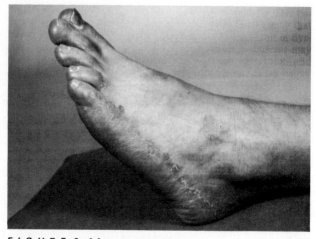

FIGURE 8-14
Tinea pedis on left foot. Note erythematous, scaly rash on solar aspect of the foot. Can have vesicles and be moderately pruritic.

T A B L E   8 - 8
Selected Topical Glucocorticoids

Agent	Fluorinated	Potency

Hydrocortisone
    Cream: 0.25%, 0.5%, and 1%
    Ointment: 0.5% and 1%
    Lotion: 0.25%, 0.5%, and 1%
	No	Low

Triamcinolone (Kenalog)
    Cream: 0.1%
    Lotion: 0.1%
	Yes	Low to
		    moderate

Triamcinolone (Aristocort) Cream: 0.5%	Yes	Moderate

Fluocinonide (Lidex)
    Cream: 0.05%
    Ointment: 0.05%
	Yes	Moderate

Amcinonide (Cyclocort) Ointment: 0.1%	Yes	Moderate
Betamethasone dipropionate (Diprolene) Ointment: 0.05%	Yes	High

NOTE: Topical glucocorticoids that are **fluorinated** should not be used on the face, as they are associated with the development of telangiectasias and other cosmetic sequelae.

Urticaria

I. **Overall manifestations**

The **overall manifestations** of urticaria include the development of intensely pruritic wheals, commonly called hives, on any area of the skin. The lesions may be local or generalized. Often dermatographism is present. **Dermatographism** is demonstrated by **gently** scratching the skin surface with a pen cap or gloved fingernail. The scratching results in local erythema; therefore, one can actually "write" symbols or letters on the skin. The patient may have a past or present history of angioedema. **Angioedema** is a phenomenon in which there is swelling of the deep tissues, often manifested as a swelling of the lips and other mucous membranes, usually of the oropharyngeal area. In severe cases, angioedema can result in upper airway dysfunction.

II. **Classification of urticaria**

Urticaria may be classified into two categories, acute and chronic.

A. **Acute urticaria**

1. **Manifestations**

The **specific manifestations** of acute urticaria include the sudden onset of urticaria, which is invariably and intimately related temporally to a precipitating event. The patient may have a past history of urticaria or of allergies to certain entities. Associated manifestations include hypotension, angioedema, and wheezing and shortness of breath as a result of bronchospasm.

2. **Pathogenesis**
   The **underlying pathogenesis** is anaphylaxis. It is usually an **IgE-mediated** event in which the allergen stimulates production of IgE from B-lymphocytes. The IgE, which is specific to that allergen, is incorporated into the plasma membrane of mast cells. If and when the allergen is presented again to the patient, it binds to the IgE on the **mast cell surface,** which induces the release of histamine from the mast cell. **Histamine** acts on the smooth muscle of the airways and vasculature to cause the specific manifestations of **anaphylaxis**—i.e., urticaria, angioedema, bronchospasm, hypotension, and airway compromise.

3. **Precipitants**
   The list of precipitants of acute urticaria is long.
   a. **Medications.** Virtually any medication can cause acute urticaria. Medications most commonly associated with urticaria include the β-lactam class of antibiotics (e.g., penicillin), the sulfa class of antibiotics, and the angiotensin-converting enzyme inhibitor class of antihypertensive agents. The urticaria is usually generalized.
   b. **Insect bites.** Virtually all insect bites will result in local urticaria; however, certain patients experience generalized urticaria and even anaphylaxis. A **bee** or **wasp bite** will result in a localized urticarial reaction at the bite site in virtually all patients, and in a small but significant minority of patients a generalized urticarial reaction occurs. **Mosquito bites** result in a localized solitary urticarial lesion but virtually never a generalized urticarial reaction.
   c. **Foods** and **food additives,** including dyes and preservatives, can result in localized angioedema and generalized urticaria.

4. **Evaluation**
   The **specific evaluation** includes that described in Box 8-3 and making the clinical diagnosis.

5. **Management**
   Management includes determining the precipitating factor and identifying the patient as **allergic** to that factor. A **Med-Alert bracelet** stating this allergy should be prepared for the patient. If allergic to in-

---

B O X 8 - 3

Overall Evaluation and Management of Urticaria

Evaluation

1. ABCs, i.e., maintain the patient's airway, breathing, and cardiac function via CPR and ACLS protocol.
2. Take a thorough **history** and perform a **physical examination** looking for the specific manifestations described in text.

Management

1. If there is any evidence of **anaphylaxis**, i.e., any bronchospasm, airway compromise, or hypotension, institute the following measures.
   a. Administer 0.3 mL **epinephrine 1:1000 SC.** This can be repeated 2–4 times at intervals of 15–20 minutes.
   b. Administer the H_1 receptor antagonist **diphenhydramine** (Benadryl), 25–50 mg PO or IM or IV. Repeat in 30 minutes and every 4–6 hours thereafter as needed.
   c. **Provide IV fluids with normal saline.**
   d. Administer **steroids** in the form of a bolus of Solumedrol, 125 mg IV, unless there is a contraindication.
   e. If there is any evidence of wheezing, administer a β_2 **receptor agonist topically,** e.g., metoproterenol (Alupent) or albuterol (Proventil), either by hand-held nebulizer.
   f. Administer an H_2 **receptor antagonist,** e.g., cimetidine, 300 mg IV, or ranitidine, 50 mg IV, at the outset.
2. Admission for observation for 24 hours is indicated.

---

sect bites, the patient or a family member should obtain an **Epi-Pen** and be educated as to its use. Finally, all of these patients should have an allergy consult for long-term follow-up.

B. Chronic urticaria

  1. Manifestations

    The **specific manifestations** of chronic urticaria include the fact that it is present for more than 2 weeks. The patient is unable to cite, even after extensive questioning, any overt precipitating event. The urticaria is usually generalized and can have associated angioedema. The patient may experience components of an acute anaphylactic reaction **at any time** during this process.

2. **Pathogenesis**

   The **underlying pathogenesis** is a mediator-related effect on the smooth muscle of the bronchial airways or vasculature. The mechanism of mediator release is multifactorial and depends on the specific mediator. The most common mediators are **histamine,** usually via the IgE mechanism described above; prostaglandins; serotonin; and/or autoimmune-mediated dysfunction of the smooth muscle.

3. **Underlying causes**

   Underlying causes include vasculitis, C_1-esterase deficiency, the prodromal phase of hepatitis B, medications, cold-induced, and idiopathic.

4. **Evaluation**

   The **specific evaluation** includes making the clinical diagnosis and performing the evaluations described in Box 8-3. Further evaluation should be directed toward ascertaining and defining the underlying cause of the urticaria. These include obtaining serum electrolytes, BUN, creatinine, and urinalysis in order to look for any concurrent renal dysfunction or glomerulonephritis. Further specific evaluation includes obtaining an ESR, ANA, RF, CH_{50}, C_3, and C_4 levels. The ESR, ANA, or RF titer may be evaluated in a vasculitis whereas the complement levels may be concurrently decreased. Further specific evaluation can include obtaining a hepatitis B panel, plasma cryoglobulins, a plasma C_1-esterase level, and a biopsy of one of the skin lesions.

5. **Management**

   The **specific management,** in addition to that described in Box 8-3, is directed toward the underlying cause. **Specific interventions** on a chronic basis include the following measures.

   a. **H_1 receptor antagonists** on an as needed or scheduled basis. These can include diphenhydramine (Benadryl), 25–50 mg PO q.i.d. PRN, or hydroxyzine (Atarax), 25 mg PO q.i.d., or astemizole (Hisminal), 10 mg/day.

   b. **H_2 receptor antagonists** on a scheduled basis. These can include cimetidine (Tagamet), 400 mg PO b.i.d., or ranitidine (Zantac), 150 mg PO b.i.d.

   c. If predominantly **cold-induced** and not as the result of a cryoglobulinemia, cyproheptadine, 4 mg

PO q.i.d., is effective. Recommend to the patient that the patient move to a warm climate and minimize exposure to cold.

d. If **severe and not related to hepatitis B, steroids,** e.g., prednisone, 40–60 mg PO q.d., can be effective.

e. If C_1-**esterase deficiency** with acute angioedema, administer methyltestosterone, 10 mg PO q.d., and an infusion of C_1-inhibitor in D5W intravenously over 10 minutes.

III. Consultation

Service	*Time*
Allergy	Urgent

IV. **Indications for admission:** Any evidence of anaphylaxis, angioedema, or airway compromise.

Viral Dermatologic Lesions

I. Herpes labialis

A. Manifestations

The **specific manifestations** of this entity include the acute onset of a unilateral, single group of vesicles on the perioral areas, including the lips. The vesicles last for approximately 2–3 days, crust over, and resolve in 7–10 days. The lesions are commonly referred to as fever blisters or cold sores. They may recur, with asymptomatic periods between episodes lasting up to several years. Events that **precipitate** these lesions include fever, any upper respiratory tract infection, trauma to the area, or generalized stress.

B. Pathogenesis

The **underlying pathogenesis** of herpes labialis is an infection of the perioral mucous membranes with the DNA virus, **HSV-I.** Most of the population becomes infected with the virus as children as the result of kissing of the child by a parent or sibling who has active infection. After the onset of vesicles, there is viral shedding for 5 days. After an initial acute vesicular lesion, the virus becomes dormant in the sensory ganglion of the dermatome involved, i.e., the **trigeminal ganglion,** only to become recurrently symptomatic at a later date.

C. Evaluation

The **specific evaluation** includes making the clinical diagnosis from the history and physical examination findings. In the vast majority of cases no further examinations are required, but if there is any question as to the diagnosis, a Tzanck smear of vesicular contents can be performed. The **Tzanck smear** will show large, bizarre, multinucleated cells, a finding consistent with HSV infection.

D. **Management**

The **specific management** is usually minimal, as the infection is usually self-limited. A 7-day course of **acyclovir 5% cream** applied to the area 5–6 times per day can be prescribed for moderately symptomatic cases.

1. If the symptoms are severe or if the group of lesions is large, systemic acyclovir, administered in a dose of 200 mg PO 5 times per day for 7 days, is effective in therapy.

2. As with other processes, **prevention** is important. Thus, someone with active herpes labialis should **never kiss anyone else** until the lesions have resolved. Parents and grandparents should be educated to this fact, so as not to transmit this viral infection to infants, toddlers, and children.

3. The clinician must monitor for and aggressively treat any **complications**. Two complications that can occur in patients with herpes labialis are keratitis and mucocutaneous herpes simplex.

   a. **Keratitis.** The acute onset of corneal inflammation concurrent with or after an episode of herpes labialis. This infection is severe and on fluorescein examination reveals a dendritic pattern of ulcerations on the cornea. If not aggressively treated, it leads to visual loss. See section on red, inflamed eyes in Chapter 13.

   b. **Mucocutaneous herpes simplex.** This occurs in patients who are immunocompromised, especially with any compromise of cell-mediated immunity, such as AIDS patients or patients undergoing chemotherapy for malignant neoplastic lesions. The infection may be unilateral or bilateral and consists of rapidly spreading vesicles of the skin and mucous membranes with concurrent painful sloughing of the superficial skin and mucosa. This can be caused by HSV-I or II and requires aggressive treatment. If the patient has no underlying reason for immunocompromise, the patient has, by definition, **AIDS.**

      i. **Specific management** includes placing the patient under blood and body fluid precautions, obtaining a serum HIV antibody, and administering acyclovir, 200 mg PO 5 times per day for 14 days or 10 mg/kg/24 hours in q.8h. dosing for 7–10 days, followed by **chronic ther-**

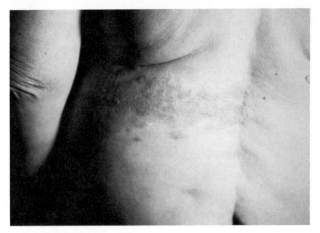

F I G U R E 8 - 1 5
Herpes zoster: unilateral, painful, vesicular rash over one dermatome.

> **apy** with acyclovir, 200 mg PO q. A.M. indefinitely.
>
> ii. Refer to section on **HIV Infection** in Chapter 6.

II. Herpes genitalis
HSV-II infection. Refer to section on Sexually Transmitted Diseases in Chapter 6.

III. Herpes zoster
A. Manifestations
The **specific manifestations** of this entity include the acute onset of erythema and vesicles unilaterally in the region of a single dermatome (see Fig. 8-15). There usually are associated hyperesthesia and significant pain. The vesicles last for 2–3 days, then crust over and slowly resolve over 3–4 weeks. **Pain** may last for a period of time after the lesions resolve and may lead to the chronic pain syndrome, postherpetic neuralgia. This entity is commonly called shingles.

B. Pathogenesis
The **underlying pathogenesis** of herpes zoster is infection with the same DNA virus that causes varicella (i.e., chicken pox). After the acute varicella infection, the varicella–zoster virus remains in the sensory ganglia of the spinal cord and cranial nerves. After a prolonged quiescent period, the virus is reactivated and the manifesta-

tions of zoster occur. Events that **precipitate** or are **risk factors** for the development of herpes zoster include increasing age, immunosuppression (e.g., with steroids, chemotherapy, or AIDS), and any generalized stress.

C. **Evaluation**

The **specific evaluation** includes making the clinical diagnosis from the history and physical examination findings. In the vast majority of cases no further examinations are required.

D. **Management**

The **specific management** includes the following measures.

1. Administer **acyclovir,** 800 mg PO 5 times per day for 7–10 days. If initiated within 48 hours of the onset of vesicles, this will decrease the duration of viral shedding and symptoms of disease.

2. Place the patient on **respiratory and contact isolation/pregnancy precautions.** During the vesicular stage it is transmissible, and anyone (including a fetus) who has not had varicella (chickenpox) is susceptible to infection.

3. The **treatment of postherpetic neuralgia** includes the administration of narcotic agents as needed and the administration of topical capsaicin (Zostrix) cream 0.075%. This agent, applied to the dermatome after the acute lesions have healed, on a b.i.d. dosing for 10 days, increases substance P, thus increasing intrinsic analgesia at the level of the nerves. Finally, if pain is intractable, referral to a **pain clinic** is necessary.

IV. **Varicella**

A. **Manifestations**

The **specific manifestations** of this entity include the acute onset of fever, malaise, mild rhinorrhea, and multiple vesicles. The **vesicles** become, in 3–4 days, **pustules,** which subsequently **rupture** and **crust over.** These then slowly **resolve** and **heal without scarring** over the next 5 days. A new group of vesicles, sometimes referred to as individual **crops,** occurs every 2–3 days until several crops of vesicles in various stages of evolution are present. The disease is usually **self-limited** and lasts for a total of 14–18 days, i.e., 4–5 crops of lesions. The lesions are usually painless but moderately pruritic in the crust stage. The **first crop** usually occurs on the trunk, with subsequent crops being progressively peripheral (see Fig. 8-16).

B. **Pathogenesis**

The **underlying pathogenesis** of this acute viral infec-

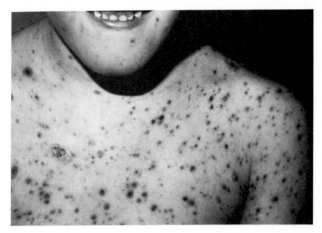

FIGURE 8-16
Varicella (chickenpox). Note various crops of papules, which evolve
into vesicles, which evolve into pustules, which then crust
over and heal.

tion is a DNA herpesvirus. The virus is **transmitted** from
another person with **acute zoster** or **varicella** by aerosol
to be inhaled by the patient. The **incubation period** is
approximately 10–14 days after exposure.

C. **Evaluation**

The **specific evaluation** includes making the clinical diagnosis via history and physical examination. In the
vast majority of cases no further examinations are required.

D. **Management**

The **specific management** is, in the vast majority of
cases, symptomatic only. The patient can be afforded
antipyretic and analgesic relief with **acetaminophen**
and topical use of **calamine lotion** applied b.i.d. The
calamine lotion will decrease any pruritus. Salicylates
should be avoided given the potential association of aspirin and viral syndrome with Reye's syndrome.

1. The clinician must watch for the development of
   complications, especially in older (>18 years) patients and those who are immunosuppressed. The
   most dramatic complication is **pneumonitis.**

   a. Varicella pneumonitis **manifests** with severe, dif-
      fuse interstitial infiltrates, an increased $A-ao_2$
      gradient, hypoxemia, and dry cough, and can
      lead to respiratory failure and death.

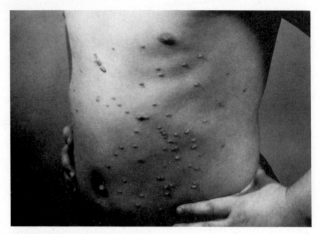

F I G U R E 8 - 1 7
Molluscum contagiosum on the trunk and abdomen.

    b. The **specific management of varicella pneumonitis** includes admission to the hospital, supportive care with oxygen, and the administration of parenteral acyclovir, 10 mg/kg/24 hours in q.8h. divided doses.

V. Molluscum contagiosum

A. Manifestations

The **specific manifestations** of this entity include the insidious onset of and slow increase in the number of firm, painless papules on the trunk, face, arms, and genitals. Each of these lesions occurs on a narrow base, i.e., each one is umbilicated (see Fig. 8-17). There are no associated systemic symptoms or signs. The lesions last for weeks to months without significantly changing and then may spontaneously resolve, especially if there is minor trauma to specific papules.

B. Pathogenesis

The **underlying pathogenesis** is a DNA virus in the poxvirus family infecting the skin. These lesions are transmitted by direct contact, either self to self, i.e., "autospread," or from one person to another.

C. Evaluation

The **specific evaluation** includes making the clinical diagnosis via history and physical examination. In the vast majority of cases no further examinations are required. If there is any question as to the diagnosis or if

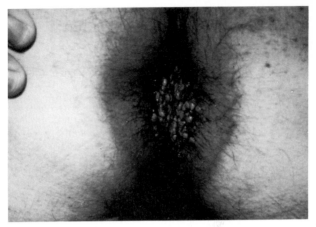

F I G U R E   8 - 1 8
Condylomata acuminata on the anal and perineal areas.

any lesion is different and/or suspicious for a malignant lesion, excisional biopsy must be performed.

D. **Management**

The **specific management** is quite simple: these lesions either spontaneously resolve or disappear after minor trauma. Thus, superficial trauma to each lesion with an **electrosurgical probe** or with **liquid nitrogen** will safely and easily cure the lesions of this viral infection. Each lesion must be individually traumatized to effect resolution.

VI. **Condylomata acuminata**

A. **Manifestations**

The **specific manifestations** of this entity include the insidious onset of single or multiple rough papules on or adjacent to the perianal, vulvar, perineal, scrotal, or penile skin. The lesions are usually asymptomatic and painless even when large (see Fig. 8-18). The lesions increase in number and slowly enlarge in size from papular lesions to large, exuberant cauliflowerlike lesions. Spontaneous regression of the lesions is uncommon. These lesions have been correlated with the development of the malignant neoplastic lesion, **squamous cell carcinoma**.

B. **Pathogenesis**

The **underlying pathogenesis** is infection of the genital

skin and mucous membranes by human papillomavirus
(HPV), especially **viral types 16 and 18.** This is one of
the most common sexually transmitted diseases in the
United States today, and its incidence is increasing. Of
concern is that a significant minority of these infections
are in patients who have subclinical disease; however,
this infection, even if not clinically demonstrable, can
be transmitted by virtually any sexual activity.

C. **Evaluation**

The **specific evaluation** includes making the clinical diagnosis via history and physical examination. If any lesion is **atypical-appearing** or suspicious for a malignant
lesion, **excisional biopsy is mandated.**

1. Often the examination should include **stereoscopic
   microscope** examinations of the affected areas. This
   technique can demonstrate smaller, earlier, and
   therefore easier to treat lesions. The stereoscope
   used is a colposcope if used to examine females or
   an androscope when used to examine male genitalia.
2. The use of **acetic acid** is another technique used to
   demonstrate the **extent** of the condylomata and to
   demonstrate small, early lesions. Gauze saturated
   with 5% acetic acid (vinegar) is placed on the skin.
   The acetic acid will turn the **condylomatous tissue
   white.** When this is used in conjunction with stere-
   oscopy, early, small lesions can be visualized and
   treated, using the schemas described below, with
   great precision.

D. **Management**

The **specific management** includes basic education on
methods of **safe sex.** Specific modalities used in the
treatment of these lesions include the following:

1. **Podophyllin 25% in benzoin.** Apply this directly to
   the lesion, dry, wash off 6–8 hours later. Anesthesia
   is not required. The **mechanism of action** is that it
   causes direct destruction/necrosis of the infected
   and normal tissue; therefore, one must be **precise
   in treatment.** Treatment can be repeated every 1–2
   weeks for 3–4 cycles. This treatment is 50%–80%
   effective, especially in small lesions.
2. **Trichloroacetic acid (TCA) 50% and 80% solution.** This is one of the best modalities in the treatment of condylomata acuminata because, with
   proper instruction, the patient can self-apply it to
   the lesions. Anesthesia is not required. This agent
   causes direct destruction/necrosis of the infected
   and normal tissues; therefore, one must be **precise
   in treatment.**
   a. The **50% solution** is applied to the lesion b.i.d.

and allowed to dry. The duration of this regimen is for 3 consecutive days per week for 3 consecutive weeks.

    b. If no improvement occurs, the same procedure and schedule is used for the **80% solution.** Because the solution causes significant necrosis of both infected and normal tissue, care must be taken to optimize **precision in treatment.**

  3. 5-fluorouracil 5% cream. Not yet approved for this entity by the FDA.

  4. α-Interferon. Applied intralesionally to the base of the lesion. There are high recurrence rates even after the aggressive use of this agent; therefore, there is no real advantage to its use over the above-described modalities.

  5. Surgery. Direct surgical resection is indicated if the lesions have not responded to 6–8 weeks of aggressive topical treatment or if there is any suspicion of a concurrent neoplasm.

    a. Direct surgical resection is effective, with a **cure rate of 90%** or more.

    b. Cryosurgery with liquid nitrogen is also effective and can be applied by the primary care physician, but is not indicated if there is any suspicion of malignancy.

    c. Electrosurgery and laser ablation are effective but **should not be performed,** given the well-documented **risk of aerosolization of the lesions** with **live virus** with the potential to cause **respiratory HPV infections,** especially laryngeal nodules, in the physician or the patient.

VII. Verruca vulgaris
A. Manifestations

The **specific manifestations** include the insidious onset of papules on the skin of the distal upper or lower extremities. The papules have a rough texture and their centers can develop minute black spots deep in the papule itself. These lesions are ubiquitous; the lifetime prevalence is virtually 100% for humans. These lesions, which are painless and virtually asymptomatic, are commonly known as **warts.** There are two major types of warts, the **common wart,** which occurs on the fingers, and the **plantar wart,** which is quite deep and occurs on the planar aspect of the feet. These lesions can slowly increase in size and number but can, quite spontaneously, resolve. An increased incidence of **squamous cell carcinoma** has been reported in warts located adjacent to the nail folds, i.e., periungual warts.

B. Pathogenesis

The **underlying pathogenesis** is an infection of keratin-ized skin on the hands or feet with the DNA virus, **human papillomavirus (HPV)**.

C. Evaluation

The **specific evaluation** includes making the clinical diagnosis via history and physical examination. If any lesion is **atypical appearing** or suspicious for a malignant lesion, **excisional biopsy is mandated.**

D. Management

The **specific management** of these lesions is to destroy the wart with minimal damage to the adjacent tissue. It requires the destruction of the tissue deep into the dermis itself. One or more of several modalities can be used.

1. **Cryosurgery with liquid nitrogen** to the wart itself. This procedure, using a cottom swab to apply the liquid nitrogen to the lesion, must be repeated on a weekly basis until the wart is completely destroyed.

2. **Trichloroacetic acid (TCA) in saturated solution.** Apply to base of wart using a cotton swab and allow to dry. Excise any destroyed tissue with a scissors in 24 hours. Repeat the process on a daily basis until the wart is completely destroyed.

3. **Salicylic acid 10% solution** (Compound W). Apply to wart using a cotton swab every evening for 7 days. Trim off the destroyed tissue each morning. This modality is clearly inferior in effectiveness relative to the above-described modalities.

VIII. Consultation

Problem	*Service*	*Time*
Any suspicious lesion	Dermatology	Urgent
Periungual wart	Dermatology	Required
Any evidence of HSV keratitis	Ophthal-mology	Emergent
Condylomata acumi-nata refractory to treatment	General surgery	Required
Varicella pneumonitis	Infectious dis-eases	Urgent
Mucocutaneous HSV	Infectious dis-eases	Urgent

IX. Indications for admission: Parenteral acyclovir, any evidence of varicella pneumonitis, or any evidence of HSV keratitis.

Bibliography

Acne Vulgaris
Bondi EE: Topical retinoid therapy. Am Fam Pract 1989;39:269–272.
Quan M, Strick RA: Management of acne vulgaris. Am Fam Pract 1988; 38:207–217.
Shalita AR, et al: Acne vulgaris. J Am Acad Dermatol 1987;16:410–412.

Blistering Diseases
Heimbach DM, et al: Toxic epidermal necrolysis. JAMA 1987;257: 2171–2175.
Imber MJ, et al: The immunopathology of bullous pemphigoid. Clin Dermatol 1987;5:81–89.
Stanley JR: Pemphigus. JAMA 1990;264:1714–1717.

Dermatitis
Buckley RH, Mathews KP: Common allergic skin diseases. JAMA 1982; 248:2611.
Hanifin JM: Atopic dermatitis. J Am Acad Dermatol 1982;6:1.
Shuster S: The aetiology of dandruff and the mode of action of therapeutic agents. Br J Dermatol 1984;3:236.

Erythemas
Horio T, et al: Potassium iodide in the treatment of erythema nodosum and nodular vasculitis. Arch Dermatol 1981;117:29.
Schosser RH: The erythema multiforme spectrum: Diagnosis and treatment. Curr Concepts Skin Dis 1985;6:6.

Neoplasia
Beacham BE: Solar-induced epidermal tumors in the elderly. Am Fam Pract 1990;42:153–160.
Greene MH, et al: Acquired precursors of cutaneous malignant melanoma. N Engl J Med 1985;312:91–97.
Koh HK: Cutaneous melanoma. N Engl J Med 1991;325:171–182.
Rhodes AR, et al: Risk factors for cutaneous melanoma. JAMA 1987; 258:3146–3154.
Tobinick EL: Basal cell carcinoma. Am Fam Pract 1987;36:219–224.

Parasitic Infestations
Brodell RT, Helms SE: Office dermatologic testing: The scabies preparation. Am Fam Pract 1991;44:505–508.
Burkhart CG: Scabies: An epidemiologic reassessment. Ann Intern Med 1983;98:498.
Witkowski JA, Parish LC: Scabies. JAMA 1984;252:1318–1317.

Scaling Diseases
Gardner SS, McKay M: Seborrhea, psoriasis, and the papulosquamous dermatoses. Primary Care 1989;16:739–763.
Truhan AP: Pityriasis rosea. Am Fam Pract 1984;29:193–196.

Fungal Skin Infections
Brodell RT, et al: Office dermatologic testing: The KOH preparation. Am Fam Pract 1991;43:2061–2065.
Pariser DM: Superficial fungal infections. Postgrad Med 1990;87:205–212.

Urticaria

Matthews KP: Urticaria and angioedema. J Allergy Clin Immunol 1983;72:1.
Zamm AV: Chronic urticaria: A practical approach. Cutis 1972;9:27.

Viral Dermatologic Lesions

Arbesfeld DM, Thomas I: Cutaneous herpes simplex virus infections. Am Fam Pract 1991;43:1655–1664.

Bolton RA: Nongenital warts: Classification and treatment options. Am Fam Pract 1991;43:2049–2056.

Carmichael JK: Treatment of herpes zoster and postherpetic neuralgia. Am Fam Pract 1991;44:203–210.

Ferenczy A: Diagnosis and treatment of anogenital warts in the male patient. Primary Care Cancer 1990;Sept:11–20.

Zazove P, et al: Genital human papillomavirus infection. Am Fam Pract 1991;43:1279–1290.

—D.D.B.

Dale Berg, Ed. *Handbook of Primary Care Medicine.* Copyright © 1993 J. B. Lippincott Company.

C H A P T E R   9

Endocrine Disorders

Diabetes Mellitus

Diabetes mellitus is quite prevalent in American culture. If uncontrolled and unchecked, it can result in significant, even life-threatening acute and chronic sequelae, all of which are preventable with early diagnosis and intervention. The overall prevalence of disease in the U.S. population is approximately 5%.

The **pathophysiology** of diabetes mellitus is quite complex and is continuing to be elucidated. Pertinent is the **physiology** of energy generation and glucose catabolism. All cells in the body require **energy** and therefore **substrates** for energy generation. Although several substrates, including proteins, amino acids, and fatty acids, can serve this function of energy generation, the most efficient and effective substrate is **glucose.** In fact, glucose is required for normal cell function, especially neuronal function.

Glucose is a monosaccharide that is absorbed from foodstuffs through the GI tract. For glucose to be utilized as a source of energy (as a substrate for energy production), it must cross **into** the cell. Cell entry is controlled by the hormone **insulin.** Insulin is a relatively small polypeptide that is secreted by the beta islet cells in the pancreas.

Once within the cells, glucose is catabolized by the **glycolytic pathway** and **Krebs cycle** and coupled with aerobic respiration to produce the basic energy molecule of the cell, **adenosine triphosphate (ATP).**

All hormones have **target cells** on which they effect change. Within the surfaces of these cells are specific **receptors,** which are requisite for hormone activity. The target cells for insulin are virtually all the cells of the body, and specific insulin receptors in the plasma membranes of these target cells are required for insulin activity and therefore the generation of energy from glucose.

The **pathophysiology** of diabetes mellitus is related to the interworking of insulin and its specific cell receptors. A deficiency in either or both can result in the basic features of diabetes mellitus, and forms the basis of the **classification paradigm** used for diabetes mellitus.

I. Pathogenesis

Two basic, interdependent features of diabetes mellitus are an **increase in glucose in the plasma** and an overall marked **decrease in glucose,** the cell's major substrate for energy production. The result is the pathophysiologic paradox of effective cellular starvation in the setting of ample amounts of glucose in the fluids bathing the cells.

The starving cells turn to other, **less optimal substrates** for energy production—proteins, amino acids, and fatty acids. These substrates not only are less efficient in energy production, but also are primarily for anabolism—i.e., the synthesis of structures—not for catabolism.

A specific outcome of the utilization of fatty acids and to a lesser extent amino acids for energy generation is the development of **ketone bodies.** These small anionic molecules, which include β-hydroxybutyrate, acetoacetate, and acetone, produce a systemic metabolic acidosis with an elevated anion gap.

II. Classification

The **classification** of diabetes mellitus is based on the physiology. There are two different pathophysiologic categories of diabetes mellitus, type I and type II.

A. Type I diabetes mellitus

Type I is a **deficiency,** either actual or relative, in the hormone insulin. The central feature is **insulinopenia.** The receptors are usually normal or even up-regulated (increased in quantity or effectiveness), but without insulin, glucose cannot enter the cell. The deficiency in insulin occurs as a result of destruction of beta islet cells within the pancreas itself. **Causes** of type I diabetes mellitus include the following conditions.

1. **Autoimmune destruction.** Certain HLA types and the coincidence of type I diabetes mellitus with other autoimmune disorders supports this pathophysiologic mechanism.

2. **Viral-mediated.** This is probably an indirect but significant mechanism in which the β-cells are damaged or destroyed by the immune system's fight against a viral infection, usually paramyxovirus.

3. **Recurrent pancreatitis.** Recurrent pancreatitis will result in destruction of the exocrine and endocrine pancreas. (See section on Pancreatitis in Chapter 2.)

B. Type II diabetes mellitus

Type II diabetes mellitus, unlike type I, is not a problem with insulin, but with the **receptor** upon which it works. It is postulated that receptors are **decreased in number or in effectiveness** at or immediately adjacent to the receptor (postreceptor level). A central feature is effective insulin resistance, usually associated with **obesity.** Obese patients have a decrease in the quantity or effectiveness of insulin receptors. This results in the ultimate paradox of effective cellular starvation in the setting of excessive glucose and excessive insulin in an obese patient. In type II diabetes, the glucose will, to certain degrees, enter the cells, and therefore the degree of intracellular starvation is less. This decreases the use of fatty acids and proteins, and therefore ketone bodies are not formed. Therefore, **type II is noninsulinopenic and nonketotic.**

III. **Overall manifestations**
   The **overall manifestations** of diabetes mellitus, type I or type II, are based on the pathophysiology.
   A. **Polyuria and polydipsia**
      Polyuria is an increased frequency and volume of urination, and **polydipsia** is an increase in the quantity of fluid ingested as a result of an increased thirst. Nocturia, or frequent urination at night, is a nonspecific manifestation that can be a marker for polyuria. In a patient who **cannot maintain thirst, intravascular volume depletion** with its specific manifestations of orthostatic hypotension and tachycardia may develop. The **underlying pathogenesis** is significant hyperglycemia with resultant glycosuria, i.e., loss of glucose, and with it water, in the urine.
   B. **Blurred vision.** The underlying pathogenesis is an increase in glucose and therefore of water within the lens itself, causing a change in the refractory profile of the lens and visual blurring.
   C. **Recurrent dermatologic fungal infections**
      1. Tinea cruris, severe.
      2. Tinea pedis with onychomycosis.
      3. Candidal balanitis (i.e., infection and inflammation of the foreskin in a male.
      4. Candidal vaginitis.
   D. **Manifestations specific to type I**
      These manifestations include the development of **ketones** with resultant acidosis (Table 9-1), acetone on the breath, and deep, rapid (Kussmaul) respiration. The patient with type I diabetes mellitus often loses weight.

IV. **Management**
   The **specific management** of diabetes mellitus is directed toward several goals: optimally **controlling serum glucose values** without precipitating hypoglycemia, monitoring and at-

T A B L E   9 - 1
Causes of High Anion Gap Metabolic Acidosis

$$\text{Anion gap} = Na - (Cl + HCO_3)$$

$$\text{Normal} = 12{-}14$$

Methanol ingestion   This toxin will form formic acid via the enzyme ethanol dehydrogenase.

Ketone bodies   The bodies, β-hydroxybutyrate, acetoacetate, and acetone, can be formed in diabetic ketoacidosis, ethanol-related ketoacidosis, and starvation.

Lactate   This anion is produced in hypoperfusion states and sepsis.

Salicylates   Overdosage or overdose.

Uremia   Fixed acids (i.e., anions) are not effectively excreted.

Ethylene glycol   Ingestion of this constituent of antifreeze will result in the formation of glyoxylic acid and oxylic acid.

Paraldehyde usage

tempting to **prevent sequelae** of diabetes mellitus, and **minimizing other concurrent risk factors** for the development of atherosclerotic vascular disease.

A. **Glycemic control**

Glycemic control is central to the management of diabetes mellitus. Although keeping serum glucose levels below 200 mg/dL minimizes polyuria, polydipsia, and other acute manifestations of hyperglycemia, the evidence is still far from conclusive that parsimonious glycemic control prevents the chronic sequelae of diabetes mellitus. Furthermore, there is always the potential of **hypoglycemia,** which can lead to morbid, even mortal events. The risk of hypoglycemia increases with the intensity of the control regimen and in patients who have problems with compliance. Therefore, **the degree of glycemic control must be tailored to the patient.** In a patient who has no sequelae and is compliant, the goal should be euglycemia, i.e., fasting glucose levels of 80–100 mg/dL and postprandial glucose levels no greater than 140 mg/dL. In a patient with multiple existing sequelae or other medical problems that will limit life span, such as metastatic carcinoma, the goal should be glucose values in the range of 150–250 mg/dL. **Regimens** for glycemic control include the following.

1. If the patient has **acutely decompensated** diabetes mellitus, emergent intervention in glycemic control is indicated. See Box 9-2 for specifics in management.

2. If the patient has **type I diabetes mellitus, insulin** is required to provide effective glycemic control.

   a. Only **human recombinant insulin** should be administered. There are various trade names of human insulin, including Humulin and Novolin.

b. The **pharmacokinetics** of **subcutaneously** administered human recombinant insulin are as follows:

Regular
    Peak effect: 2–4 hr
    Duration: 6 hr
NPH
    Peak effect: 8–10 hr
    Duration: 18–20 hr

c. The overall **total dosage** of insulin usually is approximately **0.5–1.0 unit/kg/day** of human insulin.

d. Insulin **dosing regimens** are modeled to approximate the normal physiologic secretion of insulin from the pancreas. A regimen of a long-acting agent plus boluses of short-acting insulin is optimal. Several such regimens can be used.

  i. **NPH insulin q. A.M., then a dose of regular insulin before each meal.** Glucose values must be closely monitored by a finger stick method to keep the postprandial glucose values in the range of 140–180 mg/dL with no overall glucose values below 80 mg/dL or above 180 mg/dL.

    Monitoring for glycemia should include finger sticks q.i.d.: one at **bedtime** and others ¹/₂–1 hour **after** each meal.

or

  ii. **Twice daily dosing regimen** with a mixture of NPH and regular insulin. The doses should be administered ¹/₂ hour before breakfast and ¹/₂ hour before supper. Two thirds of the total dosage is NPH and one-third is regular insulin. Two-thirds of the total dosage is taken before breakfast and one-third before supper.

    Monitoring for glycemia should include finger sticks q.i.d.: immediately **before** insulin dosing, at **noon,** and at **bedtime.**

or

  iii. **Twice daily dosing regimen** with premixed human NPH and regular insulin. Several pharmaceutical corporations make premixed NPH + regular human insulin (e.g., Novolin 70/30, which is 70% NPH and 30% regular human insulin). It is administered in a b.i.d. dosing regimen. As with other b.i.d. regimens, two-thirds of the dose is taken in the morning and one-third is taken in the evening.

Monitoring for glycemia should include finger sticks q.i.d.: immediately **before** insulin dosing, at **noon,** and at **bedtime.**

e. **Insulin adjustments** when the patient is ill (for example, the patient has gastroenteritis manifesting with nausea, vomiting, anorexia, and diarrhea) include instructing the patient to institute the following measures:

   i. Follow plasma glucose and urine ketone values closely, if possible on a q.i.d. basis.

   ii. Continue NPH at one-half to three-fourths of the baseline dose. The regular dose is resumed when the patient can resume regular oral intake of fluids and food.

   iii. Go to the hospital if **orthostatic manifestations** or **ketonuria** develop.

3. If the patient has **type II diabetes mellitus,** glycemic control is based on increasing the number and activity of the insulin receptors. This is accomplished by the following methods.

   a. **Weight reduction,** if obese, and **exercise.** These modalities are most effective for glycemic control in this type of diabetes mellitus.

   b. **Oral hypoglycemic agents.** These agents can be initiated in patients who are unable or unwilling to lose weight. The oral hypoglycemic agents of choice are glipizide (Glucotrol) or glyburide (Diabeta, Micronase). Both of these agents increase the number and effectiveness of insulin receptors and are catabolized in the liver. The range for total dosage is:

      Glipizide, 5–40 mg/day. The doses can be q. A.M. or b.i.d.

      Glyburide, 2.5–20 mg/day. The doses can be q. A.M. or b.i.d.

   c. Insulin in type II diabetes is of use in some cases. Usually after 15–20 years of untreated type II diabetes, insulin may be required to **assist** in glycemic control. The **regimen** is **NPH** insulin administered q. A.M.

   d. **Glycemic monitoring** should include **finger stick glucose determinations** every morning and **hemoglobin A_1c** determinations every 6 months. The hemoglobin A_1c is the percent of hemoglobin to which glucose is covalently bound. This is a long-term measurement of the overall glycemic control of the patient, as the life span of an erythrocyte is approximately 120 days. The hemoglobin A_1c depends on the level of glucose in the plasma and the level of hemoglobin. Hemoglobin A_1c values can be **falsely decreased** in:

   i. Anemia, owing to a decreased level of hemoglobulin.
   ii. Reticulocytosis, because these are young cells.
   iii. Hemoglobinopathies, e.g., SS/SC disease, as a result of the decreased life span of the cells.

B. **Controlling sequelae of diabetes mellitus**

   The **specific sequelae** of diabetes mellitus are diverse, and include the following.

   1. **Retinopathy**

      a. The **underlying pathogenesis** appears to relate to an overall increase in the thickness of the basement membrane in the capillaries. This abnormal thickening, referred to as microangiopathic changes, affects all of the vessels in the body, resulting in increased leakiness and even degeneration of the capillaries with consequent **exudation of fluid about the capillaries.** These effects occur throughout the body but are most evident in the retinas as **nonproliferative** retinal changes.

      A concurrent, **independent process** is **proliferative** changes in the capillaries, in which new vessels form in the capillary beds. These vessels are inherently fragile and bleed easily, resulting in small to moderate-sized hemorrhages. Although proliferative changes occur throughout the body, the bleeding is markedly symptomatic in the eyes. If there is bleeding into the vitreous humor, the blood will decrease vision, and the clot may also pull on the retina, increasing the risk of a retinal detachment.

      b. The **specific manifestations** of diabetic retinopathy include an overall loss of visual acuity. The patient is usually asymptomatic until a major event occurs, such as retinal hemorrhage. On funduscopy the **nonproliferative changes** include hard exudates, i.e., areas of protein deposition about the capillaries and mild edema in the retina itself. **Proliferative changes** include the formation of small capillaries adjacent to normal arteries, with small adjacent hemorrhages present. There can be blood in the vitreous, which may preclude complete visualization of the retina, and even retinal detachment.

      c. The **specific evaluation and management** include the steps outlined in Box 9-1 and prevention. There is increasing evidence that **tight glycemic control**

BOX 9-1

***Overall Evaluation and Management
of Diabetes Mellitus***

Evaluation

1. Take a **history** and perform a **physical examination** with emphasis on the following features.
   a. **Risk factors** for the development of diabetes mellitus, including a strong family history, obesity, a past history of diabetes during pregnancy, current pregnancy, or Native American ancestry.
   b. Current **medications,** as certain medications can result in hyperglycemia, the most common being glucocorticoids.
   c. Any **overt sequelae** of diabetes mellitus, i.e., neuropathy, or retinopathy. Query the patient and examine for any **peripheral or autonomic neuropathies,** such as carpal tunnel syndrome, ulnar tunnel syndrome, impotence, lack of sweating, or inappropriate lack of tachycardia on arising. **Funduscopy** is mandatory at baseline to look for any proliferative or nonproliferative retinal changes.
   d. Concurrent risk factors for the development of atherosclerotic disease or nephropathy. These include hypertension, a family history of atherosclerosis, a history of hyperlipidemia, and clinical manifestations of hyperlipidemia (i.e., xanthelasma or xanthomas).
2. If the patient has no overt manifestations but is at risk for the development of diabetes mellitus, determine a **screening fasting glucose level.**
   a. The screening test result is **abnormal** and **diagnostic of diabetes mellitus** if the fasting glucose level is, on two separate occasions, >140 mg/dL.
   b. The screening test result is **abnormal but not diagnostic of diabetes mellitus** if the fasting glucose level is >115 mg/dL.
3. Other diagnostic markers for diabetes mellitus include:
   a. Diabetic ketoacidosis (see text).
   b. Any random plasma glucose level >200 mg/dL.
   c. An abnormal response to a 50-g glucose oral glucose tolerance test in a pregnant female.

(continued)

B O X 9 - 1 (continued)

4. Determine **electrolyte, BUN,** and **creatinine levels** for baseline purposes. Look for a decrease in tco$_2$, potentially indicative of an acidosis.
5. Perform **urinalysis,** looking for proteinuria, ketonuria, or glycosuria.
6. Obtain a 12-lead ECG for baseline purposes.
7. Determine the **blood pressure** to look for concurrent hypertension. Hypertension is an independent risk factor for the development of nephropathy and atherosclerotic disease.
8. Obtain an ophthalmology consultation at baseline.
9. Obtain a baseline lipid panel, including triglycerides, total cholesterol, and HDL cholesterol, looking for concurrent hyperlipidemia.

Management

1. Educate the patient in **foot care,** pedicures, and so forth.
2. Institute **dietary modifications.**
   a. Obese patients should lose weight. This will reduce any concurrent hypertension and, in type II diabetes mellitus, will increase the number or activity of insulin receptors.
   b. Obese patients should decrease their overall caloric intake.
   c. The fat content should be decreased to <30% of total calories.
   d. The carbohydrates should be increased to approximately 60% of total calories.
   e. The saturated fat content should be decreased to <10% of total calories.
3. Instruct the patient to **exercise.** Exercise is an integral component of management in that it aids in weight reduction, increases the number and sensitivity of insulin receptors, and increases HDL cholesterol.
   a. **Isotonic or aerobic exercise** is recommended as it will increase cardiovascular performance, increase HDL cholesterol, and decrease hypertension. The exercise should be performed three times per week. Swimming, walking, and cycling are the best.

(continued)

B O X 9 - 1 *(continued)*

> b. **Isometric exercise** is relatively **contraindicated** as it can precipitate a retinal tear or intraocular hemorrhage in a patient with retinopathy.
> 4. A **Med-Alert bracelet** should be worn by **all** patients with diabetes mellitus. The information should include the diagnosis and the agents used in glycemic control.
> 5. Educate the patient in the **manifestations** and **acute treatment of hypoglycemia.** Both the patient and the spouse should receive this information. The manifestations of hypoglycemia include those secondary to catecholamine release, i.e., diaphoresis, tachycardia, and tremor; and those resulting from the hypoglycemia itself, i.e., confusion.
>   a. The acute intervention in hypoglycemia is intake of glucose. The best source of rapidly available sugar is **honey.** The patient should always carry some source of sugar, such as a candy bar or sugar cube, on his person.
> 6. Educate the patient in **finger stick glucose determinations.** Determining finger stick glucose values at home is useful in fine-tuning the control of diabetes mellitus and to confirm any episodes of hypoglycemia. Thus, all patients should learn the skill of glucose monitoring by finger stick and have the equipment, supplies, and glucometer readily available. Monitoring need not be done daily in all cases; in fact, in patients with type II diabetes mellitus once per week is adequate, unless the patient becomes symptomatically ill.

prevents the development of nonproliferative and proliferative retinopathy. All diabetic patients must undergo a baseline and annual retinal examination by an ophthalmologist. Any proliferative changes can be successfully treated with **laser photocoagulation.** In this procedure new, fragile vessels are destroyed before they can bleed and cause mischief.

2. Neuropathy
   a. The **underlying pathogenesis** is multifactorial and includes **ischemia** to the nerves as a result of the

(Text continues on page 528)

BOX 9-2

***Overall Evaluation and Management of Acutely
Decompensated Diabetes Mellitus, Diabetic
Ketoacidosis***

The **overall goals** include **volume repletion**, diagnosing
and treating any concurrent electrolyte disturbances, determining and treating the **underlying precipitating
event**, and **administering insulin** to decrease the glucose and, more important, to decrease the production
of ketone bodies, allowing the liver to clear them.

Evaluation

1. Admit the patient to the hospital, usually to an ICU.
2. Take a history and perform a physical examination,
   looking for an **acute precipitating factor** in the development of diabetic ketoacidosis. These factors include:
   a. The sentinel event.
   b. Poor compliance with insulin regimen.
   c. Acute coronary syndrome.
   d. Septicemia.
   e. Trauma.
   f. Acute cerebrovascular event.
3. Perform the following **baseline laboratory studies**:
   a. Determine electrolyte, BUN, creatinine, and glucose values. Often the serum glucose will exceed
      500 mg/dL; an anion gap is invariably present.
   b. Determine serum ketone values. Recall that only
      acetoacetate and acetone will be measured using
      the standard test for ketone bodies.
   c. Perform thyroid function tests to evaluate T_4,
      T_3RU, and TSH levels.
   d. Determine arterial blood gas values to evaluate
      the degree of acidosis present.
   e. Determine the CBC count with differential.
   f. Determine calcium, albumin, and phosphorus levels. Phosphorus is particularly important because,
      in the course of therapy, hypophosphatemia can
      occur.
   g. Obtain two sets of blood for cultures.
   h. Determine CK and LDH levels at baseline and ev-

(continued)

B O X   9 - 2 (continued)

ery 8 hours times three until acute myocardial necrosis is ruled out.

4. Obtain a **12-lead ECG** at baseline and every 24 hours until acute myocardial necrosis is ruled out.

5. Obtain a **chest radiograph** to look for evidence of an infiltrate or heart failure.

6. Follow **glucose, K^+, Mg^{++}, PO_4, and pH values** every 1–2 hours until the patient is stable.

7. Establish two peripheral IV catheters.

   a. One IV catheter is for fluids and electrolytes.

      i. Administer 1 liter of 0.9 normal saline at 300–500 mL/hour, then decrease to 200–250 mL/hour. Attempt to replete 50%–60% of the volume deficit in the first 24 hours.

      ii. Place a Swan–Ganz catheter as necessary to monitor volume status.

      iii. Replete **potassium** on a sliding KCl scale:

Serum level	Potassium
3.4–3.8	20 mEq KCl IV
3.0–3.3	40 mEq KCl IV
2.8–2.9	60 mEq KCl IV
<2.8	60 mEq KCl IV and call the on-call physician

      iv. Replete **magnesium** on a sliding $MgSO_4$ scale:

Serum level	Magnesium
1.4–1.8	1 g $MgSO_4$ IV
<1.4	2 g $MgSO_4$ IV

      v. Replete **phosphorus.** If <1.5, consider giving one of the potassium volutrols as K_3PO_4.

      vi. **Bicarbonate** is not indicated unless the pH is less than 7.0 or the patient is hyperkalemic (see section on Hyperkalemia, page 537).

      vii. Use this IV line for any other medications, such as antibiotics, pressors, or lidocaine.

   b. The second IV line is used **exclusively for human insulin.**

      i. Administer 5–10 units regular human insulin IV as a stat **bolus.**

      ii. Initiate a **drip** of 2–10 units human insulin per

(continued)

B O X 9 - 2 *(continued)*

hour IV. The mixture is 50 units regular human insulin in 250 mL of D5W. The goal is to decrease the glucose by a rate of 75–100 mg/dL/hr to the level of 300 mg/dL.

iii. When the **glucose reaches 300 mg/dL:**

(a) Change the IV fluids from 0.9 NS to D5 .45 NS.

(b) Administer 10 units of regular human insulin **subcutaneously** and discontinue the insulin drip in 30 min.

(c) Initiate human regular insulin on a sliding scale, based on finger stick glucose determinations made every 4 hours:

Glucose	*Insulin*
<60 mg/dL	1 ampule of D50W, and call the on-call physician
61–120 mg/dL	Status quo
121–180 mg/dL	2–3 units regular SC
181–240 mg/dL	4–6 units regular SC
241–300 mg/dL	6–9 units regular SC
301–360 mg/dL	8–12 units regular SC
>360 mg/dL	Restart the insulin drip IV

(d) It is extremely important to **continue aggressive use of human insulin** during the 24–36 hours after achieving a glucose of 250–300 mg/dL, because the patient will remain ketotic even though the glucose is under better control. Without adequate insulin replacement during this critical time, the liver is not able to clear the ketone bodies present.

iv. If the patient is ketotic, **lifelong human insulin** is necessary. Long-term dosing can be initiated with the dosing schedules and regimens described in the text.

v. It is imperative to keep the glucose level in the 250–300 mg/dL range until the ketone bodies have been catabolized, especially in the acute setting, as an acute drop of the glucose to <250 mg/dL can potentially precipitate cerebral edema.

microangiopathic (i.e., capillary basement membrane thickening) and macroangiopathic (i.e., vascular) changes. The decreased perfusion results in damage and even infarction of parts of the peripheral nerves. A concurrent process is an abnormal accumulation of the sugar **sorbitol** in the **myelin sheaths** of the peripheral nerves. The aldose reductase pathway will produce sorbitol in significant amounts in the presence of significant hyperglycemia. The sorbital is incorporated into the peripheral nerves, autonomic nerves, and probably into the nerves of the gastrointestinal tract, and results in significant and progressive neuronal dysfunction.

b. The specific manifestations of diabetic neuropathy are diverse, manifold, and dependent on what nerves are primarily involved: peripheral, autonomic, or GI tract.

    i. Peripheral neuropathies manifest with paresthesias, pain, hypesthesia, or dysthesia, usually in a stocking or glove distribution. The distribution can be variable, but usually is greater distally than proximally. There can be discrete syndromes, including carpal tunnel syndrome, ulnar tunnel syndrome, and even tarsal tunnel syndrome. The pain may be debilitating.

    ii. Autonomic neuropathies manifest with impotence, decreased sweating, and a lack of tachycardia on arising. This can preclude the development of the classic secondary manifestations of hypoglycemia, i.e., tremor, tachycardia, and diaphoresis.

    iii. Enteropathy, or dysfunction of the GI tract, will result in gastroparesis with resultant postprandial vomiting that can be quite debilitating to the patient.

c. The **specific evaluation and management** include the steps listed in Box 9-1 and the following measures.

    i. For **peripheral neuropathies,** specific management includes defining the lesions. If carpal tunnel, ulnar tunnel, or tarsal tunnel syndrome is present, one can splint the joint and administer an NSAID PRN. If the neuropathy is recurrent, surgical intervention may be indicated.

    If **no specific lesions** can be localized and the manifestations are severe, administer **amitriptyline** (Elavil), 25–50 mg PO q.H.S., or

capsaicin (Zostrix), 0.025 topically b.i.d. Capsaicin is a peripheral inhibitor of pain that interacts with the pain transmitter, substance P.

Referral to a **pain clinic** is indicated in severe cases. A pain control specialist is often an anesthesiologist with training in modalities for pain control.

ii. For **autonomic neuropathies,** define the manifestations. If they are predominantly **orthostatic hypotension** without tachycardia, instruct the patient to rise slowly from a supine position. Further modalities include above-knee hose applied to both lower extremities, and minimizing the use of medications that can exacerbate the nontachycardic hypotension. **Impotence** is managed by looking for any reversible causes, such as hypogonadism, and referral to a GU specialist.

iii. For **enteropathies,** the specific evaluation and management include defining the lesion. Two modalities for direct imaging of the pylorus are the barium swallow, which demonstrates specific anatomic lesions about the distal stomach or pylorus or problems with transit time across the pylorus, and a **radionucleotide-labeled meal,** to measure transit time across the pylorus. The **specific management** includes frequent small meals and the initiation of the agent metoclopramide (Reglan), 5–10 mg PO q.6h. PRN.

3. **Nephropathy**

a. The **underlying pathophysiology** is probably analogous to the pathophysiology of retinopathy: thickening of the basement membrane in the capillaries and microvasculature of the kidneys. This thickening is postulated to be a result of deposition of glycosylated proteins and other substances within the basement membranes. Histopathologic examination shows definite thickening of the mesangium and glomerular basement membrane. The quintessential example of this process is Kimmelstiel–Wilson kidney, or focal nodular sclerosis.

The abnormal thickening results in an abnormal leakiness of the capillaries within the kidneys, i.e., the glomeruli of albumin. Therefore, an early marker for the development of nephropathy is **albumin loss in the urine.** Several studies have demonstrated that an early and powerful marker for the development of nephropathy is **microalbuminuria,** defined as **>300 mg of albumin** in a 24-hour collection of urine. The **natural history** entails progressive increases in protein loss to the point of classic hypoalbuminemic nephrotic syndrome.

A concurrent factor in the development of nephropathy is **uncontrolled hypertension.**

b. The **specific manifestations** of nephropathy are diverse and dependent on the time of presentation. Early in the course, there are no specific manifestations. The **earliest manifestation** is microalbuminuria (i.e., >300 mg of albumin in the urine per 24 hours). This is a powerful marker for the development of nephrotic syndrome. This level of proteinuria is usually below the level of detection by dipstick analysis. Later is the natural history of the disease, **frank proteinuria** will develop. Further progression to frank nephrotic syndrome occurs with the classic manifestations of hypoalbuminemia, albuminuria and proteinuria, and edema.

c. The **specific evaluation and management** of nephrotic syndrome include prevention. **Prevention** is the cornerstone of management. It includes tight control of glucose levels and tight control of hypertension. **Hypertension** must be optimally controlled to prevent nephropathy. Furthermore, there is some evidence that prescription of a low (i.e., 80–100-g) protein diet will retard the progression of nephrotic renal failure. Once nephrotic range proteinuria (>3 g protein/24 hours) is present, renal failure will eventually occur, usually within 5 years. All patients with nephrotic range proteinuria should be referred to a nephrologist.

4. **Atherosclerotic disease** (also referred to as macrovascular disease).

a. The **underlying pathogenesis** is not completely understood. Both type I and type II diabetes mellitus are associated with an increased risk for and acceleration of atherosclerotic disease. Diabetes mellitus results in a change in the lipid profile characterized by a decrease in HDL cholesterol, an increase in LDL cholesterol, and an increase in triglycerides, all of which increase the risk of development of atherosclerotic disease. This results in the development of atheromatous plaques in the medium and large-sized arteries of the body.

b. The **specific manifestations** are few until late in the course of the disease. The manifestations are diverse and depend on where specifically the plaques occur. The most common sites for symptomatic arterial plaques (i.e., narrowing) are the **coronary arteries,** where plaques manifest with angina pectoris and acute myocardial infarction; the **cerebrovascular vessels,** where plaques manifest with TIAs and strokes; and the **peripheral arteries,** where plaques manifest with intermittent, exercise-related claudication.

  c. The **specific evaluation and management** include making the clinical diagnosis, the overall management of diabetes mellitus (see Box 9-1), and controlling any concurrent elevations of plasma lipids. Furthermore, it is important to define and then **control any concurrent risk factors** for atherosclerotic disease development: control hypertension, control the hyperglycemia, and instruct the patient to stop smoking.

V. Consultation

Problem	Service	Time
All diabetics	Ophthalmology	Required
Sudden decrease in vision	Ophthalmology	Emergent
All diabetics	Endocrinology	Elective

VI. Indications for admission: Acute decompensation of diabetes mellitus (e.g., diabetic ketoacidosis), and nonketotic hyperglycemic coma.

Hypercalcemia

The **physiology** of calcium homeostasis is relatively complex. The levels of this divalent cation are parsimoniously maintained by several interrelated and interdependent mechanisms. These involve **vitamin D,** a vitamin required for effective calcium absorption from the small intestine; the **small intestine** itself as an absorptive site; the **renal tubules,** which are under the direct regulation of the hormone parathormone (PTH), which controls the excretory loss of calcium into the urine. Finally, **bone** plays a major role in that it is the largest store of inorganic calcium in the body and will, under the direction of PTH, release calcium via osteolysis. Thus the perturbations of increased levels of vitamin D, increased levels of PTH or a PTH-like substance, or any process that results in increased osteoclastic activity (i.e., osteolysis) can result in hypercalcemia.

I. Overall manifestations

Hypercalcemia is asymptomatic in the vast majority of cases. Manifestations, when present, include the onset of moderate to marked polyuria, polydipsia, constipation, and a change in the level of consciousness (lethargy, somnolence, or even coma) that is more conspicuous than an acute confusional state (i.e., delirium). There is often evidence of **intravascular volume depletion**—i.e., orthostatic hypotension and tachycardia—which develops after the patient is unable to ingest adequate amounts of fluids to maintain hydration and indicates impending coma. There is often an antecedent history of a malignant neoplastic process, either a carcinoma or multiple myeloma.

II. Underlying causes

A. Squamous cell carcinoma of the primary site

The most common sites of squamous cell carcinoma are the lung and the head and neck.

1. Pathogenesis

The **underlying pathogenesis** is production by the tumor of a PTH-like substance that results in increased

---

B O X 9 - 3

Overall Evaluation and Management of Hypercalcemia

Evaluation

1. Determine serum **calcium and albumin levels.** Following are normal calcium values (equivalent measures):

   8.0–10.2 mg/dL, or
   4.0–5.1 mEq/dL, or
   2.0–2.6 mmol/dL.

   The corrected (true) calcium level = 0.8 (4.0 − measured albumin) + measured calcium. (Units for calcium used are mg/dL.)

2. Determine the **serum phosphorus level.** If **elevated** in the setting of hypercalcemia, it is suggestive of vitamin D intoxication, whereas if **decreased** in the setting of hypercalcemia, it is suggestive of primary hyperparathyroidism.

(continued)

B O X 9 - 3 *(continued)*

3. Obtain chest radiographs in PA and lateral views, looking for pulmonary masses.
4. Perform urinalysis to look for hematuria, an early marker for renal cell carcinoma.
5. Determine the **erythrocyte sedimentation rate (ESR),** which may be elevated in a monoclonal gammopathy.
6. Obtain a **complete blood cell count,** looking for a normochromic normocytic anemia and rouleaux, either of which is consistent with a monoclonal gammopathy.
7. If a gammopathy is suspected, perform serum protein electrophoresis **(SPEP)** and urine protein electrophoresis **(UPEP).**
8. Determine the **intact,** N-terminus **PTH (parathormone) level.** This is the biologically active form of PTH and is of most utility in measurement. Older assays for the C-terminal, nonintact PTH include the inactive catabolites of PTH and can, in the setting of renal failure, suggest false elevations of the PTH.
9. Perform thyroid function tests, especially if the patient has clinical evidence of hyperthyroidism or hypothyroidism.
10. Obtain a 24-hour urine collection for calcium determination. The normal level is 200–300 mg/24-hour urine collection. In the setting of hypercalcemia, an **elevated urine calcium level** is suggestive of a malignant neoplastic or paraneoplastic process, whereas a **decreased urine calcium level** is suggestive of primary hyperparathyroidism.
11. Determine serum vitamin D_{25}-OH and $D_{1,25}$-OH levels. Elevated levels are consistent with vitamin D intoxication.

Management

1. Volume replete the patient with 0.9 normal saline intravenously. Usually the patient has a 4–5 liter volume deficit.
2. Use a loop diuretic (e.g., furosemide [Lasix]) **if and when the patient becomes hypervolemic** from the volume repletion.
3. Further management is specific to the underlying cause of the hypercalcemia.

bone resorption and hypercalcemia with an increased urinary calcium.

2. **Manifestations**

The **specific manifestations** are referable to the elevated calcium level and to the tumor itself.

3. **Evaluation and management**

The **specific evaluation and management** include two steps outlined in Box 9-3 defining, and if possible controlling or curing the malignant squamous cell carcinoma. Unfortunately, the tumor is invariably metastatic when associated with hypercalcemia, and therefore treatment modalities are of palliative benefit at best. These modalities include:

a. **Plicamycin** (mithramycin), administered parenterally. The dose is 25 μg/kg IV, the usual dose being 1.25 mg IV for one dose. This agent has been demonstrated to inhibit osteoclastic activity.

b. **Calcitonin,** the hormone produced in the physiologic state by the parafollicular (C) cells of the thyroid gland. Calcitonin decreases levels of serum calcium and can be administered to effect a decrease in serum calcium. The dose is 0.5 mg q.d. SC.

c. **Gallium nitrate.** This rare earth metal is an exciting novel modality to decrease serum calcium. It decreases calcium levels through an undetermined mechanism. It should be used only under the direction of an oncologist.

d. **Oral phosphates,** e.g., Neutraphos. If the phosphorus is low at baseline, i.e., <4 mg/dL, oral phosphates can be administered to decrease the serum calcium. The serum phosphorus level must be closely monitored and the agent discontinued when the serum phosphorus level exceeds 5 mg/dL. This is due to the fact that, if the calcium and phosphorus reach a certain level, i.e., the double product (calcium × phosphorus) is >55, there is a high risk of metastatic calcifications in the brain and soft tissues. This is only an adjunctive therapeutic modality.

B. **Lymphoproliferative disorders**

The most common lymphoproliferative disorders are multiple myeloma and the lymphomas, either of which can manifest with hypercalcemia.

1. **Pathogenesis**

The **underlying pathogenesis** is production by the tumor of a substance that increases bone resorption and increases hypercalcemia, with an increased urinary calcium level. The substance, osteoclastic activating factor (OAF), is a lymphokine that stimulates osteo-clasts to resorb bone.

2. **Manifestations**

The **specific manifestations** are referable to the ele-vated calcium level and to the tumor itself. Recurrent pathologic fractures, bone pain, rouleaux on a periph-eral blood smear, anemia, and "B" symptoms—fevers, unintentional weight loss, and drenching night sweats—are the classic manifestations. The urinary calcium level is usually elevated.

3. **Evaluation and management**

The **specific evaluation and management** include the steps outlined in Box 9-3, defining, and if possible controlling or curing the malignant lymphoprolifera-tive disorder. Further evaluative modalities include bone marrow biopsy and referral to hematology/oncol-ogy for more definitive intervention. The hypercalce-mia is quite sensitive to therapy with steroids, e.g., methylprednisolone (Solumedrol), 60–80 mg IV q.8h., and, in patients with no contraindications to their use, a trial of NSAIDs may be of benefit. Other agents, in-cluding plicamycin and gallium nitrate, can be admin-istered when the hypercalcemia is severe or refractory to first-line therapy.

C. **Primary hyperparathyroidism**

1. **Pathogenesis**

The **underlying pathogenesis** is an autoimmune-stimulated excess secretion of PTH from the parathy-roid glands.

2. **Manifestations**

The **specific manifestations** include those referable to the hypercalcemia itself—hypercalcemia, hypophos-phatemia, and a decreased urine calcium level.

3. **Evaluation and management**

The **specific evaluation and management** include the steps outlined in Box 9-3 and referral to an endocrinol-ogist and a surgeon with expertise in parathyroid sur-gical procedures for parathyroidectomy.

D. **Vitamin D intoxication**

1. **Pathogenesis**

The **underlying pathogenesis** is ingestion of inappro-priately large amounts of vitamin D, which results in an increase in the absorption of calcium from the GI tract and a concurrent decrease in tubular excretion of calcium and phosphorus, resulting in an increase in serum calcium and phosphorus levels. People who take large quantities of vitamins are at greatest risk for this syndrome.

2. **Manifestations**

The **specific manifestations** include those attributable
to the hypercalcemia and an antecedent history of vitamin abuse. Manifestations include hypercalcemia,
hyperphosphatemia, and a decreased urine calcium
level.

3. **Evaluation and management**
The **specific evaluation and management** include the
steps outlined in Box 9-3 and discontinuing vitamin
D or A from non-food sources (recall that cod liver
oil tablets are rich in both). If severely elevated, the
administration of a short course of steroids, e.g., prednisone, 40–60 mg in a 1–2-week tapering dosage, is
helpful.

E. **Sarcoidosis**
1. **Pathogenesis**
The **underlying pathogenesis** is an increase in the activity of vitamin D by sarcoid cells, which generate
the enzyme vitamin D_1-hydroxylase, therefore resulting in hypercalcemia through a vitamin D–
mediated process.

2. **Manifestations**
The **specific manifestations** include those attributable
to hypercalcemia, as described above, and those attributable to sarcoidosis.

3. **Manifestations**
Manifestations referable to the sarcoid include interstitial infiltrates on chest radiographs, hilar adenopa-
thy on chest radiographs, a polyarticular arthritis,
erythema nodosum, and renal dysfunction. It is a systemic, idiopathic disorder which has hypercalcemia
as one of its manifestations.

4. **Evaluation and management**
The **specific evaluation and management** include the
steps outlined in Box 9-3, making the clinical diagnosis of sarcoidosis, and initiating treatment with steroids. The steroids treat not only the hypercalcemia
but also the sarcoidosis itself. The management of sarcoid is beyond the scope of this text; however, because
the most devastating manifestations are pulmonary,
referral to a pulmonologist is indicated.

III. **Consultation**

Problem	*Service*	*Time*
Primary hyperparathyroidism	Endocrine/ Surgery	Required
Malignancy	Hematology/ Oncology	Urgent
Sarcoidosis	Pulmonary	Required

IV. **Indications for admission:** Decreased levels of consciousness, evidence of intravascular volume depletion, or any concurrent electrolyte disturbances.

Hyperkalemia (Box 9-4)

The **normal range** for serum potassium in the extracellular fluids is 3.5–5.0 mEq/dL.

The **physiologic mechanisms** that maintain potassium homeostasis and prevent hyperkalemia are several.

Aldosterone (i.e., mineralocorticoids). When the serum potassium increases, the cells of the zona glomerulosa increase production of the mineralocorticoid aldosterone, which acts on the renal tubules to increase the urinary loss of potassium. This is a **coarse adjustment:** There may be an actual decrease in the total body stores of potassium. Thus, aldosterone production is central to the body's prevention of hyperkalemia.

The Renal Tubules. The kidneys act in a central role in regulating the level of potassium and adjust loss in the urine to prevent hyperkalemia. This is mainly through mineralocorticoid effects. This is a course adjustment measure in which there can be an actual decrease in the total body stores of potassium.

Catecholamines. Epinephrine and norepinephrine both drive potassium into the cells from the extracellular fluids. This is one reason why post-"code 4" patients can be hypokalemic. This is a **fine adjustment.** The total body potassium is unchanged; it is only moved from the extracellular to the intracellular compartment.

Insulin. Insulin, by driving glucose into the cell, also drives potassium into the cell. This is a **fine adjustment.** The total body potassium is unchanged; it is only moved between the extracellular and the intracellular compartment.

Acid–base status. An alkaline pH (>7) in the extracellular fluids will drive potassium intracellularly, whereas an acid pH (<7) will drive potassium from intracellular to extracellular spaces. This is a **fine adjustment.** The total body potassium is unchanged; it is only moved between the extracellular and the intracellular compartment.

I. **Underlying causes**

Underlying causes of hyperkalemia include anything that disturbs one of the physiologic mechanisms that maintain potassium homeostasis or anything that markedly increases the release of potassium into the extracellular fluids.

A. **Disturbances of physiologic mechanisms**

   1. **Primary adrenal insufficiency,** i.e., destruction or

dysfunction of either or both glands (Addison's disease) or of the zona glomerulosa, the area of the adrenal gland that produces mineralocorticoids.

2. **Acute or chronic renal failure** may contribute to or result in the development of hyperkalemia.

3. The administration of **medications,** e.g., β-blockers, NSAIDs, ACE inhibitors, and/or K-sparing diuretics, will, in certain patients, cause hyperkalemia. A patient at highest risk for the development of hyperkalemia from an ACE-inhibitor or K-sparing diuretic is one with **type IV renal tubular acidosis (RTA).** Type IV RTA is a form of tubular acidosis in which there is a non-anion gap metabolic acidosis and hyperkalemia, i.e., a syndrome quite similar to a hypoaldosterone state. This disease, which in the past was referred to as hyporeninemic hypoaldosteronism, is probably not rare, but only a rarely recognized manifestation of dysfunction associated with diabetes mellitus. The patient is often asymptomatic until an exacerbating factor is added, usually a medication such as an ACE inhibitor, at which time the potassium level significantly increases.

B. **States that increase the release of potassium from the cells into the extravascular fluids**

Hemolysis, tumor lysis syndrome, and rhabdomyolysis cause cellular disruption and release of intracellular contents, contents rich in potassium, into the extracellular fluids. **Hemolysis** can occur in the process of drawing blood and therefore is a potential source of a falsely elevated potassium level. **Tumor lysis syndrome** is a potentially catastrophic process in which a patient with a rapidly growing, usually lymphoproliferative disorder (e.g., lymphoma) receives chemotherapy. The chemotherapy destroys a significant number of tumor cells, which release large quantities of potassium, phosphorus, and purines (uric acid), resulting in severe hyperkalemia and renal failure.

II. Overall manifestations

A patient with hyperkalemia is often free of symptoms and signs until extremely elevated potassium levels are present. The first signs of severe hyperkalemia may be ECG changes, which proceed to significant dysrhythmias and even ventricular tachycardia with sudden death. The ECG changes include but are not limited to:

Diffuse flattening of the P-waves
Diffuse peaking of the T-waves

B O X   9 - 4

Overall Evaluation and Management of Hyperkalemia

Evaluation

1. **Screen patients** at risk for development of hyperkalemia, i.e., check potassium 5–7 days after starting
   an ACE inhibitor, especially in a diabetic patient or a
   patient with renal failure.
2. If hyperkalemia is present (i.e., **K^+ > 5.1 mEq/dL**),
   determine the following laboratory values:
   a. Repeat K determination within hours.
   b. Electrolytes, BUN, creatinine, and glucose, for
      baseline purposes and to look for concurrent prob-
      lems (e.g., renal failure).
   c. Urinalysis to look for evidence of renal dysfunc-
      tion (e.g., casts, hematuria).
   d. Medication profile to look for medications that
      could result in hyperkalemia.
   e. Volume status of the patient. Assess if the patient
      is hypovolemic, euvolemic, or hypervolemic.
   f. 12-lead ECG to look for any of the above de-
      scribed changes.
   g. Discontinue any exogenous source of potassium
      or any exacerbating medications (ACE inhibitors,
      NSAIDs, KCl supplements, and sodium-free salt,
      which contains KCl).
3. If the potassium level is >**6.0 mEq/dL with or without ECG changes,** or if there is any degree of hyperkalemia with ECG changes:
   a. Admit to or transfer to a telemetry bed and per-
      form all of the tests described above.
   b. Acute intervention is mandatory and is described
      in Box 9-5.

Diffuse widening of the QRS complexes
Severe, hemodynamically compromising brady/
    tachydysrhythmias

The threshold for ECG changes due to hyperkalemia is different for different patients: one patient may tolerate a potassium of 6.0 mEq/dL, whereas another will have florid ECG
changes at 5.5.

B O X 9 - 5

Acute Management of Hyperkalemia

1. Calcium gluconate

Dose:	1–3 g IV
Onset:	3–5 min
Duration:	1–2 hr
Mechanism of action:	Membrane stabilization

2. Sodium bicarbonate ($NaCO_3$)

Dose:	1–2 ampules IV
Onset:	10–15 min
Duration:	4–6 hr
Mechanism of action:	Extracellular to intracellular shift
Caveat:	Most effective if the patient has a concurrent metabolic acidosis

3. Glucose or glucose and insulin

Dose:	D10W at 100 mL/hour; add regular insulin to the infusion as needed to keep patient's serum glucose 150–200 mg%; *or* 1 ampule of D50W as an IV bolus and administer regular insulin SC to keep the serum glucose 150–200 mg/dL
Onset:	15 min
Duration:	12 hr
Mechanism of action:	Extracellular to intracellular shift

4. Loop diuretic

Dose:	Furosemide, 20 mg IV
Onset:	2–4 hr
Duration:	4–6 hr
Mechanism of action:	Loss of potassium in the urine
Caveat:	Most effective if patient has concurrent volume overload

(continued)

B O X 9 - 5 (continued)

5. Kayexalate

   Dose:
Oral:	15–30 g PO q. A.M.
Rectal:	50 g as a retention enema; must be kept in rectum/colon for >15 min
Mechanism of action:	Cation exchange of Na^+-K^+ at the colonic mucosal surface.

6. Dialysis, either hemodialysis or peritoneal dialysis

Once ECG changes due to hyperkalemia are present, the next rhythm potentially is asystole or ventricular tachycardia; therefore, any ECG changes are emergency findings.

III. **Long-term management**

Long-term management of hyperkalemia includes defining and treating the underlying cause. The clinician must be appropriately cautious in initiating any agent that may precipitate or exacerbate hyperkalemia. If such an agent is initiated, the clinician must follow, especially early on, the potassium level quite closely. If the patient has **chronic renal failure,** refer to a dietitian to educate the patient in a low potassium diet; administer $NaHCO_3$ by mouth to keep the serum HCO_3 at >15 mEq/dL; if nonacidotic or refractory to the first two interventions, administer Kayexalate, 15–30 mg PO q. A.M.; and, when necessary, initiate chronic dialysis. (See section on Renal Dysfunction in Chapter 3 for details of management.)

IV. **Management**

Problem	*Service*	*Time*
Acute renal failure	Renal	Urgent/ emergent
Addison's disease	Endocrinology	Emergent

V. **Indications for admission:** Any ECG changes, a potassium level above 6.0 mEq/dL, any evidence of acute renal failure, or Addison's disease.

Thyroid Dysfunctional States

The normal thyroid gland is located in the anterior neck and is approximately 15–20 g in total mass. The gland is soft, symmetric, bilobed, and nontender. It produces two specific hormones, calcitonin and thyroxine.

Calcitonin is produced in the parafollicular or C-cells and is involved in calcium homeostasis. An increase in plasma calcium levels will result in an increase in the production of calcitonin to decrease the calcium level back to normal. The hormone is a minor player in overall calcium homeostasis.

Thyroxine is the major endocrine product of the thyroid gland. This hormone, which requires the anion iodide for its synthesis within the thyroid gland, controls and regulates the overall baseline catabolic rate of the entire body. It is required for the sustenance of life. The hormone is produced in the tetraiodinated state (T_4), i.e., levothyroxine, in the gland. In the peripheral tissues it is deiodinated to the most active form, triiodothyronine (T_3). The thyroid gland of the average person produces approximately **150 μg of thyroxine per day.** As a result of its central and integral role to the biochemical machinery of the cells, an overall increase or decrease in the amount of this hormone produced will cause significant pathology. In this section the overall approach to thyroid dysfunction, whether or not a goiter is present, the specific manifestations, evaluation, management, and sequelae of hypothyroidism, hyperthyroidism and thyroid nodules will be discussed.

I. **Thyroid excess states (i.e., hyperthyroidism)**
   A. **Manifestations**

      The **specific manifestations** of an excess of thyroid hormone, a hormone that intimately regulates the overall catabolism of the cells within the body, include heat intolerance, diaphoresis, unintentional weight loss, fine hair, lid lag (Darymple's sign), tachycardia, atrial fibrillation, and symmetric muscle weakness, greater proximally than distally. Extreme hyperthyroidism, i.e., thyroid storm, can result in death. Manifestations that may be harbingers of such a catastrophic event include hyperpyrexia, temperatures exceeding 105 °F, and marked tachycardias.

   B. **Causes of hyperthyroidism**
      1. **Graves' disease.** This is an autoimmune disease with the constellation of **hyperthyroidism** with diffuse goiter; **dermopathy;** peau d'orange skin changes, especially on the pretibial areas; and **ophthalmopathy,** unilateral or bilateral with proptosis. The exophthalmus, i.e., proptosis, is **specific to Graves' disease** and not a part of the overall hyperthyroidism.
         a. The **specific evaluation** of Graves' disease involves making the clinical diagnosis using the tests described in Boxes 9-6 and 9-7. The TSH will be 0.0 μU/mL, and the T_4 and T_3RU will be elevated. A radioactive iodide uptake scan will show a diffuse and marked increase in the uptake of iodide, >70%

B O X 9 - 6

Overall Evaluation and Management of Suspected Thyroid Diseases

Evaluation

1. Take a history and perform a physical examination.
   a. Tachycardia, tachydysrhythmias, tremor, diaphoresis, weight loss, fine tremor, diarrhea, thin body habitus, proximal muscle weakness, and bilateral lid lag all are indicative of **hyperthyroidism.**
   b. Normocardia or bradycardia, dry skin, weight gain, constipation, obese body habitus, proximal muscle weakness, and coarse thick hair with loss of lateral eyebrow hair bilaterally (Queen Anne's sign) all are indicative of **hypothyroidism.**
   c. Further suggestive features on the history and physical examination include:
      i. A history of **antecedent radiation** to the neck, even in the distant past, which is associated with an increased risk of hypothyroidism and thyroid malignancy.
      ii. Scars about the neck. Query the patient regarding specific thyroid surgeries.
      iii. Assess and document **features of the thyroid gland** itself, including the size of the gland, the consistency of the gland, whether the gland is tender or nontender, whether any nodules are present, and, if nodules are present, their size and location within the gland.
2. Based on the clinical data gleaned from the history and physical examination, classify the patient as being clinically hyperthyroid, hypothyroid, or euthyroid.
3. Determine serum electrolyte, BUN, creatinine, and glucose levels for baseline purposes and to look for any concurrent electrolyte disturbances.
4. Determine a complete blood cell count with differential for baseline purposes.
5. Perform urinalysis and, if the patient is female, a urine pregnancy test.
6. Perform thyroid function tests, i.e., T_3RU, T_4, and TSH assays (see Table 9-2 for specifics on normal values and interpretation of any abnormal values).

(continued)

B O X   9 - 6 *(continued)*

Management

1. Specific management is discussed in the text. If the patient is **hyperthyroid,** see section I; if **hypothyroid,** see section II; if **thyroid nodules** are present, see section III; if goiter is present, see Tables 9-3 and 9-4.
2. Refer to an endocrinologist.

at 24 hours. A TRH stimulation test, if performed, will demonstrate an abnormal blunting of the TSH. A TRH stimulation test is usually unnecessary in the evaluation if a highly sensitive TSH test is performed.

   b. Specific management includes administering β-blockers, unless contraindicated. Further management includes the initiation and administration of antithyroid agents or radioactive iodine.

      i. Antithyroid medications decrease thyroid hormone synthesis and therefore, over time, decrease the levels of thyroid hormone present. They should be used for 6–12 months or until the patient is euthyroid.

B O X   9 - 7

Evaluation and Management of Hyperthyroidism

1. Perform the evaluations listed in Box 9-6.
2. Perform a urine pregnancy test.
3. Determine the underlying cause from the history and physical examination and a radioiodide uptake scan (see Table 9-4 for information on the radioiodide uptake scan).
4. Administer **β-blockers,** specifically propranolol, 40 mg PO q.i.d., unless there is a contraindication, to blunt the tachycardia and other manifestations of the hypercatabolic state.
5. Consult an endocrinologist for assistance.
6. Further management depends on the underlying cause.

T A B L E 9 - 2
Thyroid Function Tests

Test	Assay/Normal Ranges	Interpretation
T_4	Both free and bound T_4 measured in this radioimmunoassay Normal: 5–12 μg/dL	Increased: a) Hyperthyroid, or b) Elevated TBG state: 　Estrogen use 　Pregnancy 　Oral contraceptive use 　Familial 　Cirrhosis or hepatitis 　Tamoxifen use Decreased: a) Hypothyroid, or b) Decreased TBG: 　Nephrosis 　Glucocorticoids 　Familial 　Androgens
T_3RU	An indirect measurement of unbound thyroid-binding proteins using a resin technique Normal: 25%–35%	If >35%: a) Hyperthyroid, or b) Decreased TBG: 　Nephrosis 　Glucocorticoids 　Familial 　Androgens If <25%: a) Hypothyroid, or b) Increased TBG state: 　Estrogens 　Pregnancy 　Oral contraceptive use 　Familial 　Cirrhosis or hepatitis 　Tamoxifen
TSH	Highly sensitive; uses immunospecific monoclonal antibodies Normal: 0.5–6.0 μU/mL	If low: a) Primary hyperthyroidism b) Secondary hypothyroidism c) Tertiary hypothyroidism If high: a) Primary hypothyroidism b) Secondary hyperthyroidism NOTE: If low and primary hyperthyroidism is clinically suspected, can virtually rule in that diagnosis; i.e., it effectively eliminates the need to perform TRH stimulation test in workup of Graves' disease

(continued)

T A B L E   9 - 2
Thyroid Function Tests (continued)

Test	Assay/Normal Ranges	Interpretation
T_3	Direct measurement of the biologically active hormone Test is rarely needed in the workup of thyroid disease Normal: 80–200 ng/dL Radioimmunoassay Not necessary in all thyroid evaluations	Increased: a) Hyperthyroid, or b) Decreased TBG states (see above) Decreased: a) Hypothyroid, or b) Increased TBG state (see above)
Radioactive iodine uptake	Measures activity of thyroid tissue by measuring uptake of radioactive ^{131}I by thyroid tissue ^{131}I is given PO Images of uptake obtained at 6 and 24 hr Not to be confused with the clinically useless thyroid ^{99m}Tc or ^{131}I "scan" Normal: 30%–40% uptake at 24 hr	High uptake (>60%): a) Graves' disease b) Early Hashimoto's disease c) Endemic goiter d) Early postpartum Low uptake (<10%): a) Late Hashimoto's disease b) Jod Basedow c) de Quervain's disease d) After removal or ablation of thyroid tissue

(a) **Propylthiouracil** (PTU) inhibits the organification of the iodide anions, thus inhibiting T_4 synthesis. Furthermore, it blocks the peripheral conversion of the relatively inactive T_4 to T_3. Side effects are hepatitis and, rarely, agranulocytosis. The starting

T A B L E   9 - 3
Causes of Goiter

Endemic: Results from a lack of iodide salts in the diet.
   Endemic to the Great Lakes region of North America, the Balkan peninsula of Eastern Europe, the Andes region of South America, and east–central Asia.
Thyroiditis: Diffuse, symmetric goiter; see Table 9-4 for specifics.
Graves' disease: Diffuse, symmetric goiter; see text for specifics.
Plummer's disease: Multinodular, symmetric to asymmetric goiter; see text for specifics.
Solitary nodules: See III. Thyroid nodules.
Multinodular goiter: See III. Thyroid nodules.

TABLE 9-4
Thyroiditis

Disease	Presentation	Histopathology	Laboratory Findings	Radioactive Iodide Scan at 6 and 24 hr (Normal at 24 hr: 10%–40% uptake)	Natural History	Treatment
Hashimoto's disease	Nontender Diffuse goiter Hyper- or hypothyroid at presentation	Lymphocytic	Early: Increased T$_3$RU, T$_4$ Normal TSH Positive antimicrosomal antibodies Late: Decreased T$_3$RU, T$_4$ Increased TSH	Early: Increased uptake Late: Decreased uptake	Indolent, can have goiter long term; initially hyperthyroid, then hypothyroid	Early: β-blockers if symptomatic Late: Need levothyroxine replacement
de Quervain's disease	Acute onset Exquisitely tender Diffuse goiter Upper respiratory infection antedates it by 5–7 days	Granulomatous	Acutely, can be clinically and biochemically hyperthyroid; negative antimicrosomal and antithyroglobulin antibodies	No uptake diffusely	Acutely, patient is hyperthyroid, then can have 2–4 month period of hypothyroidism; long term, euthyroid	Salicylates or an NSAID If severe, can use a short course of steroids (prednisone, 60 mg PO q.d. in rapid taper)
Lymphocytic	Nontender Diffuse goiter during 2nd and 3rd trimester of pregnancy	Lymphocytic	Early: Increased T$_3$RU, T$_4$ Normal TSH Late: Normal	Contraindicated if patient is pregnant	Acutely hyperthyroid, followed by transient postpartum hypothyroidism; long term, euthyroid	Observation, symptomatic

dose is 300 mg/24 hours PO in a b.i.d. dosing schedule.

or

   (b) **Methimazole** (Tapazole) inhibits the organification of the iodide anions, thus inhibiting T_4 synthesis. Side effects are hepatitis and, rarely, agranulocytosis. The starting dose is 30 mg/24 hours PO in a once daily dosage.
 ii. **Radioactive iodide 131** is the treatment of choice in virtually all patients with Graves' disease. The only contraindication is concurrent pregnancy. The dose is 5–15 mCi (the equivalent of 4,000–20,000 rad) to the thyroid gland itself). Graham et al. reported in a long-term, longitudinal study that there is no increased risk of secondary malignancies in patients treated with the radioactive isotope iodide 131. This treatment is clearly the most efficient and effective treatment for hyperthyroidism as the result of Graves' disease.
 c. The clinician must observe the patient for the development of a **dermopathy.** The dermopathy is best treated with a topical glucocorticoid cream, e.g., triamcinolone 1% cream b.i.d.
 d. The clinician must observe the patient for the development of **ophthalmopathy.** The manifestations of the ophthalmopathy, like those of the dermopathy (specifically, unilateral or bilateral exophthalamus) can occur even after the hyperthyroidism has been successfully treated.
 e. The **specific evaluation and management** include performing ultrasonography of the orbit(s) to document thickening of the musculature and to rule out any other space-occupying lesion. **Treatment** includes administration of systemic steroids and referral to ophthalmology for specific intervention. If the process is severe or refractory to steroids, local irradiation may be indicated and is usually quite effective.
 f. Follow thyroid function tests as, after ^{131}I therapy, hypothyroidism will invariably occur. Replacement with levothyroxine is indicated.
 2. **Plummer's disease.** This is the development of a hyperthyroid state from a toxic multinodular goiter.
 a. The **specific manifestations** include the overall manifestations of hyperthyroidism and an enlarged goiter with multiple discrete nodules. The goiter

T A B L E 9 - 5
Causes of Jod Basedow

Oral ingestion of kelp
Oral ingestion of iodide tablets
Ingestion of meats with iodide or thyroid gland present, e.g., ground
    beef with strap muscle used in processing
Factitious use of thyroid hormone, either as a stimulant or as a weight
    reduction agent
Recurrent, long-term use of topical iodide-containing antiseptics.

and the nodules are nontender. There is **no associated ophthalmopathy or dermopathy.**

b. The **specific evaluation** includes the overall evaluation (see Box 9-6), a TSH of 0.0, an elevated T_4, an elevated T_3RU, and a radioactive thyroid uptake scan demonstrating several nodules with increased uptake. The **specific management** is similar to that of Graves' disease, i.e., a β-blocker and either an antithyroid agent (methimazole or PTU) or radioactive [131]I.

3. **Factitious hyperthyroidism,** including Jod Basedow syndrome. This is the surreptitious use of thyroid hormone or iodide with a resultant hyperthyroidism. See Table 9-5 for potential sources of Jod Basedow.

a. **Specific manifestations** include those of hyperthyroidism but there is invariably no goiter, ophthalmopathy, or dermopathy.

b. The **specific evaluation** includes that described in Box 9-6 and the presence of a TSH of 0.0, an elevated T_4, and an elevated T_3RU. The most specific component is a diffusely decreased uptake in the gland on radioactive iodide uptake scan.

c. The **specific management** includes discovering the source of the iodide or levothyroxine, even if it requires confronting the patient with such data. β-blockers can be administered for symptomatic relief of the hyperthyroidism; however, antithyroid agents or ^{131}I ablation are **contraindicated** as therapeutic modalities.

C. **Consultation**

Service	Time
Endocrinology	Urgent

D. **Indications for admission:** Atrial fibrillation with a rapid ventricular response, or any evidence of imminent thyroid storm. The vast majority of patients with hyperthyroidism will be managed as outpatients.

II. Thyroid deficiency states (i.e., hypothyroidism)
A. Manifestations
The **specific manifestations** of a deficiency in thyroid hormone, a hormone that intimately regulates the overall catabolism of the cells within the body, include cold intolerance, dry skin, unintentional weight gain, coarse hair, bradycardia, symmetric muscle weakness, greater proximally than distally decreased reflexes, and a delayed relaxation phase of the DTRs. Extreme hypothyroidism, i.e., myxedema can result in death. Manifestations that may be harbingers of such a catastrophic event include hypothermia, bradycardias, lethargy, and coma.
B. Underlying causes
The **underlying causes** of hypothyroidism include thyroiditides (e.g., Hashimoto's, lymphocytic, or de Quervain's; see Table 9-4), iatrogenic (e.g., antecedent radiation therapy for Graves' disease, a head and neck carcinoma, or Hodgkin's disease), or surgical removal of the gland, any of which will result in hypothyroidism. Finally, **endemic goiter** needs to be considered. This is hypothyroidism with a diffuse goiter as the result of deficiency of iodide in the diet. It was endemic to the Great Lakes basin of North America and still is endemic to the Struma River valley of Eastern Europe, east–central Asia, and the Andes region of South America.
C. Evaluation and management
The **specific evaluation and management** of the above described entities are given in Box 9-6 and Table 9-4.
D. Consultation

Problem	Service	Time
Myxedema	Endocrine	Emergent
Hypothyroidism	Endocrine	Elective

E. Indications for admission: Limited; include only impending myxedema. The vast majority of patients with hypothyroidism can be evaluated and managed as outpatients.

III. Thyroid nodules
Thyroid nodules are usually found in an asymptomatic patient during a routine physical examination. The vast majority of nodules are benign; however, malignant thyroid nodules occur in a small yet significant minority.
A. Risk factors
Risk factors for the development of thyroid carcinoma, and therefore factors that should increase the suspicion for malignant nodules, include:
1. Previous irradiation to the neck, either iatrogenic or exposure to nuclear fallout.

B O X 9 - 8

Evaluation and Management of Suspected Hypothyroidism

Evaluation

1. Take a thorough **history** and perform a **physical examination,** with emphasis on the above features/manifestations.
2. Determine serum electrolyte, BUN, creatinine, and glucose levels for baseline purposes.
3. Determine the complete blood cell count with differential analysis, looking for any concurrent anemia, usually macrocytic, if present.
4. Determine serum calcium, PO_4, and albumin levels, looking for any concurrent hypercalcemia or hypocalcemia.
5. Perform a **urine pregnancy test** at baseline.
6. Perform urinalysis, looking for concurrent proteinuria.
7. Determine creatine phosphokinase level, as it often will be elevated in patients with proximal muscle weakness, i.e., hypothyroid-related myopathy.
8. Obtain a 12-lead ECG if there is any evidence of bradycardia.
9. Determine **T_3RU, T_4, and TSH** levels (see Table 9-2).

Management

1. If consciousness is significantly depressed, suggesting impending **myxedema coma,** perform the following evaluations:
   a. Check ABCs as appropriate according to the ACLS protocol.
   b. Make finger stick glucose determinations to rule out hypoglycemia.
   c. Determine arterial blood gases at baseline to rule out hypoxemia and hypercapnia.
   d. Replete fluids IV, usually with D5 .45 NS, as appropriate.
   e. Make arrangements for admission to an ICU.
   f. If hypoglycemic, administer 1–2 ampules of D50W IV.

(continued)

B O X 9 - 8 (continued)

    g. Obtain basic core of data in Boxes 9-6 and 9-8.
    h. **Do not warm** the patient.
    i. Administer vasopressor agents (e.g., dopamine) to maintain adequate perfusion.
    j. Administer **thyroxine, 300–500 μg by IV push** over 15 minutes.
        i. Sodium levothyroxine, 500 μg/10-mg mannitol.
        ii. Mix with 5 mL of normal saline.
        iii. Administer by slow IV push (10–15 minutes).
        iv. Once mixed, it is quite unstable and must be used immediately.
    k. Hydrocortisone 80 mg IV now and q.8h. until stable, as the patient can often be concurrently adrenal insufficient.
    l. Endocrinology consultation mandated on an emergent basis.
2. If **clinically hypothyroid but not acutely ill,** or after stabilization of a myxedematous patient:
    a. Basic core of data, Boxes 9-6 and 9-8.
    b. Initiate **levothyroxine** (Synthroid), i.e., T_4. The usual repletion dose is 50–200 μg PO q.d. If the patient has a significant history of angina or ASHD, start with a very low dose, 12.5–25 μg PO q.d., and increase the dose slowly in subsequent weeks. The half-life of T_4, levothyroxine is approximately 7 days; therefore, it takes approximately 4 weeks to reach a steady state with any dose initiation or change. The dose should be titrated to a clinically euthyroid state or TSH normalization. The TSH should be checked approximately 4–5 weeks after any change in levothyroxine dosage.
    c. Check for any concurrent or concomitant autoimmune disease on a longitudinal basis.
    d. Screen for lipid abnormalities as there is a high incidence of hyperlipidemia in patients with hypothyroidism.
    e. Endocrinology consultation is recommended but not mandatory.

  2. Solitary nodule.
  3. Young age.
  4. Male sex.
  5. Firm and fixed mass.
  6. Concurrent palpable cervical nodes.
 B. **Differential diagnosis**
    The **differential diagnosis** of thyroid nodules includes **multinodular goiter,** i.e., an enlarged thyroid gland with multiple nodules, euthyroid clinically; **Plummer's disease,** i.e., multinodular goiter with hyperthyroidism; **benign adenoma,** euthyroid or hyperthyroid; and a **malignant neoplastic lesion** (see Table 9-6). Other extrathyroid causes of anterior neck masses including branchial cleft cysts and extrathyroidal lymphadenopathy must be included in the differential diagnosis but invariably may be excluded upon physical examination.
 C. **Consultation**

Problem	*Service*	*Time*
Solitary nodule	Endocrinology	Urgent
Multiple nodules	Endocrinology	Elective

B O X 9 - 9

Evaluation and Management of Thyroid Nodules

Evaluation

1. Perform an overall evaluation as described in Box 9-6.
2. Assess the clinical thyroid state of the patient: hyperthyroid, euthyroid, or hypothyroid.
3. Perform **ultrasonography** of the thyroid. This imaging study is not mandatory, as it does not differentiate benign from malignant lesions. However, it is helpful as an adjunct to physical examination in that it helps the clinician, particularly a nonendocrinologist, to define the number and size of the nodules.
4. Thyroid scans using ^{99m}Tc or ^{131}I are **useless** in the evaluation of thyroid nodules.
5. Make a **clinical judgment as to the risk that the nodule is malignant** using the basic core of data and clinical judgment.

(continued)

B O X   9 - 9 (continued)

---

   a. **High risk.** A patient with several of the above
     mentioned risk factors, e.g., a young male with a
     solitary nodule, must be referred to an endocrinol-
     ogist/thyroidologist and undergo excisional bi-
     opsy of the lesion by an experienced endocrine
     surgeon. The patient should be staged for distant
     metastases via ^{131}I body scan.

   b. **Low risk.** A patient with multiple low risk factors,
     e.g., an elderly woman with multiple nodules,
     should be followed clinically with TSH and thy-
     roid examinations.

   c. **Intermediate risk.** Usually a solitary nodule with-
     out any other high risk factors. Further evaluation
     and management of these patients include refer-
     ral to endocrinologist/thyroidologist. One of three
     approaches can be used:

     i. Excisional biopsy, *or*
     ii. Fine needle aspiration of the nodule and send
      for cytology. If cytology is **positive** for malig-
      nant neoplastic cells, refer to a surgeon and
      stage with ^{131}I body scan for distant metasta-
      ses. If cytology is **negative** for malignant neo-
      plastic cells, one cannot rule out malignancy
      and thus must use another approach listed
      here, e.g., a trial of suppression.

6. Attempt **suppression with exogenous thyroxine,** i.e.,
   100–200 μg levothyroxine q.d. PO, for 8–12 weeks.
   The theory behind suppression is that by giving the
   patient exogenous thyroxine, there is a negative
   feedback upon the hypothalamus/adenohypophysis
   and a decrease in TSH. Most **benign nodules** are
   quite dependent upon TSH and rapidly decrease in
   size when TSH is removed, whereas most malignant
   neoplastic nodules are significantly more autono-
   mous, i.e., independent of TSH for growth. Therefore, if there is a **decrease in size of the nodule,** continue levothyroxine dose/suppression; follow TFTs,
   TSH, and nodule size long term. If there is **no decrease in size of the nodule,** excisional biopsy
   should be performed.

Management

The management of thyroid malignant lesions is beyond the scope of this text.

TABLE 9-6
Thyroid Malignancies

Type	Risk Factors	Metastases	Treatment/Comments
Papillary	Past head or neck irradiation	Lymph nodes	Surgical excision of primary tumor Exogenous thyroxine, keeping the patient biochemically mildly hyperthyroid in order to suppress TSH If residual tumor is demonstrated by ^{131}I body scan, ^{131}I ablation; dose: 100–150 mC; PO; **endocrinology consultation is mandatory**
Follicular	Neck irradiation	Hematogenous Lung Bone	Essentially same as papillary; overall poorer prognosis; **endocrine consultation is mandatory**
Medullary carcinoma	Multiple endocrine neoplasia, type IIa, (Sipple's disease) Bilateral pheochromocytomas Parathyroid hyperplasia Medullary carcinoma		Surgical resection Tumor is derived from the parafollicular C-cells and can produce calcitonin, prostaglandins, and histamine
Anaplastic	Neck irradiation	Aggressive local and systemic spread	Surgical excision and chemotherapy Requires oncology and endocrinology consultations

D. Indications for admission: If and when surgical intervention is required.

Bibliography

Diabetes Mellitus

Brown MJ, Asbury AK: Diabetic neuropathy. Ann Neurol 1984;15:2.

Gerich JE: Insulin-dependent diabetes mellitus: Pathophysiology. Mayo Clin Proc 1986;61:787–791.

Gerich JE: Sulfonylureas in the treatment of diabetes mellitus—1985. Mayo Clin Proc 1985;60:439.

Harati Y: Diabetic peripheral neuropathies. Ann Intern Med 1987;107: 546–559.

Hodges D, et al: Management of the diabetic foot. Ann Fam Pract 1986;33:189–195.

Klein R, et al: Microalbuminuria in a population based study of diabetes. Arch Intern Med 1992;152:153–158.

KROC Collaborative Study Group: Diabetic retinopathy after two years of intensified insulin treatment. JAMA 1988;260:37–41.

Moller DE, Flier JS: Insulin resistance: Mechanisms, syndromes, and implications. N Engl J Med 1991;325:938–948.

Nathan DM, et al: Non-insulin dependent diabetes in older patients. Am J Med 1986;81:837–842.

National Diabetes Data Group: Classification and diagnosis of diabetes mellitus and other categories of glucose intolerance. Diabetes 1979;28:1039.

Nelson RL: Oral glucose tolerance test: Indications and limitations. Mayo Clin Proc 1988;63:263–269.

Reddi AS, Camerini-Davalos RA: Diabetic nephropathy. Arch Intern Med 1990;150:31–42.

Sherwin RS, Taborlane WV: Metabolic control and diabetic complications. In Olesky JM, Sherwin RS (eds): Diabetes Mellitus: Management and Complications. New York, Churchill Livingstone, 1985.

Singer DE, et al: Screening for diabetes mellitus. Ann Intern Med 1988;109:639–649.

Singer DE, et al: Tests of glycemia in diabetes mellitus. Ann Intern Med 1989;110:125–137.

Hypercalcemia

Boonstra CE, Jackson CE: Hyperparathyroidism detected by routine serum calcium analysis: Prevalence in a clinic population. Ann Intern Med 1965;63:468.

Levine MM, Kleeman CR: Hypercalcemia: Pathophysiology and treatment. Hosp Pract 1987;July:73–90.

Lufkin EG, et al: Parathyroid hormone radioimmunoassays in the differential diagnosis of hypercalcemia due to primary hyperparathyroidism or malignancy. Ann Intern Med 1987;106:559.

Singer FR, Fernandez M: Therapy of hypercalcemia of malignancy. Am J Med 1987;82(S2A):34–40.

Hyperkalemia

DeFronzo RA: Hyperkalemia and hyporeninemic hypoaldosteronism. Kidney Int 1980;17:118–134.

Ponce SP, et al: Drug-induced hyperkalemia. Medicine 1985;64:357–370.

Williams ME, et al: Hyperkalemia. Adv Intern Med 1986;32:265.

Thyroid Dysfunctional States

Allen ME, Braverman LE: Management of thyrotoxicosis. Compr Ther 1987;13:20–30.

Cooper DS: Antithyroid drugs. N Engl J Med 1984;311:1353–1362.

Hamberger JI: The various presentations of thyroiditis. Ann Intern Med 1986;104:219–224.

Helfand M, Crapo LM: Monitoring therapy in patients taking levothyroxine. Ann Intern Med 1990;113:450–454.

Helfand M, Crapo LM: Screening for thyroid disease. Ann Intern Med 1990;112:840–849.

Levine SN: Current concepts of thyroiditis. Arch Intern Med 1983;143: 1952–1956.

Nordyke RA, et al: Graves' disease. Arch Intern Med 1988;148:626–631.

Robbins J, et al: Thyroid cancer: A lethal endocrine neoplasm. Ann Intern Med 1991;115:133–147.

Sakiyama R: Common thyroid disorders. Am Fam Pract 1988;38:227–238.

Salman K, et al: Selection of thyroid preparations. Am Fam Pract 1989; 40:215–219.

de los Santos ET, Mazzaferri EL: Thyroid function tests. Postgrad Med 1989;85:333–351.

Wartofsky L: Guidelines for the treatment of hyperthyroidism. Am Fam Pract 1984;30:199–210.

—D.D.B.

Dale Berg, Ed. *Handbook of Primary Care Medicine.* Copyright © 1993 J. B. Lippincott Company.

CHAPTER 10

Male Genitourinary Tract

Prostate Dysfunction

The **prostate gland** is located at the inferior aspect of and immediately adjacent to the urinary bladder in males. It is an organ through which the **urethra** passes as it enters into the proximal penis. In the pelvis the prostate gland is immediately anterior to the mid-rectum. The **vas deferens** from each testis also passes through this structure as it enters the urethra. In the normal state the prostate gland produces secretions that are components of seminal fluid.

The **overall manifestations** of prostate dysfunction include those attributable to the urinary tract itself and those from the adjacent genital tract structures. Because of the location of the gland, any inflammation or enlargement of the gland may cause varied problems for the patient. Patients may present with **hesitancy,** or inability to promptly initiate a forceful urinary stream; **dribbling,** or leakage of urine after urination; **urinary tenesmus,** or the sensation of inadequate evacuation of the urinary bladder; **hematuria; pyuria; nocturia,** or frequent urination at night; **increased frequency of urination;** and even **dysuria,** or a burning sensation during urination. On rectal examination the prostate gland may be enlarged and tender, on scrotal examination the epididymides may be tender or enlarged, and in severe cases the urinary bladder may be distended with urine, as detected by percussion of the lower abdomen.

I. **Pathologic conditions affecting the prostate**

Three discrete but overlapping and quite common **pathologic conditions** are discussed here: prostatitis, benign prostatic hypertrophy, and prostatic nodules.

A. **Prostatitis**

Prostatitis, or inflammation of the prostate gland, is quite common. The **specific manifestations** of this entity include the relatively acute onset of dysuria, pyuria, increased frequency, hesitancy, and potentially rectal pain. Onset occurs from youth to old age. On **examination** the prostate gland is tender, diffusely enlarged, and boggy. There may be concurrent epididymal tenderness.

One major method of **categorizing** prostatitides is to stratify them into acute versus chronic syndromes.

1. **Acute prostatitis**
    a. In **acute prostatitis,** the manifestations listed above are present for the first time and are present for less than 1 week. **Causes** of acute prostatitis include pathogens from the **urinary tract** (e.g., gram-negative bacilli) or those from the **urethra and genitals** (e.g., *Chlamydia trachomatis, Ureaplasma* spp., and, rarely, as a solitary entity, *Neisseria gonorrhoeae*).
    b. The **specific evaluation and management** include the steps listed in Box 10-1 and, if a sexually transmitted disease (STD) is suspected, management of that disease (see section on Sexually Transmitted Diseases in Chapter 6). **Intervention** includes the initiation of antibiotics effective against the pathogens listed above. Often cultures will be negative, and therefore empirical therapy is necessary. The **duration** of therapy is 3 weeks. Regimens include:
        i. Ciprofloxacin, 500 mg PO b.i.d., *or*

B O X 1 0 - 1

Overall Evaluation and Management of Suspected Prostate Dysfunction

Evaluation

1. Take a thorough **history,** looking for any history of hesitancy, dysuria, pyuria, hematuria, increasing nocturia, or hesitancy. See text for details.
2. Perform a thorough **physical examination** with emphasis on the rectal and scrotal examinations:

(continued)

B O X   1 0 - 1 *(continued)*

    a. Evaluate the prostate size, consistency, and the presence or absence of tenderness. The **normal gland** should be smooth, without nodules, nontender, and nonboggy, but mildly firm in consistency. A marker for firmness is that the gland should be about the consistency of the flaccid belly of the biceps muscle.

    b. Examination should also include palpation of the **epididymides** and **testes** for tenderness and masses. If the gland is enlarged, check for any **urinary bladder distention** by percussing out the superior border of the bladder above the pelvis.

3. Perform a **urinalysis,** looking for any pyuria or hematuria (see Chapter 3, page 140, for specifics on the evaluation and management of pyuria and hematuria).

4. Determine the **postvoid urinary residual volume** if there is any evidence of obstruction. In this technique the patient voids, attempting to evacuate the urinary bladder completely. A sterile catheter is then inserted into the urinary bladder to obtain the residual urine. The normal residual volume is less than 50 mL. A residual volume greater than 100 mL is distinctly abnormal and consistent with urinary outlet obstruction.

5. Obtain a urine specimen for **culture** and sensitivity testing if pyuria or hematuria is present.

6. Determine serum creatinine, BUN, glucose, and electrolyte levels for baseline purposes.

Management

1. If **benign prostatic hypertrophy** is diagnosed, refer the patient to a urologist.

2. If **prostatitis** is diagnosed, initiate antibiotics for a 3-week course. Empirical regimens include:

    a. Ciprofloxacin, 500 mg PO b.i.d., *or*

    b. Trimethoprim–sulfamethoxazole (Bactrim), one tablet PO b.i.d., *or*

    c. Doxycycline, 100 mg PO b.i.d.

3. If **nodules** are present (i.e., indurated palpable lesions in the gland itself), the suspicion for prostate carcinoma should be high. Refer the patient to a urologist for transrectal prostate biopsy of the nodule.

       ii. Trimethoprim–sulfamethoxazole (Bactrim DS), one tablet PO b.i.d., *or*

       iii. Doxycycline, 100 mg PO b.i.d.

2. Chronic prostatitis

   a. In **chronic prostatitis,** the manifestations listed above are recurrently present, present for more than several weeks, and/or are refractory to first-line antibiotic regimens. The **different causes** of chronic prostatitis include the pathogens listed for acute prostatitis, i.e., from the **urinary tract** (e.g., gram-negative bacilli) and those from the **urethra and genitals** (e.g., *Chlamydia trachomatis* and *Ureaplasma* spp.). In addition, *Blastomyces* spp. or *Mycobacterium* spp. can rarely result in disease.

   b. The **specific evaluation and management** include the steps outlined in Box 10-1 and, if an STD is suspected, management of that disease. **Intervention** includes the initiation of antibiotics effective against the pathogens listed above. Often the cultures will be negative, and therefore empirical therapy is necessary. The **duration** of therapy is 6 weeks. Regimens include:

       i. Ciprofloxacin, 500 mg PO b.i.d., *or*

       ii. Trimethoprim–sulfamethoxazole (Bactrim DS), one tablet PO b.i.d., *or*

       iii. Doxycycline, 100 mg PO b.i.d.

   Referral to a urologist for chronic prostatitis is indicated.

B. Benign prostatic hypertrophy

Benign prostatic hypertrophy (BPH) is a common entity that affects all males to various degrees during their lifetimes. It is quite prevalent in the elderly.

  1. Manifestations

   The **specific manifestations** include those attributable to the obstruction, i.e., hesitancy and frequency, which are insidious and progressive in nature. The symptoms can worsen precipitously when a urinary tract infection occurs. On **rectal examination** the prostate gland is diffusely enlarged, nontender, about the consistency of the biceps muscle in contraction, and without nodules. The bladder may be distended. The **natural history** of this entity entails progression to the point of complications. **Complications** may include recurrent urinary tract infections and the development of obstructive nephropathy.

  2. Evaluation and management

   The **specific evaluation and management** include the steps outlined in Box 10-1, treating any concurrent UTI, and referral to a urologist. The agent **terazosin,** an antihypertensive agent, has been of some efficacy in decreasing symptoms and objective signs of obstruction, but surgical intervention entailing transurethral resection of the prostate (**TURP**) remains the treatment of choice.

C. **Prostatic nodules**

Prostatic nodules are also quite prevalent, especially with increasing age. These nodules may be asymptomatic until discovered on a routine **screening** digital rectal examination.

1. **Manifestations**

On **examination** these lesions are nontender, indurated (similar in consistency to the tragus of the ear), and may be single or multiple. There usually are no associated scrotal or urinary manifestations. The minimal detectable size of these lesions, i.e., the sensitivity of digital examination for nodule detection, is **1 cm.**

2. **Evaluation and management**

The **specific evaluation and management** of prostatic nodules include the steps outlined in Box 10-1 and are based on the fact that an indurated nodule is potentially a focus of prostate adenocarcinoma. Therefore, referral to a urologist for **transrectal biopsy** of the lesion is indicated. A **prostate specific antigen (PSA) assay** during the **annual digital examination** is of utility in screening (see prevention chapter) because an elevated PSA titer increases the likelihood that the nodule is prostatic adenocarcinoma, and reinforces the need for urgent invasive evaluation.

II. **Consultation**

Problem	Service	Time
Prostatic nodules	Genitourinary	Required
Benign prostatic hypertrophy	Genitourinary	Required
Chronic prostatitis	Genitourinary	Elective
Acute obstructive renal failure	Renal	Urgent
Purulent urethritis	Public Health Service	Required

III. **Indications for admission:** Renal failure, a systemic infection from urinary obstruction, or surgery. Some surgical procedures can be performed in an ambulatory surgical center, obviating an overnight in-hospital admission.

Scrotal Masses

The **scrotum** is a structure that keeps the sexual reproductive organs of the male in an extra-abdominal space. Spermatogenesis is optimal at temperatures slightly lower than 98.6 °F; therefore, it has been postulated that the scrotum evolved to keep the testes cooler by keeping them outside the abdomen and pelvis. The contents of the scrotum include the **two testes** and the **ducts** that drain the testes into the penile urethra. The **testes** in the normal state are smooth, oval, nontender structures approximately 4 cm in longitudinal dimension and 25 mL in volume. The **ducts** include the **epididymi,** which are coiled, nontender structures applied to the posterior aspect of each testis, and the **vas deferens,** a tubular structure extending from the tail of the epididymis to the prostatic urethra. The vas deferens with the spermatic vein and spermatic artery form the **spermatic cord.** The **floor** of the scrotum is made of the abdominal wall and is a site in which congenital and acquired hernias form. It is not uncommon for a male to develop a scrotal mass during the course of his lifetime.

I. Differential diagnosis

The **differential diagnosis** of scrotal masses includes the following entities:

A. Hydrocele

1. Pathogenesis

The **underlying pathogenesis** of this mass is that it is comprised of the fluid-filled congenital remnants of the processus tunica vaginalis. The **specific manifestations** include a chronic, nontender, and transilluminable lesion. The mass may wax and wane in size; an indirect hernia may be concurrently present.

2. Evaluation and management

The **specific evaluation and management** include making the clinical diagnosis by performing the steps described in Box 10-2 and referring the patient to a general surgeon for elective repair, as clinically indicated.

B. Inguinal hernia

See section on Hernias in Chapter 2, page 122.

C. Testicular carcinoma

1. Pathogenesis

The **underlying pathogenesis** of this entity is the malignant neoplastic growth of germ cells in one of the testes. A specific **risk factor** for development is cryptorchidism, or the abnormal congenital retention of one or both testes within the abdomen. **Cryptorchidism** not only decreases spermatogenesis (warmer ambient temperature) but also, through unclear means, increases the risk of development of a germ cell malignant neoplasm. The **histopathologic types** of tumors are described in Table 10-1.

2. Manifestations

The **specific manifestations** include the development

B O X 1 0 - 2

Overall Approach to a Patient with a Scrotal Mass

Evaluation

1. Take the **history,** with an emphasis on the following features:
   a. The **duration** of time that the lesion has been present. **Acute lesions** are present for less than 1 week and **chronic lesions** are present for more than 1 week.
   b. Determine the presence or absence of **pain.**
   c. Investigate the past history for trauma and sexually transmitted diseases.
2. Perform a **physical examination,** with emphasis on the following features:
   a. The mass is **tender or nontender.**
   b. The mass is **transilluminable or not.** Transillumination is checked by shining a light source such as a penlight into the mass. A mass that transilluminates is fluid-filled.
   c. The mass is **reducible or nonreducible.** If the lesion is **reducible**—i.e.; it resolves or reenters the abdominal cavity from the scrotum with application of mild force—it is consistent with an inguinal hernia.
3. Perform **urinalysis** with microscopic analysis. Determining these three variables—**acuity, tenderness, and transilluminability**—in the assessment of scrotal masses is pivotal in making the diagnosis.

Management

1. If the mass is acute, tender, unilateral, and nontransilluminable, **ultrasonography of the testes** and referral to a urologist emergently are mandatory to rule out testicular torsion.
2. If there is any evidence of concurrent purulent urethritis, manage as for a sexually transmitted disease (see Chapter 6).

TABLE 10-1
Histopathologic Types of Testicular Carcinoma

Type	Frequency	Tumor Markers	
		AFP	*β-HCG*
Seminoma	40%	Negative	Negative
Embryonal cell carcinoma	25%	Positive	Positive
Teratoma	5%	Negative	Negative
Immature teratoma	25%	Positive	Negative
Choriocarcinoma	2%	Negative	Positive

of a scrotal mass which is relatively acute, nontransilluminable, usually quite small, and usually nontender. However, if the tumor is rapidly growing it can become ischemic and, therefore, tender. Often the lesion is firm and continuous to the testis. Very often the mass is small, nontender, and **detected** only on routine physical examination or **monthly patient testicular self-examination.** When the lesion is advanced, the patient can manifest with weight loss.

3. **Evaluation and management**
   The **specific evaluation and management** include the steps outlined in Box 10-2 and referral to a urologist for further evaluation and management. If there is a suspicion for one of these neoplasms, one should obtain serum tumor markers. These markers include **α-fetoprotein** (AFP) and **β-human chorionic gonadotropin** (β-HCG). Table 10-1 summarizes the utility of these markers for different histopathologic types of testicular carcinoma.

D. **Testicular torsion**
   1. **Pathogenesis**
      The **underlying pathogenesis** is a testis abnormally twisted on its spermatic cord, thus embarrassing the venous drainage and the arterial supply to the testis, resulting in swelling, pain, and ischemia of the testes.
   2. **Manifestations**
      The **specific manifestations** include an acute, painful, tender, and nontransilluminable lesion. The condition is most common in young males, but it can occur in any age group.
   3. **Evaluation and management**
      The **specific evaluation and management** include the steps outlined in Box 10-2 and developing the clinical

suspicion clinically that torsion is the underlying lesion. Ultrasonography with Doppler flow studies should be performed to demonstrate a decreased flow of blood in the affected spermatic cord and testis. Emergent referral to a urologist for surgical intervention is indicated.

E. **Orchitis/epididymitis**
   1. **Pathogenesis**
      The **underlying pathogenesis** is a bacterial infection. The bacteria are either from a **urinary tract source,** e.g., gram-negative baccilli, or, more commonly, are sexually transmitted, i.e., *Chlamydia* spp.
   2. **Manifestations**
      The **specific manifestations** include a mass that is acute in onset, tender, and nontransilluminable. The patient can have findings of systemic infection, such as fevers and tachycardia, and often reports a past history of sexually transmitted diseases.
   3. **Evaluation and management**
      The **specific evaluation and management** include the steps listed in Box 10-2 and performing ultrasonography of the mass to look for an abscess cavity. Referral to a urologist for **surgical drainage** and the initiation of **parenteral antibiotics** are indicated. Antibiotic regimens can include intravenous trimethoprim–sulfamethoxazole or intravenous ampicillin and doxycycline.

F. **Varicocele**
   1. **Pathogenesis**
      The **underlying pathogenesis** is the formation of a venous varicosity in the spermatic vein. Because the spermatic vein on the left does not drain directly into the inferior vena cava, but on the right the spermatic vein does, there is an increased incidence of varicosities on the left side.
   2. **Manifestations**
      The **specific manifestations** include a chronic, nontender, nontransilluminable mass, usually on the **left side.** The lesion often has the consistency of "a bag of worms" and decreases in size with elevation of the scrotum.
   3. **Evaluation and management**
      The **specific evaluation and management** of this lesion entail making the clinical diagnosis by performing the steps described in Box 10-2. Usually no intervention is necessary; however, if the lesion is new and on the **right,** a thorough examination of the pelvis should be performed to rule out any new cause for obstruction to spermatic vein blood flow.

II. Consultation

Problem	Service	Time
Hydrocele	General surgery	Elective
Inguinal hernia	General surgery	
Strangulated		Emergent
Incarcerated		Urgent
Reducible		Elective
Testicular carcinoma	Urology	Urgent
Testicular torsion	Urology	Emergent
Testicular abscess	Urology	Emergent

III. Indications for admission: Strangulated or incarcerated hernia, testicular torsion or abscess, or for any elective surgical procedure.

Bibliography

Catalona WJ, Scott WWW: Carcinoma of the prostate: A review. J Urol 1978;119:1.

Lepor H: Nonoperative management of benign prostatic hypertrophy. J Urol 1989;141:1283.

O'Brien WM: Benign prostatic hypertrophy. Am Fam Pract 1991;44: 162–171.

O'Brien WM, Lynch JH: The acute scrotum. Am Fam Pract 1988;37: 239–247.

Prater JM, Overdorf BS: Testicular torsion: A surgical emergency. Am Fam Pract 1991;44:834–840.

Schwager EJ: Treatment of bacterial prostatitis. Am Fam Pract 1991;44: 2137–2141.

—D.D.B.

Dale Berg, Ed. *Handbook
of Primary Care Medicine.*
Copyright © 1993 J. B.
Lippincott Company.

CHAPTER 11

Gynecology/Breast

Breast Masses and Lumps

The female **breast** has one known physiologic purpose, the formation of milk to sustain a neonate in the postpartum time period. Milk is a complex liquid which consists of water, nutrients, vitamins, complex sugars, fats, and antibodies, specifically of the IgA class. In most cases the quantity of milk is sufficient to supply the nutritional needs of the neonate.

The **anatomy of the breast** is based upon the fact that they are skin appendages, i.e., glands within the skin itself. They consist of multiple separate exocrine glands, each with a specific duct draining into the nipple. The specific glands are composed of clumps of acini, the acini being the clumps of cells which produce the milk itself. The breast tissue is supported by strands of connective tissue, called Cooper's ligaments, located between the dermis and the underlying chest wall fascia.

The **physiology of the breasts** is such that they are under significant control of several hormones. These hormones include:

1. **Estrogens.** These hormones, which are produced by the ovaries, stimulate the proliferation of the epithelial cells in the ducts and increase the overall vascularity of the breast tissue itself. Therefore, periods of time or states which increase the level of estrogens within the physiologic milieu will result in these physiologic changes. The two physiologic times of estrogen excess are the follicular (proliferative) phase of the menstrual cycle and pregnancy.

2. **Progesterones.** These hormones which are produced by the ovaries, stimulate the proliferation of acini and will, physiologically, counter the effects of estrogens. Therefore, periods of time in which there is an increase in the level of progesterones in the physiologic milieu will result in these physiologic changes. The states in which there is an overall increase in progesterones in-

clude the luteal (secretory) phase of the menstrual cycle and pregnancy.

3. Many other hormones, including β-HCG and **prolactin,** are involved in the production and release of milk from the breast in the postpartum state. These are beyond the scope of this text.

I. Differential diagnosis

The **differential diagnosis** of breast masses includes the following lesions.

A. Fibroadenoma

1. **Pathophysiology**

The **pathophysiology** of this lesion is that it is quite probably a specific form of **fibrocystic** change. There is an increase in the fibrous and ductal epithelial tissue in the lesion itself. It is often associated with estrogen excess, the estrogens stimulating the ductal and vascular structures of the breast.

2. **Manifestations**

The **specific manifestations** of this entity include the presence of a discrete solitary lesion which quite often becomes mildly painful and tender, but will not change in size, in the follicular, i.e., high estrogen, phase of the menstrual cycle. These are invariably in a premenopausal woman, as without estrogens they will not occur.

3. **Evaluation and management**

The **specific evaluation and management** include making the clinical diagnosis by performing the examinations described in Box 11-1. The mammogram will reveal a discrete solitary mass, usually with a large clump of calcium. Once the histopathologic diagnosis is secured, no further intervention is required.

B. Intraductal papilloma

1. **Pathophysiology**

The **pathophysiology** of this lesion is that it is quite probably a specific form of FCC, involving one duct only.

2. **Manifestations**

The **specific manifestations** of this entity include the onset of serous or even bloody nipple discharge from one specific duct at the nipple. In most cases the papilloma is subareolar but nonpalpable and nontender.

3. **Evaluation and management**

The **specific evaluation and management** include making the clinical diagnosis by performing the examinations described in Box 11-1. The mammogram will reveal a solitary lesion in the subareolar area, no calcifications within the mass. Once the histologic diagno-

B O X   1 1 - 1

Overall Evaluation and Management of Breast Masses

Evaluation

1. Implement effective **screening programs** to detect masses and lumps within the breast tissue itself so that any lesion which is malignant, neoplastic, will be detected early in its clinical course. These screening programs include:
   a. **Breast self-examination (BSE).** This method should be taught to all women at the time of menarche. It should be performed by the woman on a monthly basis. A premenopausal woman should examine her breasts at approximately day 4–5 of cycle as this is the time frame in which the breast tissue is under the least hormone stimulation. A postmenopausal woman should examine her breasts on the first day of each month.
   b. **Annual breast examination by physician.** Useful in detecting any palpable lesions. Features which are positively correlated with (i.e., are attributes of) breast carcinoma include:
      i. Solitary mass.
      ii. Mass induration.
      iii. A lack of tenderness.
      iv. Concurrent axillary lymph node enlargement.
   c. **Bilateral mammograms.** Should be performed at age 35–40 for baseline, then every other year for 10 years, then annually after age 50. The mammograms complement the annual physical examination and the monthly BSE. Findings which are positively correlated with (i.e., are attributes of) a breast carcinoma include:
      i. Mass with irregular borders.
      ii. Clustered microcalcifications, especially within the mass.
      iii. Overlying skin changes.

Once a mass is discovered:

2. History is integral, including any past history of hormone-related carcinoma, endometrial and/or breast; any family history of breast carcinoma.

(continued)

B O X   1 1 - 1 *(continued)*

3. Examine the patient for any concurrent findings, i.e., any nipple discharge. If nipple discharge is present, send for cytology. Furthermore, examine for any concurrent axillary or supraclavicular lymph node enlargement.

4. Any suspicious lesion, i.e., any lesion which is solitary, or any lesion, palpable or not, which has clustered microcalcifications present, must be biopsied for histopathologic diagnosis. One of two biopsy methods can be used:

   a. Perform a needle aspiration of the mass. If fluid or cells are obtained, send the specimen for cytology. If malignant neoplastic, refer to a surgeon for definitive therapy.

      or

   b. Refer directly to a surgeon for excisional biopsy, i.e., complete resection of entire mass. A frozen section of the biopsy can easily and rapidly be performed for diagnosis of the mass. In this scenario, the patient, the primary care physician, and the surgeon should discuss the options for treatment, if indeed the lesion is malignant neoplastic, before the biopsy is performed. The surgical options include:

      i. Modified radical mastectomy, which includes the removal of the axillary lymph nodes.

         or

      ii. Quadrantectomy with concurrent axillary node dissection—mandatory for staging purposes.

sis by excisional biopsy is secured, no further intervention is required.

C. **Fibrocystic changes**

   1. **Pathophysiology**

      The **pathophysiology** of this quite common albeit diverse set of benign breast disorders has not been completely elucidated. Clearly there is a component of hormone mediation. In fact, estrogen excess states, especially those associated with luteal phase defects and dysfunctional uterine bleeding, are highly associated with fibrocystic breast disease. The estrogens result in the exuberant growth of the ductal and vascular structures, with resultant cystic and proliferative changes within the breast. The disease is quite prevalent; in fact, 90% of women will have this disorder at some time during their lifetime. In addition to the positive correlation between fibrocystic changes and dysfunctional uterine bleeding, pregnancy and oral contraceptive use appear to be negatively correlated with this disorder.

2. **Manifestations**

The **specific manifestations** of this entity include the presence of multiple, bilateral lumps within the breasts. The lumps are quite diverse in size, and can manifest marked variation in terms of tenderness and size during various portions of the menstrual cycle. Again this process is specific to the premenopausal time frame.

3. **Evaluation**

The **specific evaluation** includes making the clinical diagnosis by performing the examinations described in Box 11-1. The mammogram will reveal multiple lesions within both breasts; usually no calcifications are present. The sensitivity and specificity of mammography and of the physical examination in the detection of malignant lesions are decreased in the setting of fibrocystic changes. One caveat is that if one lesion becomes dominant or is atypical, it should be regarded as suspicious and aggressively evaluated with aspiration. Aspiration using a 20-gauge needle and syringe is an effective diagnostic tool in an atypical lesion. The lesion should be completely drained of fluid; the fluid and any tissue obtained should be sent for cytologic examination. Indications for immediate referral to a surgeon for excisional biopsy include:

a. Recurrence after lesion drainage.

b. Any atypical cells on the cytologic examination.

c. Any clusters of microcalcifications on mammography.

4. **Management**

Specific management of FCC includes instructing the patient to perform BSE on a monthly basis, and to refrain from the use of methylxanthines. Further modalities for therapy include the following:

a. Oral contraceptives. This is particularly useful in patients with concurrent dysfunctional uterine bleeding.

b. Danazol. In recurrent severe FCC. This synthetic

androgen can be administered in a dose of 100–400 mg PO q.d. (in b.i.d. dosing), and is effective in significantly decreasing the manifestations in >90% of cases. The agent is contraindicated in any woman who is pregnant or any woman who desires to become pregnant in the near future. Side effects include, but are not limited to, hirsutism, secondary amenorrhea, and hepatic dysfunction.

D. Breast carcinoma

1. Pathophysiology

The **pathophysiology** is not completely known; however, several **discrete risk factors** for the development of the most common histopathologic type of breast carcinoma, infiltrating ductile adenocarcinoma, are known. These include long-term use of estrogens unopposed, early menarche, and late menopause. Additional risk factors include a personal history of breast carcinoma in the contralateral breast, and a family history of breast carcinoma in a first-degree female relative (mother, sister, daughter).

2. Manifestations

The **specific manifestations** include the presence of a unilateral, solitary, nontender indurated lesion in the breast. It can be mobile, or if more advanced, fixed to the overlying and/or deep structures. If fixed to the overlying skin, there can be a peau d'orange appearance to the skin and/or nipple retractions, whereas if fixed to the deep fascia, it is immobile. There often is concurrent axillary and/or supraclavicular lymph node enlargement, these nodes being nontender and firm.

3. Evaluation and management

The **specific evaluation and management** include making the clinical diagnosis by performing the examinations described in Box 11-1. The mammogram will reveal a solitary lesion with irregular borders, clusters of microcalcifications, and overlying skin thickening. Clearly, referral to a surgeon for definitive therapy is indicated in an expedient manner. Staging and postsurgical therapy are discussed in the section on Breast Malignancy in Chapter 5, page 284.

II. Consultation

Problem	Service	Time
Any lesion suspicious for carcinoma	Surgeon	Urgent
Severe fibrocystic changes	Gynecology	Elective

III. **Indications for admission:** Specific only to therapeutic surgical interventions. In fact, most excisional biopsies can be
performed in ambulatory surgical suites, obviating admission
to an inpatient service.

Contraceptive Modalities

Effective and safe modalities to **prevent conception** are known at
the present time. The primary care physician is in a position to
educate patients to these modalities. Furthermore, the primary
care physician is in a position to educate patients on the specific
modalities that are effective in the prevention of sexually transmitted diseases. The modalities which will be addressed in this
discussion include abstinence, the use of condoms, the use of a
diaphragm, the use of a cervical cap, the use of oral contraceptives, and the surgical techniques of vasectomy and tubal ligation.

Although many of the modalities for contraception are designed
for women, the responsibility for contraception, prevention of
sexually transmitted disease, and of any failure of prevention rests
equally with **both sexual partners.**

I. **Contraceptive methods** (Box 11-2)

Specific modalities of contraception are quite diverse and
include one or more of the following. Specific modalities
which prevent pregnancy and prevent transmission of disease include:

A. **Abstinence**

1. **Mechanism of action**

The **mechanism of action** of this specific modality is
quite straightforward: reproduction is not possible
without heterosexual activity. This is the complete
avoidance of contact between male genitals and female genitals. The efficacy of this modality is 100%.
There are no specific adverse side effects of this modality. This is, however, in many cases an unrealistic
modality. A significant benefit of this modality is the
100% efficacy in the prevention of sexually transmitted diseases.

Although, in its pure sense, **abstinence** is straightforward, i.e., the complete inhibition of all sexual contact, this is relatively unrealistic. There are several
variants, each with varying contraceptive efficacy. The
variants include:

a. Sexual activity witnout male to female genital contact. Couples can have sexual activities which do
not require direct contact of the female to male
genitalia. Examples include cunnilingus, fellatio,
massage, and, most important, simple touching
of genital and—more important—nongenital areas.

B O X 1 1 - 2

Overall Evaluation and Management of Contraception

1. **Educate** the patient in the various modalities.
2. Encourage the patient's sexual partner to become involved in the educational process and to instruct him/her as to modalities which he/she can use that are safe and effective.
3. Obtain a **history** from the patient including:
    a. Last menstrual period.
    b. Previous pregnancies and results.
    c. Past history of STDs and of number of partners.
    d. Past or present history of hormonally stimulated malignant neoplastic lesions, e.g., endometrial carcinoma, breast adenocarcinoma, or ovarian carcinoma.
    e. Past or present history of deep venous thrombosis and/or arterial thrombosis.
    f. Previous modalities of contraception.
    g. Current knowledge base of contraceptive and modalities of "safer sex."
4. Pelvic examination, for baseline.
5. **Urine pregnancy test,** before initiating any oral contraceptive pill regimen.

The efficacy of this modality is 100% for contraceptive purposes, whereas in the prevention of sexually transmitted diseases it is of lesser efficacy.

    b. Sexual activity that involves contact of the female and male genital areas, but minimizes the risk of exposure of the ovum to sperm. One classic example is the **rhythm method.** In the rhythm method the couple abstains from direct female to male sexual contact during ovulation. This requires that the couple knows the duration of the female's cycles, that the female has regular cycles, and that the couple is able to abstain from unprotected intercourse during the period of time 10–16 days prior to the onset of menstrual flow, i.e., at the time of ovulation. Because there are normal variations in the duration of cycles, there is a significant risk for ovum-sperm interaction and, therefore, of conception using this method. **One specific variation of the rhythm method** is based on the physiologic fact that the female's temperature will increase by 1.0–1.5 °F at the time of ovulation. Therefore, if the female takes her oral temperature each morning and records it, she can attempt to predict when ovulation will occur. The couple then must abstain from unprotected intercourse during the days immediately preceding the temperature increase and during it. The overall efficacy of the rhythm method, even with fastidious recording of cycles and temperatures, is only 40%–60%. Furthermore, in a nonmonogamous relationship, there is a risk of transmission of sexually transmitted diseases.

c. Another "method" is that of **penile withdrawal.** Because there is direct female to male contact and invariably an admixture of female and male secretions, there is **no efficacy in contraception.** Furthermore, in a nonmonogamous relationship, there is a high risk of transmission of sexually transmitted diseases. The primary care physician must educate patients and the public to the risks inherent to this commonly used "method."

B. Condoms

1. Mechanism of action

The **mechanism of action** of this modality is quite straightforward. It is the application of a plastic/latex sheath over the external aspect of the penis affording a **barrier** between direct contact of female and male genital secretions. The psychomotor skills requisite for this modality are quite simple, but should be taught to the male at the outset. The condom must be placed on an erect penis and rolled up to its base. These are available over the counter without prescription. A caveat to the use of condoms is that if lubricants are used, they should be water soluble.

2. Efficacy

The **efficacy** of this modality is, when used properly, 90%–95%. There are virtually no adverse side effects. Finally, due to the fact that there is a barrier to direct contact of genital secretions, the efficacy in prevention of transmission of disease is very high.

C. Cervical cap

1. Mechanism of action

The **mechanism of action** of this modality is quite straightforward. It is the application of a plastic/latex sheath over the external aspect of the cervix affording a **barrier** between male genital secretions and the uterus, therefore precluding migration of the sperm to the ovum. The difference between this and the barrier method using condoms is that condoms afford a com-

plete barrier to contact between male and female sexual secretions, whereas a cervical cap does not. The
device is a dome-shaped plastic structure which is
fitted over the cervix. It is made in four different sizes.
The patient is fitted and instructed in the psychomotor
skills requisite to the use of this modality. It is placed
before intercourse **with** spermicidal jelly and kept in
place for up to 24–48 hours. It must remain in place
for **6 hours** after the last episode of sexual intercourse.
Caveats to use include the fact that, other than the
spermicidal jelly, no concurrent lubricant should be
used, and that another modality of contraception, e.g.,
condoms, should be used during the first several episodes of intercourse. A prescription is required for
use.
2. **Efficacy**
The **efficacy** of this modality is, when used properly,
95%. A prospective study comparing this with dia-
phragms demonstrated equal efficacy. The adverse
side effects include a disconcertingly high increase in
risk of cervical dysplasia, even when compared with
the use of a diaphragm. Therefore, a follow-up pelvic
and Pap smear should be performed at 3 months and
then yearly; if dysplasia develops the cervical cap
must be discontinued. Finally, because there is direct
contact of genital secretions, the efficacy of this modality in preventing the transmission of sexually
transmitted diseases is, in nonmonogamous relationships, low.
D. **Diaphragm**
1. **Mechanism of action**
The **mechanism of action** of this modality is not dissimilar from the cervical cap. It is the application of a
plastic/latex sheath over the external aspect of the cervix affording a **barrier** between male genital secretions
and the uterus, therefore precluding migration of the
sperm to the ovum. The difference between this and
the barrier method of condoms is that condoms afford
a complete barrier to contact between male/female
sexual secretions, whereas a diaphragm does not. The
device is a latex rubber structure with a fixed rim
which is placed in the superior vagina. The patient is
fitted for the device and is instructed in the psychomotor skills requisite to the use of this modality. The
device should snugly yet comfortably cover the entire
cervix from the symphysis pubis to the posterior for-
nix. It is placed before intercourse **with** spermicidal
jelly and kept in place for 6–12 hours. It must remain
in place for **6 hours** after the last episode of sexual

intercourse. A caveat to use is that, other than the spermicidal jelly, no concurrent lubricant should be used. A presciption is required for use.

2. **Efficacy**

The **efficacy** of this modality is, when used properly, 95%. Adverse side effects are quite minimal save for a mild vaginal odor which develops if in place for greater than 12–18 hours. The patient should have a pelvic and Pap smear performed on a yearly basis as well as refitting the diaphragm. Clearly the diaphragm should be refitted on a yearly basis, and after labor and delivery, and/or marked weight change. Finally, because there is direct contact of genital secretions, the efficacy of this modality in preventing the transmission of sexually transmitted diseases is, in nonmonogamous relationships, low.

E. **Vaginal contraceptive sponge**

1. **Mechanism of action**

The **mechanism of action** of this modality is not dissimilar from the cervical cap or diaphragm, in point of fact it is essentially a smaller, disposable model of a diaphragm. It is a polyurethane foam structure which the patient fits over the cervical os. The foam is impregnated with the spermicidal cream, **nonoxydyl-9.** It affords a **barrier** between male genital secretions and the uterus, therefore precluding migration of the sperm to the ovum, and also kills the sperm present. The difference between this and the barrier method of condoms is that condoms afford a complete barrier to contact between male and female sexual secretions, whereas the sponge does not. It is placed before intercourse and kept in place for 6–12 hours. It must remain in place for **6 hours** after the last episode of sexual intercourse. The device is available over the counter without prescription. This fact makes this modality quite convenient; however, it decreases the chance for education in its use and in overall "safer sex" techniques.

2. **Efficacy**

The **efficacy** of this modality is, when used properly, 80%–85%. Adverse side effects are quite minimal save for a mild vaginal odor which develops if in place for greater than 12–18 hours and the development of vaginal dryness during intercourse. The patient should have a pelvic examination and Pap smear performed on a yearly basis. Finally, because there is direct contact of genital secretions, the efficacy of this modality in preventing the transmission of sexually transmitted diseases is, in nonmonogamous relationships, low.

F. Oral contraceptives

  1. Mechanism of action

The **mechanism of action** of this modality is endocrinologically based. Ovulation in the physiologic setting requires the secretion of follicle-stimulating hormone (FSH) and luteinizing hormone (LH) from the adenohypophysis in general, and a midcycle surge in LH secretion in specific. The combination oral contraceptive pill, i.e., one which has both an estrogen and a progestin component, inhibits the FSH and LH secretion and the LH surge.

Although there are many different names and types of combination oral contraceptives, the dosing regimens are quite similar. The clinician should become comfortable with three or four different combination pills. There are several guidelines which one can use in dosing these agents.

    a. Ascertain **any potential contraindications** to oral contraceptive use in these patients. If any contraindication is present, they cannot be administered. **Contraindications to initiation** and indications for discontinuance include:

      i. Deep venous thromboembolism.

      ii. Thrombotic cerebrovascular accident.

      iii. Myocardial infarction.

      iv. Monocular blindness, retinal arterial occlusion.

      v. Pregnancy.

    b. Instruct patient to **discontinue smoking,** as this is an independent risk factor for the development of the adverse thrombotic effects of the oral contraceptive pill.

    c. Instruct the patient that this **will not protect her from sexually transmitted diseases,** and therefore, the principles of "safer sex" need to be described and practiced.

    d. Initiate therapy with an agent containing the minimal amount of estrogen, i.e., 35 μg of ethinyl estradiol or mestranol. Although the efficacy is unchanged if the dosing is between 35–50 μg, there are fewer side effects with the lower dose. However, there is a higher chance of spotting and amenorrhea with the lower dose; therefore, if this becomes a problem, increase the dose to 50 μg of ethinyl estradiol or mestranol.

    e. **Two first-line agents** are Ortho-Novum 1/35: 1 mg

of norethindrone and 35 μg of ethinyl estradiol; one tablet PO q.d. for 21 days, then 7 days without for withdrawal bleeding; and Ortho-Novum 7/7/7, a triphasic agent: 7 days of ethinyl estradiol 35 μg and norethindrone 0.5 mg, followed by 7 days of ethinyl estradiol 35 μg and norethindrone 0.75 mg, followed by 7 days of ethinyl estradiol 35 μg and norethindrone 1.0 mg, then 7 days off for withdrawal bleeding.

f. If the patient has a history of hypertension or significant water retention, change to an agent with lower progesterone activity, e.g., Ovcon 35 or the triphasic agent, Ortho-Novum 7/7/7.

g. If the patient develops hirsutism or acne vulgaris related to androgens, change to a progesterone agent with less androgenic activity, e.g., Demulen.

h. If the patient misses a pill, she should take it immediately. If she forgets two to three pills on consecutive days, she should take two each morning until back on schedule and use another concurrent form of contraception for the remainder of the cycle. If she misses more than three pills, she should stop completely, have withdrawal bleeding, and restart 7 days after the first pill was missed. In the latter case, other modalities for contraception should be considered and even recommended.

i. If the patient is on an agent which increases the catabolism of estrogens, e.g., phenytoin, the dose of estrogen should be increased to 80 μg of ethinyl estradiol.

2. Efficacy

The **efficacy** of this modality is 97%–98% when used appropriately.

3. Side effects

The overall risk of **serious side effects** is quite low, but the patient must know these side effects from the outset.

a. Increased risk of deep venous thrombosis.

b. Increased incidence of cholelithiasis.

c. Increased incidence of cholestatic jaundice, unrelated to cholelithiasis.

d. Increased risk of hepatic adenomas (quite rare, however).

e. Increased risk of the development of hypertension.

f. The overall effects of combination oral contraceptives on **lipids** include:

    i. Estrogens. Decrease LDL, increase HDL, and increase triglycerides.

ii. **Progestins.** Increase LDL, decrease total cholesterol, decrease HDL, and decrease triglyceride.
4. **Positive side effects.**
Potential **positive side effects** of oral contraceptives
include:
a. A decrease in risk of ovarian carcinoma.
b. A decreased risk of endometrial carcinoma.
c. A decrease in the symptoms of dysfunctional uterine bleeding and/or fibrocystic changes of the
breast.

G. **Norplant**
1. **Mechanism of action**
The **mechanism of action** of this device is quite analogous to other hormone-mediated forms of contraception. The clinician surgically inserts, intradermally, 6
Silastic capsules, each capsule containing 36 mg of
the hormone, levonorgestrol. This system continuously delivers the hormone to the patient. The capsules are effective for 5 years, after which they need
replacement.
2. **Efficacy**
The **efficacy** of this modality is virtually 100%. Adverse side effects are minimal save for a mild increase
in spotting and/or irregular vaginal bleeding. The patient should have a pelvic examination and Pap smear
performed on a yearly basis.

H. **Surgical sterilization**
A definitive modality which can be performed in men
or women, which is quite effective, but, in many cases,
irreversible. Therefore, it must be performed only in patients who know of the irreversibility.
1. **Vasectomy**
This is the surgical ligation of both of the vasa deferens, the tubes which carry sperm from the testes into
the penis. This procedure requires local anesthesia via
two small incisions in the posterior scrotum and has
few to no adverse effects. It takes approximately 2
months for the sperm already present to be absorbed;
therefore, a concurrent modality of contraception
must be used during the first 2 months after the procedure.
2. **Tubal ligation**
This is the ligation of both of the fallopian tubes, thus
preventing the sperm from reaching the proximal
tube, in effect forming a permanent barrier to sperm–
ovum interaction. This procedure can be easily performed via laparoscopy and entails tying and then re-
secting a portion of the tubes.

II. Consultation

Problem	Service	Time
Any patient	Planned Parenthood	Elective
Vasectomy	Urologist	Elective
Tubal ligation	Gynecologist	Elective

III. Indications for admission: None. Even surgical sterilization can be performed on an outpatient basis.

Menopause

The **normal reproductive system** of the human female is a complex set of organ structures and systems integrated to the goal of sexual reproduction and therefore of producing human progeny.

The **uterus** is a hollow organ located within the pelvis of the female. It is the structure into which the fertilized oocyte implants and develops until the time of parturition (delivery). The epithelial lining of the inside of the uterus is called the endometrium and is the major target of the cyclically produced hormones of the ovaries, estrogen and progesterone. This structure, under the direction of these ovarian hormones, is prepared on a monthly basis for reception and implantation of a fertilized oocyte. When estrogen and progesterone levels decrease during monthly cycles, the endometrium sloughs, resulting in menstruation.

The **ovaries** have two major functions: to produce oocytes and to produce hormones to control the uterine endometrium and prepare it for implantation of the products of conception if fertilization occurs. Estrogen and progesterone are produced in a cyclic fashion, with estrogens peaking and then plateauing early in the menstrual cycle and progesterone peaking later in the menstrual cycle.

Estrogen is produced from the follicular cells around the maturing oocytes for that cycle and stimulates the proliferation of the endometrial tissue. **Progesterone** is produced by the cells remaining after the oocyte is extruded from the ovary at midcycle. These cells are referred to as the **corpus luteum.** Progesterone results in an overall marked increase in the vascularity and secretory function of the endothelium.

If **conception** has occurred, the products of conception implant into the prepared endothelium, and hormonal control of the pregnant uterus rapidly changes from the ovaries to the embryonic structures themselves. If conception and implantation do not occur, the ovarian hormones precipitously decline, resulting in loss of hormonal stimulation for the uterine endothelium and sloughing of the endometrium with menstrual flow.

This production of hormones and oocytes begins at approximately age 11 years and manifests with the first menstrual cycle, or **menarche.** Production continues on a cyclic monthly basis for decades, usually interrupted only by pregnancy, until age 50–55

years, when ovarian failure occurs, also referred to as the **climac-
teric** or menopause. Although the central functions of these hormones include the development and support of the endometrium
and the earliest phases of pregnancy, they also have the systemic
effects of maintaining mineral and protein within bone. Furthermore, they will result in the physiologic decrease in the adenohy-
pophyseal hormones FSH and LH.

I. **Definition**
   Menopause is the loss of reproductive functioning and capacity in a previously fertile woman. Simply stated, this is the
   transition between the fertile phase of a woman's life to the
   nonfertile phase. Although many **specific manifestations** occur during and after this profound transition, the most reproducible manifestation is the acquired absence, either through
   natural or iatrogenic means, of menstruation for a period of
   greater than 1 year in a previously menstruating, currently
   nonpregnant woman. The average age at onset of natural
   menopause is 50–51 years. Iatrogenic menopause usually occurs as a result of bilateral oophorectomy with or without
   concurrent hysterectomy. Hysterectomy itself will result in
   amenorrhea but, if the ovaries are functional, not true menopause.
   A. **Natural menopause**
      This is the primary failure and atrophy of the ovaries
      as a result of the loss of oocytes produced by follicles.
      Although there are hundreds of thousands of oocytes in
      the ovaries, far too many to be used by a female, they
      rapidly decay after the age of 35 years, resulting in a loss
      of all functional oocytes and their adjacent supportive
      structures (i.e., follicles) by age 50–55 years. The ovaries
      without any oocytes results in infertility, whereas the lack
      of follicles results in inability to produce the hormones
      estrogen and progesterone.
   B. **Iatrogenic menopause**
      This will result in a syndrome of menopause depending
      on the procedure performed. If the procedure performed
      is bilateral oophorectomy, irrespective of concurrent hys-
      terectomy, there is the sudden loss of oocytes and follicu-
      lar cells; therefore it is not dissimilar from natural meno-
      pause.
      In both of these types, the hormones estrogen and proges-
   terone are no longer produced from the ovaries, resulting
   in an atrophy of the uterus in general and of the uterine
   endometrium in specific. Therefore, there is a loss of menstruation, i.e., the development of secondary amenorrhea.
   Furthermore, the deficiency of estrogen and progesterone results in a marked decrease in the feedback upon the adenohy-
   pophyseal hormones, LH and FSH.

II. Manifestations

The **specific manifestations** of ovarian failure, include an acceleration of osteoporosis, hot flashes, and atrophic vaginitis.

A. Osteoporosis

This is the loss of bone, a process of very high prevalence in the aging population. Loss of bone markedly increases the risk of fractures of the vertebral spine and the hips and results in significant morbidity.

1. Pathophysiology

The **pathophysiology** of this process is not completely understood. Although the mechanism of disease development is unclear, several descriptive features are well known.

a. It is a process of **bone loss,** both of bony matrix, i.e., the collagen and protein substrate and of the mineral component of bone, i.e., calcium phosphate. It affects the trabecular bone, i.e., the laminar, reticulated areas within the bone, to a greater extent than the cortical bone, i.e., the compact, dense areas of ossification at the periphery of the bony structures.

b. There are certain, quite specific **risk factors** for the development of osteoporosis. These include:

i. Ovarian failure, i.e., menopause. The withdrawal of chronic estrogens from the physiologic milieu increases the rate of osteoporosis.

ii. Significant long-term inactivity, i.e., a paucity of exercise and of muscle/bone use. There is an inverse correlation between the level of physical activity and the rate of osteoporosis development, i.e., exercise decreases the rate of osteoporosis development.

iii. Poor nutrition, specifically a deficiency, either absolute or relative, in vitamin D or calcium, will increase the risk of osteoporosis.

iv. Genetics. A family history of osteoporosis is strongly correlated with accelerated osteoporosis.

v. Ethanol. Excessive ingestion of ethanol is correlated with the development of accelerated osteoporosis.

vi. Tobacco smoking.

c. Once present, osteoporosis is effectively irreversible, but it is a disease process which is eminently preventable.

2. Manifestations

Osteoporosis is invariably asymptomatic until an acute event such as a fracture occurs. Fractures include compression fractures of the thoracic spine or a hip fracture. A **compression fracture of the thoracic vertebra** can manifest with a relatively diverse range, from the painless development of dowager's hump, i.e., the marked increase in kyphosis, to the development of severe pain starting at the specific vertebral body and radiating bilaterally anteriad. The specific manifestations of a **hip fracture** include the sudden onset of pain, decreased range of motion in the affected hip, and superior displacement and external rotation of the affected lower extremity at the hip itself, all precipitated by an acute fall, usually with only a modest amount of force.

3. **Evaluation**

The **specific evaluation** includes that described in Box 11-3. The overall objective is to discover patients who are at high risk for the development of accelerated osteoporosis and intervene before the process reaches the clinical level of fractures. The interventions must have as few side effects as possible. If the regimens for prophylaxis were free of side effects they could be applied to all patients, but some of the interventions, e.g., the use of estrogens, are indeed associated with side effects themselves and must be tailored to the specific patient.

B O X 1 1 - 3

Overall Evaluation and Management of Menopause

Evaluation

1. Overall history and physical must include:
   a. Date of the last menstrual period.
   b. The features of the antecedent menstrual periods, e.g., duration, regularity.
   c. The presence of any other concurrent vaginal discharge.
   d. The past history of hysterectomy and/or oophorectomy.
   e. Age of the patient.
   f. The presence of hot flashes, e.g., acute manifestation of estrogen withdrawal.

(continued)

B O X 1 1 - 3 *(continued)*

    g. The presence of dyspareunia, i.e., painful inter-
       course and atrophy of the vulvar/vaginal mucosa
       as a result of atrophic vaginitis.
    h. Pelvic examination, mandatory as a baseline ex-
       amination.
2. **Urine pregnancy test**. This is of extreme importance,
   as one must rule out pregnancy as a cause of secondary amenorrhea.
3. If hysterectomy was performed but the ovaries are
   intact, the initial manifestations of true menopause,
   i.e., ovarian failure, will be hot flashes and atrophic
   vaginitis.
4. Plasma FSH and LH levels should be obtained.
   These will be elevated in the setting of primary ovarian failure, i.e., true menopause.

Management

1. If **atrophic vaginitis** is present, the application of topical estrogens is quite effective. The agent is conjugated estrogens (Premarin) to the vulvar epithelium
   on a q.d. or b.i.d. basis.
2. If **hot flashes** are present and severe, initiate a
   course of systemic conjugated estrogen therapy. The
   dosing regimens are based on whether or not the patient has a uterus. If the patient does not have a
   uterus, the regimen is conjugated estrogens, 0.3 mg
   PO q.d. for 24 months, and then slowly wean; if the
   patient does have a uterus, the regimens must be cycled, i.e., 0.3–0.625 mg PO q.d. for 3 weeks, then no
   hormone for 1 week, all cycled for a period of 24
   months, then wean.
3. Assess the **risk for development of osteoporosis.**
   Specific intervention in evaluation and prevention of
   osteoporosis includes:
    a. Foster exercise and weight loss if obese.
    b. Initiate calcium supplementation, with calcium car-
      bonate, 1.0–1.5 g/day.
    c. Obtain baseline calcium, phosphorus, and albu-
      min levels to rule out concurrent or exacerbating
      metabolic bone disorders. If the calcium or phos-
      phorus levels are abnormal, determine the vita-

(continued)

B O X   1 1 - 3 (continued)

min D$_{25}$-OH level to rule out vitamin D deficiency (rickets). If the calcium is elevated, see section on Hypercalcemia in Chapter 9.
   d. Consider obtaining plain radiographs of any bony structures which have pain, or of the thoracic spine if "dowager's hump" is present, i.e., the abnormal accentuation of the thoracic kyphosis, in order to document any thoracic compression fractures.
   e. Consider bone densitometry imaging (see text and Table 11-1 for specifics). The density of bone as measured by bone densitometry correlates quite well with the risk of vertebral compression fracture, but not with the risk of hip fracture. This examination may assist the clinician in defining patients at high risk for the development of fractures and who would therefore benefit from estrogen prophylaxis.
   f. Initiate a multivitamin on a daily basis, 1 PO q.d.
   g. **Estrogen prophylaxis regimens** are based on the presence or absence of a uterus in the patient.
      i. If patient **does not have a uterus,** the regimen is conjugated estrogens, 0.625 mg PO q.d. for 5–10 years.
      ii. If the patient **has a uterus,** the regimen is:

Days 1–14:	Conjugated estrogens (Premarin), 0.625 mg PO q.d.
Days 15–24:	Conjugated estrogens, 0.625 mg PO q.d., and medroxyprogesterone, 2.5–10.0 mg PO q.d.
Days 25–28:	No hormones.

All cycled for 5–10 years.
4. In all cases in which estrogens are used in patients who have a uterus, **pelvic examinations are required on a regular basis,** i.e., q.6 months. Any atypical vaginal discharge and/or bleeding must be aggressively evaluated by a gynecologic consultant with endometrial biopsy and/or curettage of the uterine endometrium.
5. In all cases in which estrogens are to be used, a **baseline breast examination** and mammograms are required.

T A B L E   1 1 - 1
Bone Densitometry Imaging Techniques

Dual-energy absorptiometry (DPA)
  A radionuclide is used.
  Bone mass in spine and hip is measured.
  Total body bone mass is measured.
  Relatively low radiation dose is required.

Dual-energy x-ray absorptiometry (DXA)
  Same as DPA except that source of photons is an x-ray tube instead
    of a radionuclide.
  Significantly more precise but relatively more expensive than DPA
    technique.
  Smaller x-ray dose.
  Bone mass in spine and hip is measured.
  Total body bone mass is measured.

4. **Management**

In virtually all cases the basic **prophylactic interventions** include increased exercise, maintenance of adequate nutrition, maintenance of a nonobese weight, moderation in the ingestion of ethanol, and abstinence from smoking. The specifics can include:

a. **Walking** 1–2 miles every or every other day.

b. Prescribing a **multivitamin** on an every-day basis. This will supply adequate amounts of vitamin D to prevent concurrent vitamin D deficiency.

c. Prescribing 1.0–1.5 g of **calcium carbonate** per day. The patient should be instructed to take the calcium with meals, as the absorption of calcium is greatest in a relatively high pH (alkaline) environment.

d. **Systemic estrogens.** These agents are effective in slowing the rate of bone matrix and mineral loss in postmenopausal osteoporosis. They are, however, fraught with several quite significant side effects and therefore cannot be used in all cases. These **side effects** include but are not limited to:

i. An increased risk of **carcinoma of the uterine endometrium.** The long-term use of unopposed estrogens will result in proliferation of the endometrial tissue of the uterus. Several studies have suggested a strong correlation between the use of chronic estrogens and the development of the premalignant neoplastic lesion, cystic hyperplasia, and the malignant neoplastic lesion, uterine adenocarcinoma of the endometrium. This is a moot problem in a patient without a uterus but is a concern in all other patients on estrogens. A major method to decrease the risk of this side effect is to cycle the estrogens, using the physiologic model. This cycling of the hormones is so that there is a monthly withdrawal of the estrogens with resultant sloughing of the endometrial tissue, i.e., menstrual flow. The paradigm is one of:

Days 1–14	*Days 15–24*	*Days 24–28*
Estrogens	Estrogens Progesterone	No hormones

ii. A questionable **increase in the risk of breast adenocarcinoma.** There may be a slight increase in the risk of breast carcinoma; however, the epidemiologic evidence is far from complete. Any patient with an antecedent history of breast adenocarcinoma, a strong family history of breast adenocarcinoma, or a past or current history of dysplastic fibrocystic disease should not be prescribed estrogens.

iii. A slight increase in the risk of development of **thromboembolic disease** in premenopausal females but not in postmenopausal females. However, anyone with a past history of DVT/PTE and/or a concurrent risk of hypercoagulability should not be prescribed estrogens.

iv. Although there is evidence that the prescription of estrogens may well decrease the risk of atherosclerotic disease in females, the addition of progesterone can impact **negatively upon the lipoprotein profile of the female.** Progesterones have been demonstrated to cause a slight decrease in HDL cholesterol and a slight increase in LDL cholesterol.

e. **Indications for the administration of estrogen prophylaxis** of osteoporosis include:

   i. No contraindications to their use.

   ii. The **patient is at risk** for accelerated osteoporosis, i.e., is postmenopausal but still has adequate bone reserve, i.e., the osteoporosis has not yet resulted in significant fractures. Another method to determine bone mass using an end point before overt fractures is that of bone densitometry imaging (see Table 11-1). The mass measured can be obtained at baseline and repeated on a yearly or biyearly basis. This has the advantage in that it is an objective assessment of bone loss and therefore, when bone loss begins, i.e., a change from the previous year's mass, estrogen prophylaxis can be initiated.

iii. Dosing regimens include that described in Box 11-3 or a regimen of oral contraceptive agents containing estrogens and progesterones. These can include the cyclic use of Ortho-Novum 1/35 or Ortho-Novum 7/7/7, instead of the regimen described in Box 11-3.

iv. **Follow-up** should be a regular **pelvic examination.** If there is any abnormal vaginal discharge or bleeding, immediately refer the patient to gynecology for endometrial examination. The patient must continue with regular **breast examinations** and mammograms.

v. The patient must be told that the regimen used will effectively result in her having a "period," although she will remain in permanent ovarian failure, i.e., no longer fertile.

vi. The **duration of prophylaxis** using this regimen of estrogens should continue for approximately 10 years. It will concurrently treat any and all other acute/chronic manifestations of the menopause.

B. **Hot flashes**

These are very common acute manifestations of ovarian failure. They can be markers for the onset of true menopause, i.e., ovarian failure, in a patient who has had a previous hysterectomy without oophorectomy.

1. **Physiology**

The **physiology** of this specific process is postulated to be as the result of the sudden and precipitious decline in estrogens from the physiologic milieu. This withdrawal will actually lead to paroxysms of facial and/or body vasodilation.

2. **Manifestations**

The **specific manifestations** include the subjective feeling of flushing in the face and/or body, which can be quite frequent, quite severe, and extremely distracting to the patient. In fact, it can lead to a significant impairment in the functional ability of the patient.

3. **Evaluation and management**

The **specific evaluation and management** include the overall as described in Box 11-3 and the initiation of low-dose conjugated estrogens in the dosing regimens described in Box 11-3. Estrogens must be given in a cycle basis if the patient has a uterus. The estrogen

intervention for osteoporosis will supplant the estrogen therapy for hot flashes.
C. Atrophic vaginitis
This is a very common chronic sequela of menopause.
1. Physiology
The **physiology** of this specific process is postulated to be as the result of the significant decrease in estrogens. The loss of estrogens results in a decrease in the activity, vascularity, and thickness of the vaginal mucosa.
2. Manifestations
The **specific manifestations** include the onset of dyspareunia, i.e., painful intercourse, dry vaginal mucosa, and atrophy/kraurosis, i.e., shrinkage of the vulva and vagina. The epithelium is easily traumatized and postcoital erythema and even bleeding can occur.
3. Evaluation and management
The **specific evaluation and management** include making the clinical diagnosis, the overall as described in Box 11-3, and the use of a water-soluble jelly before intercourse and/or the application of topical estrogen cream. If the patient is on estrogens for prophylaxis of osteoporosis, this will supplant the need for topical therapy.

III. Consultation

Problem	Service	Time
Any evidence of concurrent metabolic bone disease	Endocrine	Required
Any hip fracture	Orthopedics	Urgent
Any compression vertebral fracture	Orthopedics	Elective

IV. Indications for admission: Acute hip fractures. Otherwise management is outpatient in nature.

Pelvic Masses

Masses in the uterus or adnexa may be discovered only on examination of the pelvis and abdomen by the primary care physician. A mass can be derived from any of the specific structures within the female pelvis.

I. Differential diagnosis of pelvic masses
A. Endometrial carcinoma
See section on Vaginal Discharge, page 599.

B. **Leiomyomas,** fibroids

See section on Vaginal Discharge, page 599.

C. **Pelvic inflammatory disease**

1. **Pathophysiology**

The **pathophysiology** of this entity includes the development of inflammation in the fallopian tube as the result of a bacterial infection. The infection invariably begins as cervicitis and propagates proximally to involve the endometrium of the uterus and the fallopian tubes. The underlying pathogens are usually multiple and include *Neisseria gonorrhoeae, Chlamydial* spp., and anaerobic bacteria, including peptostreptococci. **Risk factors** for the development of this entity are effectively synonymous with those of the development of any sexually transmitted disease, i.e., the practice of unsafe sex. This is particularly risky if the patient is promiscuous or has unprotected sexual activity with a promiscuous partner. Certain studies have positively correlated the risk of PID with the use of intrauterine devices (IUDs).

2. **Manifestations**

The **specific manifestations** of this entity include unilateral pain in the right or left lower abdominal quadrant, often with associated nausea, vomiting, and vaginal discharge. Furthermore, there can be the recent history of fevers and chills. Examination discloses purulent cervical discharge, quite invariably cervical motion tenderness, and a palpable and quite tender unilateral adnexal mass.

3. **Evaluation and management**

The **specific evaluation and management** include making the clinical diagnosis by using the examinations described in Box 11-4. Further evaluation and management are based on the results. An ultrasound of the pelvis in addition to obtaining a VDRL and HIV is indicated. The partner must be evaluated and treated concurrently with the patient.

a. Antibiotic regimens include:

i. Ceftriaxone, 1 g IV q.24h., and doxycycline, 100 mg IV q.12h., for 7 days or for 48 hours after the last fever spike, whichever comes first. Then, doxycycline, 100 mg PO b.i.d. for the remainder of time, so that treatment is at least a total of 14 days; or

ii. Ceftriaxone, 250 mg IM, and doxycycline, 100 mg PO b.i.d. for 10 days; or

iii. If the patient is β-lactam allergic, one can administer clindamycin, 600–900 mg IV q.8.h.,

B O X 1 1 - 4

Overall Evaluation and Management of Pelvic Masses

Evaluation

1. Query the patient regarding the time of her **last menstrual period.** This is important in determining whether the patient is premenopausal or postmenopausal. Furthermore, if the patient is premenopausal and there is an acquired absence of periods for more than one cycle, i.e., secondary amenorrhea, the suspicion for pregnancy should markedly increase.
2. **Urine pregnancy test.**
3. Query the patient regarding concurrent **vaginal bleeding** and/or other vaginal discharge. This is a very important aspect of the overall evaluation. If bleeding is present, must be evaluated as described in section on Vaginal Discharge, page 599.
4. **Pelvic examination** in all cases.
   a. Differentiate if the mass is primarily adnexal or uterine in location. Adnexal masses are more commonly the result of ovarian and/or fallopian tube processes, whereas uterine masses are more commonly either fibroids or a gravid uterus.
   b. If there is any thick and/or purulent discharge, obtain a Gram stain, culture upon Thayer–Martin medium (for *Neisseria gonorrhoeae*) and a *Chlamydia trachomatis* culture.
5. **Ultrasound of the pelvis.**
   a. This is **emergent** in the following scenarios:
      i. Tender, adnexal mass with purulent cervical discharge.
      ii. A positive pregnancy test with any adnexal mass.
      iii. Any uterine and/or adnexal mass with associated vaginal bleeding.
   b. This is **urgent** in the following scenarios:
      i. A nontender uterine mass without bleeding.

Management

1. If there is any concurrent hirsutism, refer to Table 11-2.
2. Referral to Ob/Gyn colleagues.
3. **Educate** the patient in "safer sex" methods.

TABLE 11-2
Hirsutism

Disease	Mechanism	Laboratory Findings	Treatment
Adrenal tumors (non-cortisol secreting)	Androgen dependent	Increased serum DHEAS Increased urinary 17-ketosteroids	Dexamethasone suppression with 0.5–1.0 mg dexamethasone PO q.h.s. Endocrinology consultation
Ovarian dysfunction	Androgen dependent	Decreased serum DHEAS Decreased urinary 17-ketosteroids	Endocrinology consultation Gynecology consultation Consider oral contraceptive (combination type pill)
Obesity	Androgen dependent; peripheral conversion of androstenedione to testosterone	No specific laboratory abnormalities	Weight reduction
Hypercortisolism	Androgen dependent	Abnormal lack of cortisol suppression with dexamethasone Abnormally elevated free cortisol in 24-hr urine collection	Endocrinology consultation

and a concurrent aminoglycoside, either gentamicin or tobramycin, for a total of 7–10 days.
   b. One must watch for and aggressively treat any **complications** of this infectious process. These include:
      i. Fitz–Hugh–Curtis syndrome. This is the devel-
opment of perihepatitis. Specific evaluation
and management include obtaining blood cultures, an ultrasound of the hepar, looking for
abscesses, and a longer duration of antibiotics.
      ii. Tubo-ovarian abscess. This is the development
of an actual abscess cavity in or adjacent to
the infected fallopian tube. This will usually
be quite easily demonstrable on pelvic ultrasound. It requires gynecologic consultation, a
longer duration of parenteral antibiotics, and,
if severe or refractory to treatment, surgical intervention, i.e., a unilateral adnexectomy.

D. Ovarian neoplasia—epithelial

1. Pathogenesis

The **pathogenesis** of this not uncommon etiology of
pelvic masses is not completely understood. Several
factors are correlated positively and negatively with
the development of ovarian carcinoma. The factors
which are **positively correlated** with, i.e., increase the
risk of the development of, ovarian epithelial neoplasia include being nulliparous, single, the use of talc
powders, and a history of antecedent breast carcinoma. Factors which are **negatively correlated** with,
i.e., decrease the risk of development of epithelial
ovarian carcinoma, include a history of multiparity
and the use of oral contraceptive agents.

   a. The **histopathology** of this group of epithelial neoplastic lesions is relatively diverse; however, the
most common epithelial type is adenocarcinoma.
The tumors can produce a mucinous and/or serous
discharge.

   b. The **natural history** of ovarian epithelial neoplastic
lesions in general includes the fact that it originates
in one ovary, locally enlarges, and spreads contigu-
ously to the peritoneum, with peritoneal studding
and the development of malignant neoplastic ascites. This peritoneal disease can become quite massive. When the lesion extends out of the ovary, the
prognosis, even with aggressive therapy, is very
poor, and therefore early detection is of extreme
importance in effective therapy.

2. Manifestations

The **specific manifestations** include the fact that it is
a disease process which is quite asymptomatic until

late in its course. Often the patient will present for a routine examination and have an adnexal mass and/ or abdominal mass(es) discovered. There can be a history of slow enlargement of the abdomen, thought to be adipose by the patient. The disease can occur in premenopausal or postmenopausal women. On **examination,** hirsutism can be present, as well as ascites and, on pelvic examination, nontender fixed masses in the adnexa and superior aspects of the uterus. In rare cases, the patient may have concurrent manifestations of the paraneoplastic syndrome dermatomyositis. This syndrome consists of progressive and profound muscle weakness, greater proximally than distally, a heliotropic rash (i.e., erythema about the periorbital areas bilaterally), and the erythematous papules about the dorsal aspects of the digits (i.e., Gottron's papules).

3. **Evaluation and management**

The **specific evaluation and management** include determining the clinical suspicion for the lesion based on the data gathered in the overall section, please refer to Box 11-4. Several **screening tests** have been attempted but have been woefully inadequate. One of these is the tumor marker, CA-125. This marker is measured by a monoclonal antibody to the CA-125 antigen, an antigen present in many ovarian carcinomas. It is a marker for the detection of ovarian epithelial neoplasia which does not have adequate sensitivity to be a screening tool. It can be, if elevated, at the outset, a marker to be used for follow-up of the disease.

   a. Once a mass is discovered and is suspicious for this neoplastic lesion, CT of the pelvis is indicated to further define the size and extent of the lesion. Invasive evaluation is based upon the clinical suspicion that the lesion is a malignant neoplastic process. A **low likelihood of malignancy** includes lesions that are in the ovary and <2 cm in size and without any septa or solid components. A **high likelihood of malignancy** includes lesions which are >2 cm in size, have any component of septation or solid areas, or have spread to structures extrinsic to the ovary.

   b. Modalities for **invasive evaluation and management** include:

      i. **Laparoscopy.** This procedure is performed by a gynecologist and involves the insertion of a tube with a fiber-optic imager into the peritoneum for direct visualization of the adnexae. Biopsy and therefore definitive histopathologic diagnosis using this device is possible.

  ii. **Laparotomy.** Direct surgical intervention. This is the next step if the biopsy is positive for adenocarcinoma or if laparoscopic assessment is unavailable. The surgical intervention of choice includes:

    (a) **Postmenopausal.** Total abdominal hysterectomy and bilateral oophorectomy and biopsy of adjacent lymph nodes and adjacent peritoneal structures for staging purposes. Debulking of any and all gross tumor is also required.

    (b) **Premenopausal.** Cystectomy, i.e., removal of the entire lesion, and send the entire lesion for frozen section analysis. If the lesion is benign, the procedure is complete, if the lesion is histopathologically diagnosed as malignant, total abdominal hysterectomy and bilateral oophorectomy and biospy of adjacent lymph nodes and adjacent peritoneal structures for staging purposes are necessary. Debulking of any and all gross tumor is also required.

  c. **Chemotherapeutic intervention,** including therapeutic and adjuvant regimens, as indicated for metastatic or presumed metastatic disease. A discussion of these modalities is beyond the scope of this text.

E. **Polycystic ovaries**

  1. **Pathophysiology**

  The **pathophysiology** underlying the development of this not uncommon etiology of adnexal masses in premenopausal women is based on a perturbation of the physiologic hormonal milieu of the premenopausal female.

  a. There is, as a result of **ovarian and/or adrenal** (specifically the zona reticularis) **overproduction,** a supraphysiologic and therefore abnormal overall increase in the 17-ketosteroids, especially the androgen-like agents and/or the catabolite of androgen-like agents, estrone. Adipocytes have the enzyme requisite to catabolize these 17-ketosteroids into estrone.

  b. These **ketosteroids** and their catabolites result in a negative feedback on the adenohypophysis to secrete follicle-stimulating hormone (FSH), but minimal effect upon the secretion of luteinizing hormone (LH). This results in overall abnormal levels of FSH and LH, i.e., an abnormal decrease in overall FSH and a concurrent, relative if not absolute increase in LH.

c. The overall increase in LH results in an increase in the thecal cells, a further increase in progesterone and progesterone-like hormones, and an absence of ovulation. This will result in the development of one or more ovarian cysts, i.e., polycystic ovary disease. Furthermore, this can lead, not only to anovulation and therefore, amenorrhea and infertility, but also to dysfunctional uterine bleeding (see section on Vaginal Discharge, page 599).

2. **Evaluation**

The **specific evaluation** of this entity is to make the clinical diagnosis based on the data obtained in Box 11-4 and to effectively rule out any other etiology of secondary amenorrhea. These include a primary ovarian tumor producing androgens, Cushing's syndrome (i.e., primary adrenal hypercortisolism), hypothyroidism (i.e., the overall deficiency of thyroid hormone), or secondary hypogonadism, usually as the result of a lesion in the adenohypophysis causing panhypopituitarism. Specific manifestations of panhypopituitarism include galactorrhea if prolactinoma, and secondary deficiencies in glucocorticoids and thyroxine. Therefore, in addition to the specific laboratory examinations described in Box 11-4:

a. If **Cushing's syndrome** is suspected, i.e., the patient has truncal obesity, striae, recurrent skin fungal infections, hyperglycemia, recurrent candidal vaginitis, and hypertension with hypokalemia, perform an overnight dexamethasone suppression test (see Table 11-3) and a 24-hr collection for free cortisol creatinine.

b. If **hypothyroidism** is suspected, obtain a TSH. See Thyroid Dysfunctional States in Chapter 9.

c. **Secondary hypogonadism,** usually as the result of a lesion in the adenohypophysis causing panhypopituitarism, i.e., secondary deficiencies of glucocorticoids and thyroxine and visual field defects, bitemporal hemianopsia in specific.

3. **Management**

The **specific management** includes making the clinical diagnosis and prescribing a weight loss program. An effective weight reduction program is central to management. Referral to endocrine and gynecology is indicated.

T A B L E 1 1 - 3
Overnight Dexamethasone Suppression Test

Procedure

Day 1, 7 A.M.: Obtain plasma ACTH and cortisol levels.
Day 1, 11 P.M.: Administer 1 mg dexamethasone (Decadron) PO.
Day 2, 7 A.M.: Obtain plasma cortisol level.

Interpretation

Normal response: The plasma cortisol level on day 2 suppresses to <5 µg/dL. Hypercortisolism is effectively ruled out.

Abnormal response: The plasma cortisol level on day 2 does not suppress, i.e., remains >5 µg/dL. This is a positive screen and requires further evaluation to make the diagnosis of hypercortisolism. Endocrine consultation is required.

II. **Consultation**

Problem	Service	Time
Adnexal mass in pregnant woman	Ob/Gyn	Urgent/ emergent
Adnexal mass, febrile	Ob/Gyn	Urgent/ emergent
Adnexal mass, cystic and <2 cm	Ob/Gyn	Elective
Adnexal mass, noncystic, and/or >2 cm in size	Ob/Gyn	Required, semiurgent
Polycystic ovary	Gyn	Elective

III. **Indications for admission:** Any adnexal mass in a pregnant patient, any suspicion of pelvic inflammatory disease, any evidence of hemodynamic instability, and/or any concurrent purulent or bloody vaginal discharge.

Vaginal Discharge

Every woman will have vaginal discharge at various times during her life. The normal vaginal discharge is scant and physiologic in the vast majority of cases; in fact, every nonpregnant woman will menstruate on a monthly basis. Because menstruation is the most reproducible and common form of vaginal discharge, a brief review of the physiology of menstruation is described here.

Menstruation requires the normal functioning of four specific organs, the hypothalamus, the adenohypophysis, the ovaries, and the uterus. The cycle described below occurs hundreds of times on a repeated, cyclic basis over the fertile life span of a woman.

1. At the **beginning of the cycle,** the hypothalamus produces the releasing factor for luteinizing hormone, i.e., LHRH, which results in the release of luteinizing hormone (LH) and follicle-stimulating hormones (FSH) from the adenohypophysis.

2. The FSH and LH stimulate follicles within the ovaries to develop and mature and produce the hormone estrogen. During this phase, sometimes referred to as the **follicular phase,** the oocyte develops and, under the direct influence of estrogens, results in proliferation of the endometrial tissue. Therefore, this phase has also been referred to as the **proliferative phase** and is under the direction of estrogen from the ovary.

3. At the midpoint of the cycle, i.e., on approximately day 14, the estrogens peak, which results in a surge of LH from the adenohypophysis and precipitates the forceful extrusion of the oocyte from the ovary into the abdominal cavity, i.e., ovulation.

4. At the time of ovulation and LH increase, the follicular cells remaining in the ovary evolve, under the direction of LH, into a corpus luteum, and therefore this time is called the **luteal phase.** The corpus luteum produces progesterone, a hormone which stimulates the already proliferated endometrium to evolve further and begin a secretory function, all for the goal of supporting the implantation of a fertilized oocyte. Thus this phase is also referred to as the **secretory phase.**

5. If fertilization and implantation do not occur, the LH/FSH and estrogen and progesterone will, at the end of the cycle, i.e., approximately day 27, precipitously decline. The sudden loss of hormonal support for the endometrium will result in sloughing of endometrial tissue, i.e., menstrual flow.

Any change in the quantity or quality of the vaginal discharge, the concurrent presence of vaginal or pelvic manifestations, or any changes in menstruation should be used as markers that the discharge may well be abnormal, i.e., the result of a pathologic process. Although there is significant overlap between the two groups, there are two specific categories of vaginal discharge, bloody and nonbloody.

I. Causes of abnormal vaginal bleeding
A. Fibroids, i.e., leiomyomas of the uterus
1. Pathophysiology

The **pathophysiology** of this disorder is not completely known. It has a high prevalence, i.e., 30% of women will develop these benign uterine neoplastic lesions. They are the most common neoplastic lesion involving the uterus. They are single or multiple and can occur anywhere in the uterus itself. If they occur immediately deep to the endometrium, i.e., submucosal in location, they have a high propensity of bleeding.

2. **Manifestations**

   The **specific manifestations** include the development of menorrhagia and menometrorrhagia and the presence of nontender masses within the body of the uterus. Iron deficiency anemia is not an uncommon manifestation or sequela, especially if the leiomyomas are submucosal in location.

3. **Evaluation and management**

   The **specific evaluation and management** include making the clinical diagnosis using the evaluative tools described in Box 11-5. Ultrasound will confirm the presence of intrauterine masses. If the patient is iron deficient, place her on iron and follow hematocrits and reticulocyte counts.

   a. **Premenopausal.** If the patient no longer desires to be fertile, the treatment of choice is total hysterectomy without oophorectomy. If the patient wants to have children, other modalities can be used in the treatment of fibroids. One of these procedures, performed by a gynecologic surgeon, is myomectomy, i.e., selective and specific removal of a uterine fibroid. This procedure can effectively remove the fibroid while maintaining uterine competence. If the fibroids are asymptomatic and pregnancy is not desired, follow-up every 6 months is indicated.

   b. **Postmenopausal.** A total abdominal hysterectomy is the intervention of choice.

B. **Pregnancy**

   Vaginal bleeding in a pregnant female requires immediate obstetric consultation and intervention. The three most common reasons for bleeding during pregnancy are a normal delivery (i.e., labor), a spontaneous abortion, or an ectopic pregnancy. The first cause, labor, is usually expected and quite easily diagnosed; the other two can be more vexing and fraught with potentially mortal complications.

   1. **Pathophysiology**

      The **pathophysiology** of an ectopic pregnancy and of a spontaneous abortion are quite different. A **ruptured ectopic pregnancy** is one in which the fertilized oocyte, i.e., the products of conception, implants in a site different from the uterine endometrium. The sites of implantation include the abdomen and the fallopian tube. The risk of this entity increases if there has been any scarring of the fallopian tubes. This scarring can be as the result of a past episode of pelvic inflammatory disease or an incomplete tubal ligation procedure. A **spontaneous abortion,** commonly re-

B O X 1 1 - 5

Overall Evaluation and Management of Vaginal Discharge Suspected To Be Abnormal

Evaluation

1. **History**
   a. Menstrual history
      i. Last menstrual period (LMP).
      ii. Features of the menstrual cycles and of the menstruation itself.
         (a) Polymenorrhea—multiple short episodes of menstrual bleeding, each self-limited but abnormal in frequency.
         (b) Metromenorrhagia—excessive or prolonged menstrual bleeding occurring at irregular intervals.
         (c) Menorrhagia—excessive or prolonged menstrual bleeding at the normal time.
         (d) Epimenorrhea—menstrual bleeding of various amounts between normal periods.
      iii. Para and gravida; i.e., the total number of antecedent deliveries and conceptions.
      iv. If postmenopausal, when menopause occurred, and if it was natural or iatrogenic. If iatrogenic, if the surgical procedure was a hysterectomy, i.e., not true menopause, or bilateral oophorectomy with or without hysterectomy.
   b. Current medications including systemic anticoagulants, oral contraceptives, and aspirin.
   c. History of systemic manifestations of bleeding, e.g., epistaxis, hematuria, hematemesis, easy bruising.
   d. Current method of contraception, if any. Query the patient regarding use of IUD.
2. **Physical examination,** looking for evidence of a systemic coagulopathy, e.g., petechiae, purpura, ecchymosis; and examination of the neck for goiter. The **pelvic examination** is central to all cases of vaginal discharge, bloody or nonbloody. The pelvic examinations must be performed on all patients. **Specific ex-**

(continued)

B O X 1 1 - 5 *(continued)*

aminations include visualization and palpation of all
pelvic structures, looking at the discharge itself and
from where it originates.

a. **Gram stain** and culture of any purulent discharge
   either from the Bartholin's gland or from the
   cervix.
b. A **wet mount** of any nonpurulent vaginal discharge, in which a freshly swabbed sample of the
   discharge is admixed in a test tube with 1–2 mL
   of normal saline, placed on a slide with a cov-
   erslip, and microscopically imaged. One can visualize *Trichomonas* organisms or the clue cells of
   Gardnerella vaginitis using this method.
c. A **KOH preparation** of the nonpurulent vaginal discharge. Using the wet mount specimen on the
   slide, place 2–4 drops of 10% KOH and warm the
   slide using a match or Bunsen burner. One can
   visualize any *Candida* organisms.
d. Papanicolaou smear of the cervix, looking for dysplastic cervical cells. One should use both the
   spatula, to obtain ectocervical cells, and the Cyto-
   brush, to obtain endocervical cells (see Fig. 11-1).
e. Describe any ulcer on the cervix.
f. Palpate and describe any uterine, adnexal, cervical, or vulvar masses.

3. β-**HCG** in the urine to rule out pregnancy. This is requisite in all premenopausal females who have a
   uterus and ovaries.
4. If any bleeding, intravascular volume depletion, pregnancy test positive, or fevers, obtain a complete
   blood count.
5. If any evidence of a coagulopathy, obtain a PT,
   aPTT, and platelet count.
6. If any suspicion for hypothyroidism, obtain T_3RU, T_4,
   and TSH.
7. Urinalysis, to look for a concurrent pyuria or hematuria, i.e., another site of bleeding.
8. Obtain an **ultrasound of the pelvis**. This is especially
   important in patients with any abnormal bleeding,
   any evidence of a pelvic mass on examination, or a
   positive β-hCG.

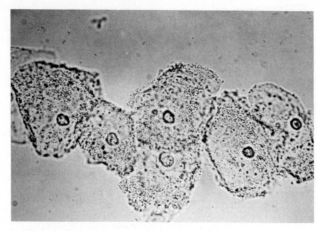

F I G U R E 11-1
Clue cells in a patient with vaginosis (nonspecific vaginitis).

ferred to as a miscarriage, is one in which the uterus extrudes the products of conception before they are viable for extrauterine existence. If in the first trimester, it usually is as the result of a gross genotypic abnormality of the fetus, whereas if in the second trimester, it usually is as the result of an abnormality of the uterus or cervix itself.

2. **Manifestations**

The **specific manifestations** include a history of "missing a few periods" and the onset of crampy abdominal pain and bloody vaginal discharge. In most cases the patient knows or suspects that she is pregnant. Often there will be left or right shoulder pain. This pain is referred and usually indicates peritoneal irritation. The patient can be intravascularly volume depleted and hemodynamically unstable, i.e., hypotensive and tachycardic, at the time of presentation.

a. If a **ruptured ectopic pregnancy,** the vaginal discharge is usually scant, but pain with radiation into the shoulder can be marked. Concurrent findings include the development of Grey Turner's sign, i.e., ecchymosis about the flank, or Cullen's sign, i.e., ecchymosis about the umbilicus. If a spontaneous abortion, there is often the passage of tissue, i.e., the products of conception, concurrent with the vaginal bleeding.

3. **Evaluation and management**

The **specific evaluation and management** include making the clinical diagnosis by using the data derived from Box 11-5. In both cases the β-hCG is positive and ultrasound will reveal no intrauterine gestational sac. In an **ectopic pregnancy** there often will be an asymmetry of the fallopian tubes with a unilateral mass. In a **spontaneous abortion,** some tissue will pass. This tissue must be saved and sent to pathology for assessment. In both cases, immediate referral to an obstetrician is clearly indicated as well as initiating intravenous access and performing preoperative laboratories, including typing and screening of blood. **Surgical intervention** on an emergency basis is indicated for a ruptured or nonruptured ectopic pregnancy, whereas observation and potential uterine dilation and curettage (D&C) are indicated for a spontaneous abortion. If the spontaneous abortion is in the second trimester, an assessment of uterine competence is indicated.

C. **Cervical carcinoma**

As a result of effective screening programs, the mortality from this specific entity has precipitously decreased.

1. **Pathophysiology**

The **pathophysiology** of this type of carcinoma has been outlined to the point that there are certain specific risk factors in its development. These **risk factors** include infection with human papillomavirus, i.e., condylomata acuminata, infection with herpes simplex virus, a history of smoking tobacco, and multiple sexual partners. The **natural history** is one of dysplasia isolated to the cervical epithelium which slowly, usually over the course of months, invades into the deeper structures of the cervix. The dysplastic cells within the cervical epithelium actually are carcinoma in situ.

2. **Manifestations**

The **specific manifestations** of this type of vaginal bleeding include postcoital spotting and dyspareunia. The bleeding is intermittent and relatively scant and usually in the premenopausal age group. Upon pelvic examination there can be and often is an indurated area, with or without ulceration, adjacent to or in the os of the cervix.

3. **Evaluation and management**

The **specific evaluation and management** of this entity includes making the clinical diagnosis using the techniques described in Box 11-5. Specific evaluation includes the Pap smear, which will demonstrate atypi-

---

B O X   1 1 - 6

*Specific Evaluation and Management
of an Abnormal Pap Smear*

1. If the smear is **positive for dysplasia,** send for colposcopy and biopsy.
2. If the smear has **atypical cells** and there are any antecedent manifestations of pain or postcoital discharge, send for colposcopy and biopsy.
3. If the test was for **screening,** i.e., no antecedent manifestations of disease:
   a. **Atypical cells** present on smear and patient < 45
      years of age: Perform **cervicography.** A micro-
      scopic photograph of the cervix is taken by either
      the primary care physician or a gynecologic spe-
      cialist and reviewed by the gynecologist. If the cer-
      vicography is interpreted as abnormal, send for
      colposcopy and biopsy; if normal, repeat the pel-
      vic and Pap smear in 3 months.
   b. **Atypical cells** present and patient > 45 years of
      age: Repeat the Pap smear in 3 months. If the
      Pap is atypical again, then refer to a gynecologist
      for colposcopy and/or endometrial examination,
      i.e., dilation and curettage.

cal and/or dysplastic cells (see Box 11-6). Referral to
a gynecologist for cervicography and/or colposcopy
is clearly indicated. **Cervicography** is a microscopic
photograph of the cervix looking for any abnormal areas consistent with carcinoma; **colposcopy** is the direct microscopic imaging of the cervix and the performance of biopsies in areas suspicious for cervical
carcinoma. If any evidence of carcinoma, the procedure of choice is **conization of the cervix,** i.e., the
removal of a cone of tissue of the cervix itself—a procedure which is curative in the vast majority of cases.

D. Endometrial carcinoma
1. Pathophysiology
The **pathophysiology** is primarily the result of abnormal proliferation of the endometrium itself. **Risk factors** for development include those which stimulate
the growth of the endometrium, including the chronic
unopposed use of oral estrogens, and states in which

the patient would have relatively high levels of endogenous estrogens on a chronic but physiologic basis. These **factors** include but are not limited to:

a. Early onset of menarche.

b. Late onset of menopause.

c. Nulliparity, i.e., never having been pregnant.

2. **Manifestations**

The **specific manifestations** include the fact that this occurs in older, usually postmenopausal woman. Often the bleeding is relatively scant, but in the postmenopausal setting, very disconcerting. In all cases, any postmenopausal vaginal bleeding must be aggressively and definitively addressed and defined.

3. **Evaluation and management**

The **specific evaluation and management** include making the clinical diagnosis and/or having a relatively high clinical suspicion as based upon the overall evaluation as described in Box 11-5. In all cases, referral to a gynecologist is indicated for endometrial biopsy and assessment. The procedure of choice is D&C of the uterine endometrium and concurrent direct imaging with a hysteroscope to look for endometrial polyps. These procedures are performed by a gynecologist.

E. **Dysfunctional uterine bleeding**

A relatively common form of abnormal vaginal bleeding.

1. **Pathophysiology**

The **underlying pathophysiology** is based upon the fact that the patient can, for whatever reason, have one or several consecutive cycles in which ovulation does not occur. Ovulation can be stymied by many different factors, including severe stress, malnutrition, anorexia nervosa, or the perimenopause. Each cycle that occurs without an effective ovulation results in several hormonal modifications.

a. The follicular cells remain intact and functional for a longer than normal period of time. This results in a longer follicular phase and overall longer duration of high levels of estrogens, causing significant proliferation of the uterine endometrium.

b. A lack of evolution of the follicular cells into a corpus luteum, resulting in a want of progesterone production. Thus the luteal phase is markedly abbreviated, if present.

c. The next cycle begins without a significant change in estrogen levels, and because there is little to no progesterone production, there is no marked decline and therefore no significant decline in the hormone levels; therefore, no sloughing of the endometrium, i.e., no menstrual flow, which manifests as a skipped period, i.e., secondary amenorrhea.

d. The next normal cycle, one in which ovulation does occur, there is the development of a normal corpus luteum and, with it, normal production of progesterones. If conception does not occur, there will be, at the end of the cycle, the normal decline in estrogens and progesterones, with a resultant sloughing of the endometrium from this cycle and the excess endometrium that had accumulated from previous anovulatory cycles. This manifests with **menorraghia,** i.e., an extremely heavy menstrual flow of long duration.

2. Manifestations

The **specific manifestations** of this cause of bloody vaginal discharge are based on the pathophysiologic description, above. They include irregular periods, both in terms of duration and amount of flow, with intermittent intervals of secondary amenorrhea in which one to three cycles are missed, followed by an inordinately heavy menses. The patient is infertile even when she is aggressively attempting to conceive. Manifestations of the underlying cause are commonly present.

3. Evaluation and management

The **specific evaluation and management** of dysfunctional uterine bleeding include making the clinical diagnoses based on the tests described in Box 11-5. Once the clinical diagnosis has been made and other, more malignant causes of vaginal bleeding have been excluded, therapy can be instituted. Therapy can include:

a. If **pregnancy is not desired** at present, the initiation of oral contraceptive agents. These agents will essentially take over the hormonal regulation of the menstrual cycles and iatrogenically make the menstrual cycles regular. Any oral contraceptive regimen is acceptable. One example is Ortho-Novum 7/7/7.

b. If **pregnancy is desired** in the near future, an attempt to make the periods regular by controlling one cycle with exogenous hormones is indicated. The specific regimen includes Ethinyl estradiol, 0.05 mg PO 1–3 times per day for 14 days (i.e., days 1–14), followed by medroxyprogesterone (Provera), 10 mg PO q.d. for 7 days (i.e., days 15–21), followed by withdrawal of hormones. The withdrawal should result in a period of menstrual flow. The next and subsequent periods can then, if the treatment was effective, be regular.

II. Causes of abnormal vaginal discharge, nonbloody (i.e., vaginitis). See also Table 11-4.

A. *Trichomonas vaginalis*

1. **Pathophysiology**

   This eukaryotic parasitic organism is transmitted only by sexual contact. It is specific to the male and female genitourinary tracts and results in superficial infection of the urethral and vaginal mucosa. Risk factors include unsafe sex with multiple sexual partners.

2. **Manifestations**

   The **specific manifestations** include the onset of dyspareunia, pruritus, and intermittent dysuria. Pelvic examination discloses copious amounts of frothy fluid with a "fishy" odor. There is concurrent evidence of cervicitis, sometimes referred to as "strawberry" cervicitis. In many patients, however, the process is relatively asymptomatic.

3. **Evaluation and management**

   The **specific evaluation and management** include making the clinical diagnosis using the techniques described in Box 11-5 and performing a wet mount preparation. The wet mount will clearly demonstrate the trichomonads swimming; their activity can be increased by warming the slide. **Specific treatment** includes treatment of the patient and her sexual partner(s) with a single 2-g dose of metronidazole (Flagyl). Metronidazole is contraindicated in pregnant females. There is a >90% cure rate if the patient and partner are concurrently treated. Further treatment includes educating the patient in "safe sex" techniques, i.e., the use of condoms or abstinence.

B. *Candida* species

1. **Pathophysiology**

   There is an abnormal overgrowth of this fungal organism, which normally colonizes the vagina. The organisms are either *Candida albicans* or *Candida glabrata*. The organism is not transmitted sexually. It is symptomatically present only if a change occurs in the normal vaginal milieu. **Risk factors** for development include the use of oral contraceptive agents, systemic glucocorticoids, or broad-spectrum antibiotics, and diabetes mellitus. The two most common reasons for an overgrowth of *Candida* are an increase in vaginal glucose levels, e.g., as the result of diabetes and/or glucocorticoids, or a decrease in the normally present bacillary bacteria, lactobacilli.

TABLE 11-4
Syndromes of Vaginal Inflammation

Cause	Discharge	Wet Mount	Treatment
Trichomonas	Clear Frothy Copious	Mobile trichomonads present	*Metronidazole, 2 g PO once; concurrently treat partner
Candida	Malodorous Whitish	Negative until KOH is added, then budding yeasts are present	Clotrimazole, 100 mg per vagina q.d. for 7 consecutive nights
Vaginosis	Clear Malodorous	Clue cells—epithelial cells coated with bacteria	*Metronidazole, 500 mg PO b.i.d. for 7 days, *or* Clindamycin, 300 mg PO b.i.d. for 7 days
Atrophic	Scant Dyspareunia Postmenopausal	No specific findings	Premarin 0.1% cream b.i.d.

*Metronidazole is contraindicated during pregnancy.

2. **Manifestations**

   The **specific manifestations** include vaginal pruritus, classically worse immediately before the onset of menstruation. There can be dyspareunia and a discharge which is thick, white, almost curdled in appearance, and even has whitish, thrushlike plaques.

3. **Evaluation and management**

   The **specific evaluation and management** include making the clinical diagnosis based on the examinations outlined in Box 11-5. The wet mount will reveal few findings; therefore, the KOH is performed, which will demonstrate yeast. Once the diagnosis is clinched, the initiation of antifungal agents should be made. The basic tenets of therapy include:

   a. Check for and reverse any and all risk factors for development.

   b. The initiation of clotrimazole (Lotrimin), 100-mg vaginal suppositories in a regimen of one per vagina q.h.s. for 7 nights; or clotrimazole, 300-mg vaginal suppositories q.h.s. for 3 nights.

   c. If recurrent, one can use systemic antifungal agents, e.g., fluconazole or ketoconazole. The regimen for fluconazole is 200 mg PO q.d. for 7 days; the regimen for ketoconazole is 200 mg PO b.i.d. for 7 days.

   d. If pruritus is severe, the concurrent administration of a low-dose corticosporin cream, e.g., hydrocortisone 1% cream t.i.d., can be administered to the vulva for the first 2–3 days.

C. **Vaginosis** (i.e., nonspecific vaginitis)

   1. **Pathophysiology**

      The **pathophysiology** is an abnormal overgrowth of anaerobic bacterial organisms and the nonspecific organism, *Gardnerella vaginalis,* concurrent with an overall decrease in the presence of lactobacilli—the anaerobic, gram-positive bacillary bacteria normally present in the vagina. The overgrowth results in a very superficial inflammatory response. The process is not transmitted sexually. It is symptomatically present only if there is a change in the normal vaginal milieu.

   2. **Manifestations**

      The **specific manifestations** include mild vaginal pruritus and a grayish to clear vaginal discharge which has a unique, almost fishy odor. There is often the presence of diffuse, mild erythema.

   3. **Evaluation and management**

      The **specific evaluation and management** include making the clinical diagnosis based on the examinations outlined in Box 11-5. The wet mount will demonstrate clue cells, vaginal epithelial cells with a stippled appearance on the cell surface (see Fig. 11-1). Management includes the initiation of oral antibiotics. The patient and her partner should be treated concurrently with one of the following regimens:

    a. Metronidazole, 500 mg PO b.i.d. for 7 days; or, if the patient is pregnant,

    b. Clindamycin, 300 mg PO b.i.d. for 7 days.

D. Atrophic vaginitis

See section on Menopause, page 582.

III. Consultation

Problem	Service	Time
Vaginal bleeding in a pregnant patient	Ob/Gyn	Emergent
Fever with purulent vaginal discharge	Ob/Gyn	Emergent

IV. Indications for admission: Any hypotension; vaginal bleeding in a pregnant female; peritoneal signs; a tender adnexal mass and discharge from the vagina, with or without concurrent fever.

Bibliography

Breast Masses and Lumps

Ernster VL: The Epidemiology of benign breast disease. Epidemiol Rev 1981;3:184.

Mushlin AI: Diagnostic tests in breast cancer. Ann Intern Med 1985;103:79.

Odenheimer DJ, et al: Risk factors for benign breast disease: A case control study of discordant twins. Am J Epidemiol 1984;120:565.

Wilkinson S, Forrest AP: Fibroadenoma of the Breast. Br J Surg 1985;72:838.

Contraceptive Modalities

Centers for Disease Control Cancer and Steroid Hormone Study: Long Term Oral Contraceptive Use and the Risk of Breast Cancer. JAMA 1983;249:1591.

Centers for Disease Control Cancer and Steroid Hormone Study: Long Term Oral Contraceptive Use and the Risk of Endometrial Cancer. JAMA 1983;249:1600.

Centers for Disease Control Cancer and Steroid Hormone Study: Long Term Oral Contraceptive Use and the Risk of Ovarian Cancer. JAMA 1983;249:1596.

Mishell DR: Contraception. N Engl J Med 1989;320:777.

Rietmeijer CAM, et al: Condoms as physical and chemical barriers against human immunodeficiency virus. JAMA 1988;259:1851.

Stadel BV: Oral contraceptives and cardiovascular disease. NEJM 1981;305:612.

Vaginal contraceptive sponge. Med Lett 1983;25:73.

Menopause/Osteoporosis

American College of Physicians: Guidelines for counseling postmenopausal women about preventive hormone therapy. Ann Intern Med 1992;117:1038–1041.

Ballinger CG: Psychiatric morbidity and the menopause: Clinical features. Br Med J 1976;1:1183.

Grady D, et al: Hormone therapy to prevent disease and prolong life in postmenopausal women. Ann Intern Med 1992;117:1016–1037.

Leiblum S, et al: Vaginal atrophy in the postmenopausal woman. JAMA 1984;252:63.

Lufkin EG, Ory SJ: Estrogen replacement therapy for the prevention of osteoporosis. Am Fam Pract 1989;40:205–212.

Naessen T, et al: Hormone replacement therapy and the risk for first hip fracture. Ann Intern Med 1990;113:95–103.

Riggs BL, Melton LJ: Involutional Osteoporosis. NEJM 1986;314:1676–1686.

Riis B, et al: Does Calcium supplementation prevent postmenopausal bone loss? NEJM 1987;316:173–177.

Stampfer MJ, et al: Postmenopausal estrogen therapy and cardiovascular disease. NEJM 1991;325:756–762.

Zilkoski M, Morrow LB: Osteoporosis. Am Fam Pract 1987;36:178–185.

Pelvic Masses

Barber HRK: Ovarian carcinoma. CA 1986;36:149.

Crum CP, et al: Human papillomavirus type 16 and early cervical neoplasia. NEJM 1984;310:880.

Eschenbach DA, et al: Polymicrobial etiology of acute pelvic inflammatory disease. NEJM 1975;293:166.

Helfer EL, Rose LI: Drug therapy for hirsutism. Am Fam Pract 1987;36:196–198.

Richardson GS, et al: Common epithelial cancer of the ovary. NEJM 1985;312:415.

Rittmaster RS, Loriaux L: Hirsutism. Ann Intern Med 1987;106:95–107.

Wasserheit JN, et al: Microbial causes of proven pelvic inflammatory disease and efficacy of clindamycin and tobramycin. Ann Intern Med 1986;104:187.

Vaginal Discharge

Brunham RC, et al: Mucopurulent cervicitis. NEJM 1984;311:1.

Friedrich EG Jr: Vulvar pruritis: A symptom, not a disease. Postgrad Med 1977;61:164.

Goldfarb JM, Little AB: Abnormal vaginal bleeding. NEJM 1980;302:666.

Pheifer TA, et al: Nonspecific vaginitis: Role of *Hemophilus vaginalis* and treatment with metronidazole. NEJM 1978;298:1429.

Richard RM: The patient with an abnormal Pap smear. NEJM 1980;302:729.

Sobel JD: Vulvovaginal candidiasis. Ann Intern Med 1984;101:390.

—D.D.B.

Dale Berg, Ed. *Handbook
of Primary Care Medicine.*
Copyright © 1993 J. B.
Lippincott Company.

CHAPTER 12

Diseases of the Ear, Nose, and Throat

Epistaxis (Box 12-1)

The nose has a rich supply of arterial and venous drainage. It is covered with mucosa, which is stratified squamous epithelium, and is easily traumatized, leading to epistaxis. Epistaxis is bleeding from the nose. Nosebleeds can occur in the anterior or posterior aspect of the nasal passages and in either or both nasal passages.

I. Anterior epistaxis

A. Description

Anterior epistaxis manifests with bleeding mainly from the anterior nasal passages. The bleeding may be bilateral. Anterior epistaxis is much more common than posterior epistaxis. Although the bleeding is anterior, there may be some oozing of blood posteriorly, especially when the patient is supine. The bleeding is invariably venous, usually from the rich venous plexus termed Kisselbach's plexus.

B. Causes

Underlying causes of anterior epistaxis include the following:

1. **Minor trauma** to the mucosa, usually associated with or resulting from nosepicking. Although denied by patients, this habit, which has negative societal connotations, is a universal habit and a risk factor for anterior epistaxis.

2. **Nasal trauma,** most commonly a fracture of the nasal bone itself, with resultant soft tissue and vascular damage.

3. **Dry nasal mucosa,** especially in the winter or in dry

B O X 1 2 - 1

Overall Evaluation and Management of Epistaxis

Evaluation

1. Take a thorough history and perform a physical examination, including a history of coagulopathy or recent trauma to head or face.
2. Attempt to define the site of bleeding, anterior or posterior (see Table 12-1).

Management

1. **Anterior site**
   a. Patient should sit upright.*
   b. The patient or caregiver should firmly pinch the **nasal ala** together for 10–15 minutes.*
   c. After bleeding stops, the patient should apply sterile petrolatum gel to the nares to aid in lubrication for several days and, as a long-term measure, should use a humidifier, especially during the winter or dry season.*

   *These are commonsense measures that the patient can be taught to perform at home.

   d. **Examine the skin** for concurrent ecchymotic or petechial lesions.
   e. **Directly visualize** the nasal mucosa, using a nasal speculum and appropriate lighting, to determine the specific site of bleeding. An assistant may hold the light source or the clinician may use a headset reflector.
   f. Apply 2–3 drops of an **α-agonist** (e.g., phenylephrine [Neosynephrine]) to a cotton swab and apply it to the affected nasal mucosa, followed immediately by 10–15 minutes more of nasal alar compression. This agent acutely vasoconstricts the vessels, thereby decreasing blood flow to the area and increasing the ability to form thrombus.
   g. If bleeding continues, directly **cauterize** the specific sites of bleeding under direct visualization. Cauterization is accomplished by applying **silver nitrate sticks** to the mucous membranes.
   h. If bleeding continues, apply a **5% cocaine spray** to

(continued)

B O X   1 2 - 1 *(continued)*

the nasal mucosa, **and** recauterize, using either silver nitrate or a heat probe, **and** pack the anterior
nasal cavity with petrolatum gauze for 24 hours.
Cocaine is an effective α-agonist and thus vaso-
constrictor, and is also a superb local anesthetic
for the nasal mucosa, thus affording the patient effective local anesthesia when placing the **anterior
packing,** a procedure which is quite painful. The
packing is **cotton gauze,** which is placed into the
anterior nasal chamber with some force. The packing is removed in 24 hours.
  i. If a **coagulopathy** is suspected, perform laboratory tests including a complete blood count, PT,
aPTT, and platelet count, looking for any elevation in the coagulation parameters or thrombocytopenia (see section on Excessive Bleeding States
in Chapter 5, page 275).
2. **Posterior site**
  a. Obtain radiographs of the face, head, and cervical
spine to rule out concurrent fractures.
  b. Place the patient in a cervical collar until a cervical spine fracture has been ruled out radiographically.
  c. Expedient referral to an ENT consultant is clearly
indicated.

---

climates. The dry mucosa is easily traumatized and
may also spontaneously crack and bleed.
  4. An **acquired or genetic coagulopathy.** The development of significant anterior epistaxis may **herald** a significant bleeding disorder. These bleeding disorders
include thrombocytopenia, DIC, and iatrogenic excessive therapeutic anticoagulation with heparin or warfarin. If a coagulopathy is present, the patient usually
has concurrent symptoms and signs of bleeding dysfunction, including menorrhagia, easy bruising, petechiae, purpura, or gingival bleeding.

II. **Posterior epistaxis**
  Posterior epistaxis is uncommon and significant, usually requiring emergency evaluation and management. It usually
occurs as a result of or associated with acute trauma to the

TABLE 12-1
Anterior versus Posterior Epistaxis

Type	Characteristics	Site	Management
Anterior	Common Mild trauma Blood from anterior nares, unilateral or bilateral	Venous Kisselbach's venous plexus	Patient should sit up and lean forward Topical α-agonists Cautery with silver nitrate Anterior nasal packing with petrolatum gauze See text
Posterior	Rare Facial trauma, usually associated with facial bone fractures	Arterial	Airway Rule out concurrent head or cervical spine trauma ENT consultation Admission

facial bones, especially trauma causing fracture. The bleeding is usually **arterial** and requires **acute management of the airway,** ruling out concurrent cervical spine or head trauma, admission to the hospital's ENT service for surgical intervention, and/or the placement of a posterior pack.

III. Consultation

Problem	Service	Time
Uncontrolled anterior epistaxis	ENT	Emergent
Posterior epistaxis	ENT	Emergent

IV. Indications for admission: Severe coagulopathy or posterior epistaxis.

Oral Diseases (Box 12-2)

The oral cavity is the anatomic space immediately anterior to the pharynx. For the most part it is lined with stratified squamous epithelium. Several structures in the oral cavity assist in basic functions. These unique structures are the teeth and the tongue. Although many disease states can affect the mouth, the three most common ones are dental caries, gingivitis, and oral carcinoma.

I. Simple caries
A. Manifestations
The **manifestations** of this common entity include acute or subacute pain referrable to one area of the mouth and

---

B O X   1 2 - 2

Overall Evaluation and Management of Oral Diseases

Evaluation

Perform a **thorough examination** of the oral structures, including direct visualization of the entire surface, including the sides of the tongue, and palpation of the mucosa of the mouth.

Management

1. Referral to dentist for any carious teeth.
2. Referral to dentist for **semiannual prophylactic care.**
3. Referral to ENT for any indurated lesions, especially if painful.

even to a specific tooth. Often the decayed area will be small, but it is not uncommon to see gross decay of the tooth with parts of the tooth actually broken. It is in teeth with such significant caries that local complications can and do occur.

B. **Pathogenesis**

The **underlying pathogenesis** is bacteria (anaerobic) production of enzymes and a slightly acid milieu that result in absorption of calcium from the tooth enamel. Once the integrity of the enamel, the hard protective covering of the tooth, is broken, a cavity forms. The **natural history** of the disease once the cavity forms is slow, irreversible progression with dentine, the softer middle layer of the tooth, being resorbed. The cavity eventually reaches the pulp cavity, the structure that supplies blood and nervous supply to the tooth. When adjacent to the pulp cavity, pain begins; when involving the pulp cavity, complications including abscess formation occur.

C. **Evaluation and management**

The **specific evaluation and management** of simple caries entail referral to a dental professional for corrective therapy and underscoring to the patient the importance of regular dental visits.

D. **Consultation**

Problem	Service	Time
All	Dentist	Required

II. **Complicated caries**

A. **Manifestations**

The **specific manifestations** of complicated caries include the onset of severe pain and loss of chewing function on the entire side of the mouth ipsilateral to the involved tooth. The pain is dull, throbbing, aching, quite severe, and is often referred to other ipsilateral trigeminal nerve roots. The patient often has concurrent intolerance to hot and cold. **Examination** reveals palpable swelling at the base of the tooth and in the adjacent gingival area, fevers, chills, and ipsilateral swelling of the face. There is, invariably, reproducible discomfort on **percussion,** i.e., tapping the diseased tooth. This is a direct result of inflammation involving the periodontal ligament.

B. **Pathogenesis**

The **underlying pathogenesis** is untreated caries that extends into the pulp cavity, resulting in **infection, ischemia,** and **necrosis** of the pulp chamber with resultant abscess formation and osteolysis at the periapical area. Causative organisms include **anaerobes** (i.e., peptostreptococci), *Bacteroides*, and **gram-positive aerobic bacteria** (i.e., streptococci, including those of the viridans group).

C. **Evaluation**

The **specific evaluation** includes examination, making the clinical diagnosis, and urgent referral to a dentist or endodontist for a drainage procedure. A **radiograph** of that tooth for confirmation of the diagnosis is indicated. This radiograph, obtained by the dental professional, will show lysis and/or sclerosis of the apical tooth area or of the adjacent bone.

D. **Management**

The specific management is drainage of the tooth itself, by the classic **root canal** (i.e., opening the roots through the crown of the tooth and debriding the tissue) or by extraction of the tooth itself.

1. All patients should receive **periprocedure antibiotics** for 5 days, starting 6 hours before the procedure. The antibiotic schedule is either penicillin, 500 mg PO q.i.d. for 5 days, or erythromycin, 500 mg PO q.i.d.

2. If there is any evidence of **cellulitis** (swelling, purulent discharge, or fevers), the antibiotics should be initiated immediately and continued for several days before the procedure for a total duration for 7–10 days. Finally, as the patient will be in significant distress, analgesics, including narcotic analgesia, should be prescribed until the procedure can be performed. Tylenol no. 3 q.6h. PRN may be effective in pain management.

E. **Consultation**

Problem	Service	Time
All	Dentist	Urgent

III. **Gingivitis**

A. **Manifestations**

The **specific manifestations** of this common oral disorder include bleeding from the gums when the teeth are brushed. There usually is no associated pain until late into the course of the disease. The patient may be unaware even of significant disease. **Examination** discloses mild swelling of the gingiva adjacent to the tooth and recession of the gingiva on the teeth, thus exposing the superior aspects of the teeth (see Fig. 12-1).

B. **Pathogenesis**

The **underlying pathogenesis** of this inflammation of the gingiva adjacent to the teeth is plaque. Plaque is an acquired, abnormal material coating the teeth that is quite hard and consists of bacteria. These bacteria invariably are anaerobic. The presence of plaque results directly in inflammation of the gingiva. The **natural history** is one of progressive loss of gingiva, increased risk of caries, especially adjacent to the gingiva, and tooth loss. Further-

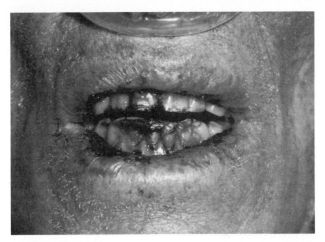

F I G U R E   1 2 - 1
Severe gingivitis. Note recession of the gingivae and purulent material on the periodontal surfaces. The gingivae bleed easily.

more, there is an increased risk of gravitational pneumonias in patients with a history of loss of gag reflex and/or decreased level of consciousness, e.g., patients with an antecedent cerebrovascular accident or ethanol abuse.

C. **Evaluation and management**
The **specific evaluation and management** include referral to a dental professional for therapeutic and prophylactic professional dental hygiene sessions every 4–6 months and instructing the patient to floss every day.

D. **Consultation**

Service	*Time*
Dental	Required

IV. **Carcinoma**
A. **Manifestations**
The **specific manifestations** of this disorder include a painless lump in the mouth, tongue, or neck. There is invariably a personal history of smoking tobacco (pipes, cigars, or cigarettes) or the chewing of tobacco, or ingestion of ethanol, especially in large quantities. The lesions can be asymptomatic until large. **Examination** includes direct visualization of the oral mucosa, palpation of the mucosal surfaces, and palpation of the cervical lymph nodes. Any lesion that is increasing in size, painless, ul-

cerated, indurated, or in a patient with risk factors for the development of carcinoma should be suspicious for a malignant neoplastic lesion.

B. Pathogenesis

The **underlying pathogenesis** is unclear. Risk factors associated with development include smoking or chewing tobacco products and ethanol abuse.

C. Evaluation and management

The **specific evaluation and management** including having an appropriate clinical suspicion that a lesion may be malignant and, at that time, expedient referral to an ENT specialist for biopsy. The use of tobacco is proscribed.

D. Consultation

Problem	*Service*	*Time*
Any suspicious lesion	ENT	Urgent

V. Indications for admission: Virtually all of these conditions can be evaluated and managed on an outpatient basis.

Otalgia/Otitis

The ear is anatomically divided into three areas, the external ear, the middle ear, and the inner ear. This division is somewhat arbitrary, but each area contributes in a different way to the overall sensory activity of the ear.

The **external ear,** also referred to as the outer ear, includes all of the structures peripheral to the tympanic membrane. These structures include the auricle, the helix, the tragus, and the external auditory canal. It is composed mainly of cartilage covered with nonkeratinizing stratified squamous epithelium. The **function** is to aid in receiving sound waves from the ambient environment.

The **middle ear** is the discrete area between the tympanic membrane and the internal auditory canal. It contains the three bones used for transmission of auditory waves, the stapedius, the incus, and the malleolus. The space is immediately anterior to the mastoid air cells, immediately superficial to the inner ear structures, and connected to the nasopharynx by the eustachian tube. The **function** of this structure is to transmit sound waves to the inner ear.

The **inner ear** is the area immediately deep to the middle ear and contains several fluid-filled canals: the cochlea for auditory sensation reception and three semicircular canals for position sensation reception. The **function** is thus both auditory and position sensation. It is innervated by cranial nerve VIII.

I. Otitis externa

A. Manifestations

The usual **manifestations** include unilateral pain in the external canal, commonly referred to as an earache. At times, the pain will extend into the ipsilateral tragus. **Examination** may reveal a significant amount of cerumen in the canal or swelling of the external canal precluding direct visualization of the tympanic membrane. Although pain and tenderness are the most common manifestations, erythema and pruritus of the affected areas are not uncommon. There may be a purulent discharge with crusting in the involved auditory canal.

A specific severe type of otitis externa is **otitis externa maligna.** This manifests with a diffusely swollen and markedly tender auricle and can progress to a severe life-threatening infection of the face and head.

B. **Pathogenesis**

The **underlying pathogenesis** is a superficial infectious inflammation of the external auditory canal. Overall risk factors for development include ceruminous impaction, trauma due to patient attempting to clean his ears, and swimming in lake water or nonchlorinated swimming pools. This entity is most common during the summer months. **Organisms** that can cause otitis externa include *Staphylococcus aureus, Pseudomonas* spp., or fungi, *Candida* or *Aspergillus.* Staphylococcal infections specifically manifest with a yellow crusty exudate; pseudomonal infections manifest with a greenish exudate. Fungal infections specifically manifest with a fine fluffy material overlying the affected skin.

In **otitis externa maligna,** risk factors include those listed above and the processes of diabetes mellitus or immunosuppression. The disease process is significantly more virulent, involves deeper structures, and the etiologic organism is invariably *Pseudomonas aeruginosa* (see Fig. 12-2).

C. **Evaluation**

The **evaluation** of otitis externa includes that listed in Box 12-3.

D. **Management**

The specific management includes, after thoroughly **cleaning and drying** the external canal, the use of topical agents. The **topical agent** is Corticosporin (Neomycin 0.5%, Hydrocortisone 1%, and Polymyxin B 10,000 units/mL) solution or suspension in a dose of 2 drops b.i.d. to t.i.d. for 10–14 days, to the external canal. If the canal is completely obstructed, a 2–3-cm ribbon of cotton gauze (e.g., Nu Gauze packing strip) can be gently inserted into the canal. This forms a wick to which the topical agents are applied. If a **fungal etiology** is suspected, clotrimazole (Lotrimin 1%) solution applied t.i.d. to the affected ear canal is indicated. **Prevention** via prohibiting the insertion of objects into the ear canal (e.g., Q-Tips) and the use of earplugs when swimming is indicated.

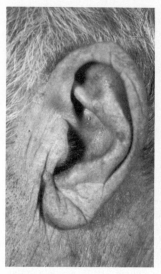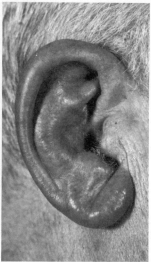

FIGURE 12-2
Left and right ears, showing otitis externa maligna in the right. Note diffuse erythema and swelling.

Otitis externa maligna mandates aggressive evaluation and management, for its natural history is one of rapid spread to adjacent tissues, bacteremia with resultant gram-negative rod septicemia, and mortality. These patients uniformly require admission, ENT and infectious disease consults, and the initiation of an intravenous aminoglycoside, e.g., gentamicin, 2 mg/kg IV **stat, and** an antipseudomonal penicillin **or** a third-generation cephalosporin.

E. Consultation

Problem	Service	Time
OEM	ENT	Emergent
OEM	Infectious diseases	Emergent

II. Serous otitis media
A. Manifestations
The **specific manifestations** of this common entity include a mild decrease in auditory acuity bilaterally or unilaterally with an associated "popping" sensation in the affected ear(s). There may be modest pain in the affected ear(s). Often there are concurrent symptoms of

B O X   1 2 - 3

Overall Evaluation and Management of Otalgia/Otitis

Evaluation

1. Take a **history** and perform a **physical examination,** including palpation of the auricle and adjacent lymph nodes and visualization of the tympanic membrane looking for erythema and swelling.
2. **Remove all cerumen** from the canal. This is best accomplished with otologic lavage with warm normal saline or sterile water or even warm tap water. The patient is placed in an upright position and, using a syringe with a "Christmas tree" top, the water is gently yet firmly injected into the external ear canal until cerumen is flushed out.
3. Query the patient regarding auditory and position sensation, including dizziness or vertigo, as these indicate more of an inner ear dysfunctional state.
4. Document **auditory acuity,** at least grossly, using a ticking watch or rubbing fingers adjacent to the ear to ascertain any gross auditory deficit.

Management

1. If concurrent vertigo is present, see section on Vertigo in Chapter 14, page 732.
2. If an auditory deficit is present after treatment of common external and middle ear dysfunctional states, refer the patient to an audiologist for formal testing.

---

nasal congestion, frontal headaches, and nonproductive cough. On **examination,** the tympanic membrane (TM) of the affected ear will demonstrate mild erythema and some air bubbles and fluid behind the affected tympanic membrane. On direct visualization, the landmarks of the TM are not embarrassed, as one can clearly see the umbo, the pars tensa, and the pars flaccida. The reflex **cone of light,** however, is often decreased.

B. **Pathogenesis**

The **underlying pathogenesis** is nonpurulent inflammation of the middle ear as a result of (i.e., concurrent with) allergic rhinitis or a viral upper respiratory tract infection.

The disease is self-limited and will resolve when the underlying process, either the allergy or the viral URI, has resolved.

C. **Evaluation**

The **evaluation** is as described in Box 12-3 and making the clinical diagnosis.

D. **Management**

The **specific management** is directed toward the underlying associated condition and the relief of symptoms. Acetaminophen PRN and/or decongestants and/or antihistamines are clinically indicated (see Table 12-5).

Mycoplasma pneumoniae can cause a specific form of serous otitis media, bullous myringitis. **Myringitis** is inflammation of the TM without concurrent effusion. This form is usually associated with an atypical interstitial pneumonitis and requires, in addition to decongestants and acetaminophen, a 10-day course of erythromycin.

III. **Purulent otitis media**

A. **Manifestations**

The **specific manifestations** of this relatively common disorder include the acute onset of unilaterally decreased auditory acuity, modest to severe pain in the affected ear (otalgia), and occasionally otorrhea (the discharge of material, usually purulent, from the affected ear when the TM ruptures). Headaches and fevers may be concurrent with this process. There usually is a several-day antecedent history of rhinorrhea and scratchy sore throat. On **examination** and direct visualization, the TM has decreased mobility to air movements, and very often there is a bulging of the TM with loss of bony landmarks and a marked decrease in the cone of light reflex. Furthermore, the TM often is very erythematous and can have evidence of a perforation. Finally, the patient will often have tender unilateral lymphadenopathy ipsilateral to the infected ear.

B. **Pathogenesis**

The **underlying pathogenesis** is a bacterial infection of the middle ear. It is not uncommon for the patient to have an antecedent serous otitis media. The pathogens that cause this disease process include *Streptococcus* spp., *Hemophilus influenzae,* and *Branhamella catarrhalis.* The **complications** of this entity, if untreated, include the local suppurative complications of leptomeningitis, purulent labyrinthitis, brain or intracranial abscesses, and purulent mastoiditis.

C. **Evaluation**

The **evaluation** includes those items described in Box 12-3 and making the clinical diagnosis.

D. **Management**
   Specific management includes the initiation of antibiotics. Antibiotic regimens include amoxicillin, 250–500 mg PO t.i.d. for 7–10 days; TMP–sulfa (Bactrim DS), 1 tablet PO b.i.d. for 7–10 days; or Augmentin, 250 mg PO t.i.d. for 7–10 days. Any one of these regimens will effectively treat an infection due to these pathogens. Further therapy includes the PRN use of antihistamines, decongestants, and acetaminophen. It is rare that consultation with ENT is necessary unless there is evidence of recurrent disease, lack of resolution after standard first-line therapy, or perforation of the TM.

E. **Consultation**

Problem	Service	Time
Any complications	ENT	Urgent
Recurrent disease	ENT	Elective
Complications	Infectious diseases	Urgent

IV. **Indications for admission:** Complications of acute purulent otitis media, or any evidence of otitis externa maligna.

Pharyngitis (Box 12-4)

The **pharynx** is the anatomic space that connects the oral cavity anteriorly, the nasal chambers superiorly, and the esophagus and larynx inferiorly. It is artificially subdivided into three specific zones, the **nasopharynx,** the **oropharynx,** and the **hypopharynx.** The basic elements of sustenance pass through the pharynx into the body. The pharynx is lined with mucosa, which is stratified squamous epithelium and has a rich supply of lymphoid tissue, predominantly in the tonsils. Because the pharynx is centrally located, infectious processes quite commonly affect this area and result in pharyngitis.

I. **Manifestations**
   The **overall manifestations** of pharyngitis include the acute onset of sore throat, pain on swallowing (odynophagia), fevers to varying degrees, diffuse erythema of the tonsils and posterior pharynx, varying degrees of cervical lymph node enlargement, varying degrees of rhinitis and cough, and symptoms and signs specific to the underlying cause.

II. **Causes**
   The causes of acute pharyngitis include bacterial and viral agents. A list of these along with their specific manifestations and natural history follows.
   A. *Streptococcus pyogenes*
      1. **Manifestations**
         The **specific manifestations** of this common cause of pharyngitis include the acute onset of sore throat,

present from the outset of the disease process, with concurrent fevers, chills, and intermittent night sweats. The sore throat can be of such magnitude as to cause significant odynophagia, potentially leading to mild intravascular volume depletion. Often, nausea with mild intermittent vomiting is present, but rhinorrhea, cough, and otalgia are uncommon. On **examination,** the tonsils and posterior pharynx are erythematous and covered with exudative material. The cervical nodes at the angle of the mandible, i.e., the jugulodigastric nodes, are invariably enlarged and tender bilaterally.

2. **Natural history**

The vast majority of cases are self-limited and resolve spontaneously within 7–10 days. There are, however, complications from this specific infectious entity. Complications occur in a small minority of patients but are potentially mortal and, with appropriate intervention, are preventable. The complications can be local or systemic.

   a. **Local** (i.e., head and neck) **complications** include the formation of a peritonsillar abscess (quinsy) or the formation of an abscess in, or spread of local infection to, the retropharyngeal space (Ludwig's angina).

   b. **Systemic complications** include the development of **rheumatic fever,** characterized by erythema marginatum, subcutaneous nodules, chorea (spontaneous large motor involuntary movements), pancarditis (valvulitis/myocarditis/endocarditis/pericarditis) with resultant aortic insufficiency and/or mitral stenosis, and polyarticular arthritis (see Table 12-2 and the section on Polyarticular Arthritis

T A B L E 1 2 - 2
Jones' Criteria in the Clinical Diagnosis of Rheumatic Fever

Major
   Pancarditis
   Chorea
   Polyarticular arthritis
   Subcutaneous nodules
   Erythema marginatum
Minor
   Increased ASO titer (Todd units)
   Increased Streptozyme titer (DNase–antideoxyribonuclease B)
   Increased C-reactive protein

in Chapter 7). A final complication is the development of immune complex–mediated **glomerulonephritis.**

B. Viral causes

1. Manifestations

The **specific manifestations** include a mild to moderate sore throat, usually preceded by rhinorrhea, otalgia, cough (productive or nonproductive), myalgias, and a low-grade fever. On **examination** the posterior pharynx is often erythematous with minimal amounts of exudative material; furthermore, there often are some shotty, mildly tender cervical lymph nodes present.

2. Natural history

The **natural history** is somewhat specific to the individual viral agent but, overall, is usually self-limited, with complete resolution in 3–5 days. Specific viral agents include **enteroviruses, adenoviruses,** and **coxsackieviruses. Coxsackievirus A** infection manifests as a distinctly painful pharyngitis with vesicles on and localized to the posterior pharynx. It is also known as **herpangina.** There are few complications of viral pharyngitis.

C. Epstein–Barr virus

1. Manifestations

The **specific manifestations** of this relatively common cause of pharyngitis include a prodromal phase of malaise and constitutional symptoms for 2–5 days, followed by the acute onset of a severe sore throat, usually with significant odynophagia. This **DNA virus** causes a syndrome that is also known as infectious mononucleosis, (kissing disease). It is spread by saliva and occurs in epidemics among adolescents and young adults. On **examination** there are an exudative, approaching purulent, pharyngitis with associated petechiae on the mucous membranes of the mouth, and diffuse, tender lymphadenopathy, both cervical and generalized. Other associated findings may include a mild amount of icterus and splenomegaly.

2. Natural history

The **natural history** usually entails complete resolution in 10–20 days. Complications can include splenic rupture, hepatitis, Coombs-positive hemolytic anemia, intravascular volume depletion due to inability to effectively swallow, and thrombocytopenia as a result of sequestration associated with splenomegaly. Approximately 5% of patients develop one of these acute complications of EBV infection.

D. *Corynebacterium diphtheriae*
   1. Manifestations
      The **specific manifestations** of this rare cause of pharyngitis include severe sore throat and fevers. On **examination** there are discrete whitish plaques on the tonsils and posterior pharynx that bleed if they are traumatized or removed. These lesions are sometimes referred to as pseudomembranes. Further manifestations include significant and quite marked bilateral cervical lymph node enlargement. This lymphadenopathy can be so extensive as to give the patient a "bull's neck" appearance. Because the number of people who are not immunized against this pathogen is increasing, the incidence of this eminently preventable infectious disease may also be increasing.
   2. Natural history
      The **natural history** is one of severe sore throat that may progress to systemic disease with the development of toxin-mediated cardiomyopathy and even death.
E. *Neisseria gonorrhoeae*
   1. Manifestations
      The **specific manifestations** of this rare form of pharyngitis, which can occur in patients who are at risk, i.e., those practicing fellatio or cunnilingus on an infected partner, include the acute onset of a severe sore throat. **Examination** reveals an exudative pharyngitis with multiple ulcer-type lesions and tender bilateral cervical lymphadenopathy. Often there is evidence of concurrent urethritis or cervicitis. For a further discussion of sexually transmitted diseases in general and *Neisseria gonorrhoeae* in specific, see Chapter 6, page 342.

III. Evaluation and management
   The **specific evaluation and management** are based on the degree of clinical suspicion that *Streptococcus pyogenes* is causing the pharyngitis.
   A. High suspicion of *S. pyogenes*
      In the **high suspicion group,** i.e., patients with the classic findings listed in the discussion on streptococcal pharyngitis, those with a past history of rheumatic fever, or those in close contact with people with documented β-hemolytic streptococcal infections, treatment should be initiated. Treatment regimens include penicillin VK, 500 mg q.i.d. for 7–10 days, or erythromycin, 500 mg PO q.i.d. for 7–10 days. There rarely is any need for pharyngeal cultures in these cases. The only indication for a pharyn-

B O X 1 2 - 4

Overall Evaluation and Management of Acute Pharyngitis

Evaluation

1. Take a thorough **history** and perform a **physical examination,** including direct visualization of the tonsils, posterior pharynx, and nasal mucosa and palpation of the cervical lymph nodes. A history of family members being diagnosed with specific entities in the recent past is also quite useful.

2. Formulate a **ranked differential diagnosis** and, based on the data gleaned from the history and physical examination, a clinical suspicion for the organism which has the greatest risk of complications, usually *Streptococcus pyogenes.*

3. Categorize the patient into one of **three overall groups** in regard to suspicion for *Streptococcus pyogenes*—**high, low,** and **intermediate suspicion**—before undertaking any further laboratory and therapeutic interventions. See text for specifics.

geal culture would be to document the disease in order to treat household contacts of the patient.

The treatment of streptococcal pharyngitis with PCN or erythromycin **will decrease** the development of local complications (i.e., abscesses), decrease the period of communicability, and decrease the risk of rheumatic fever. It **will not decrease** symptoms or the duration of the symptoms, nor will it decrease the risk of development of glomerulonephritis.

B. Low suspicion of *S. pyogenes*

If the **suspicion is low,** i.e., viral or EBV (infectious mononucleosis) is the probable cause, treat supportively. There is essentially no need for pharyngeal bacterial culture. Specific evaluation and management for this group include the following measures.

1. Provide **analgesia** and **antipyretics.** Acetaminophen, 500 mg PO q.4–6h., as a tablet or as an elixir is best.

2. Perform a **Monospot antibody test,** i.e., the heterophile antibody test. This test measures an antibody associated with EBV infection but does not directly measure the IgM antibody increase that occurs early in the

course of EBV. The patient's serum is mixed with horse RBCs. If agglutination occurs, it is positive and due to the presence of a heterophile antibody in the patient's serum. This test has a specificity of 99% and a sensitivity of 85% for EBV pharyngitis.

3. Provide **fluids** PO. If severe odynophagia is present, IV hydration may be required.

4. Determine the **CBC with differential,** as often there is an absolute and relative lymphocytosis with >40% **atypical lymphocytes.** This finding of >40% atypical lymphocytes is quite specific for EBV.

5. Prescribe **rest.** It is very important for the patient to rest and refrain from any exercise or work-related activities.

6. If EBV is diagnosed, **follow the hematocrits** and perform a baseline Coombs test to follow for the development of a Coombs-positive hemolytic anemia.

7. If EBV is diagnosed and there is severe pain in pharynx or inability to swallow even fluids, **initiate prednisone, 40–60 mg,** in a rapid taper.

8. If EBV is diagnosed, closely monitor for the development of splenomegaly. The patient should be **proscribed from any activity** that may traumatize the abdomen during and immediately after the infection. These activities include contact sports, as the spleen in EBV-related splenomegaly can easily rupture.

C. **Intermediate suspicion of *S. pyogenes***

If the suspicion for streptococcal pharyngitis is **intermediate,** pharyngeal cultures or rapid streptococcal antigen techniques for diagnosis come into play (see Table 12-3). These diagnostic techniques include the following.

1. **Pharyngeal culture.** The swab must be placed in or on the posterior pharynx and should, if possible, be **plated onto medium** at the time of the examination. This test has a sensitivity of 90% and a specificity of 75%–80%; however, it requires 24–48 hours to complete. Therefore, begin penicillin or erythromycin if and when the cultures become positive for β-hemolytic *Streptococcus* spp.

2. **Rapid antigen detection techniques.** These are novel and effective assays for the detection of the Group A carbohydrate antigen in the streptococcal cell wall. Two of these techniques are latex agglutination and ELISA. Both are commercially available and applicable and have a sensitivity of 80%–90% and a specificity of 85%–100%. The test requires 20 minutes to complete. If positive, penicillin or erythromycin can be initiated. If negative, treat as viral infection (see above discussion). If there is any indication of gonococcal

T A B L E 12-3
Evaluative Tests for Streptococcal Infections

Test	Sensitivity	Specificity	Time to Perform	Advantages	Disadvantages
Culture	90%	99%	24–48 hr	Easy to learn technique Minimal discomfort to patient	Time Cannot differentiate acute from chronic, i.e., infection from colonization
Rapid screens	95%	99%	15–20 min	Time	Cost Cannot differentiate acute from chronic infection Special laboratory setup required

T A B L E 1 2 - 4
Rhinitis Syndromes

Type	Precipitating Factors	Mechanism	Treatment
Viral	Adenoviruses Rhinoviruses Enteroviruses	Viral infection of upper respiratory tract	Decongestants Acetaminophen
Atopic	Allergens	IgE-mediated histamine release results in vasodilation and increased mucus production	Avoidance Desensitization Antihistamines Decongestants Topical steroids
Vasomotor	Odors Tear gas	Parasympathetic stimulation	Avoidance

pharyngitis, perform a pharyngeal swab with streaking of the swab on Thayer–Martin or NYC agar media. Treatment is discussed in the section on Sexually Transmitted Diseases in Chapter 6, page 342.

D. Diphtheria

If **diphtheria** is suspected, administer diphtheria antitoxin and treat with penicillin or erythromycin. Referral to infectious diseases and contacting the CDC are mandatory. Any patient with suspected diphtheria must be **quarantined** from the general population.

IV. Consultation

Problem	*Service*	*Time*
Quinsy or Ludwig's angina	ENT	Emergent
Rheumatic fever	Infectious diseases	Urgent

V. Indications for admission: Any local complications of streptococcal infections, including quinsy and Ludwig's angina; rheumatic fever; intravascular volume depletion; and any decreased hematocrit in EBV, either as a result of hemolysis or of splenic rupture.

Rhinitis

The nose is a symmetric structure with two nares or openings through which air can freely move. The nose **functions** as a conduit for air moving into and out of the respiratory tree and as a filter and humidifier of this air. To fullfil these functions, the internal aspects of the nose are richly supplied with blood vessels and lined with ciliated, pseudostratified columnar epithelium. Because of its location, functions, and recurrent exposure to viral and atopic agents, the mucosa can often become inflamed. This inflammation is referred to as **rhinitis.**

I. Viral rhinitis

A. Manifestations

The **specific manifestations** of viral rhinitis, also known as the **common cold,** include the acute onset of bilateral rhinorrhea with concurrent sore throat, boggy mucous membranes, sneezing, nonproductive cough, mild watery eyes, a popping sensation in the ears, and overall malaise. It is rare to have any significant gastrointestinal manifestations, and, with the exception of viral rhinitis due to Coxsackievirus A or B, these viruses rarely cause myalgias. **Examination** usually reveals serous otitis, a low-grade fever, usually no higher than 101.0 °F, mild erythema of the posterior pharynx, usually without exudate, and bilateral shotty, mildly tender cervical lymph node enlargement.

B. Pathogenesis

The **underlying pathogenesis** is direct infection of the mucosal surface of the nose and the entire pharyngeal area. **Viral agents** that cause this include **enteroviruses** (which include echovirus and coxsackievirus), **coronaviruses,** and **rhinoviruses.** The mucous membranes provide the source and terminus of transmission. Typical mechanisms of **transmission** of the virus include kissing, coughing, or sneezing, which spreads the infected particles of mucus. The infected particles of mucus can transmit the disease via contact with surfaces such as doorknobs or tissue paper containing the mucus. An example is tissue paper with nondissecated mucus present. The **incidence** of these infections increases in the winter or spring, and epidemics often occur in families, nursing homes, schools, and dormitories. The **natural history** is one in which the classic manifestations are self-limited, i.e., last for a period of 2–5 days, followed by complete resolution.

C. Evaluation

The **specific evaluation** includes that described in Box 12-5.

D. Management

The **specific management** is twofold, prevention and symptomatic relief. **Prevention** cannot be overemphasized. Prevention includes good hygiene, i.e., washing the hands, covering the mouth and face when coughing or sneezing, immediately **disposing of tissues after use,** and washing clothes and handkerchiefs in **hot water.** Although there is no known effective modality to shorten the natural course (i.e., cure the common cold), symptomatic relief can be afforded. Specific modalities include the use of decongestants, acetaminophen, and cough suppressants as necessary (see Table 12-5). The patient should be instructed to ingest adequate amounts of fluids and get adequate rest. The medications listed above **do not shorten the disease course** and can have side effects. Therefore, patients should use the agents sparingly and discontinue them if any side effects occur.

E. Consultation

None indicated.

II. Atopic/allergic rhinitis

A. Manifestations

The **specific manifestations** of this common disease, also known as hay fever in the fall and rose fever in the spring, include a relatively wide variety of upper respiratory tract

B O X   1 2 - 5

Overall Evaluation and Management of Rhinitis

Evaluation

1. Take a thorough **history** and perform a **physical examination,** including querying the patient as to the onset of symptoms, any new pets, any seasonal component, and any associated lower respiratory tract manifestations.
2. Attempt to determine the underlying cause, whether viral or allergic in nature.

Management

1. Instruct the patient in **basic hygiene,** such as covering the nose and mouth when sneezing or coughing, washing and drying hands before touching items, and disposing of tissues with sputum or mucus on them.
2. If a new pet is in the household, perform a trial of a **"pet holiday"**; remove the pet from the household and observe the patient for symptomatic relief.
3. Prescribe acetaminophen and/or a decongestant PRN for viral rhinitis (see Table 12-5).
4. Prescribe an antihistamine and/or a decongestant PRN for atopic rhinitis (see Table 12-5).

---

symptoms of varying degrees of intensity and severity. All of the symptoms and signs occur on a recurrent or even chronic basis, whenever the **allergen** is present. The onset of allergic-mediated rhinitis usually occurs during late childhood, adolescence, or early adulthood. Onset in neonates, toddlers, and the elderly is rare. The patient has bilateral rhinorrhea; bilateral conjunctivitis; watery, itchy, red eyes; sneezing; and nasal congestion. Rarely, if ever, are there any associated fevers, cough, myalgias, arthralgias, or gastrointestinal symptoms.

B. **Pathogenesis**

The **underlying pathogenesis** is a classic allergen IgE-mediated mechanism. In this mechanism, the patient is exposed to an **allergen,** a specific protein that causes **IgE** production from lymphocytes. The IgE then coats the plasma membrane of mast cells within the nasal mucous

T A B L E 12 - 5
Upper Respiratory Tract/Rhinitis Medications

Agent	Indications/ Effects	Side Effects	Dosage
Entex LA (phenylpropanolamine and guaifenesin)	Decongestant Expectorant	Tachycardia Tremor	One tablet PO q.12h. PRN
Drixoril (Pseudoephedrine and brompheniramine)	Decongestant Antihistamine	Dry mouth Tachycardia Urinary retention Drowsiness	One tablet PO q.12h. PRN
Benylin DM syrup (dextromethorphan and ammonium chloride)	Antitussive Expectorant	Drowsiness (contains 5% ethanol by volume)	1–2 teaspoons q.4–6h. PRN
Contac cough and sore throat liquid (acetaminophen, dextromethorphan, and guaifenesin)	Antitussive Expectorant	Contains no ethanol Tachycardia	1–3 teaspoons q.4–6h. PRN
Benadryl (diphenhydramine)	Antihistamine	Drowsiness Dry mouth	25–50 mg PO q.6h. PRN
Hismanal (astemizole)	Antihistamine	Minimal drowsiness Dry mouth	10 mg PO q. A.M.

membranes. The initial exposure to the allergen will cause no mediator release and thus is asymptomatic. The next exposure, however, causes the release of IgE from lymphocytes, and the allergen cross-links with two IgE molecules on the mast cell surface to cause the mast cell to release the mediator, **histamine.** Histamine causes vasodilation and an increase in mucus production, the classic manifestations of allergic rhinitis.

1. The **allergens** can be any inhaled protein material but are commonly pollens, molds, dusts, hair, or danders. The specific time when the rhinitis occurs is pivotal in the diagnosis. Patients in whom disease occurs seasonally are likely to be allergic to pollens or molds. If manifestations occur in the spring or fall, the allergen is likely to be a pollen, whereas if manifestations occur in the summer, the allergen is likely to be a mold or dust. Finally, if manifestations are mainly at a specific site, e.g., at home or after obtaining a new animal, the likely allergen is a hair type, a dander, or a form of hair spray.

2. The **prevalence** of this disease is between 15% and 20% of the population in the United States. The **natural history** is one of recurrence of symptoms whenever the allergen is present.

C. Evaluation

The **evaluation** of this disorder includes the steps outlined in Box 12-5 and making the clinical diagnosis. Further evaluation entails referral to an allergist for skin testing.

Skin testing is not required for all patients. Specific **indications** for skin testing include a questionable history, young age, severe symptoms that significantly affect a patient's life, or when a specific allergen needs to be diagnosed and documented in order to optimize avoidance or attempt desensitization. The methods of skin testing are described below.

1. The **scratch test** is the first one performed. Very dilute extracts of various potential allergens are placed over individual superficial scratches in the skin. A **positive reaction** is the development of a local wheal and flare. If positive, the patient has an IgE-mediated response to that protein. If negative or equivocal, and the clinical suspicion for that substance as an allergen to the patient is still present, an intradermal test is necessary.

2. The **intradermal test** is more sensitive than the scratch test. The specific protein extract is placed intradermally. A positive reaction is a wheal and flare.

3. These tests have a small risk of precipitating a severe allergic/anaphylactic reaction and therefore must be

performed under the direction of a physician and with epinephrine readily available. Please refer to Table 4-1 for specifics in the management of anaphylaxis.

D. Management

   Specific management includes the following basic principles and modalities and can be based on the clinical diagnosis. Skin test confirmation is not necessary to initiate any of the following except desensitization.

   1. **Avoidance** of the allergens. This commonsense modality is effective but underutilized by patients with allergies.

      a. **Avoidance techniques** for allergens that mainly occur **outdoors,** such as pollens and molds, include the use of central air conditioning, changing all clothes and taking a shower before retiring each night, shutting the windows in the house as much as possible, and staying indoors as much as possible, especially on windy days when pollen counts are high.

      b. **Avoidance techniques** for allergens that mainly occur **indoors,** such as dust and mites, include installing a dehumidifier in the home, the installation and use of high-efficiency particle air cleaners, keeping the bed linen clean, and covering the mattress with a plastic sheet. If the allergen is due to a **household pet,** giving the pet away is truly effective.

   2. Prescribe **antihistamines.** These agents are quite effective in the treatment of atopic/allergic rhinitis.

      a. The **mechanism of action** of these agents involves competition for H_1 receptors on the target cells for histamine. Thus, histamine is still released from mast cells, but it is not allowed to act on its target cells in and about the upper respiratory mucosa. Therefore, it is important to give the agent before histamine is released, i.e., before exposure to the allergen has occurred.

      b. Many **agents** are available over the counter and via prescription. Some of these agents include **chlorpheniramine** and **diphenhydramine,** both which cause sedation as a significant **side effect,** and **astemizole,** which is available only by prescription and causes less sedation. (See Table 12-5 for specifics on agents, doses, and side effects.)

   3. Prescribe **decongestants.** These agents afford symptomatic relief of rhinorrhea.

      a. The **mechanism of action** of these agents involves α-adrenergic receptor agonism, resulting in local **vasoconstriction.**

b. These **agents,** which are all available in over-the-counter preparations, can be applied topically as nasal sprays or taken as oral agents. **Side effects** include tachycardia and, especially if the spray is overused for more than 3–4 consecutive days, a paradoxical exacerbation of the rhinitis, **rhinitis medicamentosa.** Therefore, these agents should be used for acute treatment and with caution by patients with hypertension or heart disease (see Table 12-5).

4. Prescribe **intranasal steroids.** These newer agents are now available by prescription and are quite effective in the treatment of allergic rhinitis.

a. The **mechanism of action** of these agents involves suppression of the release of mediators and thus, on a local level, prevention of IgE- and histamine-mediated responses.

b. A commonly used **agent** is **beclomethasone** (Beconase, Vancenase) in a dose of two puffs in each nostril b.i.d. These agents are effective when used on a chronic basis during the season when the allergen is present and are especially effective if started a week or two prior to the season. **Side effects** include mucosal atrophy and an increased risk of epistaxis.

III. Vasomotor rhinitis

A. Manifestations

The **specific manifestations** of this quite common form of rhinitis include the acute onset of unilateral or bilateral nasal edema and copious rhinorrhea that is acutely precipitated by specific odors or perfumes. Associated manifestations are the onset of watery eyes and, occasionally, a cough and scratchy throat. There virtually are never any concurrent fevers, dyspnea, or otalgia. The manifestations resolve rapidly when the inciting agent is removed from the environment.

B. Pathogenesis

The **underlying pathogenesis** is direct stimulation of the parasympathetic ganglia by the agent, which results, via a completely different mechanism from that of viral or atopic rhinitis, in local vascular dilation and rhinorrhea. The classic example is tear gas.

C. Evaluation

The **specific evaluation** includes making the clinical diagnosis, usually from the history alone.

D. Management

The **specific management** is not only straightforward and easy, but it is also effective: the patient must **avoid the**

inciting agent. No further evaluation or therapy is necessary.

E. **Consultation**

No consultations are required.

Sinus Disease

The **paranasal sinuses** are normal air-filled cavities in the facial and skull bones. They are variously sized, from the large maxillary sinuses to the tiny ethmoid sinuses. Although there is variation between individuals, there are normally two sinuses in the frontal bones, two in the maxillary bones, multiple small ones in the ethmoid bone, and one in the sphenoid bone. Each sinus is lined with respiratory mucosa and is connected to the nasal chamber and/or the nasopharynx by relatively small openings, or **meati.** Although many different disease processes can affect the paranasal sinuses, only **acute sinusitis** is described here.

I. **Pathogenesis**

The **underlying pathogenesis** of sinusitis relates to the anatomical communication of the sinuses with the ambient environment via relatively small-caliber passages in the nasopharynx. Thus, any process that affects the upper respiratory system in general and the nasopharynx in specific can result in sinus dysfunction. These structures can become infected by any viral or bacterial pathogens that have infected the other portions of the upper respiratory tract. Moreover, atopic disease can directly and indirectly affect them.

A. **Risk factors**

Specific **risk factors** for the development of acute sinusitis include (1) a **recent upper respiratory tract infection** or active atopic disease, both with resultant increased formation of mucus, direct effects on the sinus respiratory mucosa, and the potential for temporary sinus obstruction; and (2) a **history of trauma** or the presence of a foreign body, either of which can obstruct drainage and thus increase the risk of infection.

B. **Causative pathogens**

The bacterial **pathogens** that cause acute purulent sinusitis include *Streptococcus pneumoniae, Hemophilus influenzae,* and *Branhamella catarrhalis.*

II. **Overall manifestations**

The **overall manifestations** of acute sinusitis include the acute onset of nasal congestion, greenish yellow nasal discharge, unilateral or bilateral facial pain that is exacerbated by leaning forward, and fever. There invariably is an antecedent history of symptomatic viral or atopic rhinitis. Other manifestations are specific to the sinus involved and include the following.

A. Frontal sinusitis
Characterized by pain and tenderness to percussion over the lower forehead, unilaterally or bilaterally. There is opacification of the involved sinus on transillumination with a speculum. On nasal examination, purulent material drains from the **meatus in the middle nasal turbinate.**

B. Maxillary sinusitis
Characterized by pain and tenderness to percussion over the cheek bones, unilaterally or bilaterally. The pain is often referred to the ipsilateral maxillary teeth as a result of trigeminal innervation. There is opacification of the involved sinus on transillumination with a speculum. On nasal examination, purulent material drains from the **meatus in the middle nasal turbinate.**

C. Ethmoid sinusitis
Pain is present in the retro-orbital area with associated erythema and tenderness to percussion over the upper lateral nose. Transillumination of this sinus is impossible. On nasal examination, purulent material drains from the **meatus in the superior nasal turbinate,** although the superior turbinate is difficult to visualize.

D. Sphenoid sinusitis
This form of sinusitis is exceedingly rare unless concurrent with other sinusitides. The pain is present in the retro-orbital area with associated erythema and tenderness to percussion over the upper lateral nose. On nasal examination, purulent material drains from the **meatus in the superior nasal turbinate,** although the superior turbinate is difficult to visualize unless a nasopharyngoscope is used.

III. Evaluation
The **specific evaluation** includes making the clinical diagnosis using the basic techniques described in Box 12-6. Further evaluation is by radiography and CT.

A. Radiography
Sinus radiographs can be of use in acute sinusitis. The films must include the Waters view—a PA view of the head with the patient's eyes looking upward—as this view is excellent for demonstrating the maxillary sinus. Other views include the Caldwell view, an AP view of the head with the neck slightly flexed, and the Chamberlain–Towne view, which is excellent for demonstrating the frontal sinuses. Evidence of sinusitis on these radiographs includes the following findings:
1. Opacification of the involved sinus.

B O X   1 2 - 6

Overall Evaluation and Management of Acute Sinusitis

Evaluation

1. **Percuss** over the symptomatic sinus. If it is tender, inflammation is present.
2. Perform nasal examination with a speculum.
3. Consider obtaining radiographs of the sinuses, including the Caldwell and Waters views, looking for opacification or mucosal thickening (see text).

Management

1. Initiate **antibiotics,** either TMP–sulfa or amoxicillin (see text).
2. Initiate a decongestant (see text).
3. If the process is recurrent or the patient is immunocompromised, referral to ENT and/or head CT are indicated.

---

    2. Air–fluid levels within the sinus.

    3. Abnormally thick mucosa (i.e., >5 mm).

  B. CT

    CT of the sinuses is rarely required in the acute setting, but if there is any evidence of complications, or if the disease process is recurrent, or if the host is an immunocompromised host, this is the optimal imaging modality to visualize the sinuses for any underlying anatomic defect.

  C. Radionuclide scintigraphy

    Bone and gallium scans are obtained if there is any suspicion of the complication, Pott's puffy tumor. The scans are quite intense in the affected area, with gallium uptake greater than uptake in the bone scan.

  D. Complications

    The **evaluation** and **definitions** of specific **complications** include the development of **osteomyelitis** of the frontal bone, sometimes referred to as Pott's puffy tumor, in which the patient has fever, pain, swelling over the frontal bone, an increased ESR, and bone and gallium scans consistent with osteomyelitis (i.e., showing increased uptake). A further complication is **orbital cellulitis:** the patient presents with ptosis, eyelid edema, proptosis, conjunctivitis, and decreased range of motion of the extraocular musculature. This can rapidly progress and lead to erysipelas and death if not treated. Finally, the most dramatic complication is **cavernous sinus thrombosis,** manifested by unilateral lid edema, ptosis, proptosis, and palsies of cranial nerves III, IV, and VI.

IV. **Management**

The **specific management** includes antibiotics, decongestants, antihistamines, and monitoring for the development of any complications. The **antibiotics** should be a 14-day course of one of the following: either amoxicillin, 500 mg PO t.i.d., or TMP–sulfa (Bactrim DS), 1 tablet PO b.i.d., or Ceftin (a second-generation cephalosporin), 500 mg PO b.i.d., or Ciprofloxacin, 250–500 mg b.i.d., or Augmentin, 250 mg PO t.i.d. The use of a **decongestant** on a short-term basis to decrease mucus production and to decrease any swelling and obstruction about the meatus is useful. An **antihistamine** is of benefit if there is any evidence of allergic rhinitis. The antihistamine can be used acutely or on a chronic prophylactic basis (see Table 12-5). If there is any evidence of **complications,** the patient will require emergent consultation with ENT and infectious disease colleagues and admission to the hospital for parenteral antibiotics and surgical drainage of the involved sinus.

V. **Consultation**

Problem	Service	Time
Any complication	ENT	Emergent
Recurrent disease	ENT	Elective
Complication	Infectious diseases	Urgent

VI. **Indications for admission:** the development of any complication of acute sinusitis, or sinusitis occurring in an immunosuppressed host.

Bibliography

Epistaxis

Juselius H: Epistaxis: A clinical study of 1724 patients. J Laryngol Otol 1974;88:317–327.

Kirchner JA: Epistaxis. N Engl J Med 1982;307:1126.

Randal DA, Freeman SB: Management of anterior and posterior epistaxis. Am Fam Pract 1991;2007–2014.

Oral Diseases

Herr RD, et al: Serious soft tissue infections of the head and neck. Am Fam Pract 1991;44:878–888.

Hubbard TM: Periodontal disease and the family physician. Am Fam Pract 1991;44:487–491.

Johnson WT: Managing odontogenic infections. Am Fam Pract 1984;29:167–172.

Morse DR, et al: Infectious flare-ups and serious sequelae following endodontic treatment: A prospective randomized trial on efficacy of antibiotic prophylaxis in cases of asymptomatic pulpal-periapical lesions. Oral Surg Oral Med Oral Path 1987;64:96–109.

Otalgia/Otitis

Bluestone CD: Otitis media in children: To treat or not to treat. N Engl J Med 1982;306:1399.

Eichenwald H: Developments in diagnosing and treating otitis media. Am Fam Prac 1985;31:155–164.

Pharyngitis

Bisno AL: Group A streptococcal infections and acute rheumatic fever. N Engl J Med 1991;325:783–793.

Brandfonbrener A, et al: Corticosteroid therapy in Epstein-Barr virus infection. Arch Intern Med 1986;146:337–339.

Centor RM, et al: Throat cultures and rapid tests for diagnosis of Group A streptococcal pharyngitis. Ann Intern Med 1986;105:892–899.

Murray BJ: Medical complications of infectious mononucleosis. Am Fam Pract 1984;30:195–199.

Raz R, Bitnun S: Dilemmas in streptococcal pharyngitis. Am Fam Pract 1987;35:187–192.

Rhinitis

Demichiei ME, Nelson L: Allergic rhinitis. Am Fam Pract 1988;37:251–263.

Druce HM, Kaliner MA: Allergic rhinitis. JAMA 1988;259:260–263.

Gwaltney JM Jr, et al: Symposium on rhinovirus pathogenesis: Summary. Acta Otolaryngol 1984;413(S):43–45.

Sinus Disease

Axelson A, Brorson JE: The correlation between bacteriological findings in the nose and maxillary sinus in acute maxillary sinusitis. Laryngoscope 1973;83:2003.

Evans FW, et al: Sinusitis of the maxillary sinus antrum. N Engl J Med 1975;29:3735.

Stool SE: Diagnosis and treatment of sinusitis. Am Fam Pract 1985;32:101–107.

—D.D.B.

Dale Berg, Ed. *Handbook of Primary Care Medicine.* Copyright © 1993 J. B. Lippincott Company.

CHAPTER 13

Ophthalmology

Acute Blindness

The **definitions** of various types of blindness include the following. Only monocular blindness will be discussed in greater detail later in this section.

Monocular denotes the complete loss of visual function of one eye, usually with dramatic results. Invariably the patient seeks immediate medical attention.

Visual field deficits

Hemianopsia is the acute or insidious onset of blindness in one half of each visual field. There are three different types of hemianopsia.

1. **Homonymous hemianopsia.** The blindness is in the **same half of both fields,** right or left. This is invariably as the result of a lesion in the contralateral optic tract.
2. **Heteronymous hemianopsia.** The blindness is in **opposite halves of both fields.** There are two types of heteronymous hemianopsia.
   a. **Bitemporal hemianopsia.** The outer (temporal) halves of both fields are blind. This is usually as the result of a pituitary tumor.
   b. **Binasal hemianopsia.** The inner (nasal) half or halves of one or both fields are blind. Quite rare and usually unilateral.
3. **Quadrantic hemianopsia.** A quarter of the visual field is blind. Usually as the result of a lesion in the contralateral occipital or temporal cerebral cortex. Recall that the optic radiation passes through the temporal lobe en route to the occipital cortex.

   ## I. Monocular blindness

   This quite dramatic loss of visual function in one eye is a medical and ophthalmologic emergency in which the patient must have aggressive and immediate evaluation and management. The causes of this process are quite diverse and are as follows.

A. Retinal detachment

1. Manifestations

The **specific manifestations** of this entity include an acute onset of monocular blindness. The patient reports the acute onset of blurred or blackened vision that over several hours progresses to complete or partial monocular blindness. The **classic description** is of a curtain being drawn over the visual field from top to bottom. The patient usually senses "floaters" and flashing lights before and at the initiation of the symptom complex. There are no concurrent pain, erythema, or conjunctival injection. **Funduscopic examination** reveals an area of the retina detached and flapping in the vitreous humor.

2. Pathogenesis

The **underlying pathogenesis** is a tear in the retina with the resultant production of "floaters." Once a tear occurs, the vitreous crosses behind the retina with a progression of the retinal detachment. The **tear** usually begins at the **superior temporal retinal area.**

Although it can happen spontaneously, certain **risk factors** for its development include **extreme myopia** as the result of an elongated eyeball length, **recent trauma** to the affected eye, and a **history** of retinal detachment.

3. Evaluation

The **specific evaluation** includes making the clinical diagnosis by performing the tests described in Box 13-1.

4. Management

The **specific management** is to obtain an emergency ophthalmology consultation, preferably with an expert in laser treatment. The patient should remain supine with the head turned to the side ipsilateral to the retinal detachment. Emergency laser or cryosurgery is indicated.

B. Central retinal vein occlusion

1. Manifestations

The **specific manifestations** of this entity include the acute onset of complete loss of vision in one eye. The loss of vision is painless. There usually are no associated prodromal symptoms. On examination, the only abnormality is a markedly edematous retina with multiple hemorrhages and dilated, tortuous veins, classically referred to as the **"blood and thunder"** appearance.

B O X   1 3 - 1

Basic Ophthalmologic Examination

1. History, including any recent exposure to agents or recent trauma.
2. Inspection of the orbits and eyes themselves, looking for any gross abnormalities, the presence of proptosis, ptosis, conjunctival injection, and/or foreign bodies in the eyes or in the palpebral surfaces.
3. Examination of the extraocular musculature.
4. Examination of the **pupillary reflex** to direct and consensual light and to accommodation.
5. If acute (closed) angle glaucoma is clinically suspected, estimate the intraocular pressure via applanation or Shiotz tonometry.
6. Visual acuity with and without refraction using the **Snellen chart,** in left eye (OS) and right eye (OD).
7. **Visual field examination** via confrontation.
8. Perform a **slit lamp** examination of the cornea, conjunctiva, and anterior chamber structures. The slit lamp examination is integral to all ophthalmologic examinations.
9. Apply **fluorescein dye** to the affected eye. The application procedure entails first applying a topical anesthetic to the eye (Table 13-1), then applying 2 drops of fluorescein to the inferior palpebral conjunctiva. The patient is then instructed to close the eye for 10 to 15 seconds and then open it for irrigation with sterile saline solution. The eye is then examined using a UV-light (e.g., a Wood's lamp). In the normal setting, no dye should be taken up by the cornea. If there is any uptake by the cornea, as manifested by a fluorescent green color, pathology is present.
10. Funduscopic examination. If any suspicion of acute glaucoma, should not use mydriatic agents.
11. Any suspected pathology mandates an **emergent referral** to an ophthalmologist.

2. **Pathogenesis**

The **underlying pathogenesis** is occlusion of the central retinal vein, often as the result of long standing **uncontrolled systemic hypertension.** Occlusion of the central retinal vein markedly impedes venous drainage from the retina, thereby increasing venous

TABLE 13-1
Ophthalmic Agents

Agent	Indications	Contraindications	Side Effects	Dosage
Timolol (Timoptic) (0.25% and 0.5% solutions)	Open angle glaucoma	Bronchospasm Left ventricular heart failure 2nd or 3rd degree AV block	Wheezing	1 drop of 0.25% solution b.i.d. OU, then increased to 1 drop of 0.5% solution b.i.d. OU, titrating to IOP.
Pilocarpine (Isotocarpine) (0.5%, 1%, 2%, 3%, 4%, and 6% solutions)	Open angle glaucoma Miotic agent	Allergy to agent	Rare	2 drops of the 1% to 4% solution in affected eye(s) b.i.d. to t.i.d., titrate the concn. of solution to the target IOP
Gentamicin (Garamycin) Ointment: 0.3% Solution: 0.3%	Dacrocystitis Hordeolum Conjunctivitis Keratitis	Allergy to agent	Rare	Ointment: apply b.i.d. to t.i.d. Solution: 1 drop q.4h.
Tobramycin (Tobrex) Solution: 0.3%	Dacrocystitis Hordeolum Conjunctivitis Keratitis	Allergy to agent	Rare	Ointment: apply b.i.d. to t.i.d. Solution: 1 drop 1.4h.
Sulfacetamide (Sulamyd) Ointment: 10% Solution: 10%, 30%	Hordeolum Conjunctivitis Keratitis Trachoma*	Allergy to agent	Rare	Ointment: apply 1–2 cm ribbon q.i.d. and q.H.S. Solution: 2 drops of the 10%–30% solution into the lower conjunctival sac q.2–3h. and q.H.S. for 5 days
Erythromycin (Ilocytin) 0.5% ointment	Conjunctivitis Trachoma*	Allergy	Rare	0.5–1.0 cm ribbon of ointment into the conjunctival sacs of the affected eye(s) q.d. or b.i.d. for 5 days

Drug	Indication	Contraindications	Side Effects	Dosage
Dexamethasone (0.1% solution)	Steroid-responsive keratitis, uveitis, conjunctivitis	HSV infections Fungal infections Viral infections	Posterior subcapsular cataracts Rupture of the globe	Should be used under direct interaction with ophthalmology
Cromolyn sodium (Opticrom 4% solution)	Atopic conjunctivitis	Allergy to agent Soft contact lenses	Rare	1–2 drops 4–6 times per day, OU
Naphcon-A (naphazoline and pheniramine) solution	Atopic conjunctivitis	Allergy to agent	Rare	1–2 drops q.4–6h. OU
Isoptotears (methylcellulose) Solution: 0.5% and 1.0%	Dry eyes	Allergy to agent	Rare	2 drops q.4–6h. PRN
Tropicamide (Mydriacyl) Solution: 1%	Mydriatic, for examination	Allergy to agent Acute (closed) angle glaucoma	Photophobia and blurred vision, acutely	1–2 drops in eye to be examined
Cyclopentolate (cyclogyl) Solution: 0.5% and 1%	Actinic keratitis	Allergy Acute (closed) angle glaucoma	Rare	2 drops OU q.6h.
Proparacaine (0.5% solution)	Topical anesthetic; lasts 15 minutes	Allergy to agent	Rare	2 drops in eye to be examined 1 min before exam
Idoxuridine (0.1% solution)	Antiviral	Allergy to agent	Rare	1 drop in affected eye q. 1–2 h. for 5–7 days. Use only under direction of an ophthalmologist

*If trachoma is suspected, the treatment includes antibiotic eyedrops, systemic antibiotics, referral to an ophthalmologist, and reporting of the case to Public Health (see page 675).

pressure in the retina, the exudation of fluids from the venous system, retinal edema, and venous dilation. The pressure can be increased to such a level as to cause arterial retinal hypoperfusion and ischemia.

3. **Evaluation and management**

The **specific evaluation** includes making the clinical diagnosis by performing the tests described in Box 13-1. The **specific management** is to obtain an emergent ophthalmology consultation.

C. **Central retinal artery occlusion**

1. **Manifestations**

The **specific manifestations** of this entity include the acute onset of monocular painless blindness. The patient usually has other sequelae of arterial thromboembolic disease in the past including CVAs and/or a past history of atrial fibrillation and/or left ventricular failure. The **funduscopic examination** reveals the presence of a cherry red spot in the macula, an optic disc which is pale relative to surrounding retinal tissue, and, when compared with the contralateral eye, the presence of retinal arteries which are significantly decreased in size. Furthermore, there is classically a "box car" appearance in the retinal veins.

2. **Pathogenesis**

The **underlying pathogenesis** is one of occlusion of the central retinal artery with resultant ischemia and infarction of the retina. This usually is as the result of an arterial thromboembolic event. The risk factors for the development of this entity include anything associated with thrombus formation in the left heart, e.g., atrial fibrillation, left-sided endocarditis, atrial enlargement, and/or plaques in the carotid artery. Of note is the fact that these are the same risk factors for ischemic embolic cerebrovascular accidents.

3. **Evaluation and management**

The **specific evaluation** includes making the clinical diagnosis by performing the tests described in Box 13-1. The **specific management** is to obtain an emergent ophthalmology consultation. Clearly, **anticoagulation with heparin** must be strongly considered. The dosage, goals, and management are quite similar to that for an ischemic embolic CVA (see section on Cerebrovascular Accidents, Chapter 14, page 683, for further discussion).

D. **Acute (narrow angle) glaucoma**

See section on Red, Inflamed Eye, page 661.

E. Temporal arteritis

1. Manifestations

The **specific manifestations** of this entity include an acute onset of painless, monocular blindness. The blindness is quite often associated with a concurrent or antecedent history of generalized, predominantly proximal muscle weakness, unilateral or bilateral jaw claudication upon mastication (chewing), and a recurrent unilateral throbbing headache ipsilateral to the affected eye. On **examination** the eye, including the fundus, is usually quite remarkable. There usually is tenderness to palpation over the ipsilateral temporal artery and objective moderate muscle weakness, greater proximally than distally.

2. Pathogenesis

The **underlying pathogenesis** is one of a systemic granulomatous vasculitis of the middle-sized arteries, especially branches of the external carotid artery.

3. Evaluation

The **specific evaluation** includes making the clinical diagnosis by performing the tests described in Box 13-1. Furthermore, an erythrocyte sedimentation rate (ESR) and biopsy of the temporal artery are indicated. The ESR will be markedly elevated, at times >100 minutes, and the biopsy will show the arterial vasculitis. Due to the fact that the results of these tests/procedures will take at least several hours to return, if this entity is clinically suspected, emergency empirical therapy with steroids is clearly indicated.

4. Management

The treatment regimen consists of **prednisone, 60 mg PO stat**, then 40–60 mg PO q.d. The dose is slowly tapered to 10–15 mg PO q.d. for the next 18–24 months, at which time further tapering is attempted. Weaning from steroids is titrated to the manifestations of weakness, blindness, and the ESR. Consultations with ophthalmology, ENT, and rheumatology at presentation are indicated.

F. Trauma

1. Manifestations

The **specific manifestations** of this entity include a marked decrease in vision after an episode of significant blunt and/or invasive trauma to the eye. Upon examination, the damage is usually quite evident upon inspection and can range from a retinal detachment to enucleation, a penetrating foreign body, or a hyphema (i.e., the presence of blood in the anterior chamber).

2. **Evaluation and management**

   The **specific evaluation and management** include making the clinical diagnosis by performing the tests described in Box 13-1. Emergency referral to ophthalmology is clearly indicated.

II. Consultation

Problem	Service	Time
Any monocular blindness	Ophthalmology	Emergent
Any visual field blindness	Ophthalmology	Emergent
Homonymous hemianopsia	Radiology, for head CT	Urgent
Temporal arteritis	Rheumatology	Urgent

III. **Indications for admission:** Monocular blindness, evidence of penetrating trauma to the eye, or any new visual field cut.

Cataracts

As the human lens ages, there are changes which, over a period of time, will result in the development of opacities. These acquired **lenticular opacities,** which are termed **cataracts,** can and do progressively worsen until the patient has significant visual impairment. There are two major types of cataracts, the **nuclear** cataract and the **posterior subcapsular** cataract. Each of these is discussed below.

I. Types of cataracts

A. Nuclear cataracts

1. **Manifestations**

   The **specific manifestations** include the insidious onset of decreased vision. The patient often reports that the visual acuity for **far** vision is affected more than for **near** vision. Upon **examination,** there is a translucent yellow discoloration in the center or nucleus of the lens. This can actually impede the ability of the examiner to visualize the fundus. One lens may be affected more than the other. The visual acuity will be objectively decreased.

2. **Pathogenesis**

   The **underlying pathogenesis** is one in which, with increasing age, the center of the lens changes from its **transparent** baseline to a **translucent** yellowish color. The major and irreversible **risk factor** for development is **increasing age:** virtually everyone over age 70 has a component of a nuclear cataract. Other, more preventable or reversible risk factors include exposure to ultraviolet light and potentially the cholesterol-lowering agent, lovastatin.

B. **Posterior subcapsular cataracts**

1. **Manifestations**

The **specific manifestations** include the insidious onset of decreased vision. The patient often reports that the visual acuity for **near** vision is affected more than for **far** vision. Upon **examination,** there is a translucent yellow discoloration in the central portion of the posterior capsule of the lens, i.e., it is located in the posterocentral aspect of the lens. This can actually impede the ability of the examiner to visualize the fundus. One lens can be affected more than the other. The visual acuity will be objectively decreased. These cataracts occur in a younger population than the nuclear cataracts.

2. **Pathogenesis**

The **underlying pathogenesis** has been postulated to be as the result of chronic abnormally increased amounts of glucose within the lens itself. The increased amounts of glucose are catabolized via an alternate pathway, using the enzyme **aldose reductase,** to the molecule **sorbitol.** Sorbitol is quite osmotically active and increases the water in the lens, making it less transparent. The **risk factors** for development are disease processes or states that result in hyperglycemia—i.e., diabetes mellitus, Cushing's syndrome, and the chronic use of glucocorticoids.

II. **Evaluation and management**

The **specific evaluation and management** of a patient with a cataract include making the diagnosis by the examination techniques described in Box 13-1. The **specific management** is referral to an ophthalmologist for surgical intervention. The surgical procedures performed are included here for the purposes of edification.

A. **Surgical intervention**

All surgical procedures are performed under local anesthesia and with mild sedation, and virtually all can be performed on an outpatient basis. There are two types of cataract surgery, **intracapsular** or **extracapsular** extractions of the cataract.

1. **Intracapsular extraction.** The entire lens is removed in one piece. Best procedure for the treatment of posterior subcapsular cataracts.

    2. Extracapsular extraction. The capsule is opened, the contents are removed, and the posterior capsule remains. Best procedure for nuclear cataracts.

Either procedure requires 6–8 weeks of **postoperative eye rehabilitation.** Rehabilitation includes the use of contact lenses or the use of intraocular implants. Intraocular implants are the rehabilitation modality of choice and must be placed at the time of surgery.

III. Consultation

Service	Time
Ophthalmology	Required

IV. Indications for admission: None.

Diabetic Retinopathy

This is a very common sequela of diabetes mellitus. It occurs in association with either **insulin-dependent** diabetes mellitus or **non-insulin-dependent** diabetes mellitus.

I. Overall manifestations
The **overall manifestations** include the insidious onset of progressive decrease in visual acuity which is painless and, until quite significant, unknown to the patient.

II. Pathogenesis
The **underlying pathogenesis** is unknown but has been postulated to be, through an unknown mechanism, a direct or indirect result of **hyperglycemia.**

III. Types
There are **two major types** of diabetes-related retinopathy, each of which has significant overlap with the other: nonproliferative retinopathy and proliferative retinopathy.
A. Nonproliferative
1. Manifestations
The **specific manifestations** include the insidious onset of decreased visual acuity. The acuity can suddenly deteriorate if there is involvement of the macula, at which time central vision is affected, and/or if bleeding into the vitreous body occurs. On **examination** there is, early in the course of disease, little to no impairment of visual acuity but, late in the course, significant impairment in the visual acuity. **Funduscopy** discloses the characteristic lesion of this group, microaneurysms. The microaneurysms result in leakage of material from the capillaries around the aneurysm into the adjacent retinal tissue

with resultant localized retinal edema. This localized retinal edema can be demonstrated on funduscopic examination as the manifestations of **retinal thickening** and **"hard exudates."**

2. **Evaluation**

   The **specific evaluation** is to make the clinical diagnosis using the examinations described in Box 13-1.

3. **Management**

   The **specific management** is to diagnose early via **screening** in all patients with diabetes.

   a. Optimize glycemic control.

   b. Once diagnosed, **laser therapy** is clearly indicated. The ophthalmologist uses the laser to stabilize the areas adjacent to the microaneurysms and prevent further deterioration. To underscore the need for early diagnosis is the fact that laser therapy is only useful in stabilizing the defects and thus in preventing damage; once present, the damage is irreversible.

B. Proliferative

1. **Manifestations**

   The **specific manifestations** include the insidious onset of decreased visual acuity. The acuity can suddenly deteriorate if and when there is bleeding into the vitreous body and/or a retinal detachment occurs. On **examination** there is, early in the course of disease, little to no impairment of visual acuity but, late in the course, significant impairment in the visual acuity. **Funduscopy** discloses the characteristic lesion of this group, retinal **neovascularization.** New vessels form in the retina, each of which is inordinately fragile and easily bleeds. This hemorrhage is into the normally clear vitreous body.

2. **Evaluation**

   The **specific evaluation** is to make the clinical diagnosis using the examinations described in Box 13-1.

3. **Management**

   The **specific management** is to diagnose early via **screening** in all patients with diabetes.

   a. Optimize the glycemic control.

   b. Once diagnosed, **laser photocoagulation** is clearly indicated. The ophthalmologist uses the laser to photocoagulate entire areas of the retina, which results in regression of the neovascular structures and the prevention of the bleeding sequelae. To underscore the need for early diagnosis is the fact that laser therapy is only useful in stabilizing the defects and thus in preventing damage; once present, the damage is irreversible.

IV. **Screening**
    Screening should be performed with **yearly** detailed fun-
    duscopic examinations by an ophthalmologist on all of the
    following patients:
    1. All **type II** patients at the time of presentation.
    2. All **type I** patients 4–5 years after diagnosis or at the
       time of presentation if nephropathy is present.

V. **Consultation**

Problem	*Service*	*Time*
Screening	Ophthalmology	Required
Acute bleed	Ophthalmology	Emergent

VI. **Indications for admission:** None.

Open Angle Glaucoma

This is a disease process which is not uncommon. It is a process
which affects **2%–3% of the population** and is asymptomatic until
advanced and irreversible damage to the visual fields has already
occurred. Although the disease shares the same name with acute
angle glaucoma and both processes have an increased IOP and, if
untreated, will lead to blindness, they have very few similarities.

I. **Manifestations**
   The **specific manifestations** of open angle glaucoma are
   quite different from acute angle glaucoma (see section on
   Red Inflamed Eye, page 661, for manifestations of acute
   angle glaucoma). They include an insidious onset of progressively deteriorating visual acuity which remains minimally symptomatic or even asymptomatic until late in the
   course of disease. There is no associated pain or redness or
   excessive watering of the eyes.
       Early in the course of disease, there are no signs, except
   for the presence of a modestly elevated IOP. Funduscopic
   and visual field examinations are quite normal.
       Late in the course, the IOP remains modestly elevated
   and, upon **funduscopic examination,** the optic cup can abnormally enlarge and deepen. Furthermore, the **visual
   fields** become constricted with loss of the temporal aspects
   of the visual field(s) first.

II. **Pathogenesis**
    The **underlying pathogenesis** of the increased IOP in open
    angle glaucoma is **unclear.** Irrespective of the mechanism,
    the increased IOP results in damage to the **optic nerve head**
    via pressure-induced enlargement of the optic cup. The in-
    creased pressure can also result in ischemia to the retina

and optic nerve and a decrease in neuronal transport flow down the dendrites and axons which comprise the optic nerve. Both of these result in the loss of axons, dendrites, and neurons in and about the optic nerve and the macula. The loss of function in the macula is temporal to nasal. Thus the increased IOP damages both the **macula** and the **optic nerve head.**

Risk factors for the development of this disease include increasing age, a family history of open angle glaucoma, male sex, African American heritage, and a past or present history of atherosclerotic heart disease or diabetes mellitus.

III. **Evaluation and management**

The **specific evaluation and management** include that described in Box 13-1 and performing **effective screening.**

A. **Screening**

This is a disease process which begs for **screening.** There is a long period of time of subclinical disease that, if untreated, results in severe visual impairment, and there are effective and relatively simple treatment modalities which prevent the development of this visual sequela. The screening techniques used include the fairly sensitive, inexpensive, and simple **Schiotz tonometry** technique (see Box 13-2) and the highly sensitive, advanced, and more expensive **direct applanation** technique. Applanation tonometry is more sensitive, and for the **purposes of screening** it is the procedure of choice.

1. **Screening** should begin at age 40 to obtain a baseline reading. Screening should be every 2–3 years until age 65–70 years, at which time the screening should be continued on an annual basis. Screening can be via either technique.

2. Normal IOP has a **mean value of 15 mm Hg,** with a range of 10–20 mm Hg.

3. If the **IOP is elevated,** i.e., >21 mm Hg, refer to an ophthalmologist for confirmation with applanation measurement. Concurrently, visual field assessment and extensive funduscopic examination are indicated.

B. **Treatment for open angle glaucoma**

1. **Topical β-blockers.** Timolol (Timoptic) solution is, unless contraindications to its use are present, a first-line agent in the therapy of open angle glaucoma. See Table 13-1 for specifics on the agent, its contraindications, and dosage.

2. **Acetazolamide (Diamox).** This carbonic anhydrase inhibitor is an effective agent in decreasing IOP by decreasing aqueous humor production. It is a second-line agent due to the fact that it has a number

B O X   1 3 - 2

Procedure to Use the Schiotz Tonometer

The tonometer comes with four different plunger mass sizes: 5.5 g, 7.5 g, 10 g, and 15 g. The higher the IOP, the greater the plunger mass size necessary to make an adequate measurement.

1. Apply local anesthetic to the eye (see Table 13-1 for a specific anesthetic agent).
2. Tell the patient the procedure.
3. Place the patient supine; open eyelid of patient.
4. Place the instrument on the cornea perpendicular to the cornea itself.
5. There should be mild denting of the cornea, increase the plunger weight until the cornea is mildly indented by the instrument. A Schiotz number of >4 indicates correct plunger weight and thus appropriate indentation. If the Schiotz number is <4, increase the plunger mass size to the next size.
6. Use the **conversion table** to determine IOP. The table is included with the tonometer.

$x : y$ z

The pair of coordinates x and y determine the value of z:

x = Schiotz number on the tonometer,
y = plunger weight,
z = IOP in mm Hg.

---

of potentially significant side effects including fatigue, the development of a normal anion gap metabolic acidosis, and the development of calcium nephrolithiasis. The dosage of acetazolamide (Diamox) is 250 mg PO 1–4 times per day.

3. **Surgical intervention.** Referral to ophthalmology for an elective laser trabeculoplasty/iridectomy using an Nd:YAG laser or an argon laser. The iridectomy forms a communication between the anterior and posterior chambers and, when performed in both eyes, is curative. This is an outpatient procedure.

IV. **Consultation**

Problem	*Service*	*Time*
All cases of increased IOP	Ophthalmology	Required

V. **Indications for admission:** None.

Red Inflamed Eye, Unilateral or Bilateral

This is not only one of the most common problems which people in day to day life develop, it is also a common reason for patients to contact a primary care physician. The overall evaluation is described in Box 13-1, the overall ophthalmologic examination.

I. **Hordeolum**

A. **Manifestations**

The **specific manifestations** of this entity include the acute onset of pain and swelling in the eyelid with increased tearing and redness in the involved eye. On examination there is a palpable, indurated area in the involved eyelid, which on visual inspection has a central area of purulence with surrounding erythema. Furthermore, there invariably is erythema in the adjacent conjunctiva. Further, quite uncommon manifestations can include redness and swelling in the periorbital area and the development of fevers and chills.

B. **Pathogenesis**

The **underlying pathogenesis** of this quite common problem is the acute development of a small abscess within a gland in the upper or lower eyelid of one eye.

1. There are two basic types of hordeola, internal and external.

   a. **Internal hordeola** are **deep from the palpebral margin** and are due to inflammation and infection of a Meibomian gland, with abscess formation in that gland.

   b. **External hordeola** are immediately adjacent to the **edge of the palpebral margin** and are as the result of inflammation and infection of the glands of Moll or Zeis, with abscess formation in one of these glands. This type of hordeolum is colloquially referred to as a **sty.**

2. The usual **pathogen** for either one of these two entities is the gram-positive coccus, ***Staphylococcus aureus.***

C. **Evaluation**

The **specific evaluation** includes making the clinical diagnosis using the information described above and the examination described in Box 13-1.

D. **Management**
   1. Apply **warm compresses** to the affected eye for 48 hours.
   2. Apply **topical antibiotics** for 5–7 days. Any of the topical drops are effective. See Table 13-1 for specific agents and dosage.
   3. If there is any evidence of concurrent **cellulitis,** systemic antibiotics are indicated. **Specific agents** include cephalexin (Keflex), 500 mg PO q.i.d. for 7 days, or dicloxicillin, 500 mg PO q.i.d. for 7 days.
   4. If there is no improvement in 48 hours, referral to ophthalmology for I&D of the hordeolum is indicated.

II. **Chalazion**
   A. **Manifestations**
      The **specific manifestations** of this entity include the presence of a painless, indurated lesion deep from the palpebral margin. This lesion may be present for months and be of only minimal concern to the patient. When symptoms are present, as they can be on an intermittent, recurrent basis, they include pruritus and redness of the involved eye and eyelid. The patient can usually recall having an internal hordeolum affecting the same eyelid in the past.
   B. **Pathogenesis**
      The **underlying pathogenesis** is chronic inflammation of an internal hordeolum involving the Meibomian gland. The chronic inflammation often becomes microscopically granulomatous but is invariably **noninfectious.** An internal hordeolum often antedates the development of a chalazion.
   C. **Evaluation**
      The **specific evaluation** includes making the clinical diagnosis using the information described above and the examination described in Box 13-1.
   D. **Management**
      Referral to an ophthalmologist for elective excision of the lesion is indicated. No further acute intervention is necessary.

III. **Blepharitis**
   A. **Manifestations**
      The **specific manifestations** of this quite common condition include **erythema** and **scale formation** on one or both eyelids. The manifestations begin and are most evident at the margin of the eyelids, involving the skin immediately adjacent to the eyelashes. There can be

some mild associated pruritus and conjunctival erythema, but virtually never any pain, edema, or fevers.

B. Pathogenesis

The **underlying pathogenesis** is an infectious or noninfectious inflammation of the palpebral edge. The inflammation is self-limited and mild. It does not progress
to a serious local or systemic process.

1. The **infectious etiology** results from superficial infection with *Staphylococcus aureus.* Unique manifestations of this cause include superficial ulcerations
   of the skin adjacent to the palpebral edge and concurrent mild to moderate conjunctivitis in the affected eye.

2. The **noninfectious etiology** results from a localized
   form of **seborrheic dermatitis.** Unique manifestations of this cause include bilateral erythema of the
   eyelid margins, with **greasy scales** present. The conjunctivitis, if present, is quite mild.

C. Evaluation

The **specific evaluation** includes making the clinical diagnosis using the information described above and the
examination described in Box 13-1.

D. Management

Specific management includes removal of the scales
and gentle scrubbing of the eyelid margins with a **moist-
ened cotton-tipped applicator** each morning, followed
immediately by application of a **topical antibiotic in
ointment form** to the eyelid margins b.i.d. for 7 days.
The solution used to moisten the cotton-tipped applicator may be tap water or baby shampoo diluted by volume 50% with tap water. See Table 13-1 for a list of the
topical antibiotics available. Consultations are rarely
necessary.

IV. Acute dacrocystitis

A. Manifestations

The **specific manifestations** of this relatively infrequent
disorder include an acute onset of unilateral pain in the
medial canthal region of the affected eye. There invariably are tenderness and warmth in the medial canthal
area and, occasionally, **purulent** discharge from the area
about the medial canthus area. There invariably are
mild to moderate conjunctivitis and a significant increase in tearing in the affected eye **(epiphora).** The
tears from the affected eye overflow.

B. Pathogenesis

The **underlying pathogenesis** is partial or total obstruction of the **nasolacrimal duct,** which then becomes sec-

ondarily infected. The nasolacrimal duct is located in the extreme lateral aspect of the medial superficial eye structures. Its orifice is in the **medial canthal area.** This duct, in the normal state, drains tears from the eye into the nasal structures.

1. **Risk factors** for the development of nasolacrimal duct obstruction and therefore of dacrocystis include **trauma** to the area, **recurrent atopic disease,** and a history of **infections** involving the area. Although there usually is an underlying reason for nasolacrimal obstruction, in some cases, especially in young children, there is a converse pathogenesis, i.e., the infection is primary with the secondary development of nasolacrimal obstruction.

2. Causative agents include the bacteria *Staphylococcus aureus, Streptococcus pneumoniae,* and the Group A streptococci.

3. **Natural history.** The process can evolve into a facial cellulitis. Furthermore, even in cases that are self-limited or effectively treated in the acute setting, there may be **scarring** of the nasolacrimal duct, which increases the likelihood of recurrence.

C. **Evaluation**

The **specific evaluation** includes making the clinical diagnosis using the information described above and the examination described in Box 13-1. Further **specific evaluation** includes performing a Gram stain and culture on any purulent discharge obtained, and clinical examination of the entire HEENT system.

D. **Management**

1. Initiate **systemic antibiotics. Specific agents** can include cephalexin (Keflex), 500 mg PO q.i.d. for 7 days, or dicloxicillin, 500 mg PO q.i.d. for 7 days, or erythromycin, 500 mg PO q.i.d. for 7 days.

2. **Topical antibiotics** in the form of **drops** can be useful as adjuvant therapy but do not replace systemic antibiotics. See Table 13-1 for specific agents and dosing schemae.

3. Referral to an **ophthalmologist** on an urgent basis is indicated for I&D of any pocket of adjacent pus and to relieve the obstruction surgically.

V. **Uveitis**

This is the **nonspecific inflammation** of any and potentially all intraocular structures. The inflammation, which can be due to a diverse array of diagnoses, can affect any structure within the eye, i.e., the iris, the ciliary body, or the choroid. This inflammatory process can be very severe and, if untreated, can lead to blindness. This process can be the result of a wide variety of underlying diseases and have a quite diverse set of disease manifestations.

A. **Classification**

As a result of these facts, several **classification models** have been developed. The classification of these disorders is either by **location** of the inflammation or by **type of precipitant** causing the inflammation.

1. The classification by **location,** as used by the Uveitis Study Group, divides uveitis into **anterior,** i.e., inflammation of the anterior chamber and adjacent structures; **intermediate,** i.e., inflammation of the vitreous humor; and **posterior,** i.e., inflammation of the choroid/retinal structures. There is a significant amount of overlap between these categories.

2. The classification by **type of precipitant** divides the processes into **nongranulomatous** and **granulomatous** precipitants. Although artificial, this is still the most useful classification model and will be used here.

B. **Nongranulomatous uveitis**

1. **Manifestations**

The **specific manifestations** of this set of uveitis include the acute onset of unilateral pain and redness of the affected eye. On **examination** there are marked conjunctival injection, a "circumcorneal flush" as a result of dilation of the limbic vessels, and an acute decrease in visual acuity. The **slit lamp examination** reveals small infiltrates in the **anterior chamber,** with sparing of the choroid and retina, i.e., the posterior structures of the eye.

2. **Pathogenesis**

The **underlying pathogenesis** of the inflammation is unclear but has been postulated to be autoimmune in nature. The **differential diagnosis** of this type of uveitis includes ankylosing spondylitis, ulcerative colitis, inflammatory bowel disease, Reiter's syndrome, Still's disease, or associated with HSV infection of the eye.

3. **Evaluation**

The **specific evaluation** includes making the clinical diagnosis using the information described above and the examination described in Box 13-1. A thorough history and physical examination, looking for evidence of underlying causes, must be performed.

4. **Management**

The **specific management** includes documenting the type of uveitis and determining and treating the underlying cause. Further treatment includes:

a. The application of topical glucocorticoids (see

Table 13-1 for specific agents and dosages). These are **contraindicated if HSV is suspected** and, in all cases, should be administered under the direct supervision of an ophthalmologist.

b. The application of **topical mydriatics** (see Table 13-1 for specific agents and doses). These should be administered under the direct supervision of an ophthalmologist.

c. If **herpes simplex** keratitis is suspected, the use of acyclovir is indicated. See **VII. Keratitis,** page 668.

d. Urgent/emergent consultation with ophthalmology is indicated.

C. **Granulomatous**

1. **Manifestations**

The **specific manifestations** of this set of uveitis include the acute onset of unilateral pain and blurred vision with only mild redness of the affected eye. This set of uveitis is much more subtle in presentation when compared with nongranulomatous uveitis. On **examination** there is mild conjunctival injection, but an acute and quite significant decrease in visual acuity. The **slit lamp examination** reveals large precipitates involving all structures within the eye, anterior, intermediate, and posterior.

2. **Pathogenesis**

The **underlying pathogenesis** of the inflammation is unclear but has been postulated to be autoimmune in nature. The **differential diagnosis** of this type of uveitis includes sarcoidosis, chronic mycobacterial disease, Vogt–Koyagnagi syndrome, lues venereum, toxoplasmosis, and leprosy.

3. **Evaluation**

The **specific evaluation** includes making the clinical diagnosis using the information described above and the examination described in Box 13-1. Further **specific evaluation** includes:

a. A thorough history and physical examination, looking for evidence of the above described underlying etiologies.

b. VDRL and FTA-abs to rule out underlying lues venereum.

c. ESR for baseline.

d. Purified protein derivative (PPD) skin tests to determine exposure to mycobacterial disease.

e. *Toxoplasma* serology in serum.

f. An angiotensin-converting enzyme (ACE) level and chest radiographs (PA and lateral) to evaluate for sarcoidosis. The ACE level can be elevated in sarcoidosis.

4. Management

The **specific management** is similar to that for non-granulomatous uveitis (refer to discussion above).

D. Sympathetic disease

A fascinating yet severe form of uveitis can be as the result of **sympathetic disease.** The **classic history** is of the development of a granulomatous, idiopathic, severe "sympathetic" uveitis in one eye, several weeks after the patient sustains significant trauma, usually of the penetrating type, to the contralateral eye. Thus the patient can become completely blind after sustaining an injury to only one eye. The **treatment** is prophylactic enucleation of the traumatized eye. The ophthalmologist needs to be intimately involved in the care of such patients.

VI. Acute (Closed) Angle Glaucoma

A. Manifestations

The **specific manifestations** of this relatively uncommon but dramatic cause of a red inflamed eye include the acute onset of a unilateral headache ipsilateral to the affected eye, and concurrent nausea and vomiting. The patient describes photophobia, severe pain, and significant redness in the affected eye. Furthermore, the patient will often report seeing halos. On **examination,** the affected eye has a moderately dilated pupil which is minimally responsive to direct or consensual light. In addition, the clinician can shine a light source (e.g., a pocket penlight or slit lamp) at an angle into the anterior chamber from the temporal side. On the "normal" setting no shadow will be demonstrated over the iris; in acute (closed) angle glaucoma a shadow is demonstrated over the nasal side of the iris. There is a markedly elevated intraocular pressure when measured by Schiotz or applanation tonometry. In point of fact, the intraocular pressure (IOP), which normally is <15 mm Hg, can be up to 40–60 mm Hg!

Because this form of glaucoma is often precipitated by items/agents which induce **mydriasis,** e.g., sudden entrance into a dark room from an area of bright sunlight, the use of topical mydriatics, the use of parenteral or enteral atropine, or the use of a scopolamine patch for motion sickness and accidently getting some of the scopolamine in the eye, the patient should be queried as to activities and medications used before the acute event.

B. Pathogenesis

The **underlying pathogenesis** is one of an underlying congenital defect in which there is an abnormally narrow angle in the anterior chamber. This results in a relative obstruction to flow of the aqueous humor out of the anterior chamber. The narrow chamber angle is present in <**1% of the population;** therefore, <1/100 of people are at risk for the development of the acute process. **Mydriasis** in and of itself decreases the angle, and therefore in a patient at risk can precipitate total obstruction to flow with the resultant marked increase in IOP. This increase in IOP will then result in decreased blood perfusion to structures, ischemia, and significant intraocular damage.

C. **Evaluation**

The **specific evaluation** includes making the clinical diagnosis using the information described above and the examination described in Box 13-1.

D. **Management**

Once the diagnosis is made or suspected, emergency therapy is indicated.

1. Discontinue the use of any precipitating or exacerbating agent.

2. Instill the **miotic agent, pilocarpine.** The dosage is 1–2 drops of pilocarpine 4% solution in the affected eye stat and repeated every 20 minutes until a surgical procedure is performed. This agent, like any miotic agent, reverses the mydriasis and decreases the degree of obstruction.

3. **Acetozolamine** (Diamox), 500 mg IV, is indicated concurrent with the above interventions. This is a weak carbonic anhydrase inhibitor which will decrease production of aqueous humor and therefore decrease IOP.

4. Emergency consultation with **ophthalmology** for emergency surgery is indicated. The surgical procedure of choice is **laser** (argon or Nd-YAG) **iridectomy** within hours of presentation. The contralateral eye should undergo this procedure prophylactically. The **iridectomy** is an acquired communication between the anterior and posterior chambers.

5. If the surgery is delayed, mannitol, **1.5 g/kg** by IV bolus, is indicated as a further temporizing therapeutic modality. This agent, by acting as an osmotically active agent in the plasma, acts not only to cause an osmotic diuresis, but also to decrease IOP.

VII. **Keratitis**

This is the **nonspecific inflammation** of the cornea. The normal function of the cornea is to act as a transparent window allowing light to enter the eye with high fidelity. It is, in the normal state, clear and avascular; however, with any inflammation, i.e., keratitis, opacity and ulcerations can develop in the cornea itself.

A. Herpes simplex

1. Manifestations

The **specific manifestations** of this uncommon but severe type of keratitis include the acute onset of unilateral pain, redness, and decreased visual acuity which often is quite marked. On **examination,** there is an extensive dendritic pattern of gray-colored corneal ulcers. On examination with fluorescein, these ulcers stain and can be clearly demonstrated using the Wood's lamp. It is not uncommon to have concurrent vesicular blepharitis, but rarely will there be any concurrent vesicular lesions in the adjacent skin.

2. Pathogenesis

The **underlying pathogenesis** is reactivation of a primary herpes simplex type I infection. The primary infection was of the oral mucosa, which then involved and remained dormant in the trigeminal ganglion. Reactivation can be precipitated by stress. Although the reactivation usually manifests as a "cold sore," a potential reactivation manifestation is of keratitis.

3. Evaluation

The **specific evaluation** includes making the clinical diagnosis using the information described above and the examination described in Box 13-1.

4. Management

Once the diagnosis is made or suspected, emergency therapy is indicated.

    a. An **emergency** consultation with **ophthalmology.** The care by the ophthalmologist will include gentle debridement of the ulcer. The material debrided should be sent for a Tzanck prep and viral culture.

    b. The initiation of **antiviral drops** and **antibiotic drops** for 14–21 days (see Table 13-1 for specific agents and dosages).

    c. Patching the affected eye.

    d. A caveat is that if there is any concurrent interstitial keratitis, i.e., an immune-mediated process, the paradoxical use of topical glucocorticoids is indicated, **under the direction of an ophthalmology colleague.**

B. Herpes zoster

1. Manifestations

The **specific manifestations** of this relatively rare form of keratitis are classic and dramatic. They include the acute onset of a unilateral keratitis and conjunctivitis with an antecedent erythematous, painful, vesicular rash on the ipsilateral skin in the distribution of the **trigeminal nerve,** specifically V_1. Furthermore, there are concurrent significant ptosis and eyelid edema. If untreated, it can progress to diffuse uveitis and blindness.

2. **Pathogenesis**

The **underlying pathogenesis** is reactivation of the DNA-containing **varicella–zoster virus.** The patient has a past history of primary varicella–zoster infection (chicken pox), which, after the acute infection, remained dormant in the dorsal ganglia. The recurrence is usually precipitated by a decrease in the immune system or increasing age. It occurs in any dermatome, but if in dermatome of V_1, can result in **herpes zoster** keratitis.

3. **Evaluation**

The **specific evaluation** includes making the clinical diagnosis using the information described above and the examination described in Box 13-1.

4. **Management**

Once the diagnosis is made or suspected, emergency therapy is indicated.

   a. The immediate initiation of **systemic acyclovir** therapy. Systemic acyclovir will decrease the period of viral shedding and the intensity of the uveitis/keratitis when initiated early in the course of disease. The dose is 600–800 mg PO 5 times per day for 10 days, or, if immmunosuppressed, 10 mg/kg IV in q.8h. dosing for 7–10 days.

   b. The patient should be placed in respiratory isolation until the rash resolves, to prevent spread to people never exposed to varicella–zoster and pregnant women.

C. **Actinic**

1. **Manifestations**

The **specific manifestations** of this not uncommon cause of keratitis include the acute onset of bilateral eye pain, photophobia, decreased visual acuity, and conjunctivitis beginning 6–12 hours after visual exposure to a source of ultraviolet light. There are usually no systemic manifestations.

2. **Pathogenesis**

The **underlying pathogenesis** is a noninfectious keratitis resulting from **overexposure to ultraviolet light.** The patient invariably was exposed to a source of UV light **without having adequate eye protection,** i.e., polarizing sunglasses. The source of UV light can be a tanning salon, arc welding flame, or sunlight. This is one of the classic problems which occurs after looking directly at the sun during a total eclipse. Recovery without sequelae occurs in 48–72 hours.

3. **Evaluation**

   The **specific evaluation** includes making the clinical diagnosis using the information described above and the examination described in Box 13-1.

4. **Management**

   Once the diagnosis is made or suspected:

   a. Initiation of **cycloplegic** agents, e.g., cyclopentolate (see Table 13-1 for specific agents and dosing).

   b. **Patching** of the affected eye(s) for 24–36 hours.

   c. Effective **prevention** with polarizing sunglasses and education on how to limit exposure to UV light.

   d. If, after 24–48 hours, there is no improvement or if at presentation there are any other abnormalities, ophthalmology should be consulted.

D. **Bacterial, specifically in contact lens wearers**

1. **Manifestations**

   The **specific manifestations** of this uncommon form of keratitis include the acute onset of unilateral pain and erythema in a patient who uses contact lenses, especially the extended-wear type. On **examination,** there is a hazy, nontransparent cornea with a central ulcer. On fluorescein examination, any ulceration present will take up the dye. On direct and slit lamp examination, pus can be demonstrated in the anterior chamber, i.e., a **hypopyon.** A hypopyon portends a poor prognosis.

2. **Pathogenesis**

   The **underlying pathogenesis** of bacterial keratitis in contact lens wearers is multifactorial. Factors include improper cleaning techniques, small areas of abrasion from the contact lenses, and the duration of the lens being in contact with the cornea.

   a. The **incidence** of bacterial keratitis in contact lens wearers is quite low. Recent studies by Poggio et al. have demonstrated that the incidence per year of bacterial keratitides is 21/10,000 users of **extended wear** contact lenses and 4/10,000 users of **soft daily contact lenses.**

   b. The **organisms** associated with contact lens keratitis are **gram-negative bacilli,** including *Pseudomonas* spp., and some **gram-positive** organisms, especially *Streptococcus* and *Moraxella*. The protozoon *Acanthamoeba* can result in contact lens–related keratitis.

c. The **natural history** is the development of a hypopyon which then results in perforation of the cornea, diffuse uveitis, and blindness.

3. **Evaluation**

The **specific evaluation** includes making the clinical diagnosis using the information described above and the examination described in Box 13-1.

4. **Management**

Once the diagnosis is made or suspected:

a. **Remove the contact lens.**

b. Obtain an emergency consultation with ophthalmology. Under the direction of the ophthalmologist, the ulcer should be scraped gently and sent for Gram stain, culture, fungal culture, and *Acanthamoeba* culture.

c. Initiate a **continuous irrigation** of the superficial surface of the eye, laterally to medially, with antibiotic solutions of a cephalosporin and tobramycin for 2 to 4 hours. This irrigation must be under the direct and intimate supervision of an ophthalmologist. This intervention is followed by administration of a **topical antibiotic ointment,** patching of the eye for 3 to 7 days, and daily follow-up with the ophthalmologist (see Table 13-1 for specific agents and dosages).

d. The major thrust of care after acute management is **prevention.**

i. Underscore the need to use **meticulous technique** when cleaning and placing the contact lenses.

ii. Instruct the patient to use commercially available sterile products for cleaning lenses. **Tap water should never be used,** as it is usually contaminated.

iii. **Remove the contact lenses** at the first signs or symptoms of irritation and wear glasses for several days, i.e., a contact lens "holiday."

VIII. Corneal abrasion

A. Manifestations

The **specific manifestations** of this relatively common problem include the acute onset of unilateral eye discomfort and erythema. The patient often will report a scratchy sensation in the affected eye. There often is an antecedent history of a foreign body on the anterior surface of the eye. The patient often will relate a history of exacerbating the symptoms by rubbing the affected eye. On **fluorescein examination,** the ulcer takes on the dye. The foreign body can be virtually any small, solid substance, including a hair, a dust particle, an eyelash, or, more ominously, a piece of metal, an insect, or a wood splinter or chip.

B. Pathogenesis

The **underlying pathogenesis** is a scratch or trauma-related erosion of the cornea. An uncomplicated abrasion resolves without sequelae in 36–72 hours.

C. Evaluation

The **specific evaluation** includes making the clinical diagnosis using the information described above and the examination described in Box 13-1. Further **specific evaluation** includes a thorough examination to look for any remaining foreign bodies. If there is any history that the particle was metal, one needs to obtain a radiograph of the eye looking for an intraocular foreign body.

D. Management

1. The **specific management** of a **simple corneal abrasion** includes flushing the eye with sterile saline for 30 minutes, the administration of topical antibiotics, usually as ointment, for 5 days (see Table 13-1), and patching the eye for 24 hours.

2. There usually is no need to consult ophthalmology unless there is a suspicion of a penetrating wound, remaining foreign body, or no improvement in 24 hours.

IX. Conjunctivitis

This is a common process that affects virtually every person one or more times during his (her) lifetime.

A. Viral

1. **Manifestations**

The **specific manifestations** of this very common form of conjunctivitis include the acute onset of unilateral or bilateral erythema of the conjunctivae, copious watery discharge, and ipsilateral preauricular lymphadenopathy. There are usually no systemic manifestations, decreased visual acuity, or any purulence unless a bacterial superinfection occurs. On fluorescein examination there is no uptake of dye.

2. **Pathogenesis**

The **underlying pathogenesis** is direct infection of the conjunctivae by a virus. The most common agents are one of three different types of **adenovirus,** types 3, 8, or 19. The **transmission** is via direct contact, usually via the fingers to the contralateral eye or other patients. It can also be transmitted in swimming pools. Adenovirus is **highly contagious** and can cause epidemics. It is most common in midsummer to early fall.

3. **Evaluation**

The **specific evaluation** includes making the clinical diagnosis using the information described above and the examination described in Box 13-1.

4. **Management**

The **specific management** includes:

a. **Eye lavage** with sterile normal saline on a twice daily basis for 7–14 days.

b. **Vasoconstrictors** are of some benefit (see Table 13-1 for specific agents and dosages).

c. Topical antibiotics are of questionable benefit unless the discharge becomes purulent, at which time the discharge must be sent for Gram stain, culture, and sensitivity.

d. Referral to ophthalmology should be made on an elective basis unless purulent discharge begins.

B. **Bacterial**

The discussion is limited to adult bacterial conjunctivitis. Neonatal conjunctivitis is extremely important, but one should refer to pediatric texts for evaluation and management of that process.

1. **Manifestations**

The **specific manifestations** of this relatively common form of conjunctivitis include an acute onset of copious, purulent discharge from both eyes. There can be some mild decrease in visual acuity and mild discomfort, but the major manifestation is marked discharge. The patient is virtually always afebrile and has few or no concurrent systemic manifestations.

2. **Pathogenesis**

The **underlying pathogenesis** is a bacterial infection of the conjunctiva with resultant purulence. **Causative agents** can be divided into two overall groups, **common pathogens** and **rare pathogens.**

a. **Common pathogens** include *Streptococcus pneumoniae*, *Staphylococcus aureus*, *Hemophilus aegytius*, and *Moraxella*.

i. The natural history is usually one of self-limited disease; however, in some cases, a secondary keratitis with visual impairment can occur.

ii. The transmission is via direct contact of secretions and/or by autoinoculation, i.e., from one eye to the other. In these cases fingers are the vehicles.

b. **Rare pathogens** include *Chlamydia trachomatis* and *Neisseria gonorrhoeae*. Although these two agents are rare in the adult population of the United States, they deserve special mention due to the following facts:

i. The **natural history** is one of severe conjunctivitis and keratitis with the development of permanent visual impairment.

ii. The **transmission** is either by direct contact of eye secretions either via fingers or via contact of the eyes with water in **nonchlorinated** swimming pools. Furthermore, it can be spread to a **neonate** via vaginal delivery from an infected mother and result in neonatal bacterial conjunctivitis. In the cases of neonatal conjunctivitis, *Chlamydia* and *Neisseria gonorrhoeae* can cause the conjunctivitis. Finally, whereas chlamydial conjunctivitis is rare in the western world, it remains endemic to the third world.

3. **Evaluation**

The **specific evaluation** includes making the clinical diagnosis using the information described above and the examination described in Box 13-1.

a. If one of the **common pathogens** is suspected, i.e., the vast majority of cases, a **Gram stain** should be performed on the discharge. The Gram stain is performed to demonstrate the presence of PMNs and a predominant organism.

i. **Specific therapy** includes the application of topical antibiotics. An especially effective topical agent is **sulfacetamide 10% solution,** 2 drops OU t.i.d. for 5–7 days.

b. If one of the **rare pathogens** is suspected, e.g., in a neonate or a patient in or from a Third World country, or if there is a concurrent gonococcal infection present, a **Gram stain** and **Geisma stain** should be performed on the discharge.

i. The **Gram stain** is performed to demonstrate the presence of PMNs. If chlamydial, no organisms will be demonstrated, whereas if *Neisseria gonorrhoeae*, intracellular/Gram-negative bacilli will be present.

ii. The **Geisma stain** should be performed looking for PMNs and, if chlamydial, i.e., trachoma, the presence of inclusion bodies.

iii. **Specific therapy** should include topical antibiotics. **Sulfacetamide 10% solution** 2 drops OU t.i.d. for 3–5 weeks, with **concurrent** systemic erythromycin, 250–500 mg PO q.i.d., for 7 days or doxycycline 100 mg PO b.i.d. for 7 days. Furthermore, the case should be reported to the CDC and a consultation with ophthalmology should be made.

C. **Atopic/Allergic rhinitis-associated**

Please refer to section Rhinitis, Chapter 12, page 635.

D. **Keratoconjunctivitis siccae**

1. **Manifestations**

The **specific manifestations** of this entity include a mild, recurrent, bilateral conjunctivitis. Patients often present with a sensation in one or both eyes of "scratchiness" and dryness. The patient can develop recurrent corneal abrasions from incessant rubbing. Furthermore, the patient is unable to produce tears when weeping or in response to noxious odors.

2. **Pathogenesis**

The **underlying pathogenesis** is a marked decrease in the production of tears. The **differential diagnosis** includes Sjögren's syndrome, a syndrome of destruction of the lacrimal glands often associated with rheumatologic disorders, or as a sequela of severe superficial eye infections or burns.

3. **Evaluation**

The **specific evaluation** includes making the clinical diagnosis using the information described above and the examination described in Box 13-1. The specifics include a thorough history for any antecedent or concurrent rheumatologic diseases, or a past history of trauma, burns, or infections of the eyes.

4. **Management**

The most **effective modalities** in treatment include the use of artificial tears (see Table 13-1 for specific agents and dosages). Referral to ophthalmology is indicated if symptoms are refractory to first-line therapy.

E. **Chemical burns**

1. **Manifestations**

The **specific manifestations** include an acute onset of pain, redness, burning, and tearing after exposure to or direct contact with a gas or liquid toxic to the eye. On **examination** there is marked erythema of the conjunctiva with the potential for ulcer formation. Visual acuity is often decreased.

2. **Pathogenesis**

The **underlying pathogenesis** of the chemical-mediated damage ("burn") is damage to the eye structures and concomitant inflammation. The chemical burn has components of both keratitis and conjunctivitis and thus, if not immediately and aggressively treated, can result in permanent visual loss and dysfunction. The most common chemical burns are the result of exposure to acids and bases. **Bases** are more malignant than **acids** and can cause more sequelae; however, both need to be aggressively managed.

3. **Evaluation and management**

   The **specific evaluation and management** include a thorough history, determining the specific agent which caused the burn, and, **as soon as possible, lavage** of the affected eye with copious amounts of tap water or, if available, normal saline. The **initial management** is quite simple: lavage, lavage, and lavage! The use of anything other than water or saline is contraindicated, for if an attempt is made to neutralize the acid or base, heat is produced, with resultant thermal injury concurrent with the chemical injury.

   a. After flushing with water or saline and **emergently contacting ophthalmology,** the remainder of the basic evaluation, as described in Figure 13-1, can be completed.

   b. If the burn is significant, one can, after **thorough flushing,** administer **mydriatic agents** and initiate **topical antibiotics** (see Table 13-1 for specifics on agents and dosages). Application of a patch to the affected eye is indicated.

   c. Close follow-up with ophthalmology is indicated.

   d. **Prevention** is key. People need to wear protective eyewear when working with chemicals or with batteries, e.g., jump starting a car. Educate patients that if an exposure does occur, immediately begin the **lavage with water!**

X. Consultation

Problem	Service	Time
Internal hordeolum	Ophthalmology	Required
Chalazion		Required
Dacrocystitis		Required
Uveitis		Emergent
Acute angle glaucoma		Emergent
Keratitis		Emergent
Corneal abrasion		Urgent

Problem	Service	Time
Conjunctivitis		Elective
Chemical burn		Urgent/
		emergent

XI. **Indications for admission:** Any evidence of herpes simplex
or herpes zoster keratitis, a penetrating wound to the eye,
acute angle glaucoma, or any significant chemical burn. All
of these admissions are to the ophthalmology service.

Bibliography

Acute Blindness
Sanders MO: Sudden visual loss. Practitioner 1977;219:43.

Cataracts
Abrahamson IA: Cataract update. Am Fam Phys 1981;24:111.

Diabetic Retinopathy
Ferris FL, et al: Photocoagulation for diabetic retinopathy. JAMA 1991;
266:1263–1265.

Raskin P, et al: The treatment of diabetic retinopathy: A view for the internist. Ann Intern Med 1992;117:226–233.

Sussman EJ, et al: Diagnosis of diabetic eye disease. JAMA 1982;247:
3231–3234.

Open Angle Glaucoma
Alguire PC: Tonometry and glaucoma screening for the primary care physician. Resident Staff Physician, 1987:6–12.

Everitt DE, Avorn J: Systemic effects of medications used to treat glaucoma.
Ann Intern Med 1990;112:120–125.

Gottlieb LK, et al: Glaucoma screening: A cost effective analysis. Surv Ophthalmol 1983;28:206.

Mosteller MW, Zimmerman TJ: The medical management of glaucoma. In:
Spoor TC, ed. Modern Management of Ocular Diseases. Thorofare, NJ:
Slack, 1985;170–188.

Quigley HA: Open-angle glaucoma. N Engl J Med 1993;328:1097–1106.

Red Inflamed Eye
Baum JL: Ocular infection. N Engl J Med 1978;299:28.

Bienfang DC, et al: Ophthalmology. N Engl J Med 1990;323:956–967.

Drugs for bacterial conjunctivitis. Med Lett 1976;18:70.

Eifrig DE: A system for examining the ocular fundus. North Carolina
Med J, October 1983, pp 631–633.

Havener WH: Synopsis of Ophthalmology, 6th ed. St. Louis, CV Mosby,
1984.

Henderly DE, et al: Changing patterns of uveitis. Am J Ophthalmol
1987;103:131.

Moutsopoulos HM, et al: Sjögren's syndrome (sicca syndrome): Current issues. Ann Intern Med 1980;92:212.
Newell SW: The management of corneal foreign bodies. Am Fam Pract 1985;31:149–156.
Shingleton BJ: Eye injuries. N Engl J Med 1991;325:408–413.
Victor WH: Watery eye. West J Med 1986;144:759.
White GL, et al: Contact lens care and complications. Am Fam Pract 1988;37:187–192.

—D.D.B.

Dale Berg, Ed. *Handbook of Primary Care Medicine.* Copyright © 1993 J. B. Lippincott Company.

CHAPTER 14

Neurology

Bell's Palsy and Other Cranial Nerve VII Disorders

Cranial nerve VII is a mixed cranial nerve in that it has both motor and sensory components. The **motor components** include the facial musculature and thus eye closing and lip movement. It also innervates the stapedius muscle in the middle ear and controls the secretion of saliva and tears from the salivary and lacrimal glands respectively. The **sensory component** is mainly of taste. The anatomy of innervation is similar to other motor nerves, **central,** i.e., upper motor neuron, and **peripheral,** i.e., lower motor neuron. A unique feature of the innervation is that the upper face and eyes receive innervation from the upper motor neuron component (central) from both sides of the brain, whereas the lower face receives innervation from the upper motor neuron component (central) from the contralateral side only. The lower motor neuron component (peripheral) innervates the entire ipsilateral side of the face. Thus the manifestations of cranial nerve VII palsy are variable and dependent on the location of the lesion. Given a set of findings, one can easily locate the lesion.

I. **Overall manifestations and causes**
   A. **Central lesions**
      A **central** (i.e., upper motor neuron) lesion will manifest with paresis (weakness) or plegia (paralysis) of the contralateral orbicularis oris muscle but not of the orbicularis oculis muscle.
      1. **Overall manifestations**
         The patient is able to easily close both eyes but being unable to completely smile. When instructed to smile, the patient is unable to normally elevate one side of the lips. This unilateral lack of a facial (nasolabial) fold on smiling is contralateral to the side of the lesion. Associated features are common and related to the underlying cause.

2. **Causes**
   Causes include the intracranial processes of intracranial tumor, head trauma, or, in the vast majority of cases, a cerebrovascular accident (see section on Cerebrovascular Accidents, page 683).

B. **Peripheral lesions**
   Peripheral (lower motor neuron) cranial nerve damage results in ipsilateral paresis or plegia of all musculature of that side of the face. Thus, in a peripheral cranial nerve VII palsy, both the ipsilateral orbicularis oris and orbicularis oculi musculature are affected.
   1. **Overall manifestations**
      Overall manifestations include, in addition to the above described defect in smiling, a concurrent inability to completely close the eye on the ipsilateral side. Other associated features include the sensation of an acute onset of ipsilateral facial stiffness, the development of hyperacusis (increased, approaching painful, sensitivity to auditory stimuli) due to the fact that CN VII can innervate the stapedius muscle, and, finally, dysgensia (dysfunctional taste) can and will occur. A further manifestation may be excessive tearing—"crocodile tears"—which occurs during the healing phase.
   2. **Causes**
      a. **Herpes simplex/zoster infection.** Involving the nucleus of CN VII (Ramsay–Hunt syndrome). This is usually quite evident given the fact that vesicles can form on the tongue and about the external ear in the disorder. It is quite rare but should be in the differential diagnosis.
      b. **Acoustic neuroma of CN VIII.** The specific manifestations include associated tinnitus and occasionally vertigo.
      c. **Facial trauma** can disrupt the nerve peripherally.
      d. **Surgical complication,** especially after a parotidectomy.
      e. **Bell's palsy.** The most common, albeit idiopathic, cause of a peripheral cranial nerve palsy, especially in young patients.

II. **Evaluation and management of CN VII palsy**
   Differentiate a central from a peripheral lesion on the basis of the physical examination.
   1. If **central,** a CT scan of the head is clearly indicated as the most likely process is a CVA. Neurology should be consulted. See section on Cerebrovascular Accidents, page 683, for further discussion.
   2. If **peripheral,** query patient regarding antecedent fa-

cial trauma, past facial surgeries, and carefully examine for any evidence of a herpes infection.

a. If due to **trauma** or **iatrogenic,** the patient should be instructed on how to patch the affected eye at night and should be prescribed lubricating eyedrops (Isotears, others).

b. If **herpes** infection is present or suspected, initiation of acyclovir, 200 mg PO 5 times per day, is indicated, as is referral to ophthalmology to evaluate for and aid in the prevention of herpes keratitis.

c. If the diagnosis is **idiopathic** peripheral cranial nerve VII palsy (i.e., **Bell's palsy**):

   i. 60% of patients will recover complete function in the proximate future without any treatment.

   ii. Patching the eye until palsy resolves is indicated to prevent trauma or severe xerosis.

   iii. If the patient presents within 5 days of onset of symptoms and there is no evidence of herpetic infection, steroids **may** be of benefit. The dose is 60–80 mg of prednisone q.d. for 5–7 days with a rapid taper. See Table 14-1 for indications and contraindications to prednisone.

III. Consultation

Problem	Service	Time
Herpes infection	Infectious diseases	Urgent
Herpes infection	Ophthalmology	Urgent
Central lesion	Neurology	Urgent

IV. Indications for admission: CVA (see page 683), and any patient with evidence of herpes infection with dissemination or a history of immunosuppression. Otherwise this can be evaluated and managed as an outpatient.

T A B L E   1 4 - 1
Prednisone in Bell's Palsy

Indications

No contraindications, as indicated below
Within 5 days of onset of syndrome
Pain associated with the syndrome
Concurrent hyperacusis

Contraindications

Greater than 5 days after onset of syndrome
Any suspicion of herpes infection
CN VII palsy

Cerebrovascular Accidents

Cerebrovascular accidents, or **strokes,** are a broad group of pathologic entities which are, by definition, death of brain tissue due to an interruption of blood flow to that area of brain. **Manifestations** can be **diverse** due to the fact that different portions of the brain control different functions and thus damage or death of a certain area will produce neurologic deficits which may be very different from the manifestations of damage/death to an area immediately adjacent. Two other reasons for differences in manifestations include the fact that there are several **different mechanisms in pathogenesis,** and that there can be some partial or even complete **reversibility** of the CVA manifestations.

I. Overall manifestations
   The **overall manifestations** of stroke syndromes are mainly dependent on the location of the brain tissue death. A thorough **physical examination** will quite often place the lesion.
   A. **Manifestations by location of brain infarction**
      1. **Occipital lobe.** Normal **function** is as the visual cortex. Therefore, damage or destruction of this area will result in blindness in the **contralateral visual field.**
      2. **Parietal lobe.** Normal **function** is as the sensory input area. Therefore, damage to this area can result in decreased ability to **perceive sensory** data and, if on the dominant side, **receptive aphasia.**
      3. **Frontal lobe.** Normal **function** is as motor cortex and a site of behaviors. Therefore, damage to this area, especially the posterior aspect, will result in **contralateral muscle weakness.**
      4. **The deep white matter, internal capsule.** Normal **function** is the axons to the spinal cord, especially from the motor cortex. Therefore, damage to this area will result in **contralateral muscle weakness.**

II. Categories of CVA by pathogenesis
   CVA (stroke) syndromes are best categorized by the mechanisms of pathogenesis as, although many of the overall manifestations are similar, each category has a different pathogenesis, some unique differentiating features, and some significant differences in specific management. The syndromes are categorized into three different groups: **ischemic thrombotic, ischemic embolic,** and **hemorrhagic** (Tables 14-2 and 14-3).
   A. **Ischemic thrombotic CVA**
      Ischemic thrombotic CVAs result from atherosclerosis of the arteries leading to the brain, carotids, and/or vertebrobasilar circulation. **Risk factors** for development are the same as for other atherosclerotic disease processes: smok-

T A B L E 1 4 - 2
Types of CVAs by Pathophysiology

Type	Risk Factors	Historical Features	TIAs
Ischemic thrombotic	Hypertension Atherosclerosis Vasculitis Hypotensive episodes Oral contraceptives	Sudden onset of deficit, progresses or improves over hours to days	Common
Ischemic embolic	Mechanical heart valves Mitral stenosis Atrial fibrillation Left-sided endocarditis	Sudden onset, fixed from outset	Uncommon
Hemorrhagic	Hypertension Berry aneurysms Arteriovenous malformations Thrombocytopenia Coagulopathy	Severe headache Nuchal rigidity Vomiting Steady, slow progression of deficits over 6 hours If intraparenchymal: CT positive If subarachnoid: CT negative, but blood on LP	Uncommon

T A B L E   1 4 - 3
Approach to Ischemic Thrombotic TIAs, RINDs, and Completed CVAs

Type	Symptoms/Signs	Acutely	Subacutely
Vertebrobasilar	Dysarthria Dysphagia Near syncope Hemiparesis	If evolving: anticoagulate with heparin for 5–7 days If fixed or resolving: aspirin, 325 mg PO q.d.	Aspirin, 325 mg PO q.d. OT/PT No surgical intervention No indications for arteriography
Carotid	Contralateral hemiparesis Amaurosis fugax	If evolving: anticoagulate with heparin and continue until definitive procedure done If resolving: aspirin If fixed: aspirin	Carotid Dopplers Carotid arteriography CEA, if stenosis present

ing, diabetes mellitus, hypertension, and hyperlipoproteinemias.

1. Manifestations

   The **specific manifestations** of this category include
   an acute onset of a neurologic deficit which can and
   will, over the next minutes, hours, or days, to various
   degrees, resolve. **Transient ischemic attacks (TIAs)**
   are deficits which resolve within the first 24 hours;
   reversible ischemia neurologic deficits (RINDs) resolve within the first 7 days. Any defect present after
   7 days is the residua of the **completed stroke.** A specific type of TIA is **amaurosis fugax,** in which the
   patient has monocular blindness which resolves in
   the first 6–24 hours.

   Acute **reversibility** is unique to this category of
   CVA. This feature is inductively reasonable if one re-
   calls that this is usually a stenosis which completely
   occludes and then can and often does reopen. In this
   model, one can compare thrombotic CVAs to acute
   coronary syndromes. The TIA would be analogous to
   unstable angina, the RIND analogous to non-Q-wave
   infarction, and the completed CVA to a Q-wave in-
   farct.

2. Evaluation and management

   The **specific evaluation and management** of these
   CVAs includes the items described in Box 14-1 along
   with the following specifics.

   a. **Maintain** the systolic blood pressure above 100
      mm Hg to keep perfusion adequate. This can be
      accomplished with fluids and, if indicated, pressor
      agents.

   b. If the **CVA is evolving clinically,** i.e., new deficits
      are developing, the patient should be, unless con-
      traindicated, **anticoagulated with heparin.** The
      dosing is a bolus of 5,000–10,000 units IV, fol-
      lowed by an 800–1,000 unit per hour drip, with a
      goal to keep the aPTT at 45–60 seconds.

   c. If the **CVA is not evolving** or is resolving, there is
      no indication for anticoagulation.

   d. Once stabilized, performance of **carotid Dopplers**
      to image for any plaques. If any **plaques** are dem-
      onstrated, carotid (two-vessel) arteriography is in-
      dicated. If stenosis of >70% is present in the carot-
      ids, carotid endarterectomy is indicated (Table
      14-4). If **no plaques** are demonstrated, the plaques
      are either intracranial or in the vertebrobasilar sys-
      tem, neither of which is amenable to surgery. Ver-
      tebrobasilar arteriography is not indicated for

B O X   1 4 - 1

Overall Evaluation and Management of Stroke Syndromes

Evaluation

1. **ABCs,** as outlined by basic and advanced life support, as necessary.
2. CBC count, for baseline purposes.
3. **Intravenous access** for fluids, as a patient with an acute CVA syndrome should be NPO during the acute event.
4. Thorough **physical examination** for baseline neurologic examination, documenting any motor, sensory, or cognitive deficits.
5. **PT, aPTT, and platelet count** to determine if there is any evidence of a coagulopathy and as baseline if anticoagulation is indicated.
6. **ESR.** If elevated, can be consistent with an inflammatory process, i.e., vasculitis.
7. **ABGs,** for baseline purposes. Supplemental O_2 should be administered to keep $Pao_2 > 65$ mm Hg.
8. **Nothing by mouth.** Very important in the acute setting, as the swallowing mechanism is often affected by a CVA.
9. **EKG—12 lead,** for baseline purposes and to look for any acute cardiac event. Furthermore, a diagnosis of the **rhythm is useful,** especially if the rhythm is one of atrial fibrillation, which is associated with embolic CVAs.
10. **CT scan without contrast,** to look for any areas of bleeding. Blood, indicative of a hemorrhagic CVA, will be demonstrable without a contrast agent. (Fresh hemorrhage is its own contrast agent.)
11. **If CT of head is negative,** but suspicion for subarachnoid bleed is still present, **lumbar puncture is indicated.** A subarachnoid bleed will often manifest with a normal head CT but a bloody CSF.

Management

1. **Maintain blood pressure** in 140–160/80–90 range.
2. **Admit** to monitored or intensive care unit bed.

(continued)

B O X   1 4 - 1 *(continued)*

3. Early and aggressive **physical and occupational therapy** is required.
4. Prevent any gravitational pneumonia by checking the gag reflex before allowing swallowing of food; refer to swallowing specialist.
5. **Enteral tube feedings** to maintain nutrition may be indicated as a temporizing measure.
6. Social services and family support required for intermediate and long-term assistance.

thombotic CVAs due to the fact that no intervention can be done based on that finding.

   e. In all cases, unless contraindicated, **aspirin,** 325 mg PO q.d., should be started.

B. Ischemic embolic CVA

   Ischemic embolic CVAs result from thrombus (clot) forming in the left atrium, left ventricle, or on the mitral or aortic valves, or as a result of bioprosthetic valves or endocarditis, and embolize to the brain and other vital organs.

   1. **Manifestations**

      The **specific manifestations** with which the patient usually presents include an acute onset of a deficit which is maximum at outset and does not resolve. Virtually never is there any TIA or RIND associated with this mechanism.

   2. **Management**

      The **specific management** of these CVAs includes the items described in Box 14-1, along with the following specifics.

      a. Maintain the systolic blood pressure about 100

T A B L E 1 4 - 4
Indications for Carotid Endarterectomy

1. High-grade (>70%) carotid stenosis with recent, documented TIA or RIND.
2. Carotid stenosis in patients who recently required heparin anticoagulation for treatment of stroke syndrome.
3. Not necessary in completed stroke if stenosis and CVA are anatomically appropriate.

mm Hg to keep adequate cerebral perfusion. This can be accomplished with fluids and, if indicated, pressor agents.

b. If there are no contraindications, the patient should be **anticoagulated with heparin.** The dosing is a bolus of 5,000–10,000 units IV, followed by an 800–1,000 unit per hour drip, with a goal to keep the aPTT at 45–60 seconds.

c. A search for the **source of emboli** should be rapidly undertaken. This entails imaging the heart with an **echocardiogram** and **monitoring** the heart rhythm for any episodes of atrial fibrillation. If no source in the heart is found, then **carotid Dopplers** looking for plaques which may have associated thrombi are indicated. If the patient is **febrile or at risk for endocarditis,** four sets of blood cultures need to be obtained, and, if clinically indicated, antibiotics initiated.

d. The patient may need **long-term anticoagulation** with warfarin after the 5–7 days of heparin. The goal is to initiate warfarin early in the heparin course and maintain an INR in the 2.0 to 3.0 range. **Long-term anticoagulation is indicated if:**

   i. Thrombus is documented in the left ventricle/atrium.

   ii. Mitral stenosis is present.

  iii. Intermittent atrial fibrillation is present.

  iv. For 3 weeks before and after electrical or chemical cardioversion of atrial fibrillation.

   v. Atrial fibrillation and left ventricular contractile dysfunction are present.

  vi. Bioprosthetic heart valve(s) are present. In this specific case the target INR is 3.0 to 4.2.

C. Hemorrhagic CVA

Hemorrhagic CVAs result from disruption or rupture of the vessels within or adjacent to the brain itself. A rupture of a vessel within the brain itself is called an **intraparenchymal bleed** and can be the result of a ruptured arteriovenous malformation or hypertension related. A rupture of a vessel immediately adjacent to the brain surface is a **subarachnoid bleed** and is usually the result of a ruptured berry aneurysm and/or hypertension. Intraparenchymal (Fig. 14-1) and subarachnoid bleeds are on a clinical continuum, with overlap between the two types.

1. Manifestations

The **specific manifestations** include a severe headache (the worst of the patient's life), nausea, vomiting, and a slow, steady progression of neurologic defects over the subsequent 2–6 hours. Virtually never is

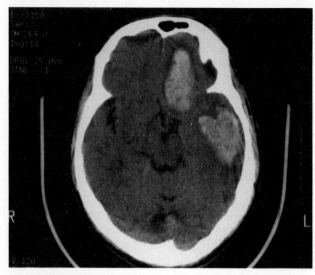

FIGURE 14-1
CT of head without contrast agent enhancement, showing large
intraparenchymal hemorrhage in the left hemisphere.

there any TIA or RIND associated with this mechanism.

2. **Management**

The **specific management** of these CVAs includes the items described in Box 14-1, along with the following specifics.

a. Any **coagulopathy** must be aggressively evaluated and corrected. See section on Excessive Bleeding States in Chapter 5.

b. If **thrombocytopenic** for any reason, transfuse platelets to keep >50,000/mm³. See section on Excessive Bleeding States in Chapter 5, page 275.

c. **Calcium channel blockers,** specifically nimopidine, 30 mg PO or NG q.6h., may be of short- and long-term benefit for intracranial bleeds, especially in subarachnoid bleeds if initiated in the first 12–24 hours.

d. The **maintenance** of a stable blood pressure is of great importance (110–140/80–90 mm Hg).

e. Further adjuvant therapy includes the initiation of stool softeners to minimize straining and the administration of acetaminophen for the relief of the headache.

f. Once the patient is stabilized, a four-vessel arteriogram is indicated. Unlike in thrombotic CVAs, it is of great importance to image the vertebrobasilar along with the standard carotid artery images to visualize the location of the ruptured aneurysm or AVM.

g. **Neurosurgical intervention** for aneurysm or AVM clipping is indicated.

III. Overall prevention

Preventive measures have dramatically decreased the overall incidence and the individual risk of cerebrovascular accidents. The impact of prevention is most clearly demonstrated in the risk factor hypertension. Unquestionably, the adequate control of hypertension has been demonstrated to decrease the risk of hemorrhagic and thrombotic CVAs. The overall prevention for all strokes includes:

1. **Atherosclerotic disease risk factor modification,** i.e., smoking cessation, control of hypertension, control of serum glucose in diabetes mellitus, and control of lipids in hyperlipoproteinemias.

2. **Anticoagulate** patients who are at high risk for **embolic CVAs.** See indications listed above.

3. **Discontinue oral contraceptives** in a woman at higher risk (smokers, hypertensives, etc.).

4. **Aspirin, 325 mg/day,** for all patients with atherosclerotic disease.

5. **Manage asymptomatic carotid bruits.** An asymptomatic carotid bruit is a prevalent finding in the older and middle-aged adult population. In all cases, unless contraindicated, aspirin, 325 mg PO q.d., should be administered. Carotid Doppler studies should be performed. If high-grade stenosis (>50%) is found, the option of carotid endarterectomy can be considered; however, recent studies by Hobson et al. reveal that carotid endarterectomy in patients with **asymptomatic carotid bruits** had **no** statistically significant improvement in the outcomes of CVA or death relative to standard medical therapy.

IV. Consultation

Problem	*Service*	*Time*
Carotid TIAs or RINDs	Vascular surgery	Urgent
Asymptomatic bruit	Vascular surgery	Elective
Any stroke	Neurology	Urgent
Any completed stroke	OT/PT	Elective

V. **Indications for admission:** Any CVA. The clinician should have a low threshold for admitting directly to the ICU unless the patient is very stable.

Delirium

This is an acute deterioration in mental status from a previously stable baseline. Simply put it is an acute confusional state. Another way to state this process is the acute loss of orientation to one or more of the parameters of person, i.e., who the patient is and how s(he) is related to others; place, i.e., where the patient is and its description; and time, i.e., what the date, season, and time is. This can be, but is not necessarily, associated with acute cognitive impairment, and/or a decrease in the level of consciousness (i.e., lethargy, somnolence). One cannot overstate the importance and gravity of this problem/diagnosis. It is truly a medical emergency which **mandates emergent** medical evaluation and management.

I. **Overall manifestations**

This is a problem/diagnosis which requires extensive history, but ironically, the patient is unable to give a good history. This is due to the very nature of delirium: the patient is a poor historian and is potentially confabulating (creating answers). Furthermore, the patient may even have concurrent aggressive, acting out type, behaviorisms. Therefore, it is important to find someone, a family member or friend, who knows the patient in order to obtain a baseline set of parameters and to determine, if possible, when the deterioration occurred. A drug and ethanol use history is also important, as is any past medical history including diabetes mellitus, and/or recent medical history, e.g., of fevers. A history of suicide attempts or any psychiatric history is also quite helpful.

II. **Differential diagnosis**

The **differential diagnosis** is based on the fundamental concept that delirium is a **medical problem,** and therefore no psychiatric diagnoses are considered. In this problem, a psychotic reaction/psychiatric dysfunction is a **diagnosis of exclusion.**

A. **Medications/drugs**

Perhaps the most common cause of delirium.

1. **Ethanol.** The ingestion of excessive quantities of ethanol can cause delirium. The **specific manifestations** include the odor of ethanol on the patient's breath, decreased inhibition, cerebellar dysfunction, and a

blood alcohol level usually greater than .10 mg/dL. **Specific management** is to have patient discontinue the binge and to rest. Driving or operating a machine are contraindicated. The patient can be sent home with a family member or friend who is sober. Further details in management are outlined in the section on Substance Abuse Syndromes in Chapter 15, page 748.

2. **Ethanol withdrawal.** Withdrawal from ethanol can result in a classic form of delirium, delirium tremens. **Specific manifestations** of delirium tremens occur after the patient abruptly discontinues ethanol ingestion after a sustained period (weeks to months) of intoxication. The patient experiences hallucinations (mainly visual) and tonic–clonic seizures during the first 48 hours, followed by delirium approximately 4 days after the initiation of abstinence. **Specific management** includes that in Box 14-2 and the initiation of benzodiazepines, e.g., lorazepam (Ativan), 1–2 mg PO/IM/IV q.6h. and watching airway. Admission to an inpatient service is required. Refer to the section on Substance Abuse Syndromes in Chapter 15, page 748 for further details.

3. **Wernicke's syndrome.** This is the acute severe deficiency of the vitamin thiamine (B_1), most often occurring in malnourished alcoholics. The **specific manifestations** include delirium, unsteady gait, nystagmus, and amblyopia (palsies of the extraocular musculature). This is a diagnosis/mechanism which can and will be concurrent with, but not the cause of, delirium tremens. The **specific management** is to replete thiamine, 100 mg IM/IV/PO q.d.

4. **Benzodiazepine (BZD) or narcotic withdrawal.** Analogous to withdrawal from ethanol, usually after abrupt cessation of BZD or narcotics after a long period of significant use/abuse. Manifestations and management are quite similar to those of delirium tremens. In addition, the agent flumazenil, 0.2 mg, should be administered IV to reverse the activity of the BZD. This agent acts by competitive inhibition of the BZD receptors and can be repeated in incremental doses of 0.3 and 0.5 mg q.3–4 minutes to a maximum of 5.0 mg. If a long-acting BZD was ingested, flumazenil in incremental of 5.0 mg.

5. **Narcotic overdose.** An overdose of narcotic agents either accidentally or as a suicide attempt can cause delirium. The **specific manifestations** include a decreased level of consciousness and bilateral miosis. The **specific management** includes that in Box 14-2

B O X 1 4 - 2

Overall Evaluation and Management of Delirium

If a known **diabetic patient** who takes insulin, check a **stat fingerstick glucose** and administer a substance high in glucose, stat. If there is complete resolution after glucose administration and the finger stick was low, i.e., <60 mg/dL, there is no need for further evaluation.

1. **ABCs,** i.e., basic and advanced life support protocol, as necessary.
2. Establish intravenous access.
3. Administer **Thiamine, 100 mg IV or IM,** to attempt to reverse any Wernicke's disease, i.e., profound thiamine deficiency.
4. Administer **one ampule of D50W IV,** to treat any hypoglycemia (after the thiamine is administered).
5. Administer one ampule of **naloxone (Narcan) IV,** to reverse any effect of a narcotic agent.
6. Perform a fingerstick glucose, stat.
7. Administer 0.2 mg of flumazenil IV to reverse any benzodiazepines ingested.
8. **Laboratory examinations.** Serum electrolytes, BUN, creatinine, glucose, calcium, albumin, phosphorus, arterial blood gas, NH_4, CBC count with differential, ethanol level, urinalysis, and urine drug screen for benzodiazepines, tricyclic agents, and/or barbiturates. Abnormalities in any of these can result in delirium; therefore, they must be checked at the time of presentation.
9. Define and treat any cause discovered above (see text).
10. If the above examinations and management **do not reveal the etiology** and/or resolve the problem, or if further investigation is clinically indicated, the following procedures, should be performed:
    a. **CT imaging of the head,** especially in any head trauma case or if any focal neurologic deficit is present.
    b. **Lumbar puncture** in every patient who has fever and delirium; this is clearly indicated.
    c. Treat the underlying cause.

and supportive measures. A continuous infusion of nalaxone is sometimes required for acute therapy. In virtually all cases admission is indicated.

6. **PCP (angel dust).** This illicit agent is associated with a delirium with the **specific manifestations** of aggressive and acting out behaviorisms. The patient can harm himself and others. Management includes benzodiazepines and restraints.

7. Virtually **every agent,** whether **medicinal** or **illicit,** can cause delirium. This is particularly germaine in the field of geriatrics. This underscores the need to carefully obtain a drug history.

B. **Electrolyte disturbances/metabolic**

Virtually every electrolyte, if abnormal to a great degree, can cause delirium, irrespective of the underlying cause of that electrolyte imbalance. These include hypoxemia, hypercapnia, hypoglycemia, hypophosphatemia, hypocalcemia, hypercalcemia, uremia (increased BUN), azotemia (increased creatinine), and hyponatremia. The **specific management** is to normalize the electrolyte imbalance and to determine and treat the underlying cause.

C. **Acute anemia**

Delirium can result from an acute anemia, irrespective of the cause. **Specific manifestations** include intravascular volume depletion, hypotension, pale mucous membranes, and pale nail beds. **Management specifics** include determining the reason for the anemia, treating that cause, and, as needed, transfusion of packed RBCs.

D. **Hepatic encephalopathy**

This is due to an accumulation of nitrogenous catabolites which cannot be further catabolized/excreted by the liver due to hepatic failure. The **specific manifestations** include a concurrent decreased level of consciousness, asterixis, and the signs of chronic hepatic failure. Refer to the section on End Stage Hepatic Dysfunction in Chapter 2, page 91, for further details.

E. **Fever**

Fever, especially a spiking fever, will cause delirium. The **specific management** is to determine and treat the underlying cause of the fever and to give the patient effective antipyretic agents, such as acetaminophen and/or acetylsalicylic acid.

F. **Leptomeningitis**

See section on Meningitis, page 717, for further discussion.

G. **Head trauma**

This is an overlooked cause of delirium, especially among patients with an increased risk of head trauma.

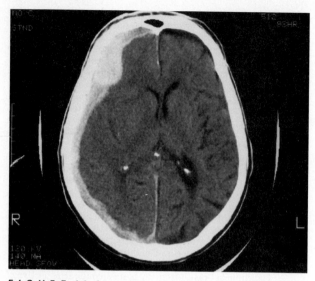

FIGURE 14-2
CT of the head without contrast agent enhancement, showing large subdural hematoma on the right side.

This is especially true in patients who were intoxicated and then went through delirium tremens. It is not uncommon for these patients to have sustained some head trauma while intoxicated. Therefore, **specific management** in these patients is to examine for any head trauma and to obtain a CT scan of the head, without contrast, in any patient with any evidence of head trauma, any focal neurologic deficits, or an inappropriate and unexplained prolonged delirium (see Fig. 14-2). The most common "silent" cause is a subdural hematoma occurring in such a scenario. If any structural defect is demonstrated on head CT, emergency consultation with neurosurgery is clearly indicated.

H. **Encephalitis**

This is a relatively uncommon cause of delirium, but one which should not be missed. Although there are many underlying causes, few are treatable. The most treatable causes are tertiary lues and herpes simplex. The **specific manifestations** of herpes simplex encephalitis include partial seizures, especially involving the temporal lobes, and a decreased level of consciousness. Often it occurs in young patients who are otherwise healthy. CSF protein will be markedly elevated without any other abnormalities. **Specific management** includes obtaining an MRI looking for temporal lobe involvement and the empirical initiation of acyclovir, 5–10 mg/kg IV q.8h. for 10–14 days.

I. **Left ventricular failure**
Heart failure, especially forward failure, can manifest with delirium owing to the diffusely decreased perfusion and oxygenation of the cerebral cortex. The specific manifestations and management are discussed in the section on Congestive Heart Failure in Chapter 1, page 9.

J. **Hypothyroidism/hyperthyroidism**
Too much or too little levothyroxine can result in delirium. Usually the diagnosis is clinically evident and specific management is directed toward the underlying cause. For specific discussion on manifestations and management, see section on Thyroid Dysfunctional States, Chapter 9, page 541.

III. **Consultation**

Problem	*Service*	*Time*
Any focal deficits	Neurology	Emergent
Meningitis/encephalitis	Infectious disease	Emergent
Subdural hematoma	Neurosurgery	Emergent
Substance abuse	Addictionologist	Urgent
Suicide attempt	Psychiatry	Emergent

IV. **Indications for admission: All** cases of delirium, unless due to a rapidly reversible process (e.g., insulin-induced hypoglycemia corrected with glucose infusion).

Dementia

This is a nonspecific, insidious, progressive deterioration in intellectual and cognitive functioning. Whereas in the majority of cases this process is irreversible, this is not necessarily always the case. The process, irrespective of the underlying cause, results in the steady loss of cortical neurons with resultant deterioration in higher brain functioning.

I. **Overall manifestations**
The **overall manifestations** are subtle early in the course of the disease and may not be recognized by family members or even by the patient. The cardinal manifestations of dementia, a deterioration in intellectual and cognitive functioning, can be demonstrated and documented by performing a thorough **mental status examination** and the **"mini-mental state"** ex-

amination. Several other salient **signs** of this process can include:

A. **Frontal release signs**

These are signs of frontal lobe cortical deterioration which, when present, usually reflect moderately advanced disease. These abnormal signs include:

1. **Grasp.** Abnormal slow flexion of the patient's fingers around the examiner's fingers when examiner places fingers on patient's palm.

2. **Snout.** Abnormal puckering and protrusion of the patient's lips when the examiner rubs on the patient's lips medially to laterally.

3. **Sucking.** Abnormal sucking activity when the lips are rubbed by an examiner laterally to medially.

4. **Apraxia.** Acquired abnormal inability of the patient to perform a motor task which he knows, wants to perform, and has no specific motor or distal neurologic defect present to prevent its performance.

B. **Loss of inhibitions**

This is a very common manifestation of dementia in which the patient performs behaviorisms (e.g., masturbation, inappropriate sexual contact) or says words (e.g., curses) which would be socially unacceptable and thus inhibited. The **frontal lobes** are the sites of learned inhibitions, and thus destruction of the frontal lobes can and does decrease these inhibitions.

C. **Inappropriate jocularity**

This is the significant increase in inappropriate verbal activity.

D. **Depression**

E. **Dementia,** irrespective of the underlying can be exacerbated by concurrent medical and/or psychiatric problems. One of the best examples of such an exacerbating process is the common major affective disorder, **depression.**

II. **Differential diagnosis**

The **differential diagnosis** of dementia includes a diverse set of disease processes. The majority of these processes are irreversible and progressive; however, some may be modifiable and even reversible. A brief discussion of the differential diagnosis with an emphasis on reversible and common causes follows.

A. **Wilson's disease**

This is a disorder of abnormal copper deposition in organs as a result of a deficiency in the copper-binding protein in plasma, ceruloplasmin. The **specific manifestations** include hepatic dysfunction, basal ganglia dysfunction, the presence of Kayser–Fleischer rings (i.e., a ring of discoloration around the limbus of the cornea), and dementia. The **specific evaluation and management** includes Box 14-3 and plasma copper and ceruloplasmin levels in addition to liver function tests, and referral to ophthalmology and gastroenterology. It is a **potentially modifiable** cause of dementia.

B. **Parkinson's disease**

See section on Gait Disturbances for specific manifestations, evaluation, and management. It is a **quite modifiable** cause of dementia.

C. **Major affective disorders**

See Chapter 15 for specific manifestations, evaluation, and management. **Depression** can present as dementia or can exacerbate the manifestations of dementia. The **specific evaluation and management** of this cause, sometimes referred to as "pseudodementia" include Box 14-3 and referral to a psychiatrist and/or a trial of an antidepressant agent. This is a **reversible** cause of dementia.

D. **Thyroid dysfunction**

Either hyperthyroidism or hypothyroidism can manifest with dementia. Hyperthyroidism in these cases is sometimes referred to as "apathetic hyperthyroidism." Refer to the section on Thyroid Dysfunctional States in Chapter 9, page 541. This is a **reversible** cause of dementia.

E. **Tertiary lues venereum**

Especially the specific entity "general paresis of the insane." See section on Sexually Transmitted Diseases in Chapter 6 for specifics. This is a **modifiable** cause of dementia.

F. **Korsakoff's syndrome**

The acquired, chronic deficiency of thiamine (B_1) will result in dementia. Although **irreversible** when present, it is **preventable** with adequate thiamine, i.e., good nutrition.

G. **Vitamin B_{12} deficiency**

The **specific manifestations** include dementia, cerebellar dysfunction, and loss of proprioceptive and vibratory sensation. There is an associated macrocytic anemia with megaloblastic changes in bone marrow. The **specific evaluation and management** are discussed in the section on Anemia in Chapter 5, page 258. This is a **reversible** cause of dementia.

H. **Heavy metal ingestion**

Usually occurs in patients who have occupational exposure or exposure in their home environment. One of the more common toxins is **lead,** which will cause the **specific manifestations** of dementia, erythrocyte basophilic stippling, renal dysfunction, and peripheral neuropathy. Common sources of lead intoxication include inhalation

B O X   1 4 - 3

Overall Evaluation and Management of Dementia

Evaluation

1. Thorough **mental status examination,** including assessment of patient's orientation to person, place, and time.
2. **Mental cognitive testing** for baseline purposes.
3. **Thyroid function tests,** to uncover any hyperthyroidism or hypothyroidism.
4. **Serum VDRL.** If reactive, may be indicative of lues venereum.
5. **Serum vitamin B_{12},** as a deficiency in vitamin B_{12} can result not only in megaloblastic anemia and neuropathy, but also in a dementing process.
6. Serum electrolytes, BUN, and creatinine for baseline purposes.
7. Serum **calcium, albumin, phosphorus,** as hypercalcemia, hyperphosphatemia, or hypophosphatemia can manifest as or exacerbate a dementing-type process.

NOTE: **No other screening tests** are indicated unless atypical features and/or concurrent findings are demonstrated on the history and physical examination.

Management

1. **Discontinue, if possible, any medications** which exacerbate dementia, e.g., the H_2 antagonist cimetidine.
2. **Screen for depression** via referral to a psychiatrist. Depression can often be an exacerbating factor or even the underlying mechanism for the patient's manifestations.
3. **Social services consultation** to outline and set in effect plans for outpatient nurse assistance and financial assistance.
4. **Referral of family to support groups.** There are several organizations which, as their primary goal, provide support to families of patients with dementing processes. The clinician must be aware of the various groups active in the community.

of paint dust when sanding/scraping, and eating of paint chips by children. The **specific evaluation and management** include obtaining serum lead levels, prevention, and treatment with chelating agents by a hematologist. This is a **reversible** cause of dementia.

I. **Chronic subdural hematoma**

This uncommon process usually occurs in a patient who has a long history of ethanol use and abuse and recurrent trauma. The **specific manifestations** include dementia and some focal neurologic findings. The **specific evaluation and management** include obtaining a CT scan of the head and referral to neurosurgery. This is a **modifiable** and potentially **reversible** cause of dementia.

J. **Normal pressure hydrocephalus**

This is the idiopathic increased size of the brain ventricles **not** secondary to an elevated intraventricular pressure. The **specific manifestations** include a wide-based gait, frontal release signs, and incontinence. The **specific evaluation and management** are to obtain a head CT scan; it is controversial if a ventriculoperitoneal (VP) shunt is therapeutic. This is a **possibly modifiable** cause of dementia.

K. **Hepatic encephalopathy**

See section on Hepatic Dysfunction in Chapter 2 for specifics in manifestations, evaluation, and management. This is a **modifiable** cause of dementia.

L. **Huntington's disease**

This is a familial form of basal ganglia and cortical destruction which is transmitted in an autosomal dominant fashion. The **specific manifestations** include the dementia along with progressive and severe choreiform movements. The **specifics in evaluation and management** include making the clinical diagnosis and prevention via genetic counseling of the patients. This is an **irreversible and progressive** cause of dementia.

M. **Alzheimer's disease**

This is the idiopathic, progressive, diffuse atrophy of the entire cerebral cortex. Variants include Pick's syndrome, in which early areas of atrophy are the frontal and temporal regions. Alzheimer's disease is the classic and most common form of dementing disease. Specifics in **evaluation and management** include that listed in Box 14-3. This is an **irreversible** cause of dementia.

III. **Management**

Chronic intervention includes support for family members and the development of schemes to manage the patient both as an outpatient and finally, when to admit the patient to a long-term care facility. In all cases the family should be intimately involved in decision making and a plan for future decisions must be formulated and formalized from the outset. These decisions include assignment of power of attorney for a family member, decisions on code status, and what criteria should be used for transfer to an extended care facility. There are many support groups throughout the United States for families of patients with dementing diseases. The families should be encouraged to avail themselves of these groups.

IV. **Consultation**

Problem	*Service*	*Time*
Huntington's chorea	Genetics counselor	Elective
Subdural hematoma	Neurosurgeon	Urgent
All cases	Support groups	Elective
Extended care facilities and plan	Geriatrician	Elective

V. **Indications for admission:** Patient is unable to care for self or family members are unable to care for patient.

Gait Disturbances

Normal gait is the activity of a person as he is walking. This is a very complex process which requires the action, interaction, and integration of many different parts of the central and peripheral nervous systems. It involves the **cerebellum,** the sense of **vision,** the senses of **proprioception** and **touch,** the **basal ganglia,** and the **sensory and motor cortex.** Due to its highly interactive and integrative mechanism, bipedal ambulation, a process which in most other animals is crude, to be streamlined and fluid, can be refined by learning new skills, and although basically the same in all normal people, has some modifications unique to each individual. An overall **description** of the normal gait is one foot in front of the other with the contralateral arm synchronously moving forward with each step.

I. **Pathogenesis**

The dark side of a process involving so many disparate sensory, motor, and integrative processes is that **damage to one area can affect the whole process** of normal ambulation. With increasing age there is an increasing incidence of damage through various mechanisms to one or more of these areas. Damage to each specific area can and will result in different gait disturbances. See Table 14-5 for specific gaits, their specific manifestations, and therapy. One gait disturbance, that of parkinsonism, is discussed in detail below.

A. Parkinson's disease and parkinsonism

This is a progressive, chronic disorder resulting from the atrophy and/or destruction of areas within the **basal ganglia.** It increases in incidence with age.

1. Pathogenesis

The underlying **pathogenesis** is a decrease in the neurotransmitter, **dopamine,** as a result of dopaminergic neuronal destruction in the **substantia nigra,** with a resultant imbalance of **acetylcholine to dopamine** within the basal ganglia. The destruction of the **substantia nigra,** a rich site of dopaminergic neurons, can result from any of the causes listed below, but, irrespective of the underlying cause, the symptoms, signs, and for the most part the prognosis are the same.

2. Causes

a. **Carbon monoxide poisoning.** High levels of CO can cause destruction of these cells and thus parkinsonism. Once present, the damage and manifestations are not reversible but will not progressively worsen.

b. **Neuroleptic drugs.** These agents, which are commonly used for major psychiatric disorders, can result in acetylcholine–dopamine imbalance and parkinsonism. This is quite reversible upon discontinuation of the agent.

c. **Postencephalitis.** This post-viral infection destruction of the basal ganglia was quite common after the influenza pandemic of 1918 and occasionally can be the presumptive cause today. This type, once present, is irreversible and progressively worsens.

d. **Idiopathic.** Idiopathic destruction of the basal ganglia and substantia nigra is the cause in the vast majority of cases. This is the true **Parkinson's disease,** also known as "paralysis agitans."

3. Manifestations

The **overall manifestations** of parkinsonism in general and Parkinson's disease in specific include the following clinical features:

a. **Gait disturbance** is the hallmark of this disorder, which is a direct manifestation of the bradykinesis (slowing of movement) inherent to parkinsonism. There is a significant bilateral decrease in arm swinging, the steps are bradykinetic, i.e., slow, shuffling, with a slightly flexed neck, and finally, the inability to quickly stop walking once initiated.

b. **Tremor** is an integral component of the manifesta-

T A B L E 1 4 - 5
Gait Disturbances

Type	Manifestations	Causes	Treatment
Spastic hemiparesis	Flexed upper extremity Arm immobile and held close to side Plantar flexed foot Circumduction of foot with foot dragging (all unilateral and contralateral to the side of the lesion)	Contralateral cerebrovascular accident (CVA) Contralateral head trauma	See CVA section PT/OT
Parkinson's	Stooped, head forward position Hips and knees flexed bilaterally Arms and wrists flexed bilaterally Rigid Bradykinetic Shuffling	Parkinson's disease Iatrogenic (neuroleptics) See text	See text PT/OT
Scissors	Stiff bilaterally Thighs cross in front Short, hesitant steps bilaterally	Bilateral CVAs to the motor cortex Bilateral head trauma	See CVA section PT/OT

Gait	Clinical Findings	Causes	Treatment/Workup
Steppage	Foot drop, unilateral or bilateral Unable to dorsiflex foot, unilateral or bilateral Unable to walk on heel(s) Needs to flex knee to lift the foot	Trauma, especially to the proximal fibula, resulting in unilateral common peroneal nerve damage Charcot–Marie–Tooth syndrome: autosomal dominant, bilateral	PT/OT
Cerebellar	Wide-based, staggering gait Patient unable to stand steady when feet are together, eyes open or closed	CVA to cerebellum Acute ethanol intoxication Multiple sclerosis Vitamin B_{12} deficiency	Discontinue ethanol CT of head B_{12} levels (serum) Treat the underlying cause PT/OT
Sensory	Wide-based gait Feet in front of body center Improves when looking at the ground Sensory deficit/neuropathy in feet Charcot joints—traumatic degenerative joint disease	Diabetes mellitus Vitamin B_{12} deficiency *Lues venereum*	Control diabetes VDRL Serum B_{12} Treat the underlying cause

BOX 14-4

*Overall Evaluation and Management of
Parkinson's Disease*

Evaluation

1. Thorough **history** and **physical examination,** to diagnose and document the type of gait and any of the concurrent manifestations described in text. Emphasis is placed on type of gait, presence of tremor, and presence of rigidity.
2. Examine patient for concurrent manifestations of **autonomic dysfunction,** i.e., lack of sweating, bladder or bowel incontinence, urine retention, orthostasis, or impotence.
3. Serum electrolytes, BUN, creatinine, and glucose for baseline purposes.
4. Serum **calcium, albumin, and phosphorus.** Abnormalities in calcium or phosphorus can exacerbate some of the features of parkinsonism.
5. If there are concurrent focal neurologic deficits, **CT of the head** is indicated to evaluate for any structural defects in the brain, e.g., CVA, subdural hematoma.

Management

1. Discontinue, if possible, **all neuroleptic agents.** Neuroleptics deplete dopamine and can exacerbate the features of Parkinson's disease. In idiopathic Parkinson's disease, any neuroleptic, e.g., haloperidol (Haldol), is effectively contraindicated.
2. Early **consultation with OT and PT** for assistance in management of the patient's mobility.
3. Initiate **antiparkinsonian agents.** The goal is to start only when symptomatic, as one will develop tolerance over time to the mainstay of therapy, levodopa. See Table 14-7 for specifics on these agents.
4. **Family support.** There are several groups in the community which provide support for family members of patients with Parkinson's disease.
5. **Neurology consultation.**

tions. The tremor is best demonstrated at **rest** and in the distal extremities and neck. It resolves with activity and is quite fine, i.e., has a frequency of 4–6 cycles/second. See Table 14-6 for other tremor syndromes.

c. **Rigidity of all musculature** is often a feature. **Rigidity** is an abnormally increased resistance to passive movement. This results in, at baseline, a slight amount of flexion at the elbows and knees. The clinician can demonstrate this rigidity by passively moving the legs and forearms. The rigidity is often bilateral and usually has component of "cogwheeling."

d. **Dementia** is an integral component.

e. **Other features** include an immobile face (mask facies), a depressed affect, and **Myerson's sign,** i.e., when the clinician taps over the bridge of the nose, an abnormally prolonged blink results.

II. Consultation

Problem	Service	Time
All cases	Neurology	Required
All cases	OT/PT	Required

III. **Indications for admission:** Very few patients require admission until very late in the course of the disease.

Headaches

Virtually everyone has headaches on an intermittent basis. The vast majority of these headaches are self-limited and/or respond to relaxation, rest and/or over-the-counter medications. Thus these headaches are, quite appropriately, not brought to the attention of the primary care physician. Several studies, however, have placed the percentage of people with **recurrent, frequent headaches at 1%–3%** of the population. Although the vast majority of these headaches are benign, a small number portend a malignant, even catastrophic, course.

I. Types of headache
A. Vascular headaches
1. Migraines
This is a quite common form of recurrent headaches. It is postulated to be due to arterial vasoconstriction followed by vasodilation, with the resultant symptomatic manifestations; the underlying reason for the vasoconstriction and vasodilation is uncertain.

T A B L E   1 4 - 6
Tremor Disturbances

Type	Manifestations	Associated Features	Mechanism	Treatment
Parkinson's	Generalized, all motor areas involved At rest Frequency of 4–6 cycles/second Exacerbated by stressors	Bradykinesis Rigidity Dementia	Decrease in CNS neurotransmitter, dopamine	See text
Essential tremor	Predominantly in hands and head; lower extremities spared At rest Decreases with ethanol ingestion Onset at any age	None	Unknown May have a hereditary component	Usually nothing is needed, but if severe, treat with β-blocker, e.g., atenolol, 25–50 mg PO q. A.M., or Primidone, 50 mg PO q.d.
Cerebellar dysfunction	Distal motor areas more affected than proximal Intention tremor, i.e., occurs during voluntary motor activity	Past pointing Decrease in fine motor skills Dysdiadochokinesis Decreased ability to perform finger to nose, heel to shin	Cerebellar CVA Multiple sclerosis Ethanol intoxication Vitamin B_{12} deficiency	Determine the cause and treat PT/OT Ethanol level as indicated
Hyperthyroid	Distal areas (hands and feet) affected more than proximal areas At rest	Weight loss Proximal weakness Goiter Eyelid lag	Elevated levels of thyroid hormone	

T A B L E 1 4 - 7
Medications for Parkinson's Disease

Agent	Indications/Activity	Mechanism	Dosing	Side Effects
Levodopa	Initiate agent when disability is imminent Improves all manifestations	Increases dopamine	To decrease side effects and increase dosage, carbidopa is added Carbidopa does not cross the blood–brain barrier and inhibits the peripheral conversion of L-dopa to dopamine by competitively inhibiting dopamine decarboxylase The carbidopa–levodopa ratio in the agent is 1:4 or 1:10, and has the trade name Sinemet (Sinemet is 25/100 or 10/100) Start at low doses, e.g., Sinemet, 25/100 t.i.d., and slowly increase dose	Dyskinesia Hypotension Tachycardia
Amantadine	Early in course, when mild	Unknown	100 mg PO b.i.d.	Restlessness
Bromocriptine	Adjunctive therapy at any time	Direct stimulation of dopamine receptors	1.25 mg PO b.i.d., increasing the dose q. 2 weeks by 2.5 mg; usual dose is 10–20 mg/day	Hypotension Tachycardia Nausea
Anticholinergic agents	Most effective in decreasing tremor and rigidity Minimally effective in decreasing bradykinesis	Unknown	Benztropine mesylate (Cogentin), 1 mg PO q.d., increase slowly to 5 mg PO q.d. Trihexyphenidyl (Artane), 2 mg PO t.i.d., increase slowly to 2–5 mg t.i.d.	Xerostomia Tachycardia Mydriasis Drowsiness Exacerbation of glaucoma

a. The **specific manifestations** include a prodromal sensation or **aura,** followed by an intense, throbbing, usually **unilateral headache** that can become generalized. The headache, without treatment, usually lasts from 2 to 8 hours and then slowly resolves. Other manifestations include nausea, vomiting, photophobia, visual "stars," **photopsia,** i.e., the patient sensing unformed light flashes, and/or **scintillating scotomas,** i.e., the transient presence of visual field defects with luminous visual hallucinations. Furthermore, the patient desires to lie flat in bed in a dark room. The **aura** symptoms are secondary to the vasoconstriction, whereas the **headache** is associated with the vasodilation phase.

b. **Past and family history** is specific for the fact that the first headache occurred during puberty and that one or more first-degree relatives also have similar headaches. The headaches are recurrent and can occur with a frequency of one time per day to one time per year. The patient may notice that specific habits or agents precipitate these headaches. These **precipitating activities** can include, but are not limited to, the ingestion of chocolate, ingestion of ethanol, a period of stress, or a menstrual cycle.

c. There are **several variants** of migraine headaches, each with specific unique manifestations. These variants include:

   i. **Classic migraine** has an antecedent aura.

   ii. **Common migraine** has no antecedent aura.

   iii. **Basilar artery migraine** is a special form of classic migraine which affects the basilar artery. The patient presents with an **aura** which consists of bilateral visual field cuts, dysarthria, tinnitus, vertigo, tingling in the trigeminal nerve (V_1, V_2, and V_3) distribution, and delirium. The **headache** is throbbing and located in the occipital regions bilaterally.

d. The specific **evaluation and management** include making the clinical diagnosis, acutely treating the pain, and, as clinically indicated, initiating prophylaxis. **Acute management** consists of placing the patient in a dark, quiet room; giving dihydroergotamine (DHE) 0.25–1.0 mg IM or IV, or the combination of ergotamine and caffeine (Cafergot), 1–4 tablets PO, at the onset of the headache; or an injection of meperidine, 50 mg (Demerol) IM, at the onset of the headache. **Ergotamines are contraindicated in pregnancy.** Furthermore, administration of the serotonin agonist **sumatriptan** in a dose of 6 mg subcutaneously has been demonstrated to be very effective in the acute management of migraine headaches. If the headache does not resolve or if any complications or focal neurologic deficits are manifest, **CT of the head** must emergently be performed to evaluate for other causes.

e. If the patient has **recurrent headaches** on a frequent basis, usually defined as more than 4 per month, prophylactic intervention should be strongly considered. Preventive measures include avoidance of precipitating factors and pharmacologic prophylactic intervention. Some agents in prophylaxis can include:

   i. **β-Blockers.** Either propranolol, 10 mg PO q.i.d., or atenolol, 25–50 mg PO q. A.M., can be effective in prophylaxis. One must not use if contraindicated (bronchospasm, heart failure, etc.) and furthermore, one must closely monitor blood pressure while using these agents.

   ii. **Calcium channel blockers.** Verapamil SR, 120–240 mg PO q. A.M., or nifedipine XL (Procardia XL), 30 mg PO q.d., can be effective. Monitor blood pressure closely.

   iii. **Amitryptiline** (Elavil), 25–50 mg PO q.H.S., is quite an effective prophylaxis.

   iv. **Ergonovine** can be very effective in prophylaxis but needs to be prescribed in low doses and with recurrent **"drug holidays."** There is a risk of **retroperitoneal fibrosis** if used in high doses and without such a drug holiday. The drug holiday is a month every 6 months in which the ergonovine is discontinued. The headaches will recur during the drug holiday.

   v. An attempt should be made every 3–6 months to **wean** the patient from any type of prophylactic therapy.

f. **Neurology consultation** should be obtained for any patient with complications or when prophylaxis is necessary. Admission to the hospital is indicated if any complications occur or if pain has not resolved with aggressive outpatient management.

2. **Cluster headaches**

   These headaches are another variant of vascular headaches.

a. The **specific manifestations** include an acute on-set, throbbing, and unilateral headaches. Rarely is there an antecedent aura. These headaches often occur at night and awaken the patient from a sound sleep. These headaches last 1–6 hours and often the patient will have several episodes in a finite period of time (1–2 weeks), followed by a period of no headaches (months to years), only to have another **cluster** of headaches occur. The patient can develop associated nasal congestion, conjunctival injection, and even a transient Horner's syndrome concurrent with the headache. In most cases the patient will be agitated and pacing the room during the headache.

b. The **specific management** includes the following features. **Acutely,** 100% Fio_2 by facial mask for 15–20 minutes is very effective. If the headache is still present, dihydroergotamine (DHE) 0.25–1.0 mg IM or IV, should be administered. Furthermore, administration of the narcotic agent meripidine, 50 mg IM, can be effective. **Ergotamines are contraindicated in pregnancy.** The **chronic management** is analogous to that for migraine headaches in that pharmacologic prophylactic intervention is not necessary unless the condition is quite frequent. One of several prophylactic agents can be used.

   i. **β-Blocker.** Same dosing as in migraine headaches.

   ii. **Calcium channel blocker.** Same dosing as in migraine headaches.

   iii. **Lithium carbonate.** Its use is indicated in severe cases which are refractory to standard therapy. In addition to closely monitoring the lithium levels, the clinician must monitor the patient for the development of any side effects of the lithium, e.g., nephrogenic diabetes insipidus.

   iv. **Prednisone.** In low doses (i.e., 10 mg PO q.d.), can be effective in prophylaxis. The disadvantage of this modality of prophylaxis is that it is fraught with the side effects of chronic glucocorticoid use.

   v. One must attempt to **wean** the patient from any prophylactic agent each 3–6 months.

c. **Neurology consultation** should be obtained for any patient with complications. Admission to the hospital is indicated if complications occur, or if pain is not resolved with aggressive outpatient management.

B. **Tension headaches**

Tension is one of the most common causes of solitary and/or recurrent headaches.

1. The **specific manifestations** include the subacute onset of a vague, potentially intense headache. The headache is quite often bilateral. Pain usually begins in the occipital area and then becomes generalized. The headaches can recur daily. There are usually no associated features except for a decreased attention span. Usually these headaches begin or are worse in the afternoon or evening. Other than tension or stress, other factors may be involved in their pathogenesis, including a **concurrent vascular** component and/or an **uncorrected myopia.**

2. The **specific evaluation and management** include querying the patient for any **refractory visual changes** and performing a visual acuity examination in order to diagnose such a problem. **Specific management** includes recommending the patient obtain a neck massage from spouse or significant other or take hot baths to relax any tense occipital muscles. **Pharmacologic intervention** can include:

   a. **Acetaminophen,** 500–1,000 mg PO now and q.4–6h. for 1–2 doses, or

   b. **NSAID—ibuprofen** (Motrin, Advil, Nuprin), 400–800 mg PO q.8h. PRN.

   c. If there is any suggestion of a vascular component to the headache, a trial injection of dihydroergotamine (DHE) 0.25–1.0 mg IM or sumatriptan 6 mg SC once may control the headache. **Ergotamines are contraindicated in pregnancy.** If there is any visual refractory dysfunction, referral to an ophthalmologist for corrective lenses is indicated.

   d. If the headaches are recurrent, even with adequate treatment, or if they progressively worsen, **biofeedback** and evaluation with neurology are indicated.

C. **CVA/Hypertensive emergency**

The mechanism of headache development in these processes is uncertain.

1. The **specific manifestations** include the acute onset of a severe, generalized headache. The headache in a **hypertensive emergency** may be the chief presenting complaint of the patient. These headaches are quite common if the hypertensive emergency is due to a pheochromocytoma. The headache of a **subarachnoid hemorrhage** is of acute onset, generalized, constant, and classically described as the worst of the patient's life.

2. The **evaluation and management** of this type of head-

ache are discussed in the section on Hypertension in Chapter 3, page 148, and in the section on Cerebrovascular Accidents, page 683.

D. Intracranial mass

These result in headaches which are thought to be secondary to the displacement of vascular structures by the intracranial mass itself.

1. The **specific manifestations** include the facts that quite often it is generalized, recurrent, and, with time, progresses in intensity and severity. This type of headache will often awaken the patient from a sound sleep and, unlike cluster headaches, is not associated with agitation. Because most intracranial masses occur in middle to late ages, an onset of generalized, recurrent headaches in any patient in these age groups should increase suspicion of an intracranial mass. This type of headache is classically **exacerbated by a Valsalva maneuver** (cough, straining with bowel movement) and eventually will manifest with concurrent focal neurologic deficits, seizures, or syncope.

2. The **differential diagnosis** of intracranial masses includes the following:

   a. **Metastatic neoplastic disease.** Usually from adenocarcinomas with primary lesions in the lungs, breast, or colon. The lesions are usually multiple, located at the border of the gray and white matter, and approximately 1–2 cm. There may be adjacent edema.

   b. **Primary neoplastic disease.** Lymphoproliferative or astrocytoma or glioblastoma multiforme. These lesions are usually unilateral, have irregular margins, and have adjacent edema.

   c. **Abscesses.** These can be single or multiple. They may be due to bacterial agents, usually anaerobic bacteria, or to the opportunistic protozoan organism, *Toxoplasma gondii*.

3. The **specific evaluation and management** include aggressive evaluation and management if an intracranial mass is suspected.

   a. **CT of the head** with and without contrast with imaging of the posterior fossa is clearly indicated. **Indications** for CT imaging include:

      i. The onset of severe, recurrent headaches in a patient more than 35 years old.

      ii. Exacerbation of the headache upon a Valsalva maneuver.

      iii. The presence of **any neurologic defects,** fevers, papilledema, or change in mental status or level of consciousness (see Fig. 14-3).

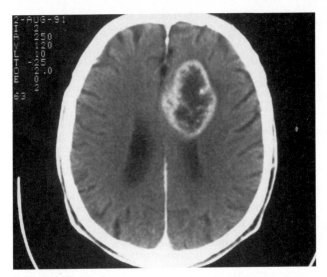

FIGURE 14-3
CT of the head with contrast showing a large contrast-enhancing lesion
in the left frontal/parietal areas. The differential diagnosis of
contrast-enhancing lesions includes abscesses, including those caused
by *Toxoplasma gondii,* lymphomas, and, as in this case, glioblastoma
multiforme.

          iv. Severe headaches in an immunocompromised
              patient.

    b. If **further imaging** is required, MRI has the highest
       sensitivity and specificity.

    c. The bottom line need is for **tissue** to diagnose the
       lesion. The easiest way is to look for the primary
       neoplastic lesion and biopsy that; however, if no
       extracranial primary lesion is found, biopsy of the
       brain lesion is indicated. The biopsy should be
       histopathologically examined and sent for Gram
       stain, bacterial cultures, and AFB cultures.

    d. If there is any **evidence of edema,** initiation of pa-
       renteral **dexamethasone** is indicated (Decadron,
       2–4 mg IV stat and then q.6h.), as is consultation
       with neurosurgery.

    e. In virtually all cases where the headache is due to
       an intracranial mass, admission to the hospital
       with neurosurgical consultation is required.

    f. If **tumor** is present, oncology consultation is indi-
       cated, whereas if an **abscess** or *Toxoplasma gondii*

is present, an HIV test should be performed and an infectious diseases consultation obtained.

E. Morning headaches

These are headaches of uncertain pathogenesis which can be due to several discrete causes.

1. The **specific manifestations** include the fact that these headaches are present at time of awakening and resolve over the course of the day. Further specifics are related to the two most common underlying causes.

   a. First, it may be due to an **ethanol-related "hangover,"** in which the patient ingests ethanol the evening before and awakens with nausea and a generalized headache. The **specific management** includes instructing the patient not to binge drink.

   b. The second disease process that can present with morning headaches is **sleep apnea syndrome.** This is a syndrome in which the patient develops abnormally prolonged periods of apnea during sleep. These episodes of apnea are usually the result of excessive pharyngeal tissue, which occurs predominantly in obese patients. These periods of apnea lead to episodes of hypercapnia, hypoxemia, and a lack of restful sleep. The associated manifestations include severe snoring and falling asleep at inappropriate times during the day. The patient can fall asleep during a routine conversation or even while driving an automobile. The **specific evaluation and management** include a formal **sleep study** and consultation with pulmonary medicine.

F. Tic douloureux (trigeminal neuralgia)

This is the dysfunction, often idiopathic, of the peripheral component of cranial nerve V. Cranial nerve V supplies sensation to the face via three branches: V_1, to the forehead; V_2, to the maxillary skin; and V_3, to the mandibular skin.

1. The **specific manifestations** include the acute onset of severe, lancing pain that begins at the mouth and radiates to the ipsilateral eye and ear. Virtually always unilateral, it usually involves V_2 and V_3 more than V_1, i.e., below the eye more than above the eye. This will spontaneously resolve only to acutely return several times in a short period of time. There can be and often are extended periods without symptoms. However, with increasing age, there is a decrease in the interval between episodes and the episodes increase in intensity, duration, and frequency.

2. The **specific evaluation and management** include making the clinical diagnosis. Further evaluation can

include MRI of the posterior fossa to look for a small glioma in that area which could be surgically resected. **Refraining from agents/activities** which can precipitate the symptoms, e.g., touching the overlying skin, chewing ice, etc., is very important. **Pharmacologic intervention** includes initiation of carbamazepine (Tegretol) PO on a chronic basis. If still symptomatic, ablation of the trigeminal nerve/ganglion may be indicated. Therefore, consultations with neurology and a pain care specialist are indicated.

G. **Carious teeth, sinusitis, and leptomeningitis**
These conditions will also cause headaches. Each is discussed in separate sections.

II. **Consultation**

Problem	*Service*	*Time*
Vascular headaches	Neurology	Urgent/emergent
Neurologic deficits	Neurology	Urgent/emergent
Intracranial masses	Neurosurgery	Urgent/emergent

III. **Indications for admission:** New focal deficits, CT-proven intracranial masses, or any evidence of leptomeningitis.

Meningitis

Leptomeningitis is the nonspecific inflammation of the **leptomeninges** themselves, including the dura mater, the arachnoid mater, and the pia mater. The **dura mater** is the thick, fibrous layer immediately adjacent (deep) to the bones of the skull and vertebral column. The **pia mater** is a thin, pliable layer of tissue which is intimately apposed to the spinal cord and surface of the brain. In between is the lacy and fine connective tissue layer of the **arachnoid mater.** There are two spaces of anatomical importance, the **subdural space,** between dura mater and bone, and the **subarachnoid space,** between the pia mater and arachnoid mater. The subarachnoid space is filled with cerebrospinal fluid (CSF) and is the space from which CSF is obtained during a lumbar puncture.

I. **Overall manifestations**
The **overall manifestations** at presentation include a decrease in the level of consciousness, even to the point of coma, delirium, convulsions, recurrent fevers, headaches, neck stiffness, nausea, and vomiting. Presenting **signs** include nuchal rigidity, **Kernig's sign** (abnormal involuntary flexion of the neck on passive extension of the knee when the patient is supine with the hip flexed), and/or **Brudzinski's sign** (abnormal flexion of the hips upon passively flexing the patient's neck with the patient supine).

II. Causes

The **causes** are quite diverse and are best divided into categories of bacterial, viral, neoplastic, and mycobacterial causes.

A. Bacterial

Bacterial etiologies cause acute leptomeningitis which, if untreated will result in the death of the patient. Each of the following organisms discussed can cause acute leptomeningitis in adults.

1. *Neisseria meningitidis.* This gram-negative coccus causes a severe meningitis and systemic illness.

   a. The **specific manifestations** include the basic findings (see above) in addition to acquired petechiae, purpura, menometrorrhagia, bleeding gingivae, and epistaxis, all as a result of an acquired consumptive coagulopathy specific to *Neisseria meningitidis.* The **natural history** of untreated disease entails sepsis and rapid death of the patient.

   b. The laboratory evaluation (Box 14-5) includes the **peripheral white blood cell** (WBC) count, which usually is elevated. If the WBC is inappropriately low, it can be a harbinger of impending septic shock. The **CSF** will have an elevated protein, a decreased glucose, and an elevated WBC, usually with predominance of polymorphonuclear (PMN) cells. **Gram stain** of the CSF shows polymorphonuclear cells and gram-negative cocci. **Latex agglutination** of the CSF will be positive for *Neisseria meningitidis* capsular antigen. A disseminated intravascular coagulation (DIC) panel (platelets, PT, PTT, and fibrinogen) should be performed to determine if a **consumptive coagulopathy** is present.

   c. **Management** includes the basics as described in Box 14-5 and aggressive, intensive, and immediate antibiotic therapy. This is a disease process which **mandates emergent antibiotics.** The essential element is time. Immediate therapy is of the essence. Regimens include:

      i. Penicillin G, 24 million units/24 hours IV (4–6 million units IV stat, then 2 million units IV q.2h.). Can be started instead of or after the dose of ceftriaxone listed in the acute management section; or

      ii. Ceftriaxone, 2 g IV q.12h.; or

      iii. **Chloramphenicol,** 100 mg/kg/day IV.

      All regimens need to be continued for 10–14 days or until patient is afebrile for 5 concurrent days (whichever is longer). Further principles of therapy include fluid management, treatment of

B O X 1 4 - 5

Overall Evaluation and Management of Suspected Leptomeningitis

Evaluation

1. **ABCs,** i.e., basic and advanced life support protocol, as needed.
2. Establish **intravenous access** in preparation for **imminent** administration of parenteral antibiotics.
3. **Blood cultures** are clearly indicated as the pathogen can be grown from the blood in a significant minority of cases.
4. **Complete blood cell count** with differential for baseline purposes. In most cases of leptomeningitis there is a significant leukocytosis and a left shift in the differential count.
5. **PT, aPTT, platelets, and fibrinogen** are important for baseline purposes as certain etiologies of leptomeningitis, specifically *Neisseria meningitidis,* can cause a severe consumptive coagulopathy.
6. Serum electrolytes, calcium, albumin, and PO_4 for baseline purposes.
7. **Lumbar puncture**—mandatory (see Table 14-8 for laboratory examinations performed on the CSF and their normal values).

Management

1. If a **bacterial etiology** is suspected:
   a. Penicillin G, 4–6 million units IV **stat,** *or*
   b. Ceftriaxone, 2 g IV **stat.**
2. **Admit** to an inpatient service.

DIC (see section on Excessive Bleeding States in Chapter 5, page 275), and placing the patient in respiratory isolation.

d. **Prevention** is of great importance as this disease can have morbid and even mortal outcomes, even with effective therapy early in the course. Prevention consists of placing patient in **respiratory isolation,** as the transmission of this pathogen is via respiratory secretions, and the prescription of **rifampin, 600 mg PO b.i.d.** for 2 days (10 mg/kg b.i.d. for 2 days in children) to any exposed con-

T A B L E   1 4 - 8
Cerebrospinal Fluid: Routine Tests and Normal Values

Test	Normal Value
Cell count with differential	0–5 WBCs per hpf, all mononuclear
Protein level	15–45 mg/dL
Glucose level	40–80 mg/dL (1/2 of serum glucose)
Gram stain	No cells, no organisms
AFB smear	No AFB
VDRL	Nonreactive
Latex agglutination for capsule antigens in *Streptococcus pneumoniae, Hemophilus influenzae,* and *Neisseria meningitidis*	None detectable
Bacterial culture	No growth
Mycobacterial culture	No growth
Cytology	No cells

tacts, e.g., members of the household, day care members, or nursing home residents.

   e. **Complications** of this specific form of meningeal infection include, in addition to death, the following entities: neurosensory deafness, which is usually transient; intracranial abscess formation; DIC; hydrocephalus; and/or adrenal insufficiency as a result of Waterhouse–Friderichsen syndrome.

2. *Hemophilus influenzae*

   This gram-negative coccobacillus, usually of the capsular type b, will cause a severe leptomeningitis.

   a. The **specific manifestations** include the basic symptoms and signs as described above after an antecedent period of upper respiratory symptoms. This form of meningitis is much more common in young children than in adults, but still needs to be considered in the differential diagnosis of adult leptomeningitis.

   b. The **laboratory evaluation** (Box 14-5) includes the **peripheral white blood cell** (WBC) count, which usually is elevated. If the WBC is inappropriately low, it can be a harbinger of impending septic shock. The **CSF** will have an elevated protein, a decreased glucose, and an elevated WBC, usually with predominance of polymorphonuclear (PMN) cells. **Gram stain** of the CSF shows PMNs and gram-negative coccobacilli. **Latex agglutination** will be positive for *Hemophilus influenzae* capsular antigen.

   c. **Management** includes the basics as described in Box 14-5 and antibiotics. Antibiotic regimens include:

     i. Ceftriaxone, 2 g IV q.12h.; or

     ii. Ampicillin, 2 g IV q.4–6h., and chloramphenicol 100 mg/kg/day IV.

     iii. Either regimen is given for 10 days.

   d. **Prevention** is also a major concern in this disease. Although it has fewer complications than *Neisseria meningitidis*, it can cause hydrocephalus and death. Preventive measures include:

     i. *H. influenzae* type b polysaccharide vaccine in **all children** ages 2–5 years (irrespective of exposure), and

     ii. **Contacts,** when <4 years of age, should be given **rifampin,** 20 mg/kg/day for 4 consecutive days.

3. *Streptococcus pneumoniae.* This gram-positive diplococcus causes an acute meningitis.

   a. The **specific manifestations** include the overall manifestations as described above along with, in virtually all cases, an antecedent otitis media, lobar pneumonitis, or upper respiratory tract infection. A specific **risk factor** for the development of this and other streptococcal infections is the presence of asplenia and/or hypogammaglobulinemia.

   b. The **laboratory evaluation** (Box 14-5) includes the **peripheral white blood cell** (WBC) count, which usually is elevated. If the WBC is inappropriately low, it can be a harbinger of impending septic shock. The **CSF** will have an elevated protein, a decreased glucose, and an elevated WBC, usually with predominance of polymorphonuclear (PMN) cells. **Gram stain** of the CSF shows PMNs and gram-positive diplococci. **Latex agglutination** will be positive for *Streptococcus pneumoniae* capsular antigen.

   c. **Management** includes the steps listed in Box 14-5 and initiation of antibiotics. Specific antibiotic regimens include:

     i. Penicillin, 24 million units IV/24 hours (4 million units IV bolus, followed by 2 million units IV/2 hours); or

     ii. Ceftriaxone, 2 g IV q.12h.

     iii. Either regimen is given for 10 days.

   d. **Prevention** is important, as severe morbidity and mortality can result, even in optimally treated cases. Observation of patient contacts and early treatment is probably the most effective.

4. *Listeria monocytogenes.* This gram-positive rod can cause a leptomeningitis in adults.
   a. The **specific manifestations** of this type of meningitis include fewer classic findings, and thus a more subacute presentation. Many patients present with mild mental status changes associated with a low-grade fever. Nuchal rigidity and the classic findings of meningeal irritation often are not present until late in the course. Groups at particularly high risk for this pathogen include alcoholics and patients on chronic steroid therapy.
   b. The **laboratory evaluation** (Box 14-5) includes the **peripheral WBC count,** which usually is elevated. If the WBC is inappropriately low, it can be a harbinger of impending septic shock. The **CSF** will have an elevated protein, a decreased glucose, and an elevated WBC, usually with predominance of polymorphonuclear (PMN) cells. **Gram stain** of the CSF shows PMNs and, rarely but diagnostically, gram-positive rods. **Latex agglutination** will be negative for capsular antigens. The diagnosis is presumptive until cultures return. The clinician must use care not to overlook this pathogen, as it can be confused with "diphtheroids," i.e., contaminants. Therefore, the clinician must interpret test results in the context of the patient.
   c. **Management** includes the steps listed in Box 14-5 and antibiotics, usually broad-spectrum antibiotics until cultures return with diagnostic confirmation. Regimens to treat *Listeria monocytogenes* include:
      i. **Ampicillin,** 2 g IV q.4–6h., and an aminoglycoside (gentamicin or tobramycin) bolus 1.5–2.0 mg/kg IV, for the first 7–10 days; or
      ii. **Chloramphenicol,** 100 mg/kg/day IV.
      iii. Either regimen is given for 6 weeks.
   d. **Prevention** is essentially having a clinical suspicion in patients with appropriate manifestations who are in high-risk groups and proscribing the use of unpasteurized products by patients at high risk.

B. **Viral meningitis**
   Also referred to as "aseptic meningitis," this can be caused by many of the RNA viruses, including enteroviruses and picornaviruses.
   a. The **specific manifestations** include an antecedent, several-day history of malaise, fever, mild neck stiffness, myalgias, and upper respiratory symptoms and signs. The neck stiffness gradually

worsens and becomes associated with headache, nausea, and intermittent vomiting. This is quite seasonal, and epidemics are not uncommon in late summer and early fall.

    b. The **laboratory evaluation** includes the steps listed in Box 14-5. In the **peripheral WBC count** there usually is a mild leukocytosis with lymphocyte predominance. The **CSF** will have a normal glucose, mildly elevated protein, and a mild increase in WBCs, all of which are mononuclear. **Gram stain** is negative for PMNs or organisms. **Latex agglutination** is negative for capsular antigens.

    c. **Management** is supportive. Antibiotics are not indicated unless suspicion of a bacterial cause is relatively high or the patient is immunosuppressed. If the patient is delirious or if HSV encephalitis is in the differential diagnoses, start acyclovir IV. This is the only form of meningitis in which the patient can, if stable, be managed as an **outpatient.**

C. Meningeal carcinomatosis

This is a type of leptomeningitis in which the infiltrate is not as a result of infection and its resultant inflammatory response but of malignant neoplastic cells.

    a. The **specific manifestations** are usually quite insidious but, once present, can consist of the classic findings of meningitis. The patient usually has acquired cranial nerve defects, especially a peripheral cranial nerve VII palsy. Many patients have an antecedent history of malignant metastatic neoplastic disease, especially adenocarcinomas of the lungs, breast, or colon, or leukemias or lymphomas.

    b. The **laboratory evaluation** includes the steps listed in Box 14-5. The **CSF** reveals a normal glucose and a markedly elevated protein. **Gram stain** of the CSF is negative for organisms, cell count usually with "atypical cells" present, and **Cytology** is positive for malignant cells. MRI is indicated, especially of the posterior fossa to demonstrate the extent of leptomeningeal and adjacent structural involvement.

    c. The **management** of this process is beyond the scope of this text. A consultation with oncology is indicated. Cranial irradiation or intrathecal chemotherapy (methotrexate) is indicated, under the direction of the oncologist.

D. Mycobacterial

This organism can spread from lungs to extrapulmonary sites either in primary (if miliary) or reactivation mycobacterial disease.

a. The **specific manifestations** of this entity can be very insidious and consist of headache, constitutional symptoms, and moderate recurrent nausea and vomiting. Nuchal rigidity and the classic features of meningeal irritation develop only late in the course of disease. Cranial nerve deficits can also develop, especially of cranial nerves VII and/or XII.

b. The **laboratory evaluation** includes the steps listed in Box 14-5. The **CSF** will have a normal glucose, a markedly increased protein, and an increase in WBCs, the majority of which are mononuclear. **Gram stain** is negative for organisms but shows mononuclear cells. **Latex agglutination** is negative. AFB smears and cultures are positive for *Mycobacterium hominis*. Urinalysis with AFB smear/culture and chest radiography are mandatory components of the evaluation, as the primary location—pulmonary or urologic—can thus be uncovered.

c. **Management** includes placing the patient in respiratory isolation if the patient has active pulmonary disease. A course of four antimycobacterial agents is indicated:

   i. Isoniazid, 300 mg PO q.d.
   ii. Rifampin, 600 mg PO q.d.
   iii. Ethambutol, 15 mg/kg/day PO.
   All three for 24 consecutive months.
   and
   iv. Streptomycin,* 1 g IM q.d. for 2 weeks, then twice per week for 10 weeks, or
   v. Pyrazinamide 25 mg/kg/day PO in a q.d. dosing for 24 months.

   If cranial nerve deficits are present or developing, steroids are indicated: prednisone, 60 mg PO q.d. As this is a chronic disease, nutritional support must be optimized.

E. **Subarachnoid hemorrhage**
This catastrophic event can manifest with acute meningeal manifestations. See section on Cerebrovascular Accidents, page 683, for further discussion.

III. **Consultation**

Problem	Service	Time
Bacterial meningitides	Infectious diseases	Urgent/ emergent
Mycobacterial	Infectious diseases	Urgent

*Streptomycin is no longer available commercially in the United States.

Problem	*Service*	*Time*

Meningeal
    carcinomatosis
	Hematology/
	    Oncology
		Urgent

IV. **Indications for admission: Bacterial** meningitis, aseptic
meningitis if unable to maintain volume orally, **mycobacterial or neoplastic** meningitis.

Seizure Disorders

A **seizure** is any uncontrolled abnormal activity of the brain. It
can present with a variety of findings ranging from a blank stare
to generalized clonic activity to repetitive, automatic movements.
The differential diagnosis, workup, and management are essentially the same for all seizure types, irrespective of the presenting
features and manifestations.

I. **Overall manifestations**
   A. **Convulsions**
      A convulsion is a specific form of seizure in which the
      manifestations include uncontrolled motor activity. The
      tonic–clonic convulsion is the classic example and is the
      type which the general public usually thinks of when
      describing a seizure.
      1. **Tonic.** A convulsion in which the major motor com-
         ponent is profound rigidity, i.e., the tone of the mus-
         culature is markedly and uncontrollably increased.
         This can occur alone or as a prelude to clonic activity.
         The classic tonic convulsion is opisthotonus, in
         which the patient is rigid and has a hyperextended
         neck. A tonic convulsive seizure is uniformly general-
         ized in nature.
      2. **Clonic.** A convulsion in which the major motor com-
         ponent is rapid repetitive uncontrolled activity. This
         often is associated with tonic activity. A clonic con-
         vulsive seizure is uniformly generalized in nature.
   B. **Epilepsy**
      The presence of recurrent seizures of any kind, classi-
      cally idiopathic. This is a colloquial term for seizures
      and/or convulsions.
   C. **Status epilepticus**
      The onset of a seizure which does not spontaneously re-
      solve, requiring **emergency medical intervention.** Any
      uncontrolled seizure, irrespective of manifestations or
      cause, must be treated aggressively as status epilepticus.
      The acute evaluation and management of this state are
      discussed below.

II. **Causes**
    The **differential diagnosis** of seizures, irrespective of mani-
    festations, is essentially the same. The most likely causes for

new onset seizures are different for young adults, i.e., 15–45 years of age, when compared with middle-aged and older adults, i.e., more than 45 years of age. Each of the following lists is by order of frequency in each age group.

A. Causes in younger adults

1. **Head trauma.** Individuals in this group are usually quite active and at risk for head trauma through contact sports, motor vehicle (especially motorcycle) accidents, and ethanol-related falls.

2. **Withdrawal** from drugs, especially withdrawal from ethanol.

3. **Acute ingestion** of agents, especially tricyclic antidepressants in a suicide attempt.

4. **Space-occupying lesions** in the cranium. These can be neoplastic (benign or malignant) or, especially in immunocompromised patients, due to infectious agents. The two most common infectious agents are anaerobic bacteria and *Toxoplasma*.

5. **Leptomeningitis.** See section on Meningitis, page 717.

6. **Idiopathic.** This is a diagnosis of exclusion, occasionally the cause of recurrent seizures (epilepsy) cannot be determined.

B. Causes in older adults

1. **Space-occupying lesions** in the cranium. These are usually neoplastic lesions, either malignant primary lesions (e.g., glioblastoma multiforme) or metastatic lesions. Lesions that commonly metastasize to the brain are colon, breast, and lung cancers and malignant melanomas.

2. **Cerebrovascular accidents** may result in a seizure disorder.

3. **Metabolic or electrolyte abnormalities.** These conditions significantly increase in frequency in the elderly population as patients are placed on medications (e.g., insulin, diuretics) that can significantly affect electrolyte balance. At baseline, patients may be at increased risk for electrolyte or metabolic disorders that can precipitate seizures. Examples of such electrolyte or metabolic causes include:

    a. Hypokalemia.
    b. Hypocalcemia.
    c. Hypophosphatemia.
    d. Hyponatremia.
    e. Hypoxemia.
    f. Hypoglycemia.

4. **Leptomeningitis.** See section on Meningitis, page 717.

5. **Withdrawal** from drugs, especially withdrawal from ethanol.

III. **Classification of seizure disorders** (modified from the International League Against Epilepsy criteria, see Table 14-10).

  A. **Partial seizures**

   These are seizures in which only a small portion of the cerebral cortex has uncontrolled activity. The manifestations can be diverse and are specific to the area involved. Any partial seizure can become, either acutely or longitudinally, a generalized seizure disorder. There are two subtypes of partial seizures, simple and complex.

   1. The **specific manifestations** of **simple partial seizures** are distinct from those of other seizures in that the patient does not lose consciousness. These seizures can manifest with focal motor activity (location: motor cortex), tactile sensation/hallucination (location: sensory cortex), perception of deja vu (perception that period of time at present has been lived or experienced before, even on a recurrent basis) (location: lower cerebral cortex), and automatic behaviorisms, e.g., snapping the fingers, mania, or delirium (location: temporal cortex).

   2. The **specific manifestations** of **complex partial seizures** include loss of consciousness. Complex partial seizures can be associated with the manifestations described for simple partial seizures either before or after the event and can, like partial simple seizures, become secondarily generalizable.

   3. Although the **evaluation and management** of these seizures are similar for all seizure types (see Box 14-6), several caveats are in order. The clinician must look for an intracranial structural defect if the seizure is partial. If a partial seizure is localized to the tempo-

---

BOX 14-6

Overall Evaluation and Management of Status Epilepticus and Seizures

Evaluation

1. ABCs—i.e., basic and advanced life support protocols, as necessary. During the seizure, maintenance of an airway is fundamental.

(continued)

B O X   1 4 - 6 *(continued)*

2. **Intravenous access** must be obtained for the potential administration of glucose, benzodiazepines, or antiseizure medications.
3. Basic laboratory studies, **stat:**
   a. Atrial blood gases.
   b. Serum calcium, albumin, magnesium, and PO_4.
   c. Serum glucose.
   d. Serum electrolytes.
   e. Antiseizure drug levels (see Table 14-9 for normal levels).
   f. Blood ethanol level.

Management

1. **Thiamine, 100 mg IV,** followed by 1 ampule of D50W IV.
2. **Benzodiazepines** to control the seizure acutely, either **lorazepam** (Ativan), 2–3 mg IV stat, repeated as necessary in 15–20 minutes; *or* **diazepam** (Valium), 5–10 mg IV stat, repeated as necessary in 15–30 minutes.
3. Initiate **chronic therapy** as clinically indicated with **phenytoin (Dilantin),** 800–1,000 mg IV loading dose, in one of the following protocols.
   a. 20 mg/min, usually by slow IV push of 8 to 10 100-mg prefilled syringes, each administered over 5 minutes, *or*
   b. 1,000 mg in 250 mL of 0.45 NS IV drip over 1 hour.
4. If patient is still **actively seizing,** add **phenobarbital,** 10–15 mg/kg (700–1,000 mg) by slow IV push at a rate of 50 mg/min.
5. **CT scan of the head** without contrast is especially important if there is any history of trauma or any evidence of papilledema or of new focal neurologic deficits.
6. **Lumbar puncture** if there is any evidence of or suspicion for leptomeningitis. See section on Meningitis, page 717.
7. **Serum VDRL** to evaluate for lues venereum. If reactive, should be performed on CSF.
8. **EEG,** to be performed under the guidance of a neurologist after admission and stabilization of patient.
9. Neurology consultation.

T A B L E 1 4 - 9
Common Antiseizure Medications: Regimens, Indications, Levels, and Side Effects

Agent	Indications	Dose	Level	Side Effects
Phenytoin (Dilantin)	Generalized tonic–clonic	100–300 mg PO q.d. (usually 300)	10–20 µg/mL	Cerebellar Nystagmus Ataxia Macrocytosis Positive ANA Peripheral neuropathy
Phenobarbital	Generalized tonic–clonic	100–200 mg PO q.d.	10–40 µg/mL	Nystagmus Ataxia Hyperactivity (exacerbation of attention deficit disorder)
Carbamazepine	Partial Generalized tonic–clonic	600–1,200 mg/24 hr (300–600 mg b.i.d.)	6–12 µg/mL	Nystagmus Hepatitis Dysarthria Leukopenia
Valproic acid	Generalized petit mal (absence) Generalized tonic–clonic	30–60 mg/kg/24° q.8h. divided doses	50–100 µg/mL	Thrombocytopenia Tremor Alopecia
Clonazepam (Clonipin)	Generalized petit mal (absence)	0.05–0.2 mg/kg/24° in b.i.d. to t.i.d. divided doses	20–80 ng/mL	Ataxia Exacerbation of generalized tonic–clonic seizures

T A B L E   1 4 - 1 0
Classification and General Management of Seizures

Type	Symptoms and Signs	Treatment

Partial
    Simple
    Complex
	Automatisms
	Mania/delirium
	Deja vu
		Carbamazepine
		    (Tegretol)

Generalized, absence (petit mal)	Acute onset of blank stare Incontinence Decreased postural tone	Valproic acid (Depakene)
Generalized, tonic–clonic (grand mal)	Aura, followed by tonic motor activ- ity, followed by clonic motor activ- ity, with a period of lethargy after cessation of motor activity	Phenytoin (Dilantin) Phenobarbital

ral region, herpes simplex encephalitis is in the differential diagnosis. Treatment specifics include the initiation of antibiotics for leptomeningitis, the use of
acyclovir in a dose of 10 mg/kg IV q.8h. for 14 days,
and MRI of the temporal lobes if herpes simplex encephalitis is suspected.

B. Generalized seizures

These are seizures in which the entire cerebral cortex is
involved. They may begin as partial seizures or may be
the first indication of a seizure disorder. In all generalized
seizures there is a loss of consciousness with amnesia for
the seizure itself. There are two major types of generalized seizures, absence type and tonic–clonic type.

1. The **specific manifestations** of **absence (petit mal) seizures** include an abrupt onset and termination, and
   lack of any prodromal aura or postictal lethargy.
   These seizures manifest with a slight decrease in pos-
   tural tone, incontinence of urine or stool, a decrease in
   the level of consciousness, and often a "blank stare"
   noticeable to people interacting with the patient.
   These seizures may last from seconds to long periods
   (status epilepticus). The EEG shows bilateral, diffuse,
   synchronous 3-Hz spikes and domes; the pattern is
   pathognomonic.

2. The **specific manifestations** of **tonic–clonic (grand
   mal) seizures** include an abrupt onset and termination, and both an antecedent aura and a significant
   period of postictal lethargy. The classic features are
   an aura of variable duration, followed by 1–2 minutes
   of tonic motor activity, followed by clonic activity for
   2–4 minutes. The patient experiences complete loss
   of consciousness, incontinence of urine and stool,
   tongue biting, and a period of postictal lethargy. If

during the postictal period there is focal weakness (paresis or plegia), the condition is described as Todd's paralysis and the cause is a structural or anatomic lesion. Laboratory findings in the postictal phase of **any** tonic–clonic seizure, irrespective of cause, include an increased serum CPK, a high anion gap metabolic acidosis (secondary to lactate), leukocytosis without a left shift, and an increase in serum prolactin levels.

3. The **evaluation and management** of generalized seizures include the steps listed in Box 14-6 and the following specific features. If a cause is determined from the overall evaluation, treatment is directed toward that cause. Specifics include antibiotics for leptomeningitis, the use of acyclovir in a dose of 10 mg/kg IV q.8h. for 14 days, and MRI of the temporal lobes if herpes simplex encephalitis is suspected, the use of dexamethasone (Decadron), 2–4 mg IV q.6h., and consultation with neurosurgery for any space-occupying lesions with adjacent edema, correction of any electrolyte disorders, the treatment of withdrawal seizures with thiamine and benzodiazepines, and consultation with neurosurgery if head trauma or a subdural hematoma is present.

In most cases in which a specific, treatable, reversible cause is demonstrated, chronic pharmacologic therapy is not necessary.

If no specific diagnosis is determined, an EEG should be performed and chronic therapy continued. Further imaging techniques including MRI should be considered if the potential for a dysmyelinating disorder (multiple sclerosis), HSV encephalitis, or small structural abnormality still exists after an initially negative evaluation.

IV. **Chronic therapy**

Chronic therapy includes antiseizure medications (see Table 14-9), support of the patient and patient's family emotionally, and instructing the patient in life style modification. These modifications may include abstinence from ethanol, phenothiazines (these agents can lower the seizure threshold), and restricting driving and pilot privileges.

A. Indications for the **withdrawal of antiseizure medications** include:

1. Ethanol-related seizures.
2. No seizure for more than 2–3 years in an otherwise stable patient. This should be performed under the guidance of a consulting neurologist and consists of a slow, careful withdrawal of the antiseizure medication(s).

V. Consultation

Problem	Service	Time
All patients	Neurology	Urgent/ emergent
Meningitis	Infectious diseases	Urgent/ emergent
Subdural hematoma	Neurosurgery	Emergent

VI. Indications for admission: New onset or **increased frequency** of seizures. All patients with **status epilepticus** need emergency admission, usually to an ICU.

Vertigo (Box 14-7)

Vertigo is the sensation by the patient of rotatory disequilibrium. The patient senses that this body or its surrounding environment is moving in a rotatory fashion. The classic example is "bed spins" described by acutely intoxicated people who lie flat in bed.

I. Pathogenesis
The **pathogenesis** involves unilateral disease or dysfunction of the inner ear, the **vestibulolabyrinthine system.** The inner ear consists of both the vestibular and cochlear apparatus. The **vestibular apparatus** is the major sensory organ for position, and dysfunction can cause vertigo; the **cochlear apparatus** is a major component of auditory sensation, and dysfunction can cause neural deafness or tinnitus, i.e., a ringing sensation in the ears. Furthermore, the same cranial nerve VIII serves both areas and functions of the inner ear. Because of its proximity to the vestibular apparatus, a patient may present with **decreased auditory acuity** and **tinnitus** concurrent with vertigo.

II. Causes
The **causes of** vertigo are diverse. The discussion here is limited to the most common or treatable/reversible causes.
A. Benign positional vertigo
Benign positional vertigo is a common, idiopathic, minimally disabling form of vertigo. It occurs when the patient acutely lies supine, with or without mild neck extension, and rapidly resolves when the patient stands up. There is some associated horizontal nystagmus, but **no** associated tinnitus or auditory dysfunction.
1. Pathophysiology
The condition may occur spontaneously or as a result of a viral infection in the upper respiratory tract.
2. Evaluation
The **evaluation** includes a thorough history and physical examination. To clinch the diagnosis, the Dix–Hallpike Bàràny maneuver can be performed (see Ta-

B O X   1 4 - 7

Overall Evaluation and Management of Vertigo

Evaluation

1. Thorough **history** and **physical examination,** with particular attention placed on duration, time of onset, exacerbating features, and concurrent features.
2. Perform the **Dix–Hallpike Bàràny maneuver** (see Table 14-11) to differentiate benign positional vertigo from other forms of vertigo.
3. Trial of specific antivertigo medications (see Table 14-12, for specific agents and their dosages).
4. **CT or MRI** of the **posterior fossa** if vertigo is recurrent or if any atypical features are present.

---

ble 14-11). If this test is positive it confirms the diagnosis. **Another strategy** useful in patients with a probable diagnosis is to **empirically treat** as such. If resolution occurs, it is not only therapeutic but quite diagnostic.

3. **Treatment**
   a. Instruct the patient to **lie flat,** as this will cause habituation of the process and a slow resolution of symptoms.
   b. Any of the agents listed in Table 14-11 may be effective for palliative therapy.
   c. If symptoms **recur** or **do not resolve** with the above modalities, CT or MRI of the posterior fossa is indicated.

T A B L E   1 4 - 1 1
Dix–Hallpike Bàràny Maneuver

---

1. The patient is placed **supine** with the head in approximately 30° of extension and turned to the right or left, for 30–90 seconds.
2. The patient assumes a sitting position for 5 minutes.
3. Repeat the test with the patient's head turned to the contralateral side.

Interpretation: This test is positive if the patient develops vertigo and nystagmus within 30 seconds of being placed in a new position. The nystagmus, which has the rapid component to the side of the head inferiorly placed, resolves within 30 seconds. A positive test is consistent with benign positional vertigo.

T A B L E   1 4 - 1 2
Medications in the Symptomatic Therapy of Vertigo

Meclizine (Antivert), 12.5–25 mg PO t.i.d. PRN
   or
Dimenhydrinate, 50 mg PO q.6h. PRN
   or
Scopolamine patch applied to skin q.24h.

B. **Meniere's disease**
The **specific manifestations** include an acute onset of vertigo that lasts for several hours and then spontaneously resolves. The vertigo is episodic, with variable intervals between episodes. The periods of vertigo are classically severe and almost always are associated with **unilateral tinnitus, a unilateral decrease in auditory acuity,** and **horizontal nystagmus** (the slow beat of nystagmus toward the symptomatic side), severe nausea and vomiting, all during the acute episode. During the acute episodes, the tinnitus invariably is **antecedent** to the vertigo itself.

1. **Natural history**
Recurrent episodes affect one or both ears. Although spontaneous remissions can occur, the patient eventually develops long-term, irreversible, bilateral, neurosensory auditory loss, especially of the low-frequency wavelengths.

2. **Pathophysiology**
The **underlying mechanism** of this disorder is an abnormal excess of endolymph in the membranous labyrinth of the vestibular and cochlear apparati of the inner ear. This results in damage to the hair cells of these structures.

3. **Evaluation**
The **evaluation** of this disorder includes a thorough history and physical examination. Usually the diagnosis is clinical, but certain tests aid in the diagnosis. One of the more important tests is **audiometry.** The hearing loss is one in which the low-frequency wavelengths are most affected. If there is any suspicion of other intracranial pathology, **CT** or **MRI of the head,** especially of the posterior fossa structures, is indicated.

4. **Management**
Management includes placing the patient on a **low-sodium diet,** i.e., 1–2 g of sodium/24 hours. Further information includes the initiation of **diuretics,** especially thiazide diuretics, e.g., HCTZ, 25–50 mg PO

q.d. Monitor volume status, potassium, and blood pressure in all patients who are placed on a regimen of sodium restriction and diuretics. Any of the agents listed in Table 14-11 can be effective for palliative therapy. Consultation with an ENT specialist with expertise in vestibulocochlear dysfunction may be indicated, especially if the process is refractory to standard therapeutic modalities.

C. Labyrinthitis

The **specific manifestations** of this not uncommon process include an acute onset of severe vertigo which lasts for 1–4 days. Associated with the vertigo are nausea, vomiting, **bilateral tinnitus,** an acute decrease in auditory acuity, and horizontal nystagmus. The process is usually self-limited and rarely results in any defect in auditory acuity. It usually **follows** an upper respiratory tract infection.

1. Pathophysiology

Although the **mechanism** of development is unknown, it has been hypothesized to result from inflammation of the vestibulocochlear apparatus.

2. Evaluation and management

The **specific evaluation and management** include audiometry and a thorough history and physical examination. Usually no intervention is necessary as the diagnosis is evident clinically. Any of the agents listed in Table 14-12 can be effective for palliative therapy.

D. Acoustic neuroma

This is a relatively uncommon cause of vertigo, even if the vertigo is chronic; however, the diagnosis which must be entertained in any case of chronic vertigo, especially in patients at high risk for von Recklinghausen's syndrome (neurofibromatosis). Furthermore, it is eminently treatable if discovered in the early phase. The location of such a lesion is about the **cerebellopontine angle** and will affect, when advanced, all of the cranial nerve roots in that area, including the trigeminal (V), facial (VII), and auditory (VIII) nerve roots, both the vestibular and cochlear components.

1. Manifestations

The **specific manifestations** include a slow, steady increase in vertigo in addition to unilateral hearing loss. The hearing loss is predominantly of **high-frequency** wavelengths. The patient may present with a cranial nerve VII palsy and dysfunction of cranial nerve V when the lesion is advanced.

2. Evaluation and management

The **evaluation and management** of this disorder include audiometry and aggressively evaluating and managing if suspicion for this lesion is high. A **high suspicion** should exist in patients who are at **high risk,** who have any **associated cranial nerve findings,** or who have significant **high-frequency hearing loss.** The imaging technique of choice is **nuclear magnetic imaging,** with specific imaging of the cerebellopontine angle. If any mass is discovered, consultation with neurosurgery is indicated. Any of the agents listed in Table 14-12 can be effective for palliative therapy, but should **not be used** unless and until a diagnosis has been made, as they can mask symptoms.

E. Brain stem infarction

This syndrome often is associated with vertigo. It is a disorder in which a CVA results in destruction of the nuclei or nerves in the brain stem unilaterally, owing to vertebrobasilar arterial insufficiency.

1. Manifestations

The **specific manifestations** make this entity easy to diagnose clinically. They include the acute onset of vertigo concurrent with diplopia, ataxia, dysphagia, dysarthria, and hemiparesis.

2. Evaluation and management

The **evaluation and management** of this form of vertigo include a history and physical examination and CT or MRI of the posterior fossa. MRI is probably the most effective imaging technique to image any infarcts. Management includes that for CVAs (see section on Cerebrovascular Accidents, page 683).

III. Consultation

Problem	Service	Time
Recurrent vertigo	Neurology	Urgent
Intracranial mass	Neurosurgery	Urgent

Bibliography

Bell's Palsy

Adour KK, et al: The true nature of Bell's palsy: Analysis of 1000 consecutive patients. Laryngoscope 1978;88:787–801.

Ohye RG, Altenberger EA: Bell's palsy. Am Fam Pract 1989;40:159–166.

Cerebrovascular Accidents

Brook RH, et al: Carotid endarterectomy for elderly patients: Predicting complications. Ann Intern Med 1990;113:747–753.

Chambers BR, Norris JW: Outcome in patients with asymptomatic neck bruits. N Engl J Med 1986;315:860–865.

Day AL, Salcman M: Subarachnoid hemorrhage. Am Fam Pract 1989; 40:95–105.

Fields WS: Aspirin for prevention of stroke. Am J Med 1983;84:61.

Fisher CM: Clinical syndromes in cerebral thrombosis, hypertensive hemorrhage, and ruptured saccular aneurysm. Clin Neurosurg 1975;22:117–147.

Hart RG, Miller VT: Cerebral infarction in young adults: A practical approach. Stroke 1983;14:110–114.

Hobson RW, et al: Efficacy of carotid endarterectomy for asymptomatic carotid stenosis. N Engl J Med 1993;328:221–227.

Meissner I, et al: The natural history of asymptomatic carotid arterial occlusive lesions. JAMA 1987;258:2704–2707.

North American Symptomatic Carotid Endarterectomy Study in Symptomatic Patients with High-Grade Carotid Stenosis: Beneficial effect of carotid endarterectomy in symptomatic patients with high-grade carotid stenosis. N Engl J Med 1991;325:445–453.

Scherokman BJ, Hallenbeck JM: Management of acute stroke. Am Fam Pract 1985;31:190–199.

Welin L, et al: Analysis of risk factors for stroke in a cohort of men born in 1913. N Engl J Med 1987;317:521–526.

Delirium

Dilsaver SC: The mental status examination. Am Fam Pract 1990;41:1489–1496.

Inouye SK, et al: Clarifying confusion: The confusion assessment method. Ann Intern Med 1990;113:941–948.

Lindberg MC, Oyler RA: Wernicke's encephalopathy. Am Fam Pract 1990;41:1205–1209.

Lipowski ZJ: Delirium (acute confusional states). JAMA 1987;258:1789–1792.

Dementia

Black KS, Hughes PL: Alzheimer's disease: Making the diagnosis. Am Fam Pract 1987;36:196–202.

Erkinjutti T, et al: Dementia among medical inpatients. Arch Intern Med 1986;146:1923–1926.

Katzman R: Alzheimer's disease. N Engl J Med 1986;314:964.

Van Horn G: Dementia. Am J Med 1987;83:101–110.

Gait Disturbances

Ahlskog JE, Wilkinson JM: New concepts in the treatment of Parkinson's disease. Am Fam Pract 1990;41:574–584.

Hallett M: Classification and treatment of tremor. JAMA 1991;266:1115–1117.

Hough JC, et al: Gait disturbances in the elderly. Am Fam Pract 1987;35:191–196.

Lees AJ: L-dopa treatment and Parkinson's disease. QJ Med 1986;59:535.

Headaches

Black PM: Brain tumors. N Engl J Med 1991;324:1471–1476.

Kumar KL, Cooney TG: Vascular headache. J Gen Intern Med 1988;3:384–395.

Linet MS, Stewart WF: Migraine headache: Epidemiologic perspectives. Epidemiol Rev 1984;6:107.

McKenna JP: Cluster headaches. Am Fam Pract 1988;37:173–143.

Schulman EA, et al: Symptomatic and prophylactic treatment of migraine and tension-type headache. Neurology 1992;42(Suppl 2):16–21.

Walling AD: Drug prophylaxis for migraine headaches. Am Fam Pract 1990;42:425–432.

Meningitis

Gellin BG, Broome CV: Listeriosis. JAMA 1989;261:1313–1320.

Gorse GJ, et al: Bacterial meningitis in the elderly. Arch Intern Med 1984;144:1603–1607.

Lefrock JL: Drugs of choice for bacterial meningitis. Am Fam Pract 1986;33:285–291.

El-Mallakh RS: CSF evaluation in neurologic disease. Am Fam Pract 1987;35:112–118.

Quagliarello V, et al: Bacterial meningitis: Pathogenesis, pathophysiology, and progress. N Engl J Med 1992;327:864–872.

Shapiro ED: Prophylaxis for bacterial meningitis. Med Clin North Am 1985;69:269.

Tarber MG, Sande MA: Principles in the treatment of bacterial meningitis. Am J Med 1984;76(Suppl 5A):224.

Seizure Disorders

Delgado-Escueta AV, et al: The treatable epilepsies. N Engl J Med 1983;1508:1576.

Drugs for epilepsy. Med Lett 1986;28:91–94.

Hopkins A, et al: The first seizures in adult life. Lancet 1988;721–726.

Jubbari B: Management of epileptic seizures in adults. Am Fam Pract 1985;31:162–172.

Ojemann LM, Ojemann GA: Treatment of epilepsy. Am Fam Pract 1984;30:113–128.

Schuer ML, Pedley TA: The evaluation and treatment of seizures. N Engl J Med 1990;21:1467–1474.

Vertigo

Drachman DA, Hart CW: An approach to the dizzy patient. Neurology 1972;22:323.

Lehrer JF, et al: Identification and treatment of metabolic abnormalities in patients with vertigo. Arch Intern Med 1986;146:1497–1500.

Snow JB Jr: Positional vertigo. N Engl J Med 1984;310:1740.

—D.D.B.

Dale Berg, Ed. *Handbook of Primary Care Medicine.* Copyright © 1993 J. B. Lippincott Company.

C H A P T E R   1 5

Psychiatry

Depression

Depression is a **very common syndrome** which can affect any human being at any time. It has been estimated that up to ¼ of patients in the outpatient setting and up to ⅓ of medical inpatients have manifestations of depression. Although quite prevalent, depression can easily be **overlooked** and therefore **undertreated.** The syndrome of depression has many different manifestations and a diverse set of etiologies, each etiology with a different pathogenesis. Furthermore, depression of any etiology exacerbates many concurrent medical problems and/or is exacerbated by concurrent medical, psychiatric, and/or substance abuse syndromes. Based upon the above, one can clearly see why depression can be a slippery syndrome to evaluate and manage.

I. **Overall manifestations**

The **overall manifestations** of depression include the presence of a **depressed mood,** i.e., the subjective manifestations of feeling "blue" or "down in the dumps," and a **despondent affect,** i.e., the objective observation of the patient by an experienced examiner. Other overall vegetative manifestations of depression include:

A. **Change in sleep pattern**

This is an often present symptom of depression. This change can be **excessive sleeping** compared with baseline or **insomnia,** classically being early morning awakening with inability to return to sleep.

B. **Change in appetite**

There is usually a **decrease** in appetite in patients with depression, which can result in weight loss.

C. **Anhedonia**

A significant **decrease** in the desire and perceived **need for pleasure** is very common in patients with depression.

D. **A feeling of hopelessness**

The patient has no aspirations and looks forward to nothing but an unchanging, bleak, cold existence.

E. **A significant decrease in libido**

The patient's interest in developing and evolving intimate interrelationships with fellow human beings, including sex, is markedly embarrassed.

F. **A significant decrease in interactions with fellow human beings**

This is a corollary to the decrease in libido, in that there can be and often is a withdrawal from others, including family members and close friends. The patient will often decrease attendance at or even completely avoid social/family gatherings. Furthermore, attendance at work and/or school can become markedly compromised.

G. **Recurrent thoughts of death, suicide, and/or homicide**

See Box 15-2 for specific risk factors in suicide.

H. **A marked increase in somatic complaints**

These complaint include but are not limited to myalgias, arthralgias, abdominal pains, and chest pains. These somatic manifestations can be severe and often the patient will have had several negative medical evaluations for these specific complaints. In patients with major depression, the somatization can be so marked as to result in **delusions** of decay or rot in the chest, muscles, or abdomen.

I. **A change in psychomotor activity**

This can be either **agitation,** i.e., irritation, restlessness, hyperactivity, or **retardation,** i.e., slow motor movements, lethargy, and increased sleepiness.

J. In severe cases there can be **delusional thoughts** which reach psychotic proportions.

II. **Causes**

The **causes** of depression are diverse and are best stratified into two groups, those that are primarily physiologic and those that are primarily psychiatric. As alluded to above, depression can be and often is multifactorial with greater than one of the following causes contributing or exacerbating the syndrome of depression.

A. **Physiologic**

Occurs as the result of a medical diagnosis. Many of these etiologies can be defined and even can be reversed. The most common of these etiologies include:

1. **Endocrinopathies.** These include hypothyroidism, hyperthyroidism, and states of hypercortisolism, either iatrogenic or as the result of Cushing's syndrome. The **specific manifestations** of these disorders as well as their specific evaluation and management are dis-

cussed in Box 15-1 and in Chapter 9. Of note is the fact that **hyperthyroidism** in the elderly can paradoxically present with weakness and depression, i.e., "apathetic hyperthyroidism."

2. **Electrolyte disturbances.** These include hypercalcemia, hypophosphatemia, hyperphosphatemia, hyponatremia, or hypernatremia. The **specific manifestations** of the most common of these disorders as well as their specific evaluation and management are discussed in Box 15-1 and in Chapter 9.

3. **Degenerative central nervous system processes.** These include dementia, parkinsonism, tertiary lues venereum, and multiple sclerosis. The **specific manifestations** of the most common of these disorders as well as their specific evaluation and management are discussed in Box 15-1 and Chapter 14 (parkinsonism, dementia) or Chapter 6 (lues venereum).

4. **Intracranial events.** These include the development of space-occupying lesions, e.g., neoplasia or any cerebrovascular accidents. The **specific manifestations** of the most common of these disorders as well as their specific evaluation and management are discussed in Box 15-1 and in Chapter 14.

5. **Chemical agents,** either illicit or iatrogenic. Virtually

---

B O X   1 5 - 1

Overall Evaluation and Management of Depression

Evaluation

1. Obtain a **history** with emphasis on:
   a. The overall manifestations of depression.
      i. Sleep disturbances.
      ii. Somatic complaints, e.g., chest pain, abdominal pain.
      iii. Delusional thoughts.
      iv. Libido disturbances.
      v. Appetite disturbances.
      vi. Depressed mood.
   b. Any **concurrent** or **antecedent events,** e.g., bad news, divorce, loss of employment, death of spouse, et cetera.

(continued)

B O X   1 5 - 1 *(continued)*

   c. A past history of mania, depression, and/or substance abuse.
   d. Current use of any therapeutic agents and agents for alteration of mood.
   e. Assess the patient for **suicide risk** potential—see Box 15-2.
2. Obtain a **physical examination** looking for objective evidence of a despondent affect, any manifestations of hyperthyroidism or hypothyroidism, any manifestations of muscle weakness/muscle atrophy, and/or any documented weight loss.
3. Obtain the following **laboratory** parameters:
   a. Serum **electrolytes,** looking for hyponatremia or hypernatremia which can exacerbate preexisting depression or manifest as a syndrome of depression.
   b. Serum **calcium,** as hypercalcemia can exacerbate preexisting depression or manifest as a syndrome of depression.
   c. Serum **phosphorus,** as hyperphosphatemia can exacerbate preexisting depression or manifest as a syndrome of depression.
   d. T_3RU, T_4, and TSH, looking for hypo-/hyperthyroidism, which can exacerbate preexisting depression or manifest as a syndrome of depression.
   e. EKG—12 lead for baseline purposes, if any antidepressant agent is considered to be initiated.
4. **Categorize** and **define** the syndrome of depression using the above data.
   a. If **major depression:** Initiate an antidepressant agent (see Tables 15-1 and 15-2) and psychotherapy.
   b. If **bipolar disorder:** Initiate lithium, an antidepressant agent (see Tables 15-1 and 15-2) and psychotherapy.
   c. **Dysthymic, cyclothymic,** and **reactive** depression: Initiate psychotherapy.
   d. If **physiologic:** Treat the underlying condition.
5. Treat any concurrent, exacerbating factors or diseases, especially any chemical abuse/dependency.
6. Admit all patients with **suicidal/homicidal ideation** or risk and any and all patients with active psychosis.

B O X   1 5 - 2

Factors in the Assessment of Suicide Risk

1. Sex of patient: Women attempt 3 times more often than men. Men are successful 3 times more often than women.
2. **Age** of patient: Highest risk in young, i.e., teenagers and in older, >50 years of age, patients.
3. The presence of a **syndrome of depression,** acute or chronic.
4. A history of previous suicide attempts.
5. A history of **substance abuse/dependency** in general and ethanol in specific.
6. The presence of a **thought process disorder,** i.e., the patient is delusional.
7. No **social support,** i.e., no job, no family.
8. The presence of an **organized plan** for completing the deed.
9. The **lack of a significant other** is a very powerful marker in increasing suicide risk.
10. The presence of an acute or **symptomatic chronic physical illness,** especially if the symptom is one of pain.

   Each factor is given 1 point.
   Any patient with a score of >5: Admit.
   2–5: Watch closely, as an inpatient or outpatient.
   <2: Watch closely, outpatient.

(From Patterson WM et al: Evaluation of suicidal patients: The SAD persons scale. Psychosomatics 1983;24:343–349.)

---

any chemical either prescribed for therapeutic purposes or used for mood-altering purposes can result in depression. The most common of these agents include benzodiazepines, β-blockers, barbiturates, and **ethanol.** The **specific manifestations** of the most common of these disorders as well as their specific evaluation and management are discussed in Box 15-1 and in the section on Substance Abuse Syndromes in this chapter.

B. Psychiatric etiologies

These are again quite diverse in manifestations, natural history, evaluation, and management.

1. Major depression

This is the quintessential etiology of depression to

T A B L E   15 - 1
Selected Antidepressant Agents

Agent	Sedation	Anticholinergic Side Effects*	Other Side Effects	Dosage, Initial/Maximal
Doxepin (Sinequan)	Strong	Mild to moderate	QRS and QTc prolongation Orthostatic hypotension	50 mg PO q.d./ 300 mg/24 hr
Amitryptyline (Elavil)	Strong	Severe	QRS and QTc prolongation Orthostatic hypotension	25 mg PO t.i.d./ 300 mg/24 hr
Desipramine (Norpramin)	Minimal	Mild	QRS and QTc prolongation Orthostatic hypotension	50 mg PO q.d./ 150 mg/24 hr
Nortryptyline (Pamelor)	Minimal	Mild	QRS and QTc prolongation Minimal orthostatic hypotension	25 mg PO q.d./ 150 mg/24 hr
Trazodone (Desyrel)	Strong	None	Little to no ECG or hypotensive changes Priapism	50 mg PO t.i.d./ 600 mg/24 hr
Fluoxetine (Prozac)	Moderate	None	No ECG or hypotensive effects Minimal side effect profile	20 mg PO q.d./ 40 mg/24 hr

*Anticholinergic side effects include tachycardia, urinary retention, xerostomia.

T A B L E 1 5 - 2
Tips on the Effective Use of Antidepressant Agents

1. Obtain a baseline ECG, if antidepressants are considered.
2. The overall side effects of tricyclic antidepressant agents include:
   Sedation
   Orthostatic hypotension with an increased risk of falls
   Anticholinergic
     Tachycardias
     Ileus
     Urinary retention, especially in male patients with prostatic
       hypertrophy
     Fevers
     Acute confusion
   ECG changes with:
     Prolongation of QRS
     Prolongation of QTc
     Increased risk of torsade du pointes and other ventricular
       tachycardias with resultant sudden cardiac death
3. The improvement of the manifestations of depression might take up
   to 2–4 weeks, in point of fact, side effects may and quite often do
   antedate the improvement.
4. The dosage of the agents in Table 15-1 (except fluoxetine) should be
   increased every 4–6 days by 25–50 mg up to the maximum dose
   and/or to the development of side effects. If there is no improvement after 4 weeks on maximal therapy, it is a treatment failure
   which requires replacement with a different agent.
5. The dosage in the elderly should be 50% that of younger adults.

which all other syndromes of depression are compared.

   a. The **specific manifestations** include those described in the overall manifestations section. In
   point of fact the patient will manifest many if not
   all of the overall manifestations. There can be and
   often are delusions, at times psychotic delusions
   and suicidal ideation is quite common. This etiol-
   ogy/syndrome of depression is quite pernicious
   in that it has a slow, insidious onset and, once
   present, the **natural history** is one of waxing and
   waning, with periods of minimal manifestations
   and normal activity to severe manifestations and
   marked embarrassment of normal activities. The
   duration is months to years and can be lifelong.

   b. The **specific evaluation and management** include
   that described in Box 15-1 and effectively ruling
   out other primary or exacerbating factors. Clearly
   an assessment of risk for suicide as described in
   Boxes 15-1 and 15-2 must be determined. **Specific
   management** includes the initiation of an antide-

pressant medication (see Tables 15-1 and 15-2) and referral of all patients to a psychiatrist for adjunctive psychotherapy. If the patient has severe depression refractory to intensive antidepressant therapy and psychotherapy including inpatient therapy, electroconvulsive treatment (ECT) should be considered.

2. **Bipolar affective disorder**

   This is a very severe affective disorder which is, when diagnosed and aggressively treated, imminently and eminently treatable.

   a. The **specific manifestations** include alternating periods of major depression with periods of severe mania. The patient will, for various periods of time, have **major depression** which then resolves only to develop into **mania.** The **mania manifests** with an increase in activity, i.e., many activities being performed, all at a harried and frenetic pace. The efficiency in performing these activities, however, is markedly compromised. The manic patient also has a rapid, forced speech and a significantly impaired judgment, going on spending sprees, taking inappropriate risks. Furthermore, the patient with mania can develop delusions, usually of grandiose schemes or of perceived increased prowess in sexual activity or business activity. Psychotic delusions can and often do occur during the depressed and the manic phases of the disease process. The **natural history** is one of recurrent alternating episodes of depression and mania of varying duration. The **duration** of the syndrome is years to lifelong.

   b. The **specific evaluation and management** include that described in Box 15-1 and effectively ruling out other primary or exacerbating factors. Clearly an assessment of **risk for suicide** as described in Boxes 15-1 and 15-2 must be determined. **Specific management** includes the initiation of lithium, an antidepressant medication (see Tables 15-1 and 15-2) and referral of all patients to a psychiatrist for adjunctive psychotherapy.

3. **Dysthymic disorder**

   a. The **specific manifestations** include some of those described in the overall manifestations, but of mild intensity. This **syndrome** is chronic, mild, and with minimal to negligible effect on appetite, sleep, energy level, motor activity, and functioning within society. The patient is chronically **morose** and can develop mild to moderate **self-pity.** The

natural history is one of chronicity; the patient usually can maintain employment. The **duration** is usually lifelong. There is little to no increased risk of suicide and the patient is never delusional.

b. The **specific evaluation and management** include that described in Box 15-1 and effectively ruling out other primary or exacerbating factors. Clearly an assessment of risk for suicide as described in Boxes 15-1 and 15-2 must be determined. **Specific management** includes the elective referral to a psychiatrist for psychotherapy. Rarely, if ever, will antidepressant agents be necessary in therapy.

4. **Cyclothymic disorder**
   a. The **specific manifestations** are a mild version of bipolar disorder, in that there are alternating periods of mild depression and mild increased activity with periods of normalcy between. The **mild depression** is identical to that described in dysthymic syndrome, above. The **increased activity** is mild and without any grossly decreased judgment. The **natural history** is one of continuing alterations between decreased and increased mood. **Duration** is usually lifelong. There is little to no increased risk for suicide and the patient is never delusional.
   b. The **specific evaluation and management** include that described in Box 15-1 and effectively ruling out other primary or exacerbating factors. Clearly an assessment of risk for suicide as described in Boxes 15-1 and 15-2 must be determined. **Specific management** includes the elective referral to a psychiatrist for psychotherapy. Rarely, if ever, will antidepressant agents be necessary in therapy.

5. **Reactive depression**
   This is the most common type of depression among all individuals. Every person will, at various times during life, experience reactive depression.
   a. The **specific manifestations** include the development of mild to severe depression after an acute stressful event in the patient's life. This event is usually one of a loss of a person near and dear to them. This **loss** can be as the result of divorce, travel, or death. The reactive depression which occurs after a loss is called **grief.** Another common event which precipitates such depression is that of a loss of one's employment or failure to attain a level long desired. There can be **significant disturbances** in libido, appetite, sleep and the manifestations can include some delusional thinking. This can be, in severe forms, not dissimilar from major

depression. The **natural history** is one of it being self-limited as the patient slowly, steadily works through the pain of the loss. **Duration** is usually less than 6 months; in point of fact, if the duration is >6 months the diagnosis of major depression must be seriously entertained. The risk of suicide is moderate.

b. The **specific evaluation and management** include that described in Box 15-1 and effectively determining the precipitating/exacerbating factor. Clearly an assessment of risk for suicide as described in Boxes 15-1 and 15-2 must be determined. **Specific management** includes the elective referral to a psychiatrist for psychotherapy. The patient must work through the grief in order to realistically recover from it. Rarely, if ever, will antidepressant agents be necessary in therapy.

III. **Consultation**

Problem	Service	Time
Major depression	Psychiatry	Urgent
Bipolar disorder		Urgent
Suicidal		Emergent
Cyclothymic		Required
Dysthymic		Required
Reactive		Elective

IV. **Indications for admission:** Suicidal or homicidal ideation or risk, mania, or psychotic delusions.

Substance Abuse Syndromes

The **syndrome of chemical substance abuse** is a problem which is endemic in the United States. This is demonstrated not only by the prevalence of substance abuse, but also by the enormous expense of this problem in economic and, most important, human terms. The **prevalence** of substance abuse has been estimated to be 10%–15%. Based upon this discussion, the syndrome of substance abuse is one of the gravest problems facing society in general and health care delivery, in specific, in the United States today. Several definitions cogent to any discussion of substance abuse syndromes must be discussed herein.

Dependence is the overt **physical** and/or **psychological,** nontherapeutic **need** for a specific substance or activity. This is a broad definition in that human beings can develop dependence upon activities or items other than chemical substances. These include compulsive gambling, eating, sexual addiction, and what will be discussed at length herein, **chemical substance abuse.** One of the integral features of these abuse syndromes is a **loss of control.** In a discussion specific to chemical substance abuse, several terms can be used to describe dependence.

Addiction, i.e., **physical dependence.** Actual physiologic changes occur in the body to make the patient require the substance to maintain a new homeostasis.

Withdrawal. The manifestations which develop upon discontinuing a chemical agent to which a patient is addicted. These are pathophysiologically as the result of abstinence from the agent. The development of a withdrawal syndrome upon abstinence from a specific chemical effectively defines addiction.

Habituation, i.e., psychological dependence. A compelling need, want of, lust for the specific substance in order to reexperience its effects. A patient can have psychologic dependence without physical dependence.

Tolerance. The need for **increasing amounts** of the specific chemical to derive the same effect. The amount increases until there is the development of significant and further dose-limiting side effects.

I. Substances of abuse

Specific substances abused today in the United States and worldwide are quite varied in chemical type, potential for physical dependence, potential for psychological dependence, and in sequelae. In all cases, however, the **natural history** of dependence on one or more of these agents, also referred to as **mood-altering drugs,** will lead to marked embarrassment in the quality of the patient's life and, in virtually all cases, markedly decrease the life span of the patient. Specific substances abused are described in Table 15-3. Ethanol, unquestionably the most commonly used and, unfortunately, abused chemical substance in the United States today, is described in Table 15-3 and expanded upon in the discussion below.

II. Ethanol abuse

Ethanol abuse and dependency are endemic in our society. Recent estimates clearly delineate the prevalence and the human and economic burden of this dependency syndrome. These estimates include the fact that in 1985, **greater than 10 million** Americans had the syndrome of ethanol dependence. Furthermore, more than \$100 billion per year is lost as the result of ethanol abuse/dependency in the United States. Finally, the human cost is enormous: **30%–40% of hospital admissions** have ethanol abuse either as the primary or a secondary diagnosis, **30%–50% of all suicides** involve patients with ethanol abuse, **50% of all motor vehicle accidents** and motor vehicle accident deaths have ethanol as a primary

T A B L E 1 5 - 3
Substances of Abuse—United States, 1993

Category	Specific Agents	Types of Dependency	Effects	Sequelae/Side Effects
Sedatives	Ethanol Benzodiazepines (BZD) Barbiturates Marijuana	Physiologic: marked Psychologic: marked	Decreased inhibitions Sense of well-being Mild euphoria Barbiturates/BZD: profound relaxation	Withdrawal syndrome upon abstinence; **death** Ethanol: a) Cirrhosis b) Pancreatitis c) Wernicke–Korsakof syndrome BZD: a) airway dysfunction Cannabis (smoked) a) increased risk of bronchogenic ca.
Narcotics	Heroin Morphine Codeine	Physiologic: marked Psychologic: marked	Euphoria Relief of tension Analgesia	Decrease in function of all physiologic drives (appetite, libido) Withdrawal syndrome upon abstinence; **death**

Stimulants	Cocaine Amphetamines	Physiologic: minimal Psychologic: marked	Perception of increased energy Euphoria Decreased appetite Decreased need for sleep Perception of increased efficiency	Marked tolerance until doses required result in severe tachycardia and hypertension Insomnia Increased aggressive behaviorisms Sudden cardiac **death**
Hallucinogen	D-lysergic acid (LSD) Phencyclidine (PCP)	Physiologic: negligible Psychologic: minimal	Vivid hallucinations, usually visual but also tactile, auditory, and olfactory are possible	"Bad trips," i.e., nightmarish hallucinations "Flashbacks," i.e., a hallucination occurring years to decades after the last use of the agent Increased aggressive/assaultive behaviorisms **Death**
Inhalants	Solvents Amyl nitrate Hydrocarbons	Physiologic: minimal Psychologic: marked	Euphoria, "head rush" Mild relaxation	Tolerance Sudden cardiac **death** Central nervous system destruction; dementia and **death**

or contributing factor, **50% of all homicides** involve ethanol as a contributing factor, and **3/1,000 live births** in the United States today have **fetal alcohol syndrome.**

A. **Reporting**

Although the numbers are striking, this remains a syndrome which is quite **underrecognized** and therefore **undertreated** by the health care profession in general and physicians in specific. This is clearly evidenced by the fact that although 30%–40% of all admissions had ethanol as a primary or major contributing factor, only a small percentage have the diagnosis of ethanol dependence described in their medical records. The **reasons for such underreporting** and/or underrecognizing are not completely known but several postulates include:

1. The social **acceptability** of ethanol as a drug.
2. The **perceived benign nature** of ethanol by society and by many health care professionals.
3. The **high prevalence** of ethanol abuse/dependency among health care professionals in general and physicians in specific.

All of these reasons decrease the physician's sensitivity in describing the problem and making the diagnosis of ethanol abuse/dependency.

B. **Pathogenesis**

The **underlying pathogenesis** for the development of an ethanol abuse/dependency syndrome is not completely clear but certain risk factors for development have been described.

1. **Genetic,** i.e., an increased propensity for ethanol abuse as the result of the patient's genetic makeup. Several studies using adopted monozygotic twins indicate that there may well be a genetic predisposition in the development of ethanol abuse syndromes.
2. **Social environment.** Adults who **grew up** in broken, dysfunctional families, and/or are **currently** in broken, dysfunctional family relationships are at higher risk of developing a syndrome of ethanol abuse/dependency. Of clear interest is the fact that individuals with healthy family relationships have a markedly lower incidence of ethanol abuse.
3. Concurrent and/or antecedent **DSM-IIIR Axis I** psychological dysfunctional states, e.g., **bipolar affective** disorder, **major depression,** or **schizophrenia.** It has been estimated that up to $\frac{1}{3}$ of all patients with ethanol abuse syndromes have such diagnoses.
4. Concurrent and/or antecedent abuse or **dependency upon other chemical agents** (see Table 15-3). Clearly, dependence on one substance is a risk factor for the development of dependence on another substance. In

point of fact, **any syndrome of addiction,** whether it be to a chemical or to an activity, e.g., compulsive gambling, all of which have central to them a loss of self-control and of self-esteem, is a **risk factor** in the development of **concurrent dependency** states.

5. Certain professions have a higher prevalence of ethanol abuse than other professions. A profession with one of the **highest prevalence** rates of ethanol abuse/ dependency is that of **physicians** themselves.

C. **Evaluation**

The **overall evaluation of an ethanol abuse/dependency syndrome** is to make the diagnosis. Making the diagnosis is clearly pivotal to therapy, as the earlier the diagnosis is made, the better the chances for effective therapy and of ethanol-related sequelae prevention. The diagnosis is made best by performing a thorough history and physical examination.

1. The **history** must be from various sources, not only the **patient** himself or herself, but also **collateral sources,** e.g., spouse, significant other, other family members, friends and roommates. Not only can **collateral sources** of information provide objective data regarding the patient's substance abuse potential, they also can provide the clinician with insight into the patient's social milieu and to what extent the ethanol abuse/dependency is affecting that social milieu.

2. Several screening instruments have been developed to detect ethanol abuse/dependency syndromes. Two of the best and both internally and externally valid instruments include the CAGE and MAST screening tests.

   a. **CAGE screening tool.** CAGE is a mnemonic for four specific questions, all of which should be asked of all new patients in order to readily screen for an ethanol abuse syndrome (see Table 15-4). A positive response to any **one** of the CAGE queries correlates well with ethanol abuse. In point of fact, the **positive predictive value** for ethanol abuse/dependency of **two positive responses is 82%,** of **3 positive responses is 99%,** and of **four, 100%.**

   b. **Michigan Alcoholism Screening Test (MAST)** uses a moderately short questionnaire to assess the patient for ethanol abuse/dependency. The questions are tailored to assess any decreased control of ethanol intake, problems with employment, and/or problems with social relationships including family and the law. The MAST has a standardized scoring system and can, with other information, be used to **screen for** and even **diagnose** ethanol dependency and abuse syndromes.

3. **Ethanol dependence** is diagnosed from:
   a. Consumption of **0.135 ounces of pure ethanol/kg/ day,** i.e., ~one fifth of hard liquor for 30 or more consecutive days, *and/or*
   b. A MAST **score of 6 or greater,** *and/or*
   c. The development of any **physiologic disease** as the result of ethanol (see Table 15-5), *and/or*
   d. The **continued use** of ethanol in the face of a medical **contraindication,** *and/or*
   e. The development of **withdrawal** upon abstinence from ethanol use, *and/or*
   f. The development of **tolerance** to ethanol, as manifested by:
      i. Blood alcohol level (BAL) of >**0.15 mg/dL without symptoms.**
      ii. BAL of >**0.3 mg/dL** at any time.
4. **Ethanol abuse** is diagnosed from
   a. A MAST **score of 3–5** and consumption of >2 ounces of pure ethanol per day, i.e., ~**5 ethanol beverages/day,** or
   b. A MAST **score of 2** or more and consumption of >4 ounces of pure ethanol per day, i.e., ~**10 ethanol beverages/day.**

D. **Management**
The **overall management** of a patient with an ethanol abuse/dependency syndrome is extremely complicated, quite labor intensive, requires involvement from multiple disciplines, and is for the duration of the patient's life. The patient can and will relapse at any time, requiring the clinician to, in effect, start from scratch. The **management schemas** can best be stratified into acute and chronic phases.

1. **Acute.** The patient is acutely intoxicated and/or acutely abstaining after a significant binge of ethanol. These patients are at high risk for withdrawal and require inpatient therapy. Please refer to Box 15-3 and Table 15-5 for specifics in acute evaluation and management.

2. **Chronic, rehabilitative.** The patient is no longer intoxicated and has had resolution of any withdrawal syndrome. This is very complex, long term, and labor intensive. Although there can be frustrations inherent to chronic therapy of such patients, the rewards of success can be marvelous to the patient, to his family, to society and therefore are quite gratifying to the clinician. The discussion here is only a brief description of some of the basic tenets of chronic ethanol dependence rehabilitative therapy.
   a. Treatment is **most effective** in patients who are **di-**

B O X 1 5 - 3

***Overall Evaluation and Management of Suspected
Ethanol Abuse/Dependency***

Evaluation

1. Obtain a thorough **history.** This must include a history from the **patient** and from **collateral** (e.g., family, friends) sources. Specific details should include:
   a. The patient's **present ethanol** consumption habits, including quantity and duration.
   b. The patient's **past ethanol** consumption habits.
   c. Any past history of **withdrawal.**
   d. Any history of admission for an **ethanol-related** disease.
   e. Any past history of **blackouts** (the patient cannot recall anything of a specific binge), and/or **brownouts** (the patient can recall events during a binge but they are fuzzy).
   f. Any history of **driving under the influence** of ethanol or ethanol-related motor vehicle accidents.
   g. Any history of **morning tremors** which resolve with ethanol use.
   h. Any history of **recurrent falls** and/or **fractures.**
   i. Any history of **abusive behavior** to family members and/or to others.
   j. The current relationships the patient has and how **constructive,** i.e., supportive, or **destructive,** i.e., detrimental, the relationships are.
   k. If the patient is not currently intoxicated, perform a CAGE (Table 15-4) and/or MAST evaluation.
2. Perform a thorough **physical examination,** with emphasis upon:
   a. The presence of **tremor** and **tachycardia** at rest are indicative of impending withdrawal.
   b. Examine for palsies of extraocular muscles, ataxic gait, bilateral nystagmus, and confusion, all of which are manifestations of **Wernicke's encephalopathy,** i.e., acute thiamine deficiency related.
   c. Examine the **odor of breath** as the presence of ethanol can be easily detected by an experienced examiner.
   d. Examine patient for any signs of chronic hepatic

(continued)

B O X   1 5 - 3 *(continued)*

disease/dysfunction (see section on End-Stage
Liver Disease, Chapter 2, page 91).

3. Categorize the patient into one of three groups, one
group being those patients who are **acutely intoxicated or acutely abstaining** from ethanol after a long
binge, a second group being those who have **ethanol dependence,** and a third group being those patients who have **ethanol abuse.**

a. **Acutely intoxicated or acute abstinence.** These patients require acute intervention. In virtually all
cases, this intervention must be as an inpatient.
The reason for inpatient intervention is based
upon the fact that the **risk for development of a
withdrawal syndrome** is quite high. The **specific
manifestations of withdrawal** are diverse and can
range from a mild tremor to hallucinations to generalized tonic–clonic seizure activity. Although
withdrawal can occur anywhere between 36
hours and 14 days after ingestion of the last ethanol beverage, the vast majority of cases occur in
the 36–72 hour range. The **specific evaluation and
management** of withdrawal include:

i. Administer **thiamine** (vitamin B_1) 100 mg IM/
IV stat to replenish thiamine stores and to
treat and prevent Wernicke's encephalopathy.

ii. Perform the following **laboratory tests:**

(a) **Serum glucose.** Patients can be hypoglycemic after a binge as the result of a shut-
down of gluconeogenesis in the liver.

(b) **Serum electrolytes,** especially **potassium,
magnesium,** and **phosphorus.** The patient
is quite often deficient in these specific
ions and will require repletion.

(c) **ECG—12 lead,** if any significant tachycardia is present.

(d) **Liver function tests,** if the patient has any
evidence of hepatic dysfunction, e.g., any
signs of hepatic disease or **icterus,** looking for gross elevations of enzymes
which would be consistent with acute eth-

(continued)

B O X 1 5 - 3 *(continued)*

          anol hepatitis. (See section on Hepatitis in Chapter 2 for specifics on hepatitides.)

    (e) **Urine for drug screen** for other chemicals of abuse.

  iii. Initiate therapy with **benzodiazepines.** These agents will **decrease the intensity** of the excitatory manifestations including tachycardia, tremor, and anxiety. They will, furthermore, **decrease the risk of withdrawal seizures.** There are many different agents on the market, two of which are described in Table 15-5. The agent of choice is **lorazepam** (Ativan). The dosage should be **scheduled** and modified to keep the patient comfortable and sleepy, but without compromise of airway. The usual dosage is ~**2 mg** lorazepam PO/IM/IV q.4–6h. **scheduled.** The patient is then weaned from the lorazepam by decreasing the dose by 25% each day. Therefore, by day 5 the patient is on lorazepam in an as needed dosage.

  iv. **Adjuvant therapy** including β-blockers or clonidine may have a role in some mild to moderate cases but certainly these are not first-line agents.

  v. Phenytoin is required only if the patient has another reason for seizures, i.e., **phenytoin is not necessary** in the treatment of seizures exclusively as the result of ethanol withdrawal.

  vi. **Nutrition** should be optimized. Consultation with a dietician may be of benefit, as well as prescription of a **multivitamin,** one tablet per day, and **thiamine,** 100 mg PO q.d.

  vii. When **sober** and through withdrawal, one can initiate ethanol **rehabilitation** therapy, best performed by referral to an addictionologist.

b. **Alcohol dependent/abuser**

  i. Initiate inpatient or outpatient ethanol **rehabilitation** with the assistance of or by referral to an addictionologist.

T A B L E 1 5 - 4
CAGE Queries

C: Attempting to **cut back** on drinking?
A: **Annoyed** at criticisms regarding drinking habits?
G: Feeling **guilty** about drinking habits?
E: Using ethanol as a morning, **"eye-opener"**?

(From Mayfield D, et al: The GAGE questionnaire. Am J Psychiatry 1974; 131:1121.)

agnosed early, who have **strong family support,** and who have a tangible **acute loss if ethanol is restarted,** or, better still, a tangible, reproducible, and **positive gain if abstinence is continued.** An **employer** who is supportive is clearly of benefit to the therapy.

  b. Successful therapy is taking **each day as it comes** for the rest of the patient's life. The patient must be motivated for the rest of his (her) life to maintain successful therapy, i.e., abstinence from all chemicals. One of the best methods to reinforce this and to keep motivation optimal is to have the patient interact on a regular basis with other patients with alcohol dependency. The best example of this is **Alcoholics Anonymous (AA).**

  c. The clinician must **confront,** with an empathic yet firm method, any and **all defenses,** e.g., **denial,** i.e., denying that there is a problem, and **projection,** i.e., blaming someone else for what the patient is doing. One method is to gently but firmly confront the patient with evidence from collateral sources regarding the ethanol habit and effects.

  d. The social supportive environment in general and the **patient's family** in specific must be **integrated** into the **treatment scheme.** A **social worker** with experience in treating alcoholics and the families of alcoholics is extremely important in the overall therapy. Another useful support group is **Alanon,** a group for family members of ethanol and substance abuse patients.

  e. Disulfiram (Antabuse) is a modality which may be useful in a **small select group** of patients. This is **aversion therapy** in which the agent disulfiram causes severe flushing, nausea, and vomiting immediately after the ingestion of any ethanol.

    i. The mechanism of action of the agent is via inhibiting the enzyme, **hepatic aldehyde NAD-oxidoreductase.** The inhibition of this enzyme results in abnormal concentrations of the mole-

TABLE 15-5
Agents Used in the Treatment of Acute Withdrawal from Ethanol

Agent	Half-life	Catabolites	Mechanism of Action	Dosage Regimen
*Lorazepam (Ativan) * Lorazepam is the agent of choice in the treatment of withdrawal syndromes.	14–16 hr	Conjugated, inactive	Binds to BZD receptors in CNS which act to release chloride anion into the neurons and inhibit activity; this is mediated by the molecule γ-aminobutyric acid (GABA) Decreases activity throughout the entire CNS, including cortical and autonomic systems Prevents seizures, decreases autonomic activity	2 mg PO/IM/IV q.4–6h., scheduled
Chlordiazepoxide (Librium)	6–18 hr	Oxidized, active Half-life of the active catabolites is 50–100 hr	Same as lorazepam	25–100 mg PO/IV q.6h., scheduled
β-Blockers (atenolol)	6–10 hr	Not catabolized, excreted intact in urine	Competitive antagonist of β-catecholamine receptors Decreases effects of catecholamines from autonomic nervous system Decreases tremor, tachycardia Adjunctive to BZD, if no contraindication to its use: a) 2° or 3° AV nodal block b) Reversible airway disease c) Systolic heart failure	50 mg PO q.d. for duration of withdrawal
Clonidine (Catapres)	6–24 hr	Hepatic, inactive	A central α₂-receptor antagonist which decreases the release of norepinephrine from the autonomic nervous system Mild sedation	0.1 mg PO q.d. for duration of withdrawal

cule **acetylaldehyde** in the serum whenever any ethanol is ingested. The acetylaldehyde will result in remarkable **flushing, nausea,** and **vomiting.**

    ii. This therapy can only be attempted in a **select group of patients** who have ethanol dependency states. These include:

        (a) Total sobriety.

        (b) Total commitment to therapy.

        (c) Intelligent patient who understands the ramifications of the therapy.

        (d) A patient **without any major affective disorder,** as disulfiram can exacerbate depression.

    iii. Dose: 250 mg PO q.h.s.

   f. Referral to and/or consultation with an **addictionologist,** i.e., an internist, family practice physician, or psychiatrist with postresidency training in the field of addiction/substance abuse is indicated in virtually all cases.

III. Consultation

Problem	Service	Time
Any concurrent Axis I* diagnosis	Psychiatrist	Urgent
All cases of substance abuse	Addictionologist	Urgent

IV. Indications for admission: hypotension as the result of tachydysrrhythmias, problems with airway maintenance, acute alcohol-related hepatitis, acute ethanol-related pancreatitis, hepatic encephalopathy, cocaine-related chest pain, any BAL of greater than 300 mg/dL, or any evidence of impending severe withdrawal. In all cases admission should be to an **inpatient internal medicine service.** Indications for admission to a **detoxification unit** include evidence of acute intoxication, i.e., BAL 100–300 mg/dL and/or evidence of mild withdrawal.

Bibliography

Depression

Green SA, et al: Management of acute grief. Am Fam Pract 1986;33:185.

Koenig HG: Depressive disorders in older medical inpatients. Am Fam Pract 1991;44:1243.

Patterson WM, et al: Evaluation of suicidal patients: The SAD PERSONS scale. Psychosomatics 1983;24:343–349.

* **Axis I diagnoses:** Schizophrenia; major affective disorder, including bipolar disorder or major depression.

The Medical Letter: Choice of an Antidepressant. 1993;35:25–26.

Wise MG, et al: Anxiety and mood disorders in medically ill patients. J Clin Psychiatry 1990;51(suppl 1):27–32.

Substance Abuse Syndromes

Jellinek E: The Disease Concept of Alcoholism. Hillhouse Press, New Jersey, 1960.

Lerner WD, et al: The alcohol withdrawal syndrome. N Engl J Med 1985; 313:951.

Mayfield D, et al: The CAGE questionnaire. Am J Psychiatry 1974;131:1121.

Petrakis PL, ed: Sixth Special Report to the Secretary of Health and Human Services. Rockville, Md, National Institute on Alcohol Abuse and Alcoholism, 1987.

Selzer ML: The Michigan alcoholism screening test. Am J Psychiatry 1971; 127:1653.

—D.D.B.

Dale Berg, Ed. *Handbook
of Primary Care Medicine.*
Copyright © 1993 J. B.
Lippincott Company.

C H A P T E R   1 6

Prevention in Primary Care

Gustavo Heudebert, M.D.

Prevention, in the context of clinical medicine, can be conceptualized as an intervention that will prevent a morbid event from occurring in a patient's future life. These interventions are typically performed in individuals who are **asymptomatic** for the disorder that we are trying to prevent. Examples of preventive interventions include immunizations, screening tests, modification of and counseling in unhealthy behaviors (e.g., smoking, drinking, sedentary lifestyle). Preventive interventions can be targeted to large segments of the population (e.g., screening for phenylketonuria and hypothyroidism among all newborns, childhood vaccinations, sickle cell tests in African Americans, breast and colorectal cancer screening) as well as to special segments of the population. Examples of tests for specific populations include tests in patients at high risk for complications of an existing condition (e.g., yearly fundoscopy for the early detection of retinopathy in diabetics), tests for the carrier state of a transmissible disease in people at high risk (e.g., PPD among immigrants), or tests for people in occupations that require perfect health (e.g., electrocardiogram for airplane pilots).

Depending on when the intervention happens, the target disorder might have not occurred at all (vaccination for the prevention of polio and measles, smoking cessation for the prevention of lung cancer and heart disease), in which case the intervention is considered **primary prevention.** If the intervention uncovers a disease in its asymptomatic stage (e.g., breast and colorectal cancer screening), it is considered **secondary prevention.** Finally, if the intervention is aimed at preventing progression of a disorder that has already manifested clinically (e.g., the use of β-blockers and ACE inhibitors for post-myocardial infarction or aspirin for patients with symptomatic carotid artery disease), then it is considered **tertiary prevention.** Further specific discussion of primary, secondary, and tertiary preventive measures will follow in this chapter.

The implementation of preventive interventions is variable. Certain interventions are mandated by law; examples are the fluoridation and chlorination of water, wearing seat belts while driving, and using helmets. Other preventive interventions are done in physician offices, commonly as a consequence of recommendations by medical organizations. Examples include cervical, breast, and colorectal cancer screening recommendations promulgated by the American Cancer Society and the American College of Physicians, among other organizations. Finally, preventive interventions can occur in public spaces, such as mass screening for hypertension, hyperlipidemia, and glaucoma at shopping malls.

Practicing physicians can implement preventive interventions in a number of ways. The **periodic health examination** refers to a comprehensive history and physical examination accompanied in the same visit by counseling if unhealthy behaviors are detected, immunizations if required, and performance of indicated screening procedures such as a cervical Papanicolaou smear, breast examination, or flexible sigmoidoscopy. A second approach, endorsed by the Canadian Preventive Task Force, entails performing a limited number of preventive interventions at each patient visit; this strategy is known as **case finding.** Advocates of the latter strategy believe that a primary care physician's patient load is too high to allow the physician to perform a periodic health examination adequately in a large number of patients, and that the general population visits a physician office often enough that preventive interventions can be provided over time at several office visits.

Physicians practicing in primary care specialties (internal medicine, family medicine, ob-gyn, pediatrics) have the unique opportunity to implement a variety of primary, secondary, and tertiary preventive interventions, depending on what segment of the population they treat. This chapter reviews interventions applicable to the adult population.

Primary prevention is truly the quintessential form of disease prevention. It actually goes to the known or suspected factor in the pathogenesis of a disease and attempts to remove or modify that factor before the disease develops. Examples include **immunizations** to prevent infectious diseases (see Table 16-1), **cessation of cigarette smoking** to prevent atherosclerotic disease and carcinomas (see Box 16-1), the use of **safety belts** in motor vehicles and **cessation** of the use of **chewing tobacco** in the prevention of oral carcinomas.

Secondary preventive strategies (see Table 16-1) are usually accomplished by the use of **screening tests.** A **screening intervention** is one that allows the discovery of a disorder in its asymptomatic stage. An effective screening intervention should sati

T A B L E 1 6 - 1
Immunizations in Adults

Influenza vaccine: Should be offered to all individuals over age 65 and to patients at high risk for significant morbidity and mortality. The latter category includes patients with diabetes mellitus, heart disease, pulmonary disease, renal disease, and immunocompromised patients. Health care personnel should also receive this vaccine. An absolute contraindication to the vaccine is a history of allergy to egg yolk. The vaccine is usually available in the fall and should be administered on a yearly basis. Side effects of the vaccine are the same as for placebo injection.

Pneumococcal vaccine: Similar indications as for influenza vaccine. Major differences include patients with asplenia (anatomical or functional), sickle cell disease, Hodgkin's disease, nephrotic syndrome, or alcoholism, all of whom clearly benefit from pneumococcal vaccine. The vaccine is available yearlong and is given once in the lifetime of the individual. There is no contraindication to vaccination in patients who are allergic to egg yolk.

Tetanus toxoid: All adults every 10 years.

Hepatitis B vaccine: Mandatory for individuals at high risk for exposure, including health care workers, individuals working in research laboratories, homosexually active men, and intravenous drug abusers. The currently available vaccine is produced by recombinant technology. Three doses are required to achieve immunity. The duration of immunity has not been clearly defined.

Measles: Individuals born after 1956 who lack evidence of immunity. Patient must agree not to become pregnant in the following 3 months. Pregnancy is an absolute contraindication. The Centers for Disease Control (CDC) also recommends vaccination of health care workers, military recruits, and college students.

Rubella: Women of childbearing age who lack proof of immunity. Patient must agree not to become pregnant in the following 3 months. Pregnancy is an absolute contraindication. The Centers for Disease Control (CDC) also recommends vaccination of health care workers, military recruits, and college students.

the following conditions: the targeted disorder should be relatively prevalent; the screening test must be reasonably safe, inexpensive, and acceptable by the patient; the test utilized for screening is capable of recognizing the vast majority of patients with the target disorder (high sensitivity) while mislabeling few patients as having the target disorder (high specificity); follow-up confirmatory tests should be safe, ideally noninvasive, and affordable; treatment of the target disorder in its asymptomatic stage will improve patients' prognosis compared to those patients with a similar disorder that are treated only when the disease becomes symptomatic; and the ultimate outcome of the target disorder has grave consequences for the well-being of patients, in terms of either morbidity or mortality. Of these desirable characteristics, the two most difficult to evaluate and quantify are the characteristics of the candidate screening test (sensitivity and specificity) and the efficacy of available interventions for disease diagnosed in an asymptomatic stage.

Examples of interventions that have been shown not to benefit

B O X 1 6 - 1

Outline of Cigarette Smoking Cessation Technique

Background

1. Cessation of cigarette smoking is **essential to the primary prevention** of:
   a. Atherosclerotic disease in general and coronary and cerebrovascular atherosclerotic disease in specific.
   b. Bronchogenic carcinoma.
   c. Low birth-weight infants in pregnant mothers.
2. Cessation of cigarette smoking is **essential to the primary prevention** of disorders attributable to **passive,** i.e., second-hand, smoke:
   a. Respiratory infections in children.
   b. Bronchogenic carcinoma in family members and coworkers.

Management

1. The physician must state clearly and unequivocally to each and every patient who smokes cigarettes that the patient **must stop cigarette smoking.** Several tips to make this statement more effective include:
   a. State the **negative outcomes** that may occur if smoking cessation is not effected. These may be general items such as an increased risk of heart attack, stroke, or lung and other cancers. The clinician must attempt to make this **personal** and **tangible** to the patient; e.g., if one of the patient's parents had a heart attack at a young age, stress the fact that smoking puts the patient at an extremely high risk for a heart attack.
   b. **Educate** the patient about the untoward outcomes of passive smoke. They should understand that their habit is not only directly jeopardizing their own life but also **negatively impacting** on the health of their coworkers, roommates, and family members.
   c. State the **positive outcomes** of the cessation of cigarette smoking. These include the decrease in risk of heart attacks, strokes, lung and other can-

(continued)

B O X 1 6 - 1 *(continued)*

cers, and the prolongation of life expectancy.
Again the clinician must attempt to make this **personal** and **tangible** to the patient; e.g., if the patient has chronic cough, the cessation of smoking may decrease the cough; if the patient has small children at home, cessation of smoking will decrease the risk of respiratory illness in these children.

d. Stress the importance of this behavioral modification and emphasize that, although it will be difficult, the **benefits of cessation are enormous.**

e. Describe the **withdrawal symptoms** the patient may feel after cessation of smoking, e.g., increased irritability, increased weight, and an intense craving for nicotine. Stress the fact that these are transient, that they are an investment in better health for the individual and his or her family, and that they can be **minimized** by exercise, fluids, and the short-term use of a nicotine substitute, i.e., the **transdermal nicotine patch.**

The **dosage** of the transdermal nicotine is Habitrol or Nicoderm, one 21-mg patch each day for 30 days, followed by one 14-mg patch each day for 15 to 30 days, followed by one 7-mg patch each day for 15 to 30 days; or Nicotrol one 15-mg patch each day for 30 days followed by one 10-mg patch each day for 15 to 30 days followed by 5-mg patch for 15 to 30 days. The Habitrol and Nicoderm patches are applied for 24-hour time periods, whereas the Nicotrol patches are applied for 16-hour time periods, i.e., applied in the morning and removed at night. The patch must be used **only** in the setting of an intense and committed effort of smoking cessation.

f. Instruct the patient to **set a date for cessation** and to resolve to abstain from cigarette smoking from that day hence.

2. Complement the discussion with **written materials** regarding the cessation of cigarette smoking. These can be written by the clinician himself or herself for distribution or they can be brochures that are ob-

(continued)

B O X   1 6 - 1 *(continued)*

> tained free or at a nominal fee from various health
> organizations. Examples of these include *Calling It
> Quits,* by the American Heart Association, and *Smart
> Move,* by the American Cancer Society.
> 3. Finally, select a nurse in the clinic to spend some
>   time on the same day to provide **reinforcement** of
>   the points made by the clinician and to make fol-
>   lowup appointments and telephone calls with the
>   sole purpose of longitudinal support for cessation of
>   cigarette smoking.

patient outcome include the following: yearly chest x-ray for the
screening of lung cancer, carcinoembryonic antigen (CEA) assay
for colorectal cancer screening, a battery of blood tests in asymptomatic individuals, complete routine urinalysis in nonpregnant
or nondiabetic patients, and electrocardiograms in otherwise
healthy individuals. Strategies currently being investigated as potentially useful screening strategies include the prostate specific
antigen (PSA) assay alone and in combination with transrectal
ultrasonography for the early diagnosis of prostatic cancer, fecal
occult blood testing for colorectal cancer screening, and serum
markers for ovarian cancer (CA-125), along or in combination
with transvaginal ultrasonography.

Numerous preventive interventions other than the ones reviewed in this chapter are suggested in the report issued in 1989
by the U.S. Preventive Task Force. The scientific merit of each of
those recommendations is beyond the scope of this book but is
discussed in the report.

Tertiary preventive interventions, i.e., those used to prevent
further progression of disease that is already extant, include the
use of aspirin in patients with atherosclerotic heart disease and
cerebrovascular disease, the use of beta-blockers and ACE inhibitors in the postmyocardial infarction period, and the cessation of
smoking in a patient with chronic obstructive pulmonary disease.

In summary, primary care providers are ideally positioned to
provide preventive services to large segments of the population.
What preventive measures are appropriate to institute depend on
the characteristics of the disease to be prevented (prevalence
morbidity, mortality), currently available technology for diagnos
and treatment, cost, and the availability of screening and con
matory tests.

T A B L E   1 6 - 2
Recommendations for Cancer Screening

Breast cancer: Breast examination by a physician every 1–2 years, starting at age 40. Annual mammography starting at age 50. Stop screening by age 75. We also recommend monthly breast self-examination (to be done at midcycle). For women with a family history of breast cancer, yearly mammography should be started at age 35. The American College of Obstetricians and Gynecologists recommends annual or biannual mammography **and** annual breast examination by a physician, starting at age 40.

Colorectal cancer: Currently the U.S. Preventive Task Force recommends screening only in patients at high risk for colorectal cancer (positive family history), starting at age 50. We recommend the performance of flexible sigmoidoscopy every 3–5 years, starting at age 50. The utility of fecal occult blood testing (FOBT) is under investigation. The American Cancer Society recommends yearly FOBT, starting at age 40, and flexible sigmoidoscopy performed in two consecutive years starting at age 50 and every 3 years thereafter if the initial flexible sigmoidoscopy results are normal.

Cervical cancer: Papanicolaou smears every 1–3 years from the beginning of sexual activity. Screening can be stopped by age 65 if the smears are consistently normal. Other organizations recommend starting screening at age 18 or at the beginning of sexual life, performing Pap smears annually for 3 years, and then every 3 years if three prior Pap smears were normal.

Prostate cancer: The U.S. Preventive Task Force does not recommend either digital rectal examination, serum marker assays (PSA) or transrectal ultrasonography for asymptomatic men. The American Cancer Society recommends yearly rectal examination starting at age 40.

Skin cancer: Thorough complete skin examination recommended only for patients at high risk: family or personal history of skin cancer, precursor lesions (i.e., dysplastic nevi). The American Academy of Dermatology recommends annual complete examination for all patients as well as monthly self-examination.

Ovarian cancer: No specific recommendation other than examining carefully the uterine adnexae when performing pelvic examinations. The role of serum marker assay and (CA-125) transvaginal ultrasonography is still under investigation. Patients with a family history of ovarian cancer or breast cancer in first-degree relatives might benefit from serum marker assays and transvaginal ultrasonography done sequentially as a screening modality.

Testicular cancer: Routine examination only for patients at high risk for testicular cancer: testicular atrophy, cryptorchidism, orchiopexy. The American Cancer Society recommends testicular examination as part of the periodic health examination **and** monthly self-examination in postpubertal men.

Bibliography

Guide for Adult Immunization, Second Edition. Philadelphia: American College of Physicians, 1990.

Kramer SE, Graham KE: Helping your patients who smoke quit for good. Postgrad Med 1991;90:233–246.

Lawrence RS, et al: Preventive services in clinical practice: Designing the periodic health examination. JAMA 1987;257:2205–2210.

United States Preventive Services Task Force: Guide to Clinical Preventive Services. Baltimore: Williams and Wilkins, 1989.

Index

Note: Numbers followed by an f indicate a figure; t following a page number indicates tabular material.